Controversial Issues in Implant Dentistry

Federico Hernández Alfaro

Associate editors:
Hugo Campos Leitão, Cristina Porta Ferrer, Vanessa Ruiz Magaz

Controversial Issues in Implant Dentistry

QUINTESSENCE PUBLISHING

London, Berlin, Chicago, Tokyo, Barcelona, Beijing, Istanbul, Milan,
Moscow, New Delhi, Paris, Prague, São Paulo, Seoul, Singapore and Warsaw

"To my parents
To my daughter Alicia"

A CIP record for this book is available from the British Library.
ISBN: 978-1-85097-234-1

QUINTESSENCE PUBLISHING

Quintessence Publishing Co. Ltd,
Grafton Road, New Malden, Surrey KT3 3AB,
United Kingdom
www.quintpub.co.uk

Editing: Quintessence Publishing Co. Ltd, London, UK
Layout and Production: Quintessenz Verlags-GmbH, Berlin, Germany
Printed and bound in Germany

Foreword

It is always an important event in our academic and professional communities in Europe when the release of a new book enlarges our scientific culture and promotes the training of our professionals and students. These books frequently introduce new knowledge and above all, new technologies that improve our preventive and therapeutic capabilities. Less frequently, new books deal with controversial and practical aspects of a specific therapeutic field, which directly affect our daily professional activity and, therefore, become an important source of relevant information.

It is precisely a book of these characteristics I have the honor to present. *Controversial issues in Implant Dentistry* provides excellent coverage of these aspects of implant dentistry where we do not have clear scientific evidence or fully validated protocols. These important areas of implant dentistry are covered in this book with high scientific rigor, clarity and with the support of excellent images and illustrations. They will undoubtedly make this book an important reference source for those professionals involved in implant dentistry.

The author and editor, Professor Federico Hernández Alfaro, together with the associate editors and authors, comprise a team that have an important knowledge base in Europe in the areas of maxillofacial surgery, implant dentistry and periodontology. The prestige of Professor Hernández Alfaro does not rest only on his successful academic career – being the Professor and Chairman of the Department of Oral and Maxillofacial Surgery at the International University of Catalonia – but also on his prestige as a highly reputed surgeon, with vast clinical experience in the treatment of the most complex patients requiring oral and maxillofacial surgery. Throughout his career, Professor Hernández Alfaro has left a legacy of excellent surgeons, both at the University and at the Teknon Medical Center. This legacy is clear when evaluating this book, which demonstrates his dedication to implant surgery, as well as his academic soul.

In summary, I have the honor to present an excellent book that combines scientific rigor with highly relevant practical information that will be of great interest to the readers.

Mariano Sanz
Professor of Periodontology
Complutense University of Madrid, Spain

Preface

Dental implantology has seen a revolution in the last decade. Reasons for this include the universal incorporation of 3D tools for diagnosis and planning, new surfaces and macro designs of implants, bioactive materials, tissue engineering techniques, and minimally invasive surgical procedures. This new paradigm is still evolving, and will doubtless change the way we treat edentulous patients in the forthcoming years.

There are, however, a number of issues that either remain unanswered or are subject to discussion, mainly due to the lack of scientific evidence. In this book we have focused on several controversial topics in implant dentistry. A comprehensive approach, combining existing evidence with authors' experience and skills, will hopefully shed light on questions that most of us, as clinicians, face in daily practice. Controversial Issues in Implant Dentistry is aimed at the clinician who deals with implant therapy and needs deep insight into topics that are still the subject of debate.

I want to thank all the contributing authors, most of them members of the Department of Oral & Maxillofacial Surgery at the International University of Catalonia, which I have the privilege to chair. Thanks also to our colleagues from the Periodontics Department, and my very special thanks to Professor Alberto Sicilia from Oviedo University, and Manuel Sancho from the University of Zurich, who honored me with his collaboration.

Federico Hernández Alfaro MD, DDS, PhD, FEBOMS
Editor

Editors and Authors

EDITOR
Federico Hernández Alfaro MD, DDS, PhD, FEBOMS

ASSOCIATE EDITORS
Hugo Campos Leitão DDS
Cristina Porta Ferrer DDS
Vanessa Ruiz Magaz DDS

AUTHORS
Maher Al Atari DDS, PhD
Associate Professor, Department of Oral & Maxillofacial Surgery, International University of Catalonia, Barcelona, Spain.
Director, Laboratory for Regenerative Dentistry, International University of Catalonia, Barcelona, Spain

Pau Altuna
Pau Altuna DDS, MS
International Masters in Oral Implantology: Oral Surgery and Prosthetics, International University of Catalonia, Barcelona, Spain.
Assistant Professor, Department of Oral & Maxillofacial Surgery, International University of Catalonia, Barcelona, Spain.

Patricia Anguis Martín DDS, MS
Masters in Oral Implantology: Oral Surgery and Prosthetics, International University of Catalonia, Barcelona, Spain.

Jorge Bertos DDS
Masters in Oral Implantology: Oral Surgery and Prosthetics, International University of Catalonia, Barcelona, Spain.
Assistant Professor, Department of Oral & Maxillofacial Surgery, International University of Catalonia, Barcelona, Spain.

Hugo Campos Leitão DDS
Certificate in Periodontics, International University of Catalonia, Barcelona, Spain.
Advanced Education Program in Implant Dentistry, Loma Linda University, California, United States.
Associate Professor, Department of Periodontology, International University of Catalonia, Barcelona, Spain.

Punjamaporn Chatakun DDS
Masters in Oral Implantology: Oral Surgery and Prosthetics, International University of Catalonia, Barcelona, Spain.

Isabel Cuesta MD, DDS, PhD
Doctor in Medicine, Specialist in Stomatology.
Clinical Professor, Masters in Periodontology, University of Oviedo, Spain.

Elvira Ferres Amat DDS, PhD
Associate Professor, Department of Oral & Maxillofacial Surgery, International University of Catalonia, Barcelona, Spain.
Director, Ferres-Amat Institute, Barcelona, Spain

Eduard Ferres Padró MD, DDS, PhD
Chief, Department Oral and Maxillofacal Surgery, Children's Hospital, Barcelona, Spain.
Former Chief, Department Oral & Maxillofacial Surgery, International University of Catalonia, Barcelona, Spain.

Susana García González DDS, MS
International Masters in Oral Implantology: Oral Surgery and Prosthetics, International University of Catalonia, Barcelona, Spain.
Assistant Professor, Department of Oral & Maxillofacial Surgery, International University of Catalonia, Barcelona, Spain.

Raquel Guijarro Martínez MD, DDS
Oral and Maxillofacial Surgeon, Craniofacial Center, Hirslanden Medical Center Aarau, Aarau, Switzerland.
Fellow, Institute of Maxillofacial Surgery, Teknon Medical Center, Barcelona, Spain.

Federico Hernández Alfaro MD, DDS, PhD, FEBOMS
Professor and Chairman, Department of Oral & Maxillofacial Surgery, International University of Catalonia, Barcelona, Spain.
Chief, Department Oral & Maxillofacial Surgery, Teknon Medical Center, Barcelona, Spain.

Jose M Lluch MD
Oral and Maxillofacial Surgeon
Former Assistant Professor, Department of Oral & Maxillofacial Surgery, International University of Catalonia, Barcelona, Spain.

Anna Mañes Medina DDS, MsC
Masters in Oral Implantology: Surgery, Prosthodontics and Periodontics, International University of Catalonia, Barcelona, Spain.
Assistant Professor of International University of Catalonia, Barcelona, Spain.

Javier Mareque Bueno MD, DDS, PhD, FEBOMS
Oral & Maxillofacial Surgeon, Teknon Medical Center, Barcelona, Spain.
Associate Professor, Department of Oral & Maxillofacial Surgery, International University of Catalonia, Barcelona, Spain.

Santiago Mareque Bueno DDS
Masters in Oral Implantology: Surgery, Prosthodontics and Periodontics, Assistant Professor, Master of Periodontics, International University of Catalonia, Barcelona, Spain.

Jose Nart DDS, PhD
Diplomate, American Board of Periodontology.
Chairman and Program Director, Department of Periodontology, International University of Catalonia, Barcelona, Spain.

Natália Oliveira DDS, MsC
Masters in Oral Implantology: Surgery, Prosthodontics and Periodontics, International University of Catalonia, Barcelona, Spain.
Private Practice, Oporto, Portugal.

Jordi Ortega Martínez DDS, MS
Masters in Oral Implantology: Surgery, Prosthodontics and Periodontics, International University of Catalonia, Barcelona, Spain.
Assistant Professor, International University of Catalonia, Barcelona, Spain.

Octavi Ortiz Puigpelat DDS, MS
Postgraduate advanced fellowship in implant dentistry, New York University, NY, USA,
Assistant Professor, Department of Oral & Maxillofacial Surgery, International University of Catalonia, Barcelona, Spain.

Andres Pascual La Rocca DDS
Master in Periodontics.
Co-Chairman, Masters in Periodontology, International University of Catalonia, Barcelona, Spain.

Tania Perez Pascual DDS, MS
Masters in Oral Implantology: Oral Surgery and Prosthetics, International University of Catalonia, Barcelona, Spain.

Marc Quevedo Pou DDS, MS
Masters in Oral Implantology: Oral Surgery and Prosthodontics, International University of Catalonia, Barcelona, Spain,
Assistant Professor, Masters in Implant Dentistry, International University of Catalonia, Barcelona, Spain.

Alberto Rodríguez DDS
Master in Periodontology, University of Oviedo, Spain.
Clinical Professor, Masters in Periodontology, University of Oviedo, Spain.

Vanessa Ruiz Magaz DDS
Masters in Periodontics, , International University of Catalonia Barcelona, Spain.
Postgraduate in Clínical Implantology, International University of Catalonia, Barcelona, Spain.
Assistant Professor, Periodontology Department, International University of Catalonia, Barcelona, Spain.

Eva Salvan Garcia DDS, MS
Masters in Oral Implantology: Oral Surgery and Prosthetics, International University of Catalonia, Barcelona, Spain.
Assistant Professor, Department of Oral & Maxillofacial Surgery, International University of Catalonia Barcelona, Spain.

Victoria Sanchez D'Onofrio DDS, MS
Postgraduate Certificate in periodontics by EPAO (Houston-Bilbao), 2007.
International Masters in Oral Implantology: Oral Surgery, Periodontics and Prosthodontics, International University of Catalonia, 2013.

Manuel Sancho Puchades DDS
Master Degree in Oral Surgery and Orofacial Implantology, University of Barcelona, Barcelona, Spain.
Postgraduate Program in Fixed and Removable Reconstructive Dentistry and Implant Dentistry, University of Zurich, Zürich, Switzerland.

Alberto Sicilia MD,DDS, PhD
Professor of Periodontology, University of Oviedo, Spain.
Medical Director, Clínica Sicilia, Oviedo, Spain.
Board Director, European Association for Osseointegration.

Estefania Solans DDS, MS
Masters in Oral Implantology: Oral Surgery and Prosthetics, International University of Catalonia, Barcelona, Spain.

Contents

Chapter 1

What is the best possible implant when it comes to design and surface?

Manuel Sancho Puchades, Raquel Guijarro Martínez, Federico Hernández Alfaro

1.1 Introduction

Dental implant success relies on the conjunction of optimal esthetic and mechanical parameters. These, in turn, depend on the characteristics and stability of the bond created between the implant and its surrounding bone.[1] More than 30 years ago, Albrektsson et al.[2] described the six factors that influence the interfacial bone–implant bonding: surgical technique; host bed; implant design; implant surface; material biocompatibility; and loading conditions. Thereafter, the standards of each factor have evolved, but the relevance of each of the six points persists.

The implant itself determines three of these factors: design; surface; and material biocompatibility. The rate and quality of osseointegration is directly related to these properties.[3] Implant topography can be further characterized as macro-, micro- and nanoroughness according to the scale of evaluation. The characteristics of the implant at each of these levels have specific consequences on wound healing and osseointegration (Fig 1-1).

Implant macroroughness, or design, refers to features that range from millimeters to tens of micrometers. Therefore, this scale is directly related to implant geometry, which includes body shape and thread design. Implant geometry determines both primary implant fixation and long-term mechanical stability due to force transmission modulation at the implant–bone interface. The implant–abutment connection can also be considered a design trait. It has an influence both in marginal bone level changes and in stability and durability of the prosthodontic connection.[4]

Microroughness, in turn, describes features in the range of 1 to 10 µm. These play an important role in the initial phases of bone healing, influencing the quality

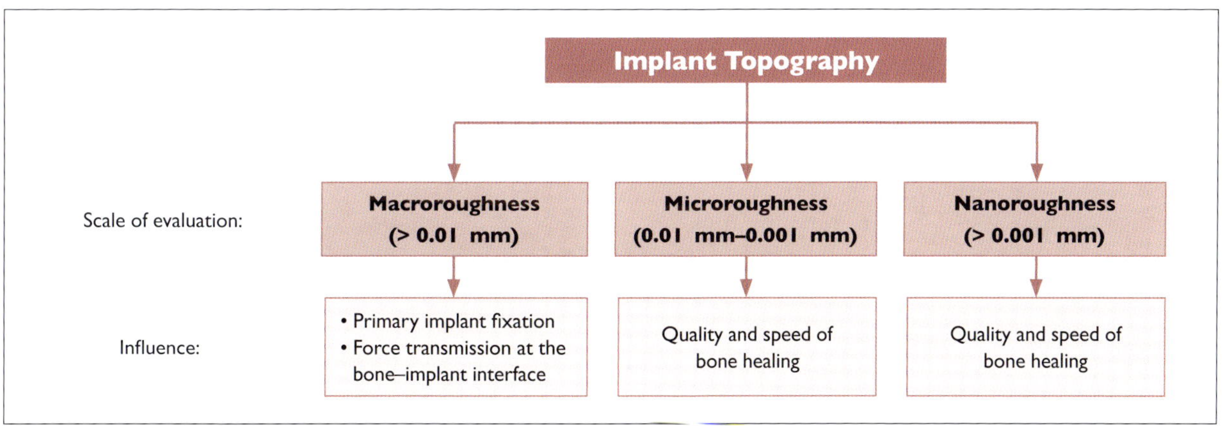

Fig 1-1 Influence of implant topography on wound healing and osseointegration.

and speed of osseointegration and therefore modulating loading protocols. They also maximize the interlocking between mineralized bone and implant surface, leading to stable and rigid osseointegration.

Although microroughness is still considered the most important factor for improved bone behavior, current thinking is that the nanoscale topography could also have an influence.[5] Nanometer roughness (between 1 and 100 nm) is a key factor in protein adsorption and cell adhesion. Therefore, it is expected that improved nanometer roughness may enhance the rate of osseointegration.[6] Future studies aimed at surface development also include chemical and/or physical modifications such as newly developed calcium-phosphate (CaP) coatings, hydrophilic surfaces, and the incorporation of ions or biological drugs that accelerate bone healing in the peri-implant area.

This chapter will review the current scientific literature on implant topography and offer a critical analysis of the influence of these factors on peri-implant bone formation and maintenance. The following topics will be addressed:

- 1.2 Implant design
  - 1.2.1 Background
  - 1.2.2 Is there an ideal implant shape?
  - 1.2.3 Is implant morphology relevant in implant performance?
  - 1.2.4 How does the implant's crest module modulate marginal bone resorption?
  - 1.2.5 Conclusions
- 1.3 Implant surface
  - 1.3.1 Background
  - 1.3.2 How should an implant surface be characterized?
  - 1.3.3 What surface treatments are available?
  - 1.3.4 Are modern surfaces better than their predecessors?
  - 1.3.5 What can we expect from the future?
  - 1.3.6 Conclusions

1.2 Implant design

1.2.1 Background

Implant design, or macrodesign, describes an implant's macroscopic characteristics. It comprises features in the range of millimeters to tens of micrometers. This scale directly relates to implant geometry. Evidence exists that macrodesign influences initial stability of the implant and the transmission of forces from the implant to the bone during and after osseointegration. The underlying mechanism may be the mechanical interlocking between the macroscopic surface features and the surrounding bone profile.[7] A lot of effort has been put into the improvement of implant design so as to enhance initial implant stabilization, upgrade osseointegration, improve force transmission to bone, and maintain bone levels over time.

Bone remodels under the influence of external stimuli. Wolff[8] observed a direct association between bone morphology and mechanical loading. He established that every change in function leads to a change in bone configuration. His theory entails that bone formation occurs when increasing stresses apply, while decreased stress leads to bone loss. However, it has also been shown that bone loss can also occur under extreme stresses.[9,10] Frost[11] hypothesized that bone cells respond to local bone deformation (strain) produced by mechanical stress. With slightly increased strain, the bone becomes slightly overloaded and responds with new bone formation. If the strain is intense and surpasses a specific threshold, fatigue fracture may occur. Finally, if strains are very low, disuse of the bone results in net bone loss.

Frost[11] described four microstrain zones in compact bone that lead to different bone reactions. These are the pathologic overload zone, the mild overload zone, the adapted window zone, and the acute disuse zone. Both the pathologic overload zone and the acute disuse zone represent the two extremes of bone reaction to strain and lead to bone loss. The most desirable state of peri-implant bone is the adapted window zone, where slow bone turnover takes place. High bone turnover leads to immature bone formation, which implies a lower bone quality. This occurs mostly in the mild overload zone.

Bone remodeling rate is defined as the time needed for new bone to replace existing bone and can be expressed as a percentage or volume of new bone for a specific period of time.[12] Slow bone remodeling leads to the predominant formation of lamellar bone. This type of bone is strong, well organized and highly mineralized. Woven bone can also be found around implants, and is immature, less organized, and less mineralized. Lamellar bone remodels at a rate of 1 to 5 µm per day, while woven bone does so at 60 µm per day.[13] Lamellar bone is better prepared to sustain bone loading and is more desirable around implants.

The predominant formation of a specific bone type around an implant is highly influenced by how the latter transmits the forces to the bone interface. Implant design modulates stress transmission by dissipating and distributing forces to the surrounding peri-implant tissues.[12] In other words, implant macrostructure can modify both the magnitude and direction of the force received.

Excessive forces beyond the bone's resistance capacity may lead to bone resorption.[14] Hence, an increase in the surface area upon which the force is applied is one possibility to reduce the stress transmitted to the bone. Bone-to-implant contact (BIC) is a quantitative way of measuring the surface area of an implant that is in contact with bone. It is essentially linked to the implant's microtopography, but macrotopography may also have an influence.[1] This is especially true in the crestal region of the implant body, since it has been shown that the majority of stress accumulates here. Consequently, the design of this area is particularly significant. Some manufacturers have introduced microthreads in the crestal module in order to improve force transmission in this critical area. This point will be further discussed later.

Misch et al.[12] believe that not all the bone contacting the implant is at work during occlusal load. They describe a functional surface area, which represents the portion of the thread that participates in compressive load transmission under the action of an axial occlusal load (Fig 1-2). The relevance of thread shape in force direction modulation is emphasized. In this sense, an 8 mm-long square-threaded implant would have a greater functional surface area than a 14 mm V-shaped or reverse buttress, due to the improved loading transmission capacity of the square-shaped thread.

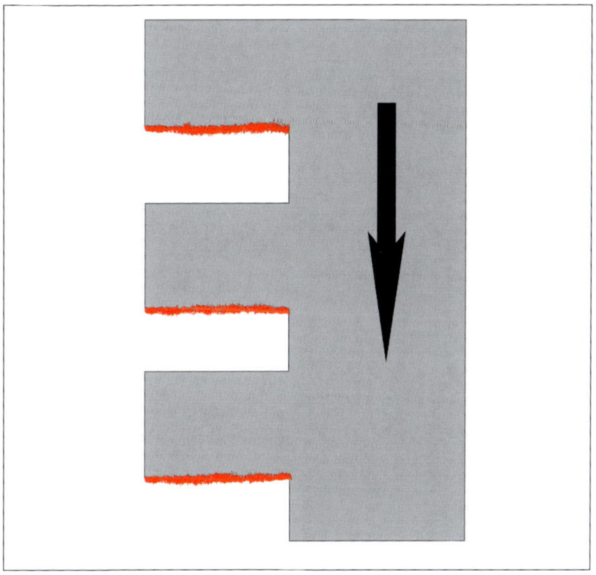

Fig 1-2 Functional surface area: portion of the thread that participates in compressive load transmission under axial loading.

Three types of forces have been described at the bone–implant interface: compressive (pushing); tensile (pulling); and shear (twisting) forces (Fig 1-3).[12,15] It is generally believed that compressive forces exert the best influence on the bone–implant boundary.[12] These forces increase bone density around implants, thereby increasing the strength of the interface.[12] On the other hand, tensile and, especially, shear forces are thought to generate weaker bone responses.[12] The ideal implant design should provide a balance between compressive and tensile forces while minimizing shear force generation.[1] Both implant shape and thread design have an influence on functional surface area and the type of force that is generated.

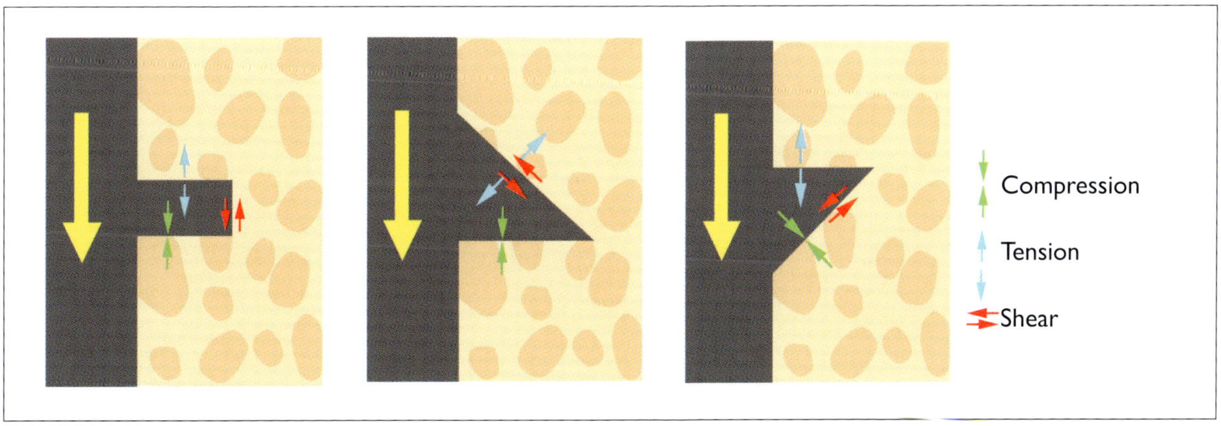

Fig 1-3 Force types at the implant–bone interface resulting from axial loading with different thread designs.

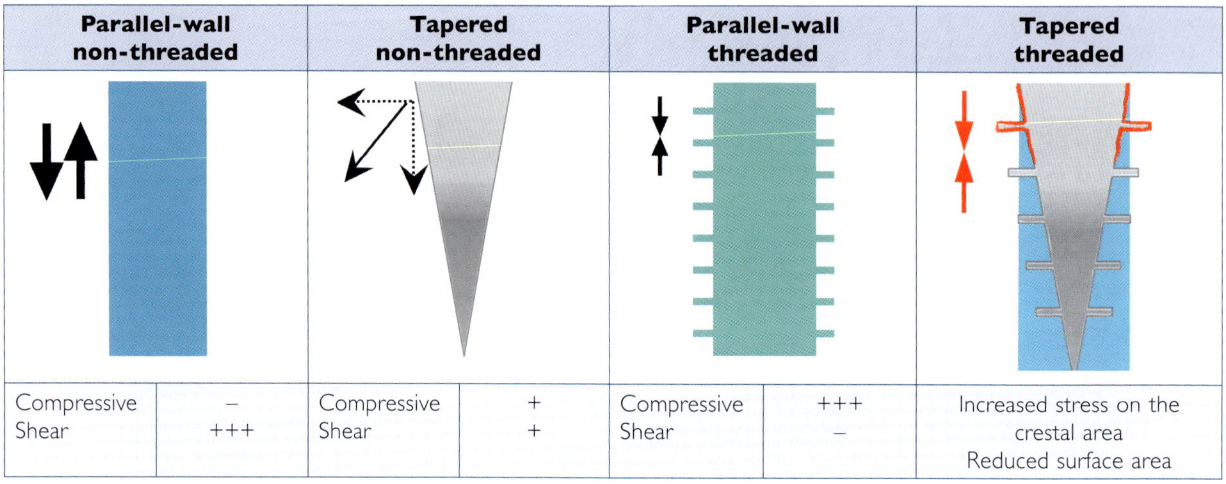

Fig 1-4 Influence of implant shape on force transmission at the bone–implant interface.

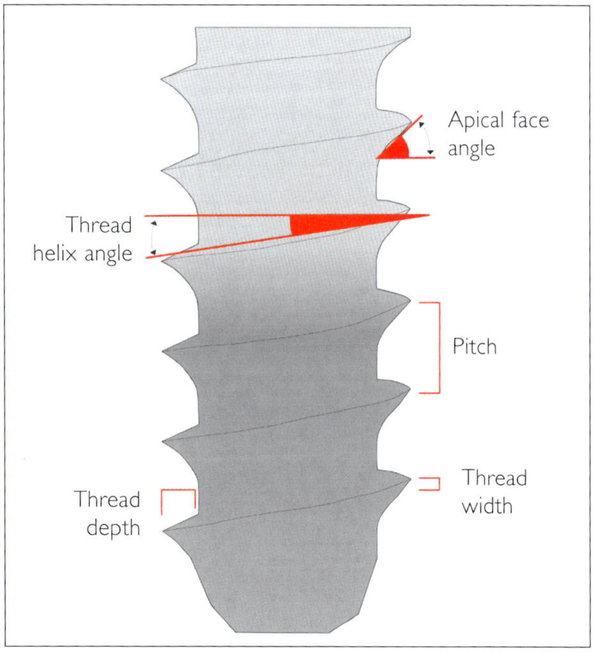

Fig 1-5 Basic implant design features: face angle, thread helix angle, thread pitch, thread depth, and thread width.

1.2.2 Is there an ideal implant shape?

Implant shape has undergone numerous variations in accordance to prevailing theories and innovations. The initial parallel-wall non-threaded implant design was far from optimal, since a considerable component of shear forces was transmitted to the bone. The tapering of these implants introduced a beneficial compressive vector on the bone–implant interface.[16] Nonetheless, force transmission to bone was still improvable, since a considerable component of shear forces persisted. The introduction of screw-shaped implants gave way to better force modulation thanks to the threads. These act as stress transfers to the bone, creating predominantly compressive vectors. Adding a taper geometry to these implants represents little mechanical advantage due to the fact that surface area is reduced and the amount of stress at the crestal portion of the implant is increased (Fig 1-4).[17]

1.2.3 Is implant morphology relevant in implant performance?

Thread morphology – described by thread shape, pitch, lead, depth, and width – plays an important role in BIC and bone distribution as a result of the modulation of force transmission to surrounding tissues (Fig 1-5).[12] Under loading, bone remodels and adapts to the stress transferred by the threads' geometry. In an animal model, Duyck et al.[18] observed a shift in bone distribution around the implant's threads with loading. After the initial healing period, equal distribution of bone over and under the implant threads was present. Dynamic loading resulted in greater amounts of bone under the thread face angle. Bolind et al.[19] reported similar findings after implant retrieval in humans. The greatest amount of bone was located under the thread face angle and the least at the tips of the threads. Kohn[20] hypothesized that less bone was present at the threads' tips due to the accumulation of greater strains.

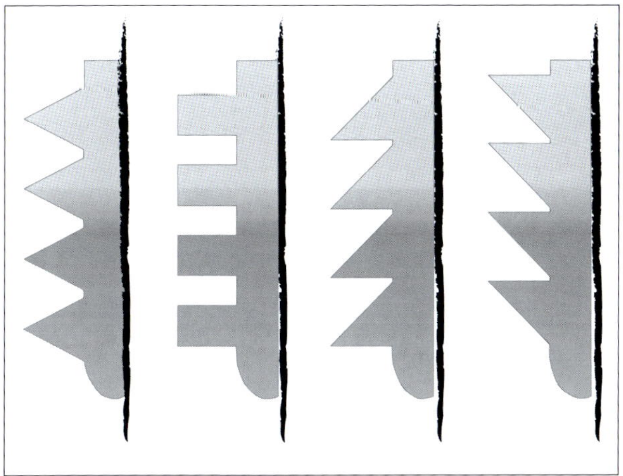

Fig 1-6 Thread shape (from left to right): V-shaped, square, buttress, and reverse buttress.

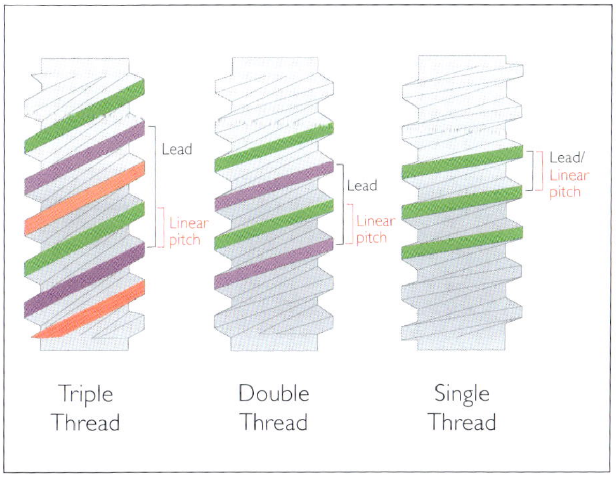

Fig 1-7 Thread configuration in relation to thread number, pitch, and lead. Single-threaded implants have an equal thread pitch and lead. Double- and triple-threaded implants have a lead that is double or triple the pitch.

Thread shape

Currently, four types of thread shape exist: square, V-shaped, buttress, and reverse buttress (Fig 1-6). Since occlusal loads have an overall intrusive effect on teeth, thread design in dental implantology should focus on optimizing force transmission to bone when intrusive loads are applied. Therefore, the critical part of the thread is the lower face angle, which opposes to intrusion. Contrarily to this principle, V-shaped and reverse buttress geometries are aimed to counteract pullout loads. Their apical face angle is not intended to bear intrusive loads. Shear forces are transmitted to the bone when intrusive loads are applied. These unfavorable forces are ten times greater in a 30 degree V-shaped thread than in a square-shaped thread.[12] When loaded, square threads deliver compressive forces to the bone. Kim and Oh[21] studied thread shape through a 3-dimensional (3D) finite element analysis (FEA) study. They compared identical implants with square, buttress and V-shaped threads and found that the square shape delivered the least stress, both in the compressive and shear components. This favorable distribution of stress may lead to enhanced osseointegration. In fact, Steigenga et al.[22,23] observed improved BIC and reverse torque test values with square thread implants when compared to buttress and V-shaped implants.

Thread pitch

Thread pitch refers to the distance from the center of a thread to the center of the next thread, measured parallel to the axis of the implant.[1] It can be calculated by dividing the unit length by the number of threads.[12] Considering implants with equal length, the smaller the pitch the greater the number of threads. Thread pitch is the geometric parameter with the greatest influence on surface area.[12] It is particularly relevant when there is limited bone height or poor bone density.[1] In these cases, an implant design with a smaller pitch, that is, with more threads, will provide an increased initial fixation and a greater surface area with loading.[12,13,23]

In any case, in the context of adequate bone quantity and quality, the role of pitch distance in primary stability and stress distribution may be minor when compared to other parameters such as implant length.[24] Moreover, a smaller pitch could be a disadvantage in these cases, since implant insertion is hindered due to the high resistance offered by the greater number of threads. This could be particularly relevant in denser bone areas.

Thread lead

Thread lead is the distance from the center of a thread to the center of the same thread after one turn. It is the distance that a screw would advance in the axial direction if turned one complete revolution.[1] In a single lead implant, lead is equal to pitch. However, some implants have a double or triple thread lead, which means that lead is double or triple the pitch (Fig 1-7). These are manufactured using two or three blades, which produce two or three threads running parallel to each other along the

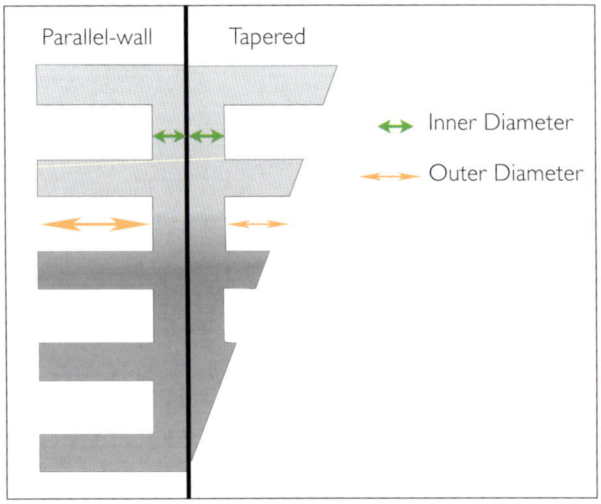

Fig 1-8 Thread depth decreases towards the apical region in tapered implants, but remains constant in parallel-wall implants..

implant body. Their main characteristic is a faster speed of insertion, with the theoretical maintenance of a favorable pitch distance.[1] An implant with double thread lead would insert twice as fast as a single-threaded implant, and three times as fast if a triple thread is considered.

However, thread lead increase could have negative effects on implant stability. By increasing the number of threads running parallel to each other, the thread helix angle changes. The helix angle is defined as the angle between the flank lead and a plane perpendicular to the long axis of the implant on its right.[25] Ma et al.[26] compared identical implants with different thread helix angles (single-, double-, or triple-threaded). Although all implants had a 0.8-mm constant pitch, the helix angle of double- and triple-threaded implants was double and triple that of single-threaded implants, respectively. FEAs showed implant stability decreased as helix angle increased. These findings suggest faster insertion may compromise implant stability. Misch et al.[12] state that thread lead increase only affects insertion speed and has no positive influence in surface area.

Thread depth and width

Thread depth (height) is the distance between the major and minor diameter of the thread. Thread width (thickness) is the distance between the most coronal and most apical parts of the tip of a single thread in the same axial plane.[1] Parallel-wall implants provide a uniform thread depth throughout the implant length, while depth decreases toward the apical region in tapered implants. The latter tend to have similar minor diameters but their outer diameter varies in relation to the tapering (Fig 1-8). Therefore, tapered implants are less capable of fixating bone in the apical region, a factor that could reduce initial stability. Moreover, thread depth decrease entails surface area reduction as well. On the other hand, shallow threads facilitate insertion.

Each manufacturer provides a specific thread depth; this tends to remain constant despite changes in implant diameter. According to Misch et al.,[12] since implant walls are thicker in greater diameter implants and there is no risk of thinning the implant wall between the inner diameter and the abutment screw, thread depth could be increased (Fig 1-9). This would translate to an increase in surface area. When diameter increases by 1 mm in constant thread depth implants, surface area increases 15 to 20% only. However, in increased thread depth implants, surface area increases 150% for every 1 mm in diameter increase.[12]

1.2.4 How does the implant's crest module modulate marginal bone resorption?

The crest module (or neck) of an implant is the part that extends coronally from the implant body, emerging from the bone cortex and soft tissues. It often incorporates the anti-rotational components of the implant–abutment connection.[12] This area has a great influence on crestal bone preservation. Its particular location is biologically and mechanically crucial: first, it is in direct contact with the oral cavity, which means it represents the transition between the sterile part of the implant and the septic oral environment. Second, loading leads to high stress concentration around the crest module. FEA has shown that the application of extreme occlusal loads on an implant leads to overloading near the superior region of the contact bone.[27] Hence, the crest module plays a critical role in the establishment of a frontier between the internal and external environment and in force regulation and transmission to the bone. Nevertheless, the underlying mechanisms of bone remodeling in the crestal area are still not completely understood.

Various hypotheses for these crestal bone changes have been postulated. These include: surgical trauma;[28] location, shape, and size of the implant-abutment microgap and its microbial contamination;[29] development of a biologic width;[30] bacterial colonization of the sulcus;[31]

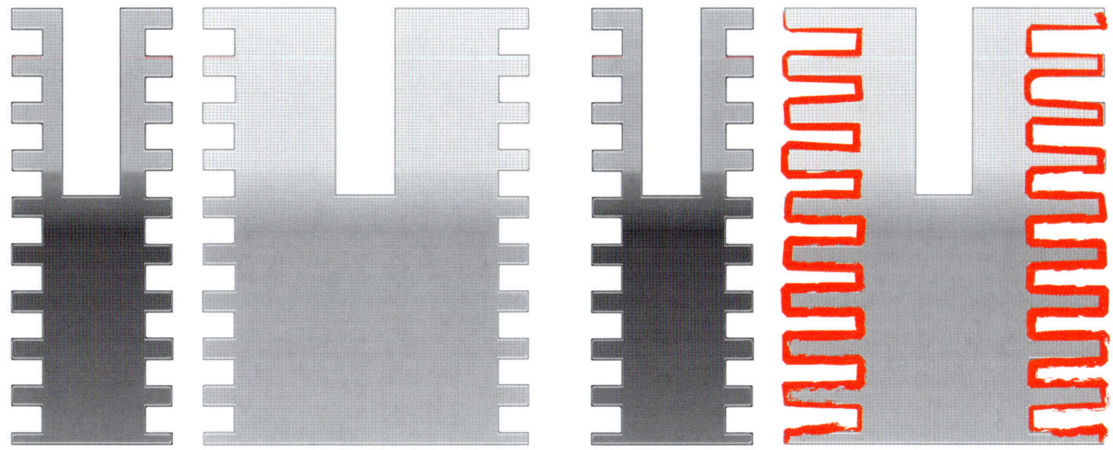

Fig 1-9 The surface area of wide-diameter implants could be increased significantly by increasing the thread depth without compromising the inner wall thickness.

micromovements of the implant and prosthetic components;[32] repeated screwing and unscrewing;[33,34] and force transmission to the crestal bone interface.[35]

Originally, the crest module of rough implants was polished in an attempt to reduce plaque accumulation. The current tendency is to roughen the entire implant body or even add microthreads to the crestal portion with the aim to improve marginal bone and soft tissue maintenance around implants.

When embedded in bone, smooth collars lead to marginal bone loss[36-38] and hence increase the risk of pocket formation. Hämmerle et al.[36] buried smooth crest implants below bone level and compared them to rough crest module implants in the same position. Rough implants maintained marginal bone levels while smooth implants lost bone down to the roughened part. A biological explanation for this is that smooth surfaces promote less contact osteogenesis and BIC during bone healing.[39] Others believe marginal bone loss around smooth-neck implants is due to disuse atrophy as a result of an absence of compressive force transmission to the bone.[40] Nevertheless, current available data indicates there is no evidence of improved marginal bone preservation for any particular surface microtopography.[41,42]

Regardless of surface treatment, several authors state that marginal bone loss in loaded implants occurs down to the first thread systematically.[36,43-46] Jung et al.[46] evaluated the bone loss around four different implant designs after 1 year of loading. They concluded that marginal bone loss stabilized at the level of the first thread no matter the time of exposure of the polished neck or the implant design. It seems the first thread changes the shear created by the crest module to a favorable component of compressive loading, maintaining the bone interface in homeostasis.[12]

In an attempt to reduce marginal bone loss and acknowledging that threads modulate force transmission to the bone, manufacturers have introduced threaded crest modules. A crest module with angled geometry or grooves may generate beneficial compressive stress on the contiguous bone, thereby decreasing the risk of bone loss (Fig 1-10).[12] Current scientific literature provides evidence that microthread incorporation at the implant's crest module can positively influence bone maintenance at a more crestal level. This is true at least during the early phases of bone healing.[47,48] However, long-term evidence of marginal bone preservation during function is still lacking.

Alternatively, sound evidence exists of other possible causes of marginal bone remodeling. The implant–abutment junction or microgap causes a local accumulation of inflammatory cells that may lead to marginal bone remodeling.[31] The relative position of the microgap to the bone crest will determine the amount of marginal bone remodeling. The closer to the bone crest the microgap is positioned, the greater the quantity of bone remodeling. The origin and nature of a persistent chemotactic stimulus remain unknown, but likely reflect the presence of microorganisms within the implant–abutment/crown interface, as demonstrated by previous clinical studies.[49,50]

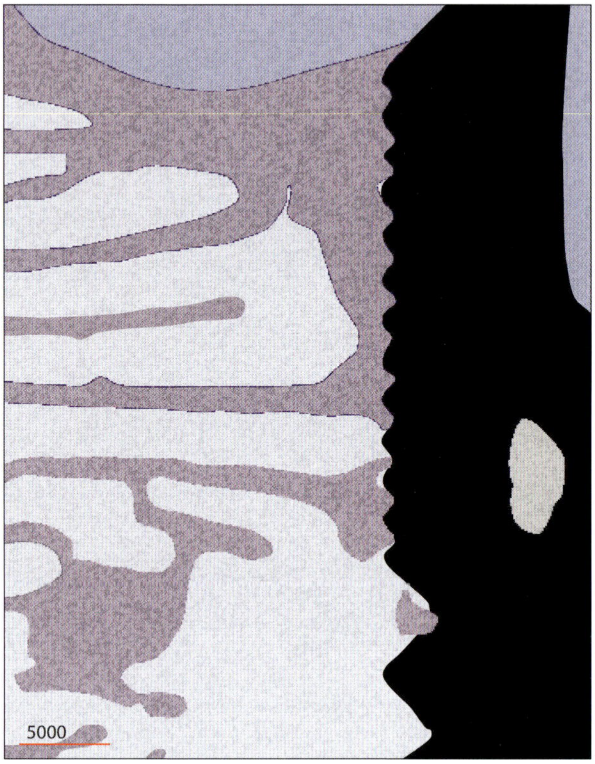

Fig 1-10 Microthreads on the implant crest module could improve marginal bone maintenance (magnification ×5000).

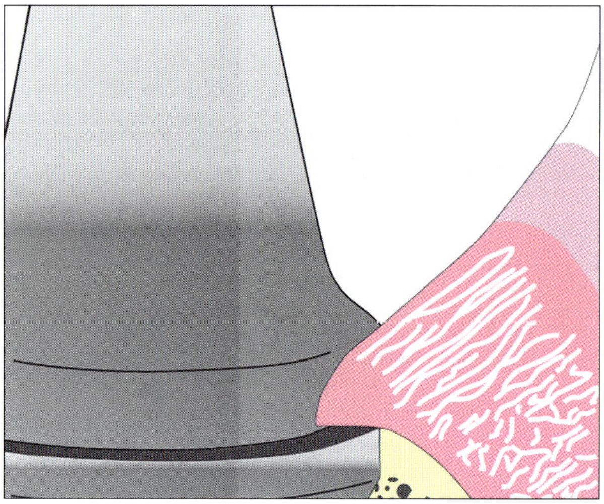

Fig 1-11 Platform switching concept: a smaller-diameter prosthetic component connected to a larger-diameter implant platform to create a 90 degree step between the implant and abutment.

In the late 1980s, wide-diameter implants were commercially introduced. Initially, the implants were restored with standard-diameter abutments due to the lack of matching prosthetic components. Contrary to what was expected, post-loading radiographic evaluation showed no changes in crestal bone levels around those implants. This finding led to the introduction of the concept of platform switching, in which a smaller-diameter prosthetic component was connected to a larger-diameter implant platform to create a 90 degree step between the implant and abutment (Fig 1-11).[4,51] Several clinical reports[52,53] demonstrated more favorable soft and hard tissue responses using implants placed with platform switching compared to standard platform-matched implants. Consequently, an increasing number of implant systems incorporated platform switching into their designs as an innovative feature for preserving peri-implant bone.[4]

Different theories were suggested to explain this phenomenon. The biomechanical theory states that connecting the implant to a smaller-diameter abutment may limit bone resorption by shifting the stress-concentration zone away from the crestal bone–implant interface and directing the forces of occlusal loading along the axis of the implant. However, several authors[52,53] showed that this modification does not significantly alter the stress generated at the marginal bone around the implants. An alternative explanation is that shifting the implant–abutment connection may medialize the location of the biologic width and minimize marginal bone resorption. However, the most accepted explanation concerns the shifting of the inflammatory cell infiltrate away from the bone. The physical repositioning of the microgap away from the outer edge of the implant and neighboring bone may limit bone resorption by restricting the inflammatory cell infiltrate to the horizontal mismatch between implant and abutment platforms.[51] The conclusions extracted from the meta-analysis performed by Atieh et al.[4] on platform switching are in agreement with this idea. The authors observed that an implant–abutment mismatch greater than 0.4 mm presented more favorable changes in marginal bone levels, due to the greater physical distance between the inflammatory cell infiltrate and the bone.

Table 1-1 Proper thread morphology according to bone quality and quantity

Bone quality and quantity	Pitch	Lead	Depth
Poor	Smaller	Simple	Increased
Adequate	Greater	Double or triple	Normal

1.2.5 Conclusions

- Implant design has its greatest influence on two factors: initial implant stability; and force transmission to the peri-implant tissues.
- The nature of the recipient bone should be taken into consideration when selecting the most appropriate implant design (Table 1-1).
- Primary implant stability depends on thread number and depth. An increase in thread pitch and depth enhances surface area, which in turn augments the mechanical implant–bone interlocking. This improvement in stability favors the implementation of immediate loading protocols.
- Thread shape plays an important role in the modulation of force transmission to the peri-implant tissues. A flat lower thread angle seems to be the ideal geometry due to the transmission of favorable compressive forces to the bone when intrusive loads are applied.
- Microthread incorporation to the implant's crest module can positively influence bone maintenance at a more crestal level. This is true at least during the early phases of bone healing. However, long-term evidence of marginal bone preservation during function is still lacking.
- Bacterial contamination at the implant–abutment junction (or microgap) promotes marginal bone remodeling due to the local accumulation of inflammatory cells. The closer to the bone the microgap is placed, the greater the quantity of bone resorption.
- Inward shifting of implant–abutment junction platform switching can be considered a desirable morphologic feature that may prevent the horizontal saucerization and preserve the vertical crestal bone levels. An additional improvement in marginal bone levels around dental implants may also be obtained with a greater degree of shifting.

1.3 Implant surface

1.3.1 Background

Implant surface characteristics are defined by topographic features below 10 µm. Early peri-implant wound healing is greatly dependent on this scale. The rate, quantity, and quality of bone response are related to implant surface properties.[3,54] This fact has led manufacturers to develop improved surfaces in order to achieve an enhanced bone response that will enable faster and stronger bone bonds, and hence an earlier loading of implants.

Immediately after implant insertion, a series of cellular reactions intended to stimulate bone apposition around the implant begins. Davies[55] divided this biological cascade into the following phases.

- Osseoconduction. This is the initial and most important stage of peri-implant bone healing. Implants' surface characteristics modulate this phase since they promote platelet activation and facilitate fibrin clot stabilization. Rough implant surfaces activate platelets, which in turn recruit osteogenic cells to migrate to the implant. However, in order for this to happen, a strong physical interlocking of fibrin fibers to the implant surface is essential, since osteogenic cells use these fibers to reach the implant surface. Textured surfaces allow the solid interlocking of fibrin fibers, which withstands initial clot retraction and hence maintains a proper matrix for cell migration (Fig 1-12).
- *De novo* bone formation. Osteogenic cells that have reached the implant surface differentiate to start new bone formation. Protein secretion to the extracellular space leads to the formation of an osteoid matrix on the implant surface that eventually mineralizes. Bone formation starting at the implant surface and moving outwards towards the opposing regenerating bony bed is known as contact osteogenesis (Fig 1-13). This healing pattern leads to the most favorable bone quality.
- Should the implant surface fail to stabilize the clot in the osseoconduction phase – as may occur with smooth surfaces – osteogenic cells would be unable to reach the implant and would differentiate a distance away from the target implant surface (Fig 1-14). As a result, this type of osseoconduction – known as distance osteogenesis – leads to the formation of a bone spicule heading towards the implant surface,

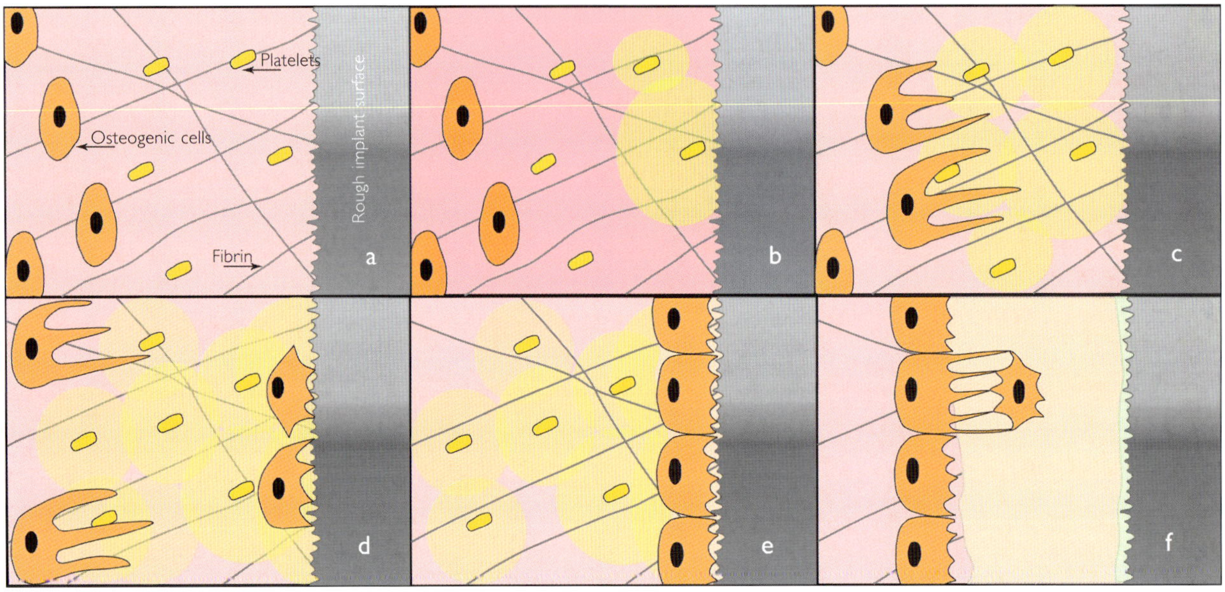

Fig 1-12a to f Osseoconduction: platelets in the wound site are activated by the implant microtopography (a and b). They secrete multiple growth factors and cytokines that recruit osteogenic cells to migrate to the implant surface (c). These cells migrate through a 3D fibrin matrix that is firmly anchored to the surface irregularities (d). When osteogenic cells reach the implant, they polarize and start secreting a collagenous bone matrix that will rapidly be mineralized (e and f).

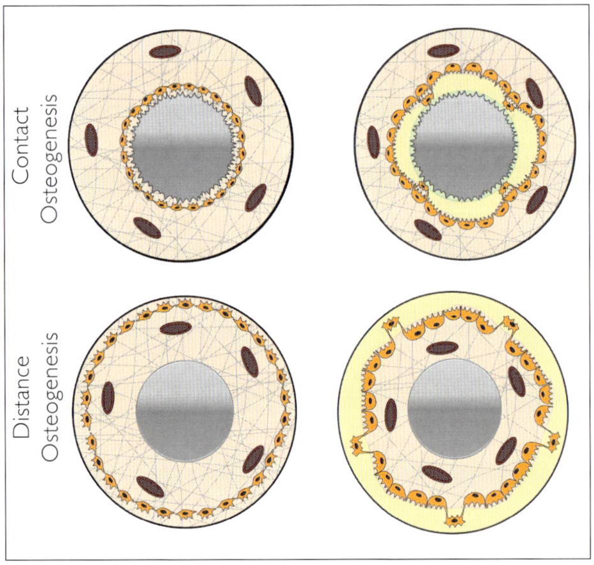

Fig 1-13 Bone formation patterns around dental implants. Rough surfaces tend to enhance the stability of the fibrin matrix, which allows osteogenic cells to start secreting bone from the implant surface towards the opposing bony bed. This healing pattern is known as contact osteogenesis. When osteogenic cells are unable to reach the implant surface and bone grows from the bony bed towards the implant, the process is called distance osteogenesis.

which results in a slower and weaker implant–bone connection.

- Bone remodeling. Remodeling entails a series of slow processes of bone turnover and specialization towards the generation of mature, highly organized peri-implant bone. As previously mentioned, bone stress derived from implant loading plays an important role in bone remodeling processes and hence in the bone type and distribution around the implant.

Although it is widely accepted that surface topography plays an important role in these phases of initial bone healing, the scientific literature fails to fully explain the underlying mechanisms of these phenomena.[3] Reviews on surface topography and bone healing have only been able to conclude that increasing surface roughness enhances bone integration.[3,56,57] This limited knowledge is mainly caused by methodological problems in implant surface topography research.

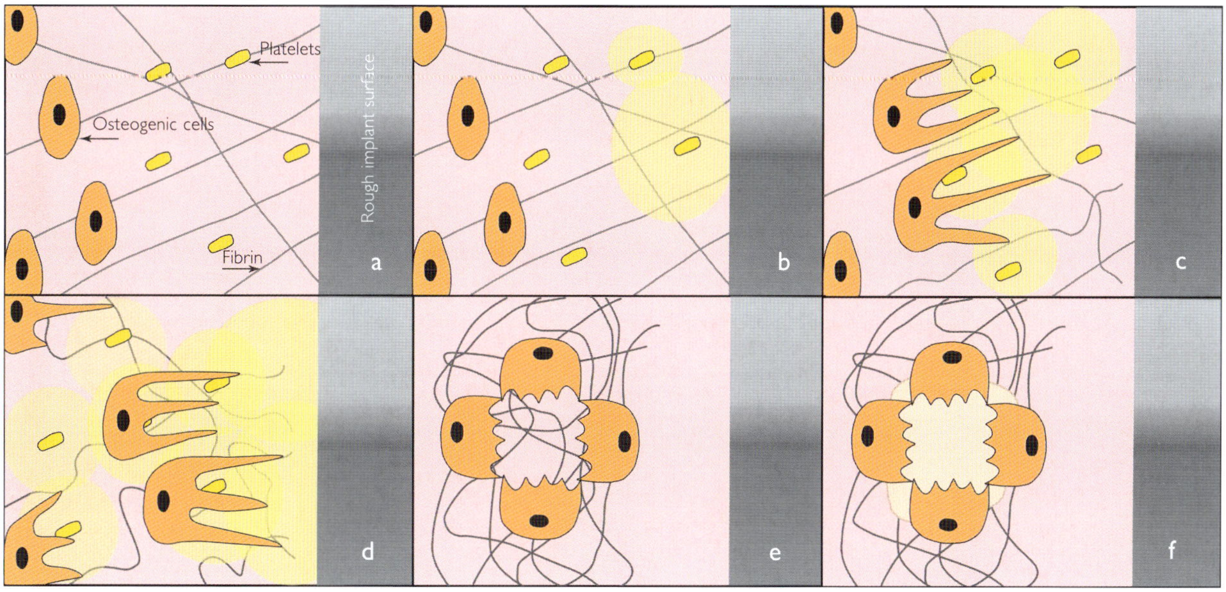

Fig 1-14a to f Distance osteogenesis. Platelets in the wound site are activated by the implant microtopography, and in turn recruit osteogenic cells to migrate to the implant surface (a and b). When these cells move through the blood clot, tension is created on the 3D fibrin matrix (c). If the physical interlocking between the fibers and the implant surface is not strong enough, the bridges for the cells to reach the implant shoulder are lost (d) and osteogenic cells differentiate (e) and start forming bone away from the implant shoulder (f).

The first methodological problem is the lack of standardized controls. Machined Bränemark implants (Nobel Biocare®, Zurich, Sweden) have been considered the gold standard in implant surface for many years. These implants have specific surface characteristics, including anisotropy and small roughness (Ra) values (Fig 1-15).[58] Many trials have used them as controls to evaluate new implant surfaces. However, the methodological problem arose when researchers started to produce their own control implants. The machining process of implants can be achieved through different techniques, which can hence lead to diverse implant topographies. In other words, "machined controls" are no longer a synonym for "machined Bränemark implants." Moreover, authors often fail to report the surface characterization of their machined controls. This inconsistency of controls makes the comparison between studies very difficult, hindering a clear interpretation of the data.

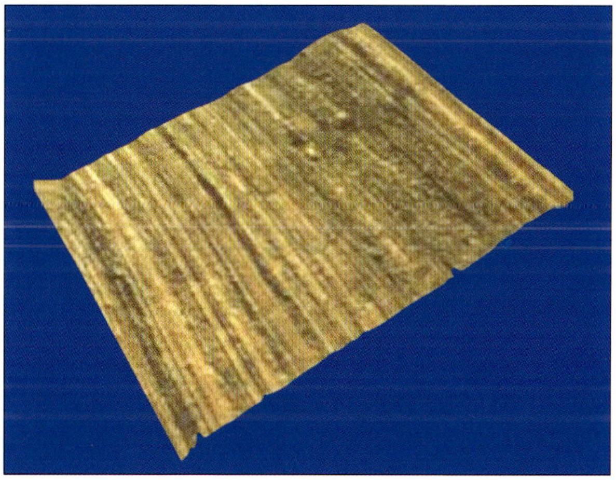

Fig 1-15 Machined Bränemark implant surface (surface 0.9 µm; surface area ratio 34%).

Other major problems in data analysis include the use of inappropriate techniques and instruments to characterize implant surface. In addition, it seems there is not a proper understanding of the concepts of form, waviness, and roughness.[59] This has led to erroneous classifications of surfaces, thereby impeding their comparison. The same surface has been described as "smooth" by some authors and as "rough" by others. Reliable quantitative surface evaluations are mandatory before any conclusions can be drawn as to which surface roughness results in the strongest bone response.[58,59] However, there is no consensus as to which parameters should be evaluated or the preferred level of resolution.

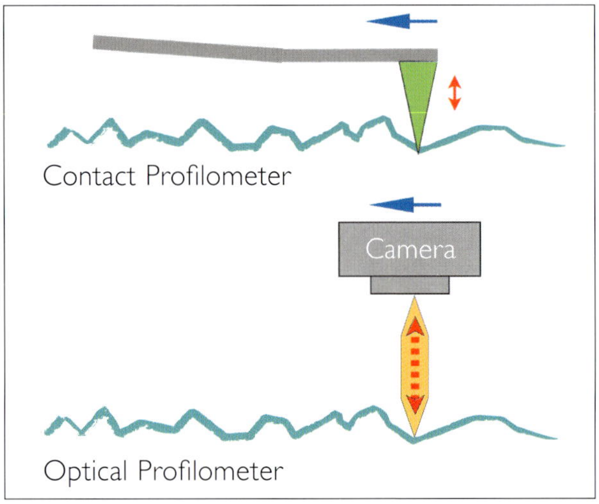

Fig 1-16 The principles of contact and optical profilometers. In contact instruments, a pick up with a stylus on its end is traversed over the study surface at a constant velocity, characterizing its roughness. In contrast, optical profilometers are non-contacting instruments that use a light beam to scan the study surface.

1.3.2 How should an implant surface be characterized?

Instruments

Three major groups of instruments have been used to provide quantitative and qualitative data for surface topographic evaluations: mechanical contact profilometers, optical profiling instruments; and scanning probe microscopes.

Both mechanical contact profilometers and scanning probe microscopes are contact systems that measure the interaction between a sharp tip and the sample surface. The fact that these systems cannot assess a threaded surface without damaging it makes them unsuitable for evaluating the most common types of oral implants. Only optical profiling instruments, such as confocal laser scanning profilometers and interferometers, are able to evaluate threaded implants, making them the only acceptable method at present. They register light reflected by the surface using an optical stylus. These instruments are generally faster and have better resolution than mechanical contact instruments (Fig 1-16).

Form, waviness, and roughness

Surface topography consists of form, waviness, and roughness (Fig 1-17).

Form is understood as the shape or design of an implant at a millimeter level of resolution. As explained earlier in this chapter, implant design has an influence on primary stability, force transmission to peri-implant tissues, and bone preservation, as shown by poor long-term levels of bone around cylindrical implants compared to screw-shaped implants.[60]

Waviness is the parameter representing repeating irregularities with spacing greater than the roughness sampling length. The filter size used determines the categorization of irregularities considered roughness and those considered waviness.

Roughness refers to the smallest scale of resolution of surface rugosities, often at a micro- or nanometer level.

For some time, waviness was considered the topographic key factor in implant surface engineering, since it was believed that bone could not invade pores smaller than 100 µm in diameter. This is true for osteonic bone with typical Haversian canals surrounded by circumferentially arranged osteocytes.[61] However, it is well known that bone tissue may nevertheless invade pores down to the 1 µm level of resolution.[58] Therefore the micrometer-scale of resolution is now considered the most relevant level in bone response generation.

Some research lines point out the relevance of the nanometer level of resolution as a modulator of cell response.[5] These nanometric-scale irregularities could be decisive in biologic bone reaction. Nevertheless, no *in vivo* studies have confirmed this hypothesis, and the micrometer level of resolution remains the gold standard in implant surface characterization. Possibly the combined effect of waviness and roughness is responsible for the biologic response of bone. In order to analyze the contribution of each factor and hence completely characterize implant surface, waviness and roughness should be reported as separate entities in every study.

Even though invalid measurement systems can lead to inconsistent values in roughness parameters, the factor with the greatest influence is the filter used to segregate roughness from waviness and form. When errors of form and waviness are filtered, roughness remains. In two-dimensional (2D) measurements, a specific length is selected and analyzed as a unit (Fig 1-18). This cut-off length, as it is called, filters errors of form. In 3D measurements, a Gaussian filter is used as a standard filter.[59]

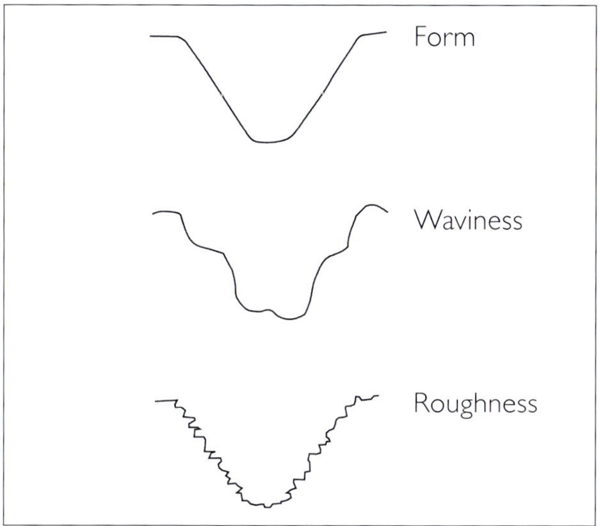

Fig 1-17 Thread of an implant demonstrating form, waviness, and roughness.

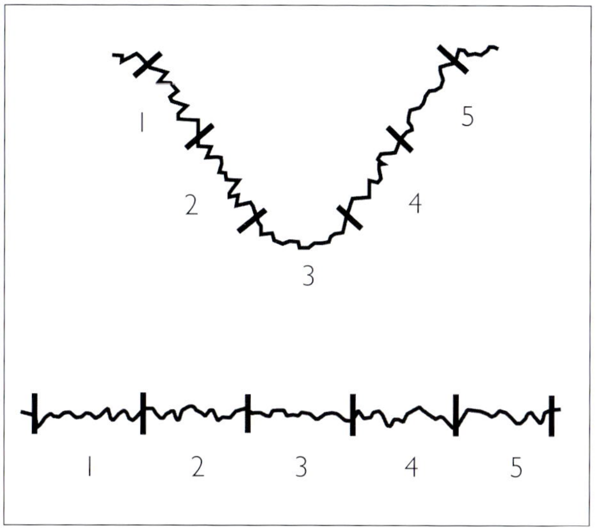

Fig 1-18 To exclude the assessment of form, a cut-off length is often used in 2D evaluation.

Parameters to be evaluated

Surface topography is described by three major groups of parameters. These are height, spatial, and hybrid parameters. Height parameters are solely descriptive of deviation in the vertical plane. Spatial or texture parameters describe the horizontal distance between irregularities. Finally, hybrid parameters include both spatial and height information.[59] In order to correctly characterize surface topography, more than a single parameter should be studied. This is even more important today, since the new surfaces developed have small (low height values) but frequent (high spatial values) irregularities. However, the ideal set of parameters to be used remains undetermined. What is indeed certain is that representative parameters from the three major groups should be included.

It is acknowledged that 3D surface evaluation is preferable to 2D analysis. Since surface topography is three-dimensional in nature, only 3D analyses can accurately represent the inherent characteristics of surface topography. For example, the average roughness of a surface (Sa) is a much more reliable parameter than the average profile roughness (Ra); it is less influenced by the measurement direction (while the profile is measured across or along the dominant direction of the irregularities), and it is considerably more consistent than its 2D counterpart.

Typical height descriptive parameters include Ra, Rq, Rz, and Rt. Their 3D spatial counterparts are Sa, Sq, Sz, and St, respectively. The arithmetic mean deviation of a profile is expressed by Ra; Sa when describing a surface. The root mean square deviation of a profile is defined as Rq; Sq for a surface. Rq gives almost the same information as Ra but is slightly more sensitive to high peaks and low valleys. Rz (Sz for 3D) is the 10-point height. It is the average of the five lowest valleys and five highest peaks within the profile (Rz) or surface (Sz). Finally, the difference between the highest peak and the lowest valley is defined by Rt in a profile and by St in a surface. It is an extreme parameter that easily varies over different measurement areas.

Most studies tend to report height parameters only. However, spatial and/or hybrid parameters are highly recommendable. Wennerberg and Albrektsson[62] showed their preference for a hybrid parameter called surface area ratio (Sdr). It informs about the number and height of the peaks of a given surface and allows the clinician to recognize the amount of surface enlargement achieved when the surface is flattened out. Both the density of peaks (Sds) and the Sa are relevant to this parameter.

Even though Ra is known to be quite stable and insensitive to occasional high peaks or deep valleys,[59] very different values have been reported for apparently similar surfaces. For example, different Ra values have been reported when evaluating machined surfaces: 0.08 μm,[63] 0.15 μm,[64] 0.35 μm,[65] 0.7 μm,[66] 1.3 μm,[67] and 4.7 μm.[68] Similarly, important discrepancies exist regarding titanium plasma-sprayed (TPS) surfaces, where Ra values vary from low values of 0.5 μm[63] to intermediate values of 2.4 μm,[68] 3.1 μm,[64] 4.0 μm,[66] or to extremely high values of 18.9 μm[69] or 37.9 μm.[65] These

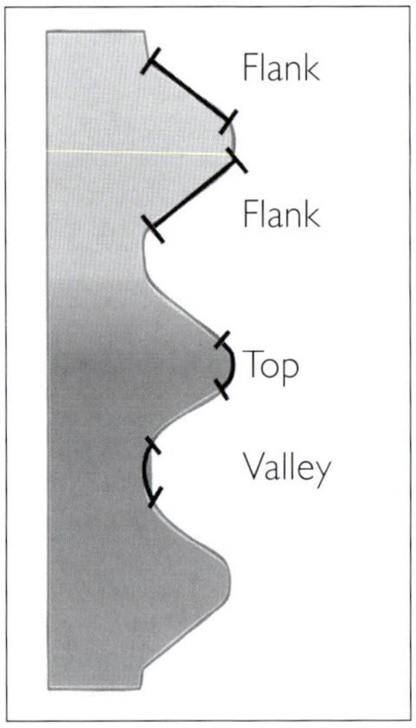

Fig 1-19 Areas of a threaded implant that need to be measured: top, flank, and valley.

variations may result from real differences between surface topographies but are most likely due to the use of different measuring equipment, different measurement lengths or filters, and the use of either 2D or 3D evaluations.[59]

Most studies lack information about the wavelength of roughness considered to be waviness. In addition, filter sizes used to separate roughness, waviness, and form vary greatly among studies. There is no accepted standard definition of when roughness becomes waviness. The limit between them is determined by the size of the chosen filter. Size selection is subject to some subjectivity but should be performed according to the roughness deemed relevant for a particular application (for example, cell differentiation or protein adhesion).[59] Different Gaussian filter sizes will lead to large variations in the descriptive parameters studied. This results in serious difficulties in data interpretation and comparison between studies, leading to the lack of reliable knowledge in surface topography.[59] To avoid this, information about filter size must be included in the description of the topographic evaluation. In fact, it is strongly recommended that roughness and waviness evaluations are presented separately for better surface understanding.

The area to be measured is also an important aspect of surface metrology. In screw-shaped implants, surface roughness measurements vary considerably between different locations of the same implant. This implies that different locations should be measured in order to obtain a reliable mean value.[58] Thread tops seem to be rougher than flanks, and valleys are the smoothest sites.[59] Wennerberg[58] observed that a mean roughness value was stable after measuring three tops, three flanks, and three valleys of a single implant (Fig 1-19).

For the purpose of overcoming these methodological differences and with the aim to achieve comparable data, guidelines have been proposed (Table 1-2).[59]

1.3.3 What surface treatments are available?

Many techniques have been developed to modify implant surfaces in order to modulate bone response and enhance osseointegration. Currently, the general trend is to roughen the surface by additive or subtractive procedures (Table 1-3). The techniques that add material

Table 1-2 Guidelines for surface characterization

Measuring method	Confocal laser scanning profilometers and interferometers are the only acceptable methods available at present able to evaluate densely threaded oral implant designs.
Suggested areas of measurement	Preferably, 3D measurements should be performed.
	On screw-type implants, tops, valleys, and flanks should be evaluated, in three different measuring areas.
	The measuring areas should be as large as possible to allow for different wavelengths inherent in the topography. Selecting only a flat portion of a screw for analysis is unacceptable.
	Cylindric implants should be measured on at least three different areas, each as large as possible. In addition, at least three samples of a batch should be evaluated.
Filtering process	The filter should be chosen in such a way that values for waviness plus roughness, and roughness could be presented separately.
	Filter size must be specified.
Parameters	For numeric evaluation, at least one height, one space, and one hybrid parameter should be presented.

to the bulk of metal lead to a convex profile, leaving a bumpy surface. On the other hand, subtractive techniques remove particles from the surface, creating a concave profile with pits and pores.[70]

Subtractive procedures (Table 1-4)

Turning/machining

In general, after machining, the implant surface presents periodic grooves that vary according to the machining equipment. This procedure typically results in a clean, minimally rough surface (Ra typically ranging from 0.4 to 0.8 μm). The original Bränemark turned, commercially pure titanium grade I machined implant has been considered the gold standard in implant surface design for decades.[71]

Currently, the use of machined implants is restricted to research purposes as a control to compare with other surfaces, usually rougher. However, controls are no longer standardized Bränemark machined implants; the surface topography of controls varies among studies as a result of customized machining processes. Therefore, the topographical description of machined implants is mandatory in order to enable comparisons between studies.

Table 1-3 Surface treatment procedures

Subtractive processes	Turning/machining
	Blasting
	Etching
	Blasting + etching
	Oxidation
Additive processes	Plasma spraying
	Sol-gel deposition
	Pulsed laser deposition sputtering coating
	Ion beam-assisted deposition
	Electrophoretic deposition
	Dip coating
	Biomimetic coating
	Hot isostatic pressing

Table 1-4 Subtractive procedures and representative surfaces

Surface treatment	Representative surface	Sa (μm)	Sdr (%)	Observations
Turned	Bränemark turned (Nobel Biocare)	0.9	34	Good clinical results for up to 20 years.[71] Restricted use as control implants for research purposes.
Blasted	TiOblast (Astra Tech)	1.1	31	Animal studies suggest blasted implants demonstrate better bone integration than turned.[74-79] Human studies do not find major differences between blasted and turned surfaces.[42,80] Limited data are available comparing blasted with other rough surfaces.
Etched	Osseotite (Biomet 3i)	0.68	27	Animal studies suggest etched implants demonstrate better bone integration than turned.[82-84]
	Prevail (Biomet 3i)	0.3	24	Human studies do not find major differences between etched and turned surfaces.[86]
Blasted + etched	OsseoSpeed (Astra Tech)	1.4	37	Animal and human studies support the superiority of blasted + etched over turned implants.[87-91,94,96]
	SLA old batch (Straumann)	1.5	34	Results are not so clear when compared with other surfaces.[97,98]
	SLA new batch (Straumann)	1.78	97	
Oxidized	TiUnite (Nobel Biocare)	1.1	37	Animal and human studies support the superiority of oxidized over turned implants.[100-103] Oxidized surfaces seem to be advantageous when implants are to be loaded during healing.[105,106]

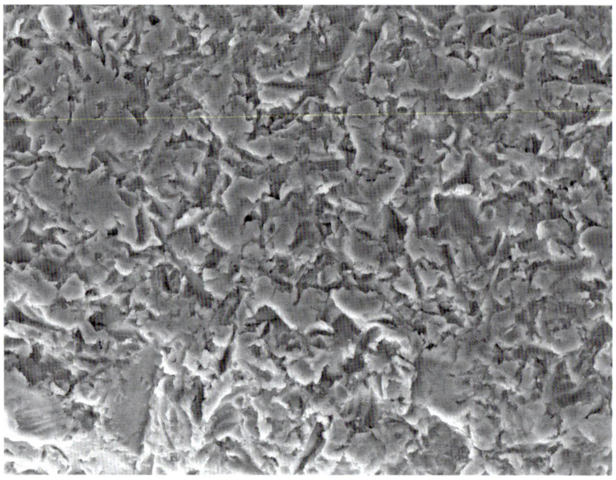

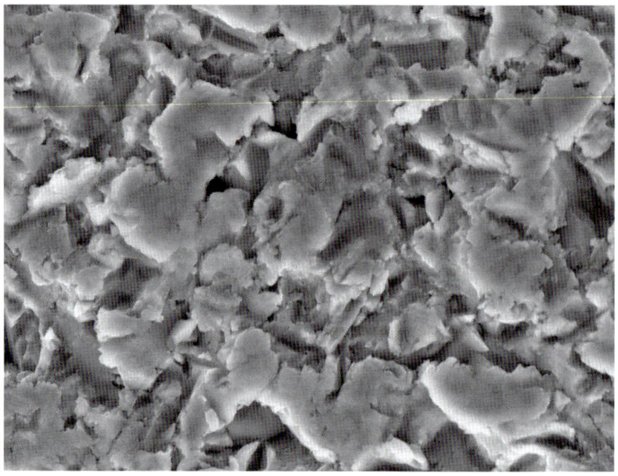

Fig 1-20a and b SEM images of a titanium oxide blasted surface: TiOblast® (Astra Tech®) [magnification: (a) ×1000, (b) ×2500].

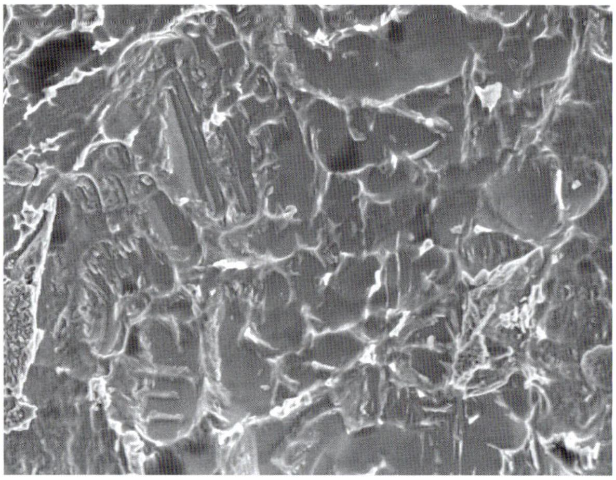

Fig 1-21 SEM image of a dual acid-etched surface: Osseotite® (Biomet 3i®) (magnification ×20,000).

Blasting

The grit-blasting procedure is generally performed via propulsion towards the implant body of particles of silica (sand blasting), resorbable bioceramic (resorbable blast media [RBM], alumina, or titanium dioxide, of different particle sizes. Depending on particle size, different surface roughness can be produced. Blasting material should be chemically stable, biocompatible, and should not hamper the osseointegration of the titanium implants.

The TiOblast® (Astra Tech®, Mölndal, Sweden) surface is blasted with small micron-sized titanium dioxide TiO_2 particles (Fig 1-20). This was the first moderately rough implant surface commercially available. Since its clinical introduction in 1993, 10 years of positive clinical data have been reported.[72,73]

Animal studies demonstrate that blasted surfaces obtain better bone integration than turned/machined surfaces. Wennerberg et al.[74-79] observed the strongest bone response in terms of peak removal torque and BIC for a blasted surface with an Sa value of 1.5 µm, an average wavelength of 11 µm, and a surface enlargement of 50%. These findings led the authors to state that moderately rough surfaces (Sa of approx. 1.5 µm, and Sdr of approx. 50%) promote the strongest bone response. Smoother and rougher surfaces produce weaker bone bonds than this hypothetical ideal roughness, indicating the existence of a threshold.[62]

Nevertheless, when blasted and turned implants are studied in human trials, differences don't seem so manifest. In a 5-year prospective study, Wennstrom et al.[41] compared implants with either a turned or a TiO_2 particle-blasted surface in periodontitis-susceptible patients. They found minor bone loss for both surface modifications, with no statistically significant differences between them. Karlsson et al.[80] compared the same two implant models and found no differences in survival rate or marginal bone loss after two years of loading. Consequently, in contrast to animal studies, clinical studies often fail to find any major advantages or disadvantages of blasted implants over turned implants.

Etching

Titanium is a corrosion-resistant metal even though some acids can be used to remove small amounts of material from the surface to create pits. Acids like hydrochloric acid (HCl), sulfuric acid (H_2SO_4), nitric acid (HNO_3),

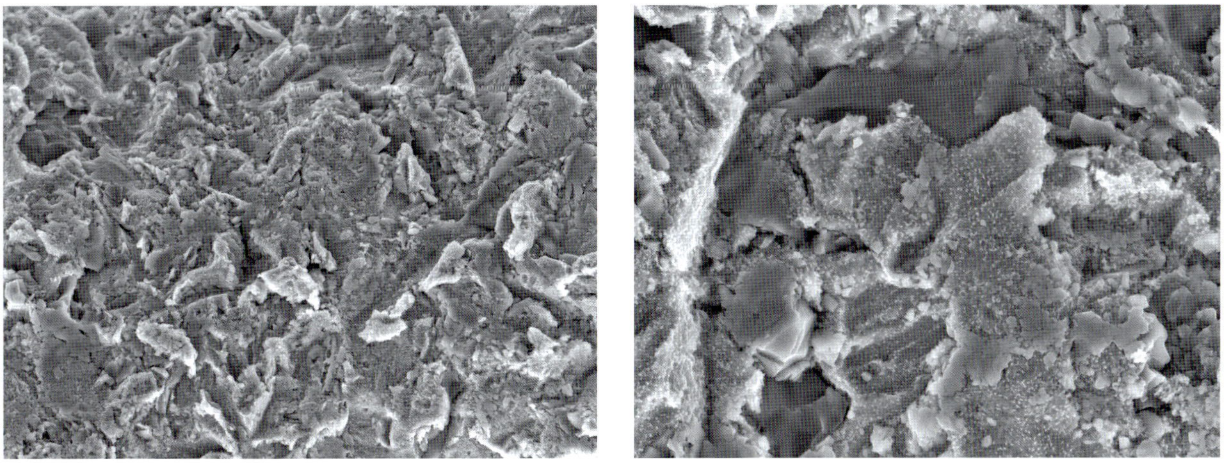

Fig 1-22a and b SEM images of a titanium oxide blasted surface with hydrofluoric acid treatment: OsseoSpeed® (Astra Tech®) [magnification: (a)×1000, (b) ×2500].

and hydrofluoric acid (HF) are examples of commonly used chemical agents for the etching of titanium. The surface area may increase, but the average height deviation may not necessarily follow; it can even decrease. Another effect of the etching procedure is to transform anisotropy (clear surface groove orientation) to isotropy (absence of groove orientation).[70]

Biomet 3i® (Palm Beach Gardens, FL, USA) produces a commercially pure titanium implant with a turned collar and a dual acid-etched (HCl and H_2SO_4) anchorage portion, the Osseotite® implant (Fig 1-21). Good results support this surface configuration after 5 years of follow-up.[81] Biomet 3i® developed another implant under the name of Prevail®. This implant exhibits lower Sa and Sdr values than its predecessor, possibly due to the fact that the core material is the titanium alloy Ti-6Al-4V. Since the alloy is harder than commercially pure titanium, the grooves left by the turning process of the implant are not so pronounced and, in addition, even though the acid treatment is the same, its influence on the surface irregularities is milder.[62]

Etched surfaces seem to demonstrate better osseointegration than machined/turned implants in animal studies.[82,83] Some researchers have even found evidence of a superior bone response when compared with rougher surfaces. Cordioli et al.[84] compared machined (Ra 0.29 μm), acid-etched (Ra 0.62 μm), blasted (Ra 1.26 μm), and TPS (Ra 9.10 μm) surfaces in rat bone. After 5 weeks, the etched surfaces demonstrated higher removal torque and BIC than the other three surface modifications. However, these findings are in disagreement with other studies. Klokkevold et al.[85] compared removal torque values of machined (Ra 185 nm), dual-etched (494 nm), and TPS (7.01 μm) surfaces at 1, 2, and 3 months in a rabbit model. Even though both etched and blasted surfaces performed better than the machined in all three time points, the TPS surface was superior to the dual-etched surface at 2 and 3 months.

Clinical trials yield minor differences when etched and turned surfaces are compared. In a retrospective clinical study, Al-Nawas et al.[86] compared double-etched implants (Osseotite®, Biomet 3i®) with turned implants (Nobel Biocare®). No difference in survival rate was found between implants. However, more turned implants were lost when bone regeneration procedures were required.

Blasting and etching

A combination of blasting and etching has been a common strategy to modify implant surfaces. The reason for this combination of methods is that the blasting procedure hypothetically achieves an optimal roughness for mechanical fixation, whereas the additional etching smooths some sharp peaks and may add a high-frequency component on the implant surface which can potentially improve protein adhesion.[70] Even though reported surface topography values vary between studies, the majority of blasted-etched surfaces are moderately rough.

OsseoSpeed® (Astra Tech®) possesses 50–100 nm structured features created by titanium oxide blasting followed by chemical modification of the surface by HF treatment (Fig 1-22).[87,88] Despite the chemical enhancement with fluoride ions, investigations show that the

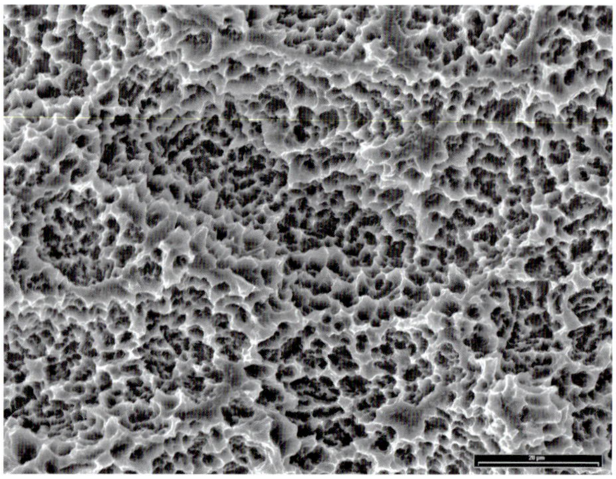

Fig 1-23 SEM image of a sand-blasted and acid-etched surface: SLA® (Straumann®) (magnification: × 1500).

remaining fluoride found in the surface is less than 1 atomic percent.[62] This surface has been clinically documented for 1 year with good results in different publications,[89,90] and one study observed positive results over a 3-year follow-up period.[91]

The SLA® (sand-blasted, large-grit, acid-etched) surface of Straumann® (Basel, Switzerland) implants has a grit-blasted and acid-etched surface. It is characterized as a hydrophobic surface due to the adsorbed hydrocarbons and carbonates from ambient air.[92,93] It has an Sa of 1.5 µm and an Sdr of 34%. However, the characterization study performed by Wennerberg and Albrektsson[62] in 2008 found that roughness of SLA® implants had increased to an Sa of 1.78 µm and an Sdr of 97% (Fig 1-23). At any rate, 5-year clinical documentation supports the positive results of this surface.[94]

The first *in vivo* study of SLA® implants was performed by Buser et al.[7] They compared electropolished, blasted-etched and hydroxyapatite (HA)-coated implants with Ra values ranging from 0.6 to 50 µm.[64,95] It seems that the surface modification caused by the acid may have a stronger influence on bone response than surface treatments with superior height deviation values. Human studies involving retrieved microimplants also support the superiority of blasted-etched over machined implants.[96]

However, when blasted-etched implants are compared to surfaces other than machined, the outcome is less certain. No differences in osseointegration capacity have been observed between minimally rough, moderately rough (oxidized or blasted-etched), and highly rough (TPS) surfaces in dog models.[97,98] Similarly, no differences in cell migration or osteogenesis were observed between etched (Ra 0.4 µm) or blasted-etched (Ra 2 µm) titanium rods in an electron microscopic evaluation.[99]

Oxidation

All titanium implants have a native oxide layer. However, this layer is thicker in oxidized implants, normally due to a caloric or electrochemical treatment. Oxidized implants are either heated or placed as anodes in a galvanic cell with suitable electrolytes; after the passage of an electric current through the galvanic cell, the surface oxide develops from the native state of around 5 nm thickness to 1 mm or even more.[70]

Nobel Biocare® implants are manufactured using this process, and the resulting surface receives the name of TiUnite® (Fig 1-24). During the process, the electrolyte used contains phosphoric acid[62] and the surface oxide grows to a 10,000 nm thick layer. When clinically introduced, the implant had a surface gradient with a thicker oxide layer in the apical area. However, the gradient has currently disappeared and the surface has turned more hydrophobic.[62] The original TiUnite® implant has been positively documented clinically for 5 years.[100] Whether clinical results of the new surface will be influenced in any way by the introduced alterations remains to be confirmed.

A positive correlation between increasing height deviation and implant incorporation has been stated for oxidized implants. Choi et al.[101] investigated oxidized implants prepared at different voltages and found that implants with higher height deviation showed higher removal torque and BIC values compared with smoother implants. Similarly, human studies using microimplants have shown oxidized implants promote superior bone responses compared with turned controls.[102,103]

In addition to topographic variations, oxidation can also modulate surface chemistry by adding particulate ions to the electrolyte during the manufacturing process. Chemically modified implants have demonstrated higher removal torque and more BIC than the control turned implants. The calcium- and magnesium-reinforced surfaces showed significantly stronger osseointegration than other modifications.[104]

Clinical studies suggest that oxidized surfaces perform better than turned surfaces in immediate or early loading protocols. Rocci et al.[105] compared implants with the

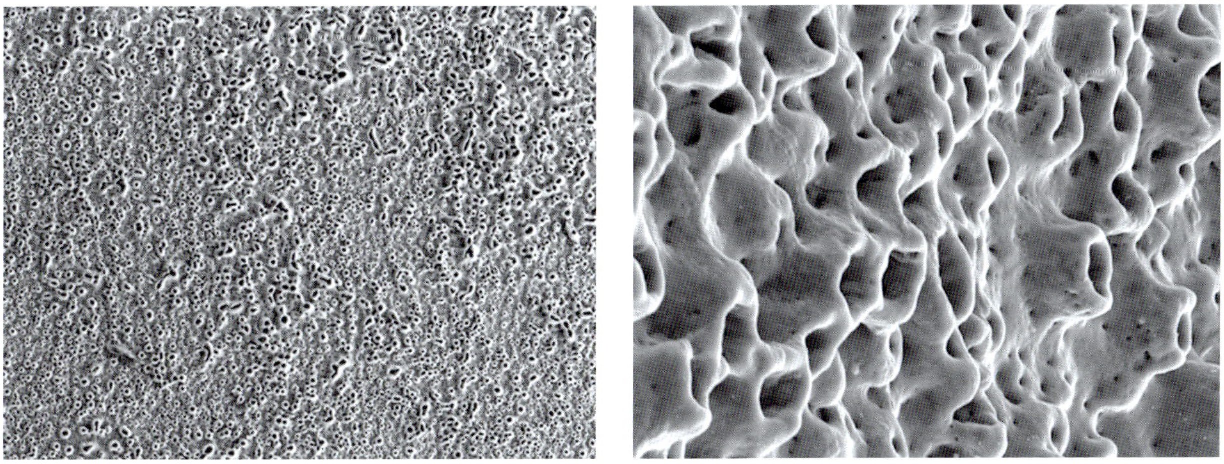

Fig 1-24a and b SEM images of an anodized surface: TiUnite® (Nobel Biocare®) [magnification: (a) ×500, (b) ×6000].

same macrodesign but with different surface treatment (turned vs. oxidized) in an immediate loading protocol. The authors found a significantly higher success rate for the oxidized implants compared with the turned. Similar results were found by Friberg and Jemt[106] when comparing the same implants in an early loading protocol. After 1 year of function, a significantly higher survival rate was confirmed with oxidized compared with turned implants.

Additive procedures

Plasma spray

Plasma spray techniques are coating procedures in which melted materials are sprayed onto a surface. Common coating precursors in implantology are titanium or calcium phosphate (HA) particles.

Titanium plasma-sprayed (TPS) coatings

The TPS method has been used to produce highly rough implant surfaces. It consists in injecting titanium powders into a plasma torch at high temperature. Titanium particles are projected onto the implant surface, where they condense and fuse together, forming a 40- to 50-µm-thick film (Fig 1-25).

Several animal studies suggest that a moderate increase in height deviation to levels ranging from 0.7 to 4.7 µm in TPS implants leads to a stronger bone response, but no effect is seen if Ra values reach 10 µm or more.[70] On the other hand, human trials seem to reflect increased marginal bone resorption around

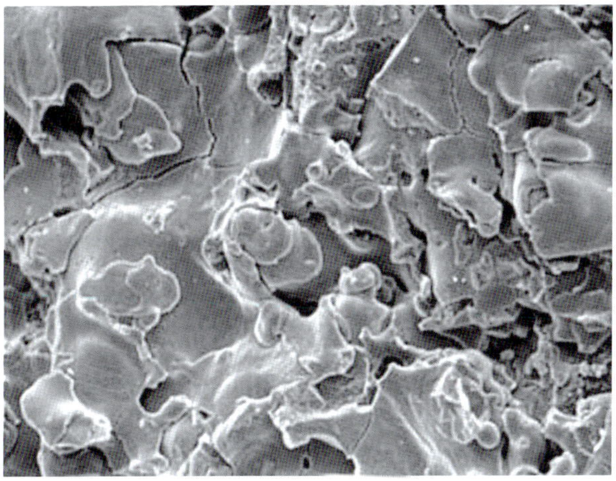

Fig 1-25 SEM image of a titanium plasma-sprayed surface: TPS (Straumann®) (magnification: ×1500).

TPS surfaces compared with other surface modifications.[107-109] Roynesdal et al.[107] compared turned, HA-coated and TPS implants placed in the anterior mandible and concluded that significantly more marginal bone loss was observed on TPS implants in comparison with the other two designs.

Another concern related to TPS surfaces is the possibility of particle detachment from the implant coating. Metallic wear particles have been detected in the bone adjacent to TPS hip implants, but also in further distant anatomical sites, such as the liver, spleen, and paraaortic lymph nodes.[110] Metal ions released from implants may be the product of dissolution, fretting, and wear. Although potentially harmful local and systemic effects have been reported for hip implants, including carcinogenesis,[3] these effects have not been described for dental implants.

Nowadays, rough TPS implants have fallen into disuse in favor of moderately rough surfaces, which have obtained better long-term results.

Plasma-sprayed hydroxyapatite (PSHA) coatings

Plasma spraying has also been used to apply ceramic coatings to metal implants. These layers of calcium phosphates (mainly HA) have demonstrated an improved healing capacity over non-coated implants.[111-114]

Some authors believe that following implantation, the release of calcium phosphate into the peri-implant region increases the saturation of local body fluids and a biological apatite precipitates onto the implant surface. This layer of biological apatite might contain endogenous proteins and serve as a matrix for osteogenic cell attachment and growth-enhancing bone attachment.[3,115,116] However, other authors[117,118] have highlighted that even though the chemistry of these surface modifications plays a role in bone response enhancement, positive results could be equally dependent on surface topography. Further studies should be performed in order to clarify this point.

Metal implant HA coating can be achieved by different methods: plasma-spraying; sputter-deposition; sol-gel coating; electrophoretic deposition; or biomimetic precipitation, among others.[119] However, only the first three methods have been used in commercial implants. The plasma-spraying method was the first and most broadly used coating method in clinical practice.[3] Hydroxyapatite ceramic particles are injected into a plasma torch at high temperature and projected onto the titanium surface, where they condense and fuse together, forming a film. Plasma-sprayed coatings can be deposited with a thickness ranging from a few micrometers to a few millimeters. In order to obtain coating retention, the surface of the metallic implant must be roughened, since the union between both materials seems entirely mechanic.[114]

Even though PSHA-coated prostheses are very popular in orthopedics, the clinical use in dental implantology is limited. The popularity of these surface modifications dropped when shortcomings of the plasma-spraying method arose. Disadvantages such as coating porosity, residual stress at the substrate-coating interface, and changes in the composition and crystallinity of the initial calcium phosphate powder were reported.[120] However, what led to the neglection of these surfaces was the delamination of the coating from the surface of the titanium implant due to failure at the implant-coating interface, despite a complete integration of the coating to the bone tissue.[121-124] The discrepancy in dissolution behavior between amorphous and crystalline calcium phosphate phases that make up the coating may explain this delamination and thus the clinical failure of implants.[54,121,123,124] Nevertheless, despite their bad reputation, a meta-analysis performed by Lee et al.[123] concluded that HA-coated surfaces have similar long-term survival rates compared with other surfaces.

1.3.4 Are modern surfaces better than their predecessors?

Recently, implant manufacturers have marketed novel surface treatments with presumably increased osseointegration capacity.[62] The Nanotite® (Biomet 3i®), OsseoSpeed® (Astra Tech®), and SLActive® (Straumann®) surfaces have been claimed to incite stronger bone responses than their respective predecessors. But which is the underlying mechanism to this superior bone response? The reality is that it is not yet completely understood. An easily acceptable explanation would be that OsseoSpeed® generates a stronger bone response than its predecessor TioBlast® due to fluoride ions in its composition, that Nanotite® generates a stronger bone response than its predecessor Osseotite® due to a particular nanotopography, or that SLActive® exerts a stronger bone response than its predecessor SLA® due to its hydrophilicity. However, it must be acknowledged that these new implants differ from their respective predecessors in several parameters, not in a single one.[70] All three have a modified microtopography, potentially different surface chemistry, and modified nanoroughness.[62]

Since these novel surfaces differ from their predecessors in surface microroughness, this could account for their better performance. Nanotite® has a greater Sdr than Osseotite® (27% vs 40%) but smaller Sa (0.5 µm vs 0.68). OsseoSpeed® has greater Sdr and Sa than TiOblast® (37% vs 31%; 1.4 µm vs 1.1 µm). And SLActive® has a greater Sdr than SLA® (143% vs 97%) but similar Sa values (1.75 µm vs 1.78 µm).[62] However, based on current knowledge in implant surface microroughness, the different bone response cannot be explained fully by differences in microroughness. For example, the Sdr values of SLActive® are theoretically considered too high, and SLA®'s lower values seem more desirable.[77,79] Moreover, in an experimental study, the OsseoSpeed® surface was manipulated down to minimal roughness (Sa 0.9 µm, Sdr 21%) and compared with the TiOblast® surface (Sa 1.1 µm, Sdr 31%). Even though OsseoSpeed® had a supposedly weaker microroughness, it obtained a significantly greater bone response than TiOblast®.[125] These facts emphasize that other surface traits, besides microtopography, may have a positive influence on bone response.

These surface enhancers may include the chemical and physical properties of the surface. The better bone response observed with the Nanotite® surface may be chemically generated by the HA in its nanotextured coating. However, Meirelles et al.[126-128] found that factors other than chemistry may explain the strong bone response to nano-HA compounds. Likewise, fluoride ions on the OsseoSpeed® surface could catalyze bone response; though, chemical analyses clearly demonstrate that the surface possesses less than 1 atomic percent of fluoride ions attached to it.[129] Consequently, the chemical effect of such a small amount is questionable. From a physical point of view, it must be pointed out that surface treatment with fluoride-containing ions generates a hydrophilic response of the surface.[130] The SLActive® implant would share this surface trait, which could account for an enhanced response on both surfaces (Fig 1-26). However, whether hydrophilia has a relevant effect in implant anchorage is questionable.[131]

Nanoroughness is the third possible mechanism behind the noted strong bone response to these three novel surfaces. Wennerberg and Albrektsson[62] characterized surface roughness at the nanoscale level in implants from the four most popular manufacturers. SLActive®, Nanotite®, and OsseoSpeed® all had nanofeatures, but the ideal nanoroughness, if any, remains undefined. The authors proposed an altered nanoroughness pattern could be a possible mechanism behind strong bone response. The different etching procedures involved in the three surfaces result in a superficial layer of titanium hydride (whether it is TiH_2, TiH_3, TiH_4, or a combination of these remains to be investigated).[132] Hydrogen is gradually replaced by oxide, resulting in the formation of nanometer-sized particles of titanium on such surfaces. These nanofeatures may be important in protein adhesion immediately after implant placement.

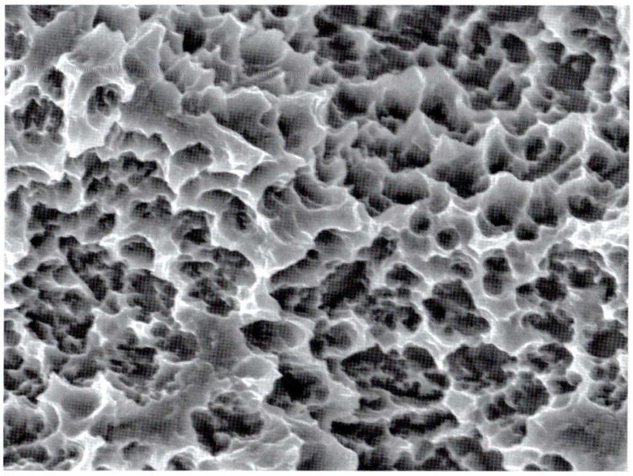

Fig 1-26 SEM image of a sand-blasted and acid etched surface rinsed under nitrogen protection and stored immersed in an isotonic NaCl solution: SLActive® (Straumann®) (magnification: × 1500).

1.3.5 What can we expect from the future?

Scientific research and technological development have given way to high-quality implant surfaces with excellent predictability and reliable bone response. These advances have broadened the spectrum of indications to include poor bone quality situations and have shortened treatment times by permitting earlier loading protocols. However, further development is still possible and desirable in order to further reduce treatment time, obtain stronger bone–implant bonding and prevent progressive bone loss over time.

With these aims, several strategies are currently under assessment. These future trends concern the modifications of surface roughness at the nanoscale level to promote protein adsorption and cell adhesion, biomimetic calcium phosphate coatings to enhance osseoconduction, and the incorporation of biological drugs to accelerate the bone healing process in the peri-implant area.[3]

Nanometer-scale roughness

Nanometer roughness is an issue under debate in current dental implant therapy. Nanotechnology involves materials with a nano-sized topography or which are composed of nano-sized materials. These materials have a size range between 1 and 100 nm.[54] Nanometer roughness may play an important role in the selective adsorption of proteins, adhesion of osteoblastic cells, and thus in the rate of osseointegration, although the optimal surface nanotopography remains undefined.[3,6] Moreover, reproducible surface roughness in the nanometer range is difficult to produce with current manufacturing.

The individual contribution of nanoroughness to bone response is extremely difficult to determine. When the topography of a surface is somehow modified, a physical and chemical change occurs at all scales. In other words, the modification of microtopography entails a simultaneous change in nanotopography and vice versa. The ideal experimental setup would be one in which microroughness and chemistry were controlled and bone responses to nanoroughness alone were investigated. Meirelles addressed this issue in various research projects.[126-128,133] By carefully electropolishing cylindrical implants, irregularities at the micron level of resolution were eliminated and only the nanotexture remained. This enabled investigations on the possible influence of such fine surface irregularities. The first trial compared polished implants with a nanocoating of HA (HA particles in a range of 20 nm) with polished non-coated controls, and obtained stronger bone responses associated to coated implants.[133] However, these findings could be associated either with the chemical effect of HA coatings or with the improved nanoroughness of coated implants.[127] To clarify this matter, a nano-textured non-coated titanium implant was introduced for comparison with the HA nanocoated implant. The former showed the strongest bone response, thereby proving that the nanotexture had a greater influence on bone response than surface chemistry. Nanotitanium implants showed increased feature density and a larger feature coverage area than nano-HA implants, thereby theoretically presenting more binding sites for proteins.[126]

At any rate, little is known beyond data from *in vitro* observations. *In vitro* results have some scientific interest indeed, but their applicability is limited, since the complex *in vivo* conditions are often not accurately reproduced. Future research should focus on *in vivo* studies in order to help clarify the role of this nanoscale roughness in bone behavior.

New calcium phosphate coatings

In an attempt to solve the problems that arose with PSHA coatings, new techniques to obtain thin-film nanostructured ceramic coatings have been developed. Some of the techniques used are sol-gel deposition,[134,135] pulsed laser deposition,[136,137] sputtering coating,[138,139] ion beam-assisted deposition,[140-142] electrophoretic deposition,[142] dip coating,[143] biomimetic coating,[144,145] and hot isostatic pressing.[145]

Desirable features of thin-film coatings include controlled composition and thickness of the coating besides enhanced adhesion to the metallic substrate (40 MPa vs < 20 MPa for PSHA-coated implants).[119,134,140,141,146] Controlled composition and thickness have also proved to influence coating dissolution *in vivo*,[119] thereby potentially increasing osseoconductivity at early implantation times. Rapid dissolution of thin films may result in the exposure of the metallic substrate soon after surgical placement. Therefore, the possibility of having close bone contact to the implant metallic substrate at the optical microscopy level after coating dissolution may be an attractive feature of thin-films. This close contact would avoid an interphase between bone, bioceramic, surface oxides, and implant metallic substrate, possibly supporting favorable conditions for implant device long-term anchorage.[15,119]

The Nanotite® surface is one of the commercially available calcium phosphate thin-coatings. This surface is created by a particulate sol-gel deposition method using discrete crystalline deposition of calcium phosphate (nominal crystal size 20–100 nm) on a minimally rough titanium alloy surface.[147] The Sa value is 0.5 µm and the Sdr is 40%.[62] The suggested nano-feature size of the coating is 20 to 100 nm.[147] Studies by Goené et al.[148] and Orsini et al.[149] confirm a stronger bone response to this implant than to its predecessor Osseotite®.

Incorporation of biomolecules and biologically active drugs

Extracellular matrix and bone morphogenetic proteins

The role of the extracellular matrix (ECM) in cell adhesion, migration, proliferation, morphological change, gene expression, and cell survival is well known.[150] In an attempt to enhance biological acceptance and function of titanium implants, the incorporation of ECM components is currently under investigation. Potential ECM components that may be used as coatings agents include the Arg–Gly–Asp (RGD) peptide sequences, type I and III collagen, chondroitin sulfate, and growth factors.[54] In particular, growth factors, such as bone morphogenetic proteins (BMPs), have been shown to promote bone formation and could also hypothetically enhance bone remodeling at the bone–implant interface.[151]

Research on this area demonstrates that biologic coatings show a tendency to improve bone response in peri-implant tissues, but the results of studies evaluating the different surface treatments are not consistent. Regarding BMPs, current findings seem to indicate they do not provide a useful strategy to coat implants since no increase in BIC is observed.[54] Further animal and human studies are needed to evaluate the suitability and efficiency of these biological surfaces.

Bisphosphonates

The addition of molecules that control the bone remodeling process to the implant surface is another promising line of investigation. The incorporation of bone antiresorptive drugs, such as biphosphonates, might be indeed very relevant in clinical cases lacking bone support, such as resorbed alveolar ridges.[3]

Recently, it was shown that a biphosphonate incorporated onto titanium implants increased bone density locally in the peri-implant region. The effect of the antiresorptive drug seemed to be limited to the vicinity of the implant.[152] Studies using PSHA-coated dental implants immersed in Pamidronic acid or zoledronic acid demonstrated a significant increase in bone contact area.[153-155] Further in vivo studies support these findings without any adverse effects being reported.[156,157] The main problem lies in the grafting and sustained release of antiresorptive drugs on the titanium implant surface. Due to the high chemical affinity of biphosphonates for calcium phosphate surfaces, incorporation of the antiresorptive drug onto dental implants could be achieved by using calcium phosphate coatings. However, the ideal dose of antiresorptive drug is still to be determined since the increase in peri-implant bone density is biphosphonate concentration-dependent.[155]

1.3.6 Conclusions

- The exact role of surface chemistry and topography on the early events of the osseointegration of dental implants remains poorly understood.
- Past methodological problems in implant surface topography characterization limit data comparison between studies.
- Literature reviews can only conclude that increasing surface roughness enhances osseointegration.
- Future research should follow recommended guidelines such as those proposed by Wennerberg and Albrektsson.[59]
- Even though most of the commercially available surfaces have proven clinical efficacy, there is no evidence to conclude that there is an optimal surface treatment.
- Novel implant surfaces, as Nanotite®, OsseoSpeed® and SLActive®, have shown improved bone responses over their predecessors. However, the mechanisms behind these effects are still to be determined since surface microroughness, chemistry, physics, and nanoroughness could be responsible.
- Future trends in surface treatment such as nanoroughness, new calcium phosphate coatings, and the incorporation of biomolecules or antiresorptive drugs, may lead to the definition of potential bone response enhancers. However, further *in vivo* research is necessary in order to prove their efficacy.

References

1. Abuhussein H, Pagni G, Rebaudi A, Wang HL. The effect of thread pattern upon implant osseointegration. Clin Oral Implants Res 2010;21:129-136.
2. Albrektsson T, Branemark PI, Hansson HA, Lindstrom J. Osseointegrated titanium implants. Requirements for ensuring a long-lasting, direct bone-to-implant anchorage in man. Acta Orthop Scand 1981;52:155-170.
3. Le Guehennec L, Soueidan A, Layrolle P, Amouriq Y. Surface treatments of titanium dental implants for rapid osseointegration. Dent Mater 2007;23:844-854.
4. Atieh MA, Ibrahim HM, Atieh AH. Platform switching for marginal bone preservation around dental implants: a systematic review and meta-analysis. J Periodontol 2010;81:1350-1366.
5. Svanborg LM, Andersson M, Wennerberg A. Surface characterization of commercial oral implants on the nanometer level. J Biomed Mater Res B Appl Biomater 2010;92:462-469.
6. Brett PM, Harle J, Salih V, Mihoc R, Olsen I, Jones FH, et al. Roughness response genes in osteoblasts. Bone 2004;35:124-133.
7. Buser D, Schenk RK, Steinemann S, Fiorellini JP, Fox CH, Stich H. Influence of surface characteristics on bone integration of titanium implants. A histomorphometric study in miniature pigs. J Biomed Mater Res 1991;25:889-902.
8. Wolff J. The Laws of Bone Remodeling. Berlin: Springer, 1892.
9. Frost HM. Skeletal structural adaptations to mechanical usage (SATMU): 2. Redefining Wolff's law: the remodeling problem. Anat Rec 1990;226:414-422.
10. Frost HM. Skeletal structural adaptations to mechanical usage (SATMU): 1. Redefining Wolff's law: the bone modeling problem. Anat Rec 1990;226:403-413.
11. Frost HM. A 2003 update of bone physiology and Wolff's Law for clinicians. Angle Orthod 2004;74:3-15.

12. Misch CE, Strong T, Bidez MW. Scientific rationale for dental implant design. In: Misch CE (ed). Contemporary Implant Dentistry, ed 3. St. Louis: Mosby, 2008:200-229.
13. Roberts WE, Smith RK, Zilberman Y, Mozsary PG, Smith RS. Osseous adaptation to continuous loading of rigid endosseous implants. Am J Orthod 1984;86:95-111.
14. Verborgt O, Gibson GJ, Schaffler MB. Loss of osteocyte integrity in association with microdamage and bone remodeling after fatigue in vivo. J Bone Miner Res 2000;15:60-67.
15. Lemons JE. Biomaterials, biomechanics, tissue healing, and immediate-function dental implants. J Oral Implantol 2004;30:318-324.
16. Lemons JE. Dental implant biomaterials. J Am Dent Assoc 1990;121:716-719.
17. Rieger MR, Mayberry M, Brose MO. Finite element analysis of six endosseous implants. J Prosthet Dent 1990;63:671-676.
18. Duyck J, Ronold HJ, Van Oosterwyck H, Naert I, Vander Sloten J, Ellingsen JE. The influence of static and dynamic loading on marginal bone reactions around osseointegrated implants: an animal experimental study. Clin Oral Implants Res 2001;12:207-218.
19. Bolind PK, Johansson CB, Becker W, Langer L, Sevetz EB Jr, Albrektsson TO. A descriptive study on retrieved non-threaded and threaded implant designs. Clin Oral Implants Res 2005;16:447-455.
20. Kohn DH. Overview of factors important in implant design. J Oral Implantol 1992;18:204-219.
21. Kim WT CY, Oh SJ. The three dimensional finite element analysis of stress according to implant thread design under the axial load. Korean J Oral Surg 2001;27:3-8.
22. Steigenga JT, al-Shammari KF, Nociti FH, Misch CE, Wang HL. Dental implant design and its relationship to long-term implant success. Implant Dent 2003;12:306-317.
23. Steigenga J, Al-Shammari K, Misch C, Nociti FH Jr, Wang HL. Effects of implant thread geometry on percentage of osseointegration and resistance to reverse torque in the tibia of rabbits. J Periodontol 2004;75:1233-1241.
24. Liang DK, Wang JH, Ma QS, Lu YP, Zhu RF. The influence of the screw thread and the height of constraints on the stress distribution around dental implants by using three-dimensional finite element analysis [in Chinese]. Shanghai Kou Qiang Yi Xue 2002;11:324-326.
25. American Gear Manufacturers A, American National Standards I. Gear nomenclature, definitions of terms with symbols: AGMA standard. Alexandria, VA: American Gear Manufacturers Association, 2005.
26. Ma P, Liu HC, Li DH, Lin S, Shi Z, Peng QJ. Influence of helix angle and density on primary stability of immediately loaded dental implants: three-dimensional finite element analysis [in Chinese]. Zhonghua Kou Qiang Yi Xue Za Zhi 2007;42:618-621.
27. Bozkaya D, Muftu S, Muftu A. Evaluation of load transfer characteristics of five different implants in compact bone at different load levels by finite elements analysis. J Prosthet Dent 2004;92:523-530.
28. Becker W, Goldstein M, Becker BE, Sennerby L. Minimally invasive flapless implant surgery: a prospective multicenter study. Clin Implant Dent Relat Res 2005;7(Suppl 1):S21-27.
29. Hermann JS, Schoolfield JD, Schenk RK, Buser D, Cochran DL. Influence of the size of the microgap on crestal bone changes around titanium implants. A histometric evaluation of unloaded non-submerged implants in the canine mandible. J Periodontol 2001;72:1372-1383.
30. Berglundh T, Lindhe J. Dimension of the periimplant mucosa. Biological width revisited. J Clin Periodontol 1996;23:971-973.
31. Broggini N, McManus LM, Hermann JS, Medina R, Schenk RK, Buser D, et al. Peri-implant inflammation defined by the implant-abutment interface. J Dent Res 2006;85:473-478.
32. King GN HJ, Schoolfield JD, Buser D, Cochran DL. Influence of the size of the microgap on crestal bone levels in non-submerged dental implants: A radiographic study in the canine mandible. J Periodontol 2002;73:1111-1117.
33. Hermann JS, Buser D, Schenk RK, Cochran DL. Crestal bone changes around titanium implants. A histometric evaluation of unloaded non-submerged and submerged implants in the canine mandible. J Periodontol 2000;71:1412-1424.
34. Hermann JS, Cochran DL, Nummikoski PV, Buser D. Crestal bone changes around titanium implants. A radiographic evaluation of unloaded nonsubmerged and submerged implants in the canine mandible. J Periodontol 1997;68:1117-1130.
35. Rangert B, Jemt T, Jorneus L. Forces and moments on Branemark implants. Int J Oral Maxillofac Implants 1989;4:241-247.
36. Hämmerle CH, Bragger U, Burgin W, Lang NP. The effect of subcrestal placement of the polished surface of ITI implants on marginal soft and hard tissues. Clin Oral Implants Res 1996;7:111-119.
37 Hanggi MP, Hanggi DC, Schoolfield JD, Meyer J, Cochran DL, Hermann JS. Crestal bone changes around titanium implants. Part I: A retrospective radiographic evaluation in humans comparing two non-submerged implant designs with different machined collar lengths. J Periodontol 2005;76:791-802.
38. Hermann JS, Buser D, Schenk RK, Schoolfield JD, Cochran DL. Biologic width around one- and two-piece titanium implants. Clin Oral Implants Res 2001;12:559-571.
39. Gotfredsen K, Berglundh I, Lindhe J. Bone reactions adjacent to titanium implants with different surface characteristics subjected to static load. A study in the dog (II). Clin Oral Implants Res 2001;12:196-201.
40. Vaillancourt H, Pilliar RM, McCammond D. Finite element analysis of crestal bone loss around porous-coated dental implants. J Appl Biomater 1995;6:267-282.
41. Wennstrom JL, Ekestubbe A, Grondahl K, Karlsson S, Lindhe J. Oral rehabilitation with implant-supported fixed partial dentures in periodontitis-susceptible subjects. A 5-year prospective study. J Clin Periodontol 2004;31:713-724.
42. Gotfredsen K, Karlsson U. A prospective 5-year study of fixed partial prostheses supported by implants with machined and TiO_2-blasted surface. J Prosthodont 2001;10:2-7.
43. Adell R, Lekholm U, Rockler B, Branemark PI. A 15-year study of osseointegrated implants in the treatment of the edentulous jaw. Int J Oral Surg 1981;10:387-416.
44. Ricci G, Aimetti M, Stablum W, Guasti A. Crestal bone resorption 5 years after implant loading: clinical and radiologic results with a 2-stage implant system. Int J Oral Maxillofac Implants 2004;19:597-602.
45. Quirynen M, Naert I, van Steenberghe D. Fixture design and overload influence marginal bone loss and fixture success in the Branemark system. Clin Oral Implants Res 1992;3:104-111.
46. Jung YC, Han CH, Lee KW. A 1-year radiographic evaluation of marginal bone around dental implants. Int J Oral Maxillofac Implants 1996;11:811-818.
47. Lee DW, Choi YS, Park KH, Kim CS, Moon IS. Effect of microthread on the maintenance of marginal bone level: a 3-year prospective study. Clin Oral Implants Res 2007;18:465-470.
48. Abrahamsson I, Berglundh T. Tissue characteristics at microthreaded implants: an experimental study in dogs. Clin Implant Dent Relat Res 2006;8:107-113.
49. Quirynen M, van Steenberghe D. Bacterial colonization of the internal part of two-stage implants. An in vivo study. Clin Oral Implants Res 1993;4:158-161.
50. Persson LG, Lekholm U, Leonhardt A, Dahlen G, Lindhe J. Bacterial colonization on internal surfaces of Branemark system implant components. Clin Oral Implants Res 1996;7:90-95.
51. Lazzara RJ, Porter SS. Platform switching: a new concept in implant dentistry for controlling postrestorative crestal bone levels. Int J Periodontics Restorative Dent 2006;26:9-17.
52. Hurzeler M, Fickl S, Zuhr O, Wachtel HC. Peri-implant bone level around implants with platform-switched abutments: preliminary data from a prospective study. J Oral Maxillofac Surg 2007;65(7 Suppl 1):33-39.

53. Canullo L, Rasperini G. Preservation of peri-implant soft and hard tissues using platform switching of implants placed in immediate extraction sockets: a proof-of-concept study with 12- to 36-month follow-up. Int J Oral Maxillofac Implants 2007;22:995-1000.
54. Junker R, Dimakis A, Thoneick M, Jansen JA. Effects of implant surface coatings and composition on bone integration: a systematic review. Clin Oral Implants Res 2009;20(Suppl 4):185-206.
55. Davies JE. Understanding peri-implant endosseous healing. J Dent Educ 2003;67:932-949.
56. Cooper LF. A role for surface topography in creating and maintaining bone at titanium endosseous implants. J Prosthet Dent 2000;84:522-534.
57. Shalabi MM, Gortemaker A, Van't Hof MA, Jansen JA, Creugers NH. Implant surface roughness and bone healing: a systematic review. J Dent Res 2006;85:496-500.
58. Wennerberg A. On surface roughness and implant incorporation. Gothenburg: University of Gothenburg, 1996.
59. Wennerberg A, Albrektsson T. Suggested guidelines for the topographic evaluation of implant surfaces. Int J Oral Maxillofac Implants 2000;15:331-344.
60. Albrektsson T. On long-term maintenance of the osseointegrated response. Aust Prosthodont J 1993;7(Suppl):15-24.
61. Albrektsson T. In vivo studies of bone grafts. The possibility of vascular anastomoses in healing bone. Acta Orthop Scand 1980;51:9-17.
62. Wennerberg A, Albrektsson T. On implant surfaces: a review of current knowledge and opinions. Int J Oral Maxillofac Implants 2010;25:63-74.
63. Cooper LF, Masuda T, Whitson SW, Yliheikkila P, Felton DA. Formation of mineralizing osteoblast cultures on machined, titanium oxide grit-blasted, and plasma-sprayed titanium surfaces. Int J Oral Maxillofac Implants 1999;14:37-47.
64. Buser D, Nydegger T, Oxland T, Cochran DL, Schenk RK, Hirt HP, et al. Interface shear strength of titanium implants with a sandblasted and acid-etched surface: a biomechanical study in the maxilla of miniature pigs. J Biomed Mater Res 1999;45:75-83.
65. Vercaigne S, Wolke JG, Naert I, Jansen JA. The effect of titanium plasma-sprayed implants on trabecular bone healing in the goat. Biomaterials 1998;19:1093-1099.
66. Suzuki K, Aoki K, Ohya K. Effects of surface roughness of titanium implants on bone remodeling activity of femur in rabbits. Bone 1997;21:507-514.
67. Kilpadi DV, Lemons JE. Surface energy characterization of unalloyed titanium implants. J Biomed Mater Res 1994;28:1419-1425.
68. Vercaigne S, Wolke JG, Naert I, Jansen JA. Bone healing capacity of titanium plasma-sprayed and hydroxylapatite-coated oral implants. Clin Oral Implants Res 1998;9:261-271.
69. David A, Eitenmuller J, Muhr G, Pommer A, Bar HF, Ostermann PA, et al. Mechanical and histological evaluation of hydroxyapatite-coated, titanium-coated and grit-blasted surfaces under weight-bearing conditions. Arch Orthop Trauma Surg 1995;114:112-118.
70. Wennerberg A, Albrektsson T. Effects of titanium surface topography on bone integration: a systematic review. Clin Oral Implants Res 2009;20(Suppl 4):172-184.
71. Bryant S. Oral implant outcomes predicted by age- and site-specific aspects of bone condition. Toronto: University of Toronto, 2001.
72. Rasmusson L, Roos J, Bystedt H. A 10-year follow-up study of titanium dioxide-blasted implants. Clin Implant Dent Relat Res 2005;7:36-42.
73. Vroom MG, Sipos P, de Lange GL, Grundemann LJ, Timmerman MF, Loos BG, et al. Effect of surface topography of screw-shaped titanium implants in humans on clinical and radiographic parameters: a 12-year prospective study. Clin Oral Implants Res 2009;20:1231-1239.
74. Wennerberg A, Albrektsson T, Andersson B, Krol JJ. A histomorphometric and removal torque study of screw-shaped titanium implants with three different surface topographies. Clin Oral Implants Res 1995;6:24-30.
75. Wennerberg A, Albrektsson T, Johansson C, Andersson B. Experimental study of turned and grit-blasted screw-shaped implants with special emphasis on effects of blasting material and surface topography. Biomaterials 1996;17:15-22.
76. Wennerberg A, Albrektsson T, Andersson B. Bone tissue response to commercially pure titanium implants blasted with fine and coarse particles of aluminum oxide. Int J Oral Maxillofac Implants 1996;11:38-45.
77. Wennerberg A, Ektessabi A, Albrektsson T, Johansson C, Andersson B. A 1-year follow-up of implants of differing surface roughness placed in rabbit bone. Int J Oral Maxillofac Implants 1997;12:486-494.
78. Wennerberg A, Hallgren C, Johansson C, Sawase T, Lausmaa J. Surface characterization and biological evaluation of spark-eroded surfaces. J Mater Sci Mater Med 1997;8:757-763.
79. Wennerberg A, Hallgren C, Johansson C, Danelli S. A histomorphometric evaluation of screw-shaped implants each prepared with two surface roughnesses. Clin Oral Implants Res 1998;9:11-19.
80. Karlsson U, Gotfredsen K, Olsson C. A 2-year report on maxillary and mandibular fixed partial dentures supported by Astra Tech dental implants. A comparison of 2 implants with different surface textures. Clin Oral Implants Res 1998;9:235-242.
81. Feldman S, Boitel N, Weng D, Kohles SS, Stach RM. Five-year survival distributions of short-length (10 mm or less) machined-surfaced and Osseotite implants. Clin Implant Dent Relat Res 2004;6:16-23.
82. Ronold HJ, Lyngstadaas SP, Ellingsen JE. Analysing the optimal value for titanium implant roughness in bone attachment using a tensile test. Biomaterials 2003;24:4559-4564.
83. Ronold HJ, Lyngstadaas SP, Ellingsen JE. A study on the effect of dual blasting with TiO_2 on titanium implant surfaces on functional attachment in bone. J Biomed Mater Res A 2003;67:524-530.
84. Cordioli G, Majzoub Z, Piattelli A, Scarano A. Removal torque and histomorphometric investigation of 4 different titanium surfaces: an experimental study in the rabbit tibia. Int J Oral Maxillofac Implants 2000;15:668-674.
85. Klokkevold PR, Johnson P, Dadgostari S, Caputo A, Davies JE, Nishimura RD. Early endosseous integration enhanced by dual acid etching of titanium: a torque removal study in the rabbit. Clin Oral Implants Res 2001;12:350-357.
86. Al-Nawas B, Hangen U, Duschner H, Krummenauer F, Wagner W. Turned, machined versus double-etched dental implants in vivo. Clin Implant Dent Relat Res 2007;9:71-78.
87. Cooper LF, Zhou Y, Takebe J, Guo J, Abron A, Holmen A, et al. Fluoride modification effects on osteoblast behavior and bone formation at TiO_2 grit-blasted c.p. titanium endosseous implants. Biomaterials 2006;27:926-936.
88. Abron A, Hopfensperger M, Thompson J, Cooper LF. Evaluation of a predictive model for implant surface topography effects on early osseointegration in the rat tibia model. J Prosthet Dent 2001;85:40-46.
89. Schliephake H, Scharnweber D, Roesseler S, Dard M, Sewing A, Aref A. Biomimetic calcium phosphate composite coating of dental implants. Int J Oral Maxillofac Implants 2006;21:738-746.
90. Oikarinen VJ, Leikomaa TM, Lindqvist K, Ylipaavalniemi P, Gustafsson B. Comparison of the effectiveness of Astra 2167 and Dolorin in the relief of pain after removal of impacted mandibular third molar. Proc Finn Dent Soc 1978;74:18-22.
91. Stanford CM. Surface modifications of dental implants. Aust Dent J 2008;53(Suppl 1):S26-33.
92. Buser D, Broggini N, Wieland M, Schenk RK, Denzer AJ, Cochran DL, et al. Enhanced bone apposition to a chemically modified SLA titanium surface. J Dent Res 2004;83:529-533.
93. Zhao G, Schwartz Z, Wieland M, Rupp F, Geis-Gerstorfer J, Cochran DL, et al. High surface energy enhances cell response to titanium substrate microstructure. J Biomed Mater Res A 2005;74:49-58.

94. Bornstein MM, Schmid B, Belser UC, Lussi A, Buser D. Early loading of non-submerged titanium implants with a sandblasted and acid-etched surface. 5-year results of a prospective study in partially edentulous patients. Clin Oral Implants Res 2005;16:631-638.
95. Buser D, Nydegger T, Hirt HP, Cochran DL, Nolte LP. Removal torque values of titanium implants in the maxilla of miniature pigs. Int J Oral Maxillofac Implants 1998;13:611-619.
96. Grassi S, Piattelli A, de Figueiredo LC, Feres M, de Melo L, Iezzi G, et al. Histologic evaluation of early human bone response to different implant surfaces. J Periodontol 2006;77:1736-1743.
97. Al-Nawas B, Groetz KA, Goetz H, Duschner H, Wagner W. Comparative histomorphometry and resonance frequency analysis of implants with moderately rough surfaces in a loaded animal model. Clin Oral Implants Res 2008;19:1-8.
98. Novaes AB Jr, Papalexiou V, Grisi MF, Souza SS, Taba M Jr, Kajiwara JK. Influence of implant microstructure on the osseointegration of immediate implants placed in periodontally infected sites. A histomorphometric study in dogs. Clin Oral Implants Res 2004;15:34-43.
99. Kawahara H, Nakakita S, Ito M, Niwa K, Kawahara D, Matsuda S. Electron microscopic investigation on the osteogenesis at titanium implant/bone marrow interface under masticatory loading. J Mater Sci Mater Med 2006;17:717-726.
100. Glauser R, Zembic A, Ruhstaller P, Windisch S. Five-year results of implants with an oxidized surface placed predominantly in soft quality bone and subjected to immediate occlusal loading. J Prosthet Dent 2007;97(Suppl 6):S59-68.
101. Choi JW, Heo SJ, Koak JY, Kim SK, Lim YJ, Kim SH, et al. Biological responses of anodized titanium implants under different current voltages. J Oral Rehabil 2006;33:889-897.
102. Ivanoff CJ, Hallgren C, Widmark G, Sennerby L, Wennerberg A. Histologic evaluation of the bone integration of $TiO_{(2)}$ blasted and turned titanium microimplants in humans. Clin Oral Implants Res 2001;12:128-134.
103. Shibli JA, Vitussi TR, Garcia RV, Zenobio EG, Ota-Tsuzuki C, Cassoni A, et al. Implant surface analysis and microbiologic evaluation of failed implants retrieved from smokers. J Oral Implantol 2007;33:232-238.
104. Sul YT, Kang BS, Johansson C, Um HS, Park CJ, Albrektsson T. The roles of surface chemistry and topography in the strength and rate of osseointegration of titanium implants in bone. J Biomed Mater Res A 2009;89:942-950.
105. Rocci A, Martignoni M, Gottlow J. Immediate loading of Branemark System TiUnite and machined-surface implants in the posterior mandible: a randomized open-ended clinical trial. Clin Implant Dent Relat Res 2003;5(Suppl 1):57-63.
106. Friberg B, Jemt T. Rehabilitation of edentulous mandibles by means of five TiUnite implants after one-stage surgery: a 1-year retrospective study of 90 patients. Clin Implant Dent Relat Res 2008;10:47-54.
107. Roynesdal AK, Ambjornsen E, Stovne S, Haanaes HR. A comparative clinical study of three different endosseous implants in edentulous mandibles. Int J Oral Maxillofac Implants 1998;13:500-505.
108. Astrand P, Anzen B, Karlsson U, Sahlholm S, Svardstrom P, Hellem S. Nonsubmerged implants in the treatment of the edentulous upper jaw: a prospective clinical and radiographic study of ITI implants – results after 1 year. Clin Implant Dent Relat Res 2000;2:166-174.
109. Becker W, Becker BE, Ricci A, Bahat O, Rosenberg E, Rose LF, et al. A prospective multicenter clinical trial comparing one- and two-stage titanium screw-shaped fixtures with one-stage plasma-sprayed solid-screw fixtures. Clin Implant Dent Relat Res 2000;2:159-165.
110. Urban RM, Jacobs JJ, Tomlinson MJ, Gavrilovic J, Black J, Peoc'h M. Dissemination of wear particles to the liver, spleen, and abdominal lymph nodes of patients with hip or knee replacement. J Bone Joint Surg Am 2000;82:457-476.
111. Geurs NC, Jeffcoat RL, McGlumphy EA, Reddy MS, Jeffcoat MK. Influence of implant geometry and surface characteristics on progressive osseointegration. Int J Oral Maxillofac Implants 2002;17:811-815.
112. Barrere F, van der Valk CM, Meijer G, Dalmeijer RA, de Groot K, Layrolle P. Osteointegration of biomimetic apatite coating applied onto dense and porous metal implants in femurs of goats. J Biomed Mater Res B Appl Biomater 2003;67:655-665.
113. Kay JF. Calcium phosphate coatings for dental implants. Current status and future potential. Dent Clin North Am 1992;36:1-18.
114. Nimb L, Gotfredsen K, Steen Jensen J. Mechanical failure of hydroxyapatite-coated titanium and cobalt-chromium-molybdenum alloy implants. An animal study. Acta Orthop Belg 1993;59:333-338.
115. LeGeros RZ. Properties of osteoconductive biomaterials: calcium phosphates. Clin Orthop Relat Res 2002;395:81-98.
116. Jarcho M, Kay JF, Gumaer KI, Doremus RH, Drobeck HP. Tissue, cellular and subcellular events at a bone-ceramic hydroxylapatite interface. J Bioeng 1977;1:79-92.
117. Wennerberg A, Albrektsson T. Structural influence from calcium phosphate coatings and its possible effect on enhanced bone integration. Acta Odontol Scand 2009;31:1-8.
118. Albrektsson T, Wennerberg A. Oral implant surfaces: Part 1: review focusing on topographic and chemical properties of different surfaces and in vivo responses to them. Int J Prosthodont 2004;17:536-543.
119. Yang Y, Kim KH, Ong JL. A review on calcium phosphate coatings produced using a sputtering process: an alternative to plasma spraying. Biomaterials 2005;26:327-337.
120. Filiaggi MJ, Coombs NA, Pilliar RM. Characterization of the interface in the plasma-sprayed HA coating/Ti-6Al-4V implant system. J Biomed Mater Res 1991;25:1211-1229.
121. Chang YL, Lew D, Park JB, Keller JC. Biomechanical and morphometric analysis of hydroxyapatite-coated implants with varying crystallinity. J Oral Maxillofac Surg 1999;57:1096-1108; discussion 108-109.
122. Wheeler SL. Eight-year clinical retrospective study of titanium plasma-sprayed and hydroxyapatite-coated cylinder implants. Int J Oral Maxillofac Implants 1996;11:340-350.
123. Lee JJ, Rouhfar L, Beirne OR. Survival of hydroxyapatite-coated implants: a meta-analytic review. J Oral Maxillofac Surg 2000;58:1372-1379; discussion 9-80.
124. Tinsley D, Watson CJ, Russell JL. A comparison of hydroxylapatite coated implant retained fixed and removable mandibular prostheses over 4 to 6 years. Clin Oral Implants Res 2001;12:159-166.
125. Ellingsen JE, Johansson CB, Wennerberg A, Holmen A. Improved retention and bone-to-implant contact with fluoride-modified titanium implants. Int J Oral Maxillofac Implants 2004;19:659-666.
126. Meirelles L, Melin L, Peltola T, Kjellin P, Kangasniemi I, Currie F, et al. Effect of hydroxyapatite and titania nanostructures on early in vivo bone response. Clin Implant Dent Relat Res 2008;10:245-254.
127. Meirelles L, Arvidsson A, Andersson M, Kjellin P, Albrektsson T, Wennerberg A. Nano hydroxyapatite structures influence early bone formation. J Biomed Mater Res A 2008;87:299-307.
128. Meirelles L, Arvidsson A, Albrektsson T, Wennerberg A. Increased bone formation to unstable nano rough titanium implants. Clin Oral Implants Res 2007;18:326-332.
129. Kang BSYT, Oh SJ, Lee HJ, Albrektsson T. XPS, AES and SEM analysis of recent dental implants. Acta Biomater 2009;5:2222-2229.
130. Jimbo R, Sawase T, Baba K, Kurogi T, Shibata Y, Atsuta M. Enhanced initial cell responses to chemically modified anodized titanium. Clin Implant Dent Relat Res 2008;10:55-61.
131. Carlsson LV, Alberktsson T, Berman C. Bone response to plasma-cleaned titanium implants. Int J Oral Maxillofac Implants 1989;4:199-204.

132. Cheng H-C LS, Chen CC, Shyng YC, Ou KL. Influence of hydrogen charging on the formation of nano-structural titania by anodizing with cathodic pretreatment. J Electrochem Soc 2007;154:E13-18.
133. Meirelles L. On nano sized structures for enhanced early bone formation. Gothenburg: University of Gothenburg, 2007.
134. Lacefield WR. Current status of ceramic coatings for dental implants. Implant Dent 1998;7:315-322.
135. Liu DM, Yang Q, Troczynski T. Sol-gel hydroxyapatite coatings on stainless steel substrates. Biomaterials 2002;23:691-698.
136. Kim H, Camata RP, Vohra YK, Lacefield WR. Control of phase composition in hydroxyapatite/tetracalcium phosphate biphasic thin coatings for biomedical applications. J Mater Sci Mater Med 2005;16:961-966.
137. Cleries L, Martinez E, Fernandez-Pradas JM, Sardin G, Esteve J, Morenza JL. Mechanical properties of calcium phosphate coatings deposited by laser ablation. Biomaterials 2000;21:967-971.
138. Vercaigne S, Wolke JG, Naert I, Jansen JA. A histological evaluation of TiO_2-gritblasted and Ca-P magnetron sputter coated implants placed into the trabecular bone of the goat: Part 2. Clin Oral Implants Res 2000;11:314-324.
139. Vercaigne S, Wolke JG, Naert I, Jansen JA. A mechanical evaluation of TiO_2-gritblasted and Ca-P magnetron sputter coated implants placed into the trabecular bone of the goat: Part 1. Clin Oral Implants Res 2000;11:305-313.
140. Ong JL, Carnes DL, Bessho K. Evaluation of titanium plasma-sprayed and plasma-sprayed hydroxyapatite implants in vivo. Biomaterials 2004;25:4601-4606.
141. Park YS, Yi KY, Lee IS, Han CH, Jung YC. The effects of ion beam-assisted deposition of hydroxyapatite on the grit-blasted surface of endosseous implants in rabbit tibiae. Int J Oral Maxillofac Implants 2005;20:31-38.
142. Han Y, Fu T, Lu J, Xu K. Characterization and stability of hydroxyapatite coatings prepared by an electrodeposition and alkaline-treatment process. J Biomed Mater Res 2001;54:96-101.
143. Choi J, Bogdanski D, Koller M, Esenwein SA, Muller D, Muhr G, et al. Calcium phosphate coating of nickel-titanium shape-memory alloys. Coating procedure and adherence of leukocytes and platelets. Biomaterials 2003;24:3689-3696.
144. Oliveira AL, Elvira C, Reis RL, Vazquez B, San Roman J. Surface modification tailors the characteristics of biomimetic coatings nucleated on starch-based polymers. J Mater Sci Mater Med 1999;10:827-835.
145. Wie H, Hero H, Solheim T. Hot isostatic pressing-processed hydroxyapatite-coated titanium implants: light microscopic and scanning electron microscopy investigations. Int J Oral Maxillofac Implants 1998;13:837-844.
146. Coelho PG, Granjeiro JM, Romanos GE, Suzuki M, Silva NR, Cardaropoli G, et al. Basic research methods and current trends of dental implant surfaces. J Biomed Mater Res B Appl Biomater 2009;88:579-596.
147. Mendes VC, Moineddin R, Davies JE. Discrete calcium phosphate nanocrystalline deposition enhances osteoconduction on titanium-based implant surfaces. J Biomed Mater Res A 2009;9:577-585.
148. Goené RJ, Testori T, Trisi P. Influence of a nanometer-scale surface enhancement on de novo bone formation on titanium implants: a histomorphometric study in human maxillae. Int J Periodontics Restorative Dent 2007;27:211-219.
149. Orsini G, Piattelli M, Scarano A, Petrone G, Kenealy J, Piattelli A, et al. Randomized, controlled histologic and histomorphometric evaluation of implants with nanometer-scale calcium phosphate added to the dual acid-etched surface in the human posterior maxilla. J Periodontol 2007;78:209-218.
150. de Jonge LT, Leeuwenburgh SC, Wolke JG, Jansen JA. Organic-inorganic surface modifications for titanium implant surfaces. Pharm Res 2008;25:2357-2369.
151. Liu Y, Huse RO, de Groot K, Buser D, Hunziker EB. Delivery mode and efficacy of BMP-2 in association with implants. J Dent Res 2007;86:84-89.
152. Josse SFC, Soueidan A, Grimandi G, Massiot D, Alonso B, et al. Chemically modified calcium phosphates as novel materials for bisphosphonate delivery. Adv Mater 2004(2004):1423-1427.
153. Yoshinari M, Oda Y, Ueki H, Yokose S. Immobilization of bisphosphonates on surface modified titanium. Biomaterials 2001;22:709-715.
154. Kajiwara H, Yamaza T, Yoshinari M, Goto T, Iyama S, Atsuta I, et al. The bisphosphonate pamidronate on the surface of titanium stimulates bone formation around tibial implants in rats. Biomaterials 2005;26:581-587.
155. Peter B, Pioletti DP, Laib S, Bujoli B, Pilet P, Janvier P, et al. Calcium phosphate drug delivery system: influence of local zoledronate release on bone implant osteointegration. Bone 2005;36:52-60.
156. Meraw SJ, Reeve CM. Qualitative analysis of peripheral peri-implant bone and influence of alendronate sodium on early bone regeneration. J Periodontol 1999;70:1228-1233.
157. Meraw SJ, Reeve CM, Wollan PC. Use of alendronate in peri-implant defect regeneration. J Periodontol 1999;70:151-158.

Chapter 2

Short implants ... short life?

Marc Quevedo Pou, Susana García González, Octavi Ortiz Puigpelat

2.1 Introduction

Oral implantology is one of the pillars of contemporary dentistry. It is a conservative therapy that avoids preparation of healthy teeth, and stimulates bone preservation with implant loading in cases where teeth have been lost.

In the last 30 years, the use of osseointegrated dental implants has resulted in increased survival rates. Some prospective studies have shown an accumulative survival rate of 94.4% with fixed prostheses, versus 95.7% with implant-retained overdentures. Oral implant therapy has become a common and accepted treatment. Patients are better informed and more demanding, and dental professionals have more tools and well-documented techniques available to them.

Some implant cases are favorable and straightforward. When sufficient bone and soft tissue is available, the treatment option could be simple surgery with a standard, non-advanced technique. On the other hand, some patients present bone and/or soft tissue atrophies, becoming a challenging case and requiring alternative techniques in terms of surgical approach. Bone reconstruction, short implants, or complete removable dentures are among the most common options in these cases. The clinician's goal is to offer a simple and predictable treatment with a satisfactory and successful result.

Short implants are an option in cases of reduced bone height, when standard or longer implants are contraindicated. Any implant under 10 mm in length is usually referred to as a "short" implant. When first introduced, reported success rates were considered low, but the development of new surfaces has increased the acceptance and credibility of short implants. This is clearly beneficial to the patient and practitioner, but there is also a need for greater understanding of the criteria used to select the best treatment for each patient.

This chapter will guide the reader through implant selection, taking into account factors such as length, diameter, surface treatment, and prosthetic connections. Prosthetic, biomechanical, and occlusal factors are evaluated so that the clinician can make important decisions when it comes to selecting the most appropriate treatment.

2.2 Background

Alveolar ridge resorption due to tooth loss, trauma, and infection can make the placement of dental implants more challenging. Several bone regeneration techniques have been described to correct such bone deficiencies. However, evaluating the relative success of each technique is hampered by a lack of reliable studies. On the other hand, for regeneration of severe vertical and horizontal defects, high complication rates have been reported. Therefore, recent literature reviews have considered short implants or distraction osteogenesis to be better treatment options for reconstruction of such severe defects.

Since the description of the osseointegration concept by Bränemark, one of the main parameters to establish the successful prognosis of osseointegrated implants has been the use of the maximum available alveolar bone.[1-5]

This has been considered a general basic principle in oral implantology.[1-5] In recent years, a trend towards the use of short implants in bone-compromised situations has been observed.

One of the important factors to achieve osseointegration is implant primary stability. Primary stability of implants not exceeding a range of micromotion between 50 and 150 µm leads to uneventful bone healing and apposition, therefore bone-to-implant contact (BIC) is increased.[5-7] Primary stability is influenced by factors such as bone density and quality, surgical technique, and implant body geometry.[2,3,8] Implant diameter and length have been considered the main parameters of the geometry of dental implants that can influence to the area of BIC.

Premature tooth loss due to trauma or periodontal disease will mean a loss of esthetics, function, and resorption and atrophy of the alveolar bone, especially in posterior regions of the maxilla and mandible.[6]

For a long time, the predictability and high survival rates of implant therapy were associated with the use of standard and long-length implants.[7,8] However, these implants are limited in their application, owing to reduced bone height or proximity to anatomical structures, such as the inferior alveolar nerve (IAN), maxillary sinus, or even the nasal cavity.[9-17] One in three dental implants requires an augmentation procedure of the alveolar ridge because of atrophy.[10]

In cases with a considerable ridge defect, the treatment of edentulism with standard or long dental implants is difficult, or even impossible. In the anterior regions the quality of permanent bone is normally good, and the quantity is usually sufficient for implant placement. However, the situation is different in the posterior regions due to poor bone quality, faster resorption, and the presence of adjacent anatomical structures.[6,9-18] Therefore, restoring function and esthetics in these cases can be challenging. Alternative techniques and materials are required for treatment of this type of patient.

Advanced surgery with reconstructive techniques is one solution. Procedures like sinus lift, guided bone regeneration (GBR), lateralization or transposition of the IAN, block grafting, or osteogenic alveolar distraction are some alternatives to achieve the correct bone volume to place standard or long implants.[6,19-21] However, the risk of morbidity and the time and cost of these treatment modalities compared with other alternatives should be taken into account.[9]

The implant industry has contributed to partially solving the problem of bone height through the fabrication of special implants,[22] such as zygomatic or pterygoid implants. These dental implants have enhanced dimensions for use in specific areas and to avoid bone defects and anatomical structures. Normally, both types of implants are longer than standard implants and have been designed for placement in maxilla buttresses like the zygomatic bone or pterygoid apophysis. Nevertheless, the surgical technique to place these implants is more challenging and has to be performed by an experienced surgeon. Another option is tilted implants,[9] for the maxilla and the mandible. This uses fewer implants, leaving the neck of the distal implant as distal as possible in an angled position, forward of the anterior wall of the sinus in the maxilla or forward of the mental nerve in the mandible, and restores the dentition by means of a full-arch prosthesis with distal cantilevers.

Short implants may also be considered a viable long-term solution in these limited situations, as well as in cases where augmentation is required, but the results still do not permit the use of standard length implants.[7,11,13,17,22,23] Short implants could reduce the need for advanced surgery in these atrophic regions.[18,24]

The minimal length for predictable success was always considered 10 mm and thus implants of this length are commonly referred to as "standard length implants." As a result, any implant under 10 mm in length has come to be referred to as a "short" implant.[22] The most controversial issues regarding short implants are discussed in this chapter.

- 2.3 General topics
  - 2.3.1 Is the length of the implant a risk factor?
  - 2.3.2 How should the surface of a short implant be treated?
  - 2.3.3 How does bone density influence treatment with short implants?
  - 2.3.4 How do occlusal forces affect short implants?
  - 2.3.5 How important is the diameter of short implants?
  - 2.3.6 Where can a short implant be placed?
  - 2.3.7 Are short implants successful?
- 2.4 Prostheses and short implants
- 2.5 Short implants and parafunctional and toxic habits
  - 2.5.1 Can short implants be placed in patients with parafunctional habits?
  - 2.5.2 Can short implants be placed in patients with toxic habits?

- 2.6 Surgical techniques for short implants
  - 2.6.1 Planning short-implant surgery
- 2.7 Complications encountered with short implants
  - 2.7.1 Treatment of complications
  - 2.7.2 Prevention of failures and complications
- 2.8 Clinical cases
- 2.9 Conclusions

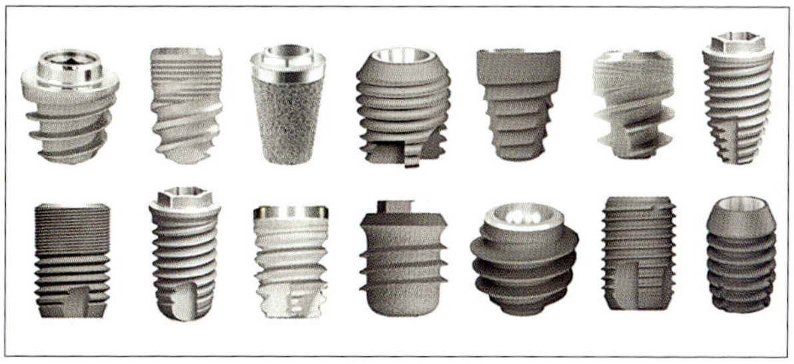

Fig 2-1 Different commercially available types of short implant.

2.3 General topics

2.3.1 Is the length of the implant a risk factor?

The success of implants placed in reduced bone quantity can be compromised. Inadequate bone height should be considered as a risk factor for implant failure.[25-32]

In cases with reduced bone quantity, there are many options and techniques available. The goal is to increase the length of the bone (by alveolar distraction, bone grafting, sinus lift, and GBR), and to avoid the adjacent anatomical structures (by IAN transposition and lateralization, zygoma and pterygoid implants, and tilted implants) in cases where standard or long implants have to be placed. Some of these advanced techniques are predictable, but others are less successful. All should be performed by an experienced surgeon, sometimes under general anesthesia, meaning high costs, high morbidity, and lengthy treatment times. Due to these reasons, many patients refuse this type of treatment.

In cases with reduced bone height, short implants can be used as an alternative, using all of the available bone and taking into account the biomechanics and biological conditions of each case. According to the review of Esposito et al.[20] short implants appear to be a better option than vertical bone grafting of resorbed mandibles.

How short is a short implant? It is generally agreed that implants less than 10 mm in length are considered short implants. A variety of short implants is commercially available (Fig 2-1). As mentioned above, the concept of a short implant is not well defined, but many combinations are possible. Short implants are available from 5 to 10 mm in length, making it possible to treat and restore resorbed ridges. Various diameters are also available, the most common being regular and wide implants (4 and 5 mm).

There is no evidence to support the idea that short implants have a worse prognosis than standard implants.

2.3.2 How should the surface of a short implant be treated?

In early modern oral implantology, the majority of implants placed were machined titanium implants. In the last 15 years, different surface treatments have emerged.

Machined screwed implants achieve functional osseointegration because of the macroscopic union between bone and implant threads. Adding a rough surface to the machined screwed implant makes it possible to increase the percentage of BIC,[33] achieving a higher insertion and removal torque[34] and improving the clinical performance. As more implant surface is in contact with the bone, less stress is transmitted to the bone and loading distribution is also improved.[35]

In long machined implants, the implant surface is important, but some crestal bone resorption can appear, and has been accepted.[36] However, in short implants all the implant threads have to be osseointegrated and loaded. There is some evidence of poor results with short or even standard machined implants.[37,38] Thus, implant surface treatment should optimize short-implant success rates.[18,35,39]

Research teams have improved implant texture and design to facilitate osseointegration. Using different techniques (acid etching, grit blasting, titanium plasma spraying, surface coating, porous sintered surfacing), implant companies today have replaced the traditional polished surfaces on implants with "rough" surfaces that have led to significantly better short- and long-term results. These techniques result in implant surface irregularities in height, thread length, and spatial dimension. Arguments in favor of rough implant surfaces include that they: increase contact area to offer better mechanical stability between bone and implant immediately following insertion; provide surface configuration that properly retains the blood clot; and stimulate the bone healing process.[22]

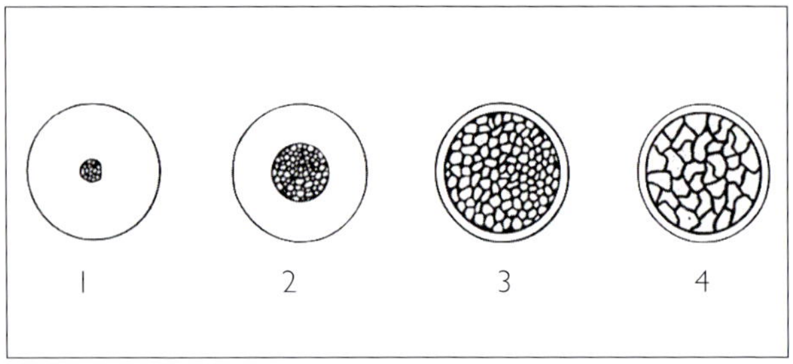

Fig 2-2 Bone density classification by Lekholm and Zarb.[52] Type 1: Essentially cortical bone. Type 2: Dense corticocancellous bone. Type 3: Low density corticocancellous bone. Type 4: Thin cortical layer and very low density trabecular bone. (Reproduced from Lekholm and Zarb[52] with permission.)

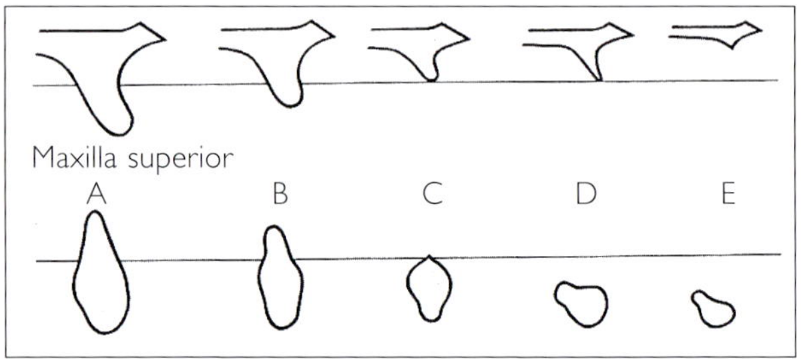

Fig 2-3 Classification of the degree of resorption of edentulous jaws, according to Lekholm and Zarb.[52] Type A: Intact alveolar ridge. Type B: Low resorption of alveolar ridge. Type C: Advanced resorption of alveolar ridge. Type D: Initial resorption of basal bone. Type E: Extreme resorption of basal bone. (Reproduced from Lekholm and Zarb[52] with permission.)

Rough surfaces contribute to a higher BIC, which results in a better distribution of forces through the implant geometry. For short implants placed where there is a reduced bone height, the use of all available bone and the increase in implant surface is crucial in terms of implant integration and BIC, in order to achieve enough support for the prosthetic restoration.

The surface area can be increased significantly simply by altering the texture configurations of rough implants. Rough implants offer extensive surface area for osseointegration and therefore allow the clinician to consider the placement of short implants.

Many recent short-implant studies have used treated surfaces,[11,13,16,23,31,40-50] since these have been proven to produce better clinical results. Besides the surface treatment, there are other factors that are crucial to avoid marginal bone loss, such as the type of connection and implant macrodesign.

Several surfaces have been studied, in line with the different short implants available. Surfaces studied include Osseotite®, Nanotite®, porous sintered surface, TPS and SLA®, TiUnite®; RBM®, HA, and OsseoSpeed®, with various processes to achieve the roughness (eg acid etching, plasma spraying, sand blasting, sustraction, and bioactivation).

To determine the best option for short-implant surfaces, further studies comparing rough surfaces in short implants are needed, and also investigations into different surfaces with different macro-designs.

Although surface treatment improves overall integration of implants, it may render the implant more susceptible to contamination. This could threaten a normal implant, but would be fatal to a short one.

2.3.3 How does bone density influence treatment with short implants?

The density of each bone reflects its own resistance. The minimum available bone length for long-term implant survival is related to the bone density of that bone. Only in cases where high-density bone is available may short implants be placed.[39] Poor quality bone, normally located in the posterior maxilla, has mechanically reduced resistance in comparison with dense bone. It is also unable to support the same forces as cortical bone, which is normally located in the interforaminal region of the mandible.[23] Thus, in implant therapy, and especially in short implants, the type of bone is a key factor in terms of forces distribution.

There are several classifications of bone quantity and density (Figs 2-2 and 2-3). In terms of type of bone density and quality, the most commonly used classifications are by Misch,[51] and Lekholm and Zarb.[52]

To overcome the anatomic difficulties, new implant designs and surface treatments have been created to improve BIC,[53] achieving better clinical results for osseointegrated implants. This is even more important when implants are placed in soft bones, as short implants do not present either a large diameter or length. High implant survival rates have been reported for implants with treated surfaces placed in the posterior maxilla.[31]

Implants with porous or rough surfaces are more successful than smooth-surfaced implants in low-density bone. This type of bone is highly vascularized, with a large number of osteoprogenitor cells that increase bone growth inside the implant surface or pores.[54]

In terms of density, when soft bones are present, special attention must be paid to additional risk factors like bruxism, smoking, or smooth-surface implants. If a combination of these factors is present with type IV bone, short implants should be avoided. For short implants, the aim should be for use within high-density, well-vascularized bone.

2.3.4 How do occlusal forces affect short implants?

Biomechanical failure is an important factor related to crestal bone loss in machined screwed implants because of the weak union between surface and bone, which gives poor resistance to tension forces during chewing. Excessive forces can cause compression of the bone in contact with the implant and, as a result, some micro-fractures and resorption could appear due to the overloading.

Compressive forces would be concentrated in a smaller area near to the coronal part of the implant. Therefore, it can be assumed that by increasing implant length these compressive forces would act on a larger bone area in contact with the implant, reducing the local stress in the crestal area and the possibility of micro-fractures.[55]

A 13-mm implant has a surface area increase of 10% compared with a 10-mm implant. The BIC interface is not influenced by this surface area increase in longer implants during functional time, but it could mean an improvement of the primary stability.

Finite element analysis studies report that when the implant is integrated, horizontal and vertical occlusal forces are mainly distributed through the crestal bone instead of being distributed towards the entire BIC interface. Consequently, implant length is not an effective factor to reduce the load on the crestal bone around the implant.[39,56,57]

Bone resorption of the jawbones is normally related to an unfavorable maxillary relationship and an increased maxillomandibular space. Consequently, prosthetic rehabilitation is designed to compensate by increasing crown length and width. It is also important to consider the position in the arch, the functional and parafunctional habits, the type of antagonist, the torsion moments, and the unfavorable distribution of the forces.[12]

Several studies have observed the direct relation between the posterior cantilever length and complications or prosthetic failures.[23] However, this relationship has not been demonstrated in unfavorable crown–implant (C/I) ratios.

Crown length is measured from the occlusal or incisal plane to the crestal ridge, and could be considered a vertical cantilever. An increase of the crown length means higher tension in the bone-to-implant interface during occlusal loading. The greater the crown length, the higher the lever arm. Furthermore, when a force acts out of the major implant axis, tension will be increased by up to 20% in the crestal bone, affecting the bone–implant interface, prosthetic screws, or the weakest point of the restoration.[23,39]

In the posterior region the occlusal forces are 400% greater than in the anterior zone. Thus, if short implants are used in posterior regions and there is an increased maxillomandibular space, which means longer prosthetic crowns, more implants should be placed. These short implants should also have large diameters, and prostheses should be designed to reduce the load on the implants and to avoid increased tension. This is based on the principle that forces will be well distributed when there is greater bone surface in contact with the implant/s, as transference of the occlusal forces is easier.[53]

Transmission of the forces is concentrated in the cortical bone around the neck of the implant, in the first threads.[58] This means that the cervical part of the implant works more than the apical part, and in terms of load distribution, the first third of the implant will be the most determinant.

Excessive C/I ratios have been cited in the literature as being detrimental to long-term implant survival.[59] However, an unfavorable C/I ratio does not mean an increased biomechanical failure risk or high peri-implant bone loss, as long as the occlusion is adequate and stable, and the maxillomandibular relationship is correct. It is important to correctly distribute the forces as axial as possible and to eliminate all the occlusal interferences. In short implants the effects of these concepts are more apparent.[12] For many years, the main argument against short implants was the C/I ratio disproportion and bone loss because of high occlusal forces. However, most studies rehabilitate short implants with single crowns with predictability.[32,60]

If the occlusal conditions are optimal, less bone surface will be necessary to distribute the forces, and short implants will be a viable and predictable therapy.[61,62] Of course, the evaluation of bone density is necessary.

Although the C/I ratio may not affect peri-implant crestal bone loss, it has been hypothesized that implant restorations with low C/I ratios may cause less overload on prosthetic components, reducing the risk of technical complications such as screw loosening, cement failure, and framework fracture.[60]

No comparative clinical data correlate C/I ratio with technical complications of implant-supported reconstructions. For this reason, future research should evaluate, through randomized controlled trials and larger sample sizes, the effect of the C/I ratio on technical complications of implant restorations functioning for more than 5 years.

In summary, controlling occlusal forces is crucial. Crown–implant ratios of implant-supported restorations do not influence peri-implant crestal bone loss. There are few data evaluating the relationship between the C/I ratios and implant survival rates or the occurrence of technical complications in implant-supported prostheses.[60]

2.3.5 How important is the diameter of short implants?

The use of wide diameter implants (>3.75 mm) has increased in the last decade, especially in the posterior area of the mandible. It is generally accepted that wider implants improve the ability of posterior implants to tolerate the occlusal forces, create a wider base for prostheses, and avoid the placement of two standard-size implants at one site to obtain a double-root prosthetic tooth.[63]

In terms of short implants, diameter is an important factor to consider, since the cervical part will be related to the initial bone resorption and other complications.[39] As previously mentioned, with increasing diameter the BIC is increased, and less stress is transmitted to the bone, improving the prognosis of the implants, especially ≥7 mm implants placed in soft bones.[18] Thus, by adding 1 mm to a cylindrical implant diameter, the total surface area will be increased by up to 20 to 30%.

In short-implant therapy, 4- and 5-mm platforms should be used, in order to increase the implant surface area in contact with the bone. However, there are reports of high percentages of bone necrosis in surgery with wider implants.[63] Therefore, the drilling protocol should be controlled in each case.[64]

Short implants should be as wide as possible, in order to increase the implant surface area and decrease the stress distribution to the bone.

2.3.6 Where can a short implant be placed?

Reviewing the literature,[11,16,31,32,43,44,46,47] the most common area where short implants are necessary is in the posterior region of both jaws, due to the related anatomic structures and the bone resorption patterns.

The placement of short implants in the analyzed studies[11,16,31,32,43,44,46,47] is more prevalent in the mandible than the maxilla, with more placed in the posterior region.

The difference between the number of implants used in the posterior and anterior regions is more significant in the maxilla than in the mandible. There is a higher percentage of failures in the maxilla than in the mandible.[13,32] This can be explained by the reduced structural quality of bone in the maxillary posterior area. Survival rates are higher in the anterior compared with the posterior regions, probably due to the bone quality.[13]

More short implants have been reported in the posterior mandible than elsewhere. This may be related to the good predictability of shorts implants when compared with vertical regeneration techniques for standard implant placement.[20] The anterior region of the mandible, based on these studies, is where fewer short implants are placed, because of reduced resorption in the interforaminal area. However, some studies[13] present higher success in anterior rather than posterior zones, probably due to bone quality characteristics.

There is a lack of information when analyzing survival, success, and failure percentages, in distinguishing clearly the maxilla from the mandible.

2.3.7 Are short implants successful?

The overall survival rate for short implants is over 95% in some studies,[11,23,27,32,42,45,47,48,50] and over 91% in others.[13,40,41,43]

Most studies demonstrate a high survival rate of short implants, well above 90%. This finding could be considered very similar to the survival rate of standard implants. However, there are some differences when it comes to restorations. In single restorations the success rates are slightly higher (98.1% to 99.2%) than in partial or total restorations (98%).[11]

Although longer follow-ups are needed, it can be stated that short implants have a similar prognosis to standard ones.

2.4 Prostheses and short implants

Several studies do not specify the type of prosthesis used.[16,32,42,49] Of those that are more specific, the most common restoration was the single fixed crown (although often it is unclear if these were cemented or screwed), followed by fixed partial dentures.[11,13,23,31,40,41,43-48,50] The latter, in the same studies, can be separated according to the number of units (more or less than five units).[13,42,44,46] Less frequently, full arch restorations are the reported prosthetic treatments using short implants.[23,43,48,49] The survival rates, when mentioned, with this type of prosthesis are high. One study reported 2,073 short implants placed, and obtained a survival rate between 98.1% and 99.2% in single crowns, and 98% in three-unit fixed splints.[11]

There are more reports of single-unit rehabilitations with short implants. There is no relationship between an unfavorable C/I ratio and increased failure rate, but it is important to avoid restoring one single-unit implant in Kennedy class I/II.[11] Furthermore, partial and total rehabilitations with short implants have favorable survival and low complication rates, but it is crucial to splint the implants.

In terms of loading time, the majority of studies mentioned short-implant loading after 4 to 6 months of osseointegration. The implants were placed in most studies with two surgical stages,[13,16,23,31,32,40-42,44,45,47,50] and in some cases in one stage.[23,32,41,44,46]

Short implants can be used to support any kind of prosthesis: single crowns (avoiding restoring in Kennedy class I/II), fixed partial dentures, fixed complete dentures, and even overdentures. The most common and predictable restorations are single crowns, followed by fixed partial dentures, fixed complete dentures, and overdentures.[41,45]

2.5 Short implants and parafunctional and toxic habits

2.5.1 Can short implants be placed in patients with parafunctional habits?

Bruxism has to be taken into account when rehabilitating with short implants, particularly in the posterior region where the occlusal bite forces are greater. Nonetheless, as yet there is no evidence for a correlation between bruxism and increased implant failure.

Isolated bruxism is not a risk factor, unless accompanied by other potential risk factors such as poor quality bone, very reduced length of the ridge, non optimal occlusion, machined implants, smoking or other toxic habits, non-splinted implants, or buccolingual or mesiodistal cantilevers.

2.5.2 Can short implants be placed in patients with toxic habits?

The majority of studies consider heavy smoking (more than 10 cigarettes per day) as an exclusion criteria, but several studies included moderate smokers (less than 10 cigarettes per day) without specifying the exact quantity of cigarettes, and reported no increased risk in terms of short-implant failures.[11,16,45]

Moderate smoking does not increase risk significantly in short-implant placement.[11,13,16,31,42,44,45,47,49] Nevertheless, since heavy smokers are not considered in any study no conclusions can be made. With that said, we would not recommend placing short implants with treated surfaces in heavy smokers, especially those with poor hygiene habits.

2.6 Surgical techniques for short implants

2.6.1 Planning short-implant surgery

Short-implant surgery is planned and performed similarly to standard- or long-implant surgery. The steps are normally the same as conventional surgery.

However, there are a few steps in terms of treatment planning that will provide accurate and successful therapy. Waxing-up the case before the surgery gives vital information of the occlusal pattern of the patient and the future crown length can be determined, as well as the presence of cantilevers and C/I ratio. As mentioned previously, a rigorous occlusal study must be performed. Most of the patients who need to receive short implants are limited cases, for example with low height in posterior areas because of the proximity to the alveolar nerve, or low height in maxillary posterior areas because of the proximity to the maxillary sinus. In this way, it is possible to avoid advanced surgeries such as sinus lifts or tooth nerve lateralizations and inlay or onlay grafts in posterior mandibular areas.

Sometimes, three-dimensional (3D) planning (guided planning) might be useful; a surgical stent may be designed to allow totally guided surgery. The quantity and quality of the bone must also be measured prior to surgery.

Bahat,[65] who reported very high success rates, considers patient selection and treatment planning fundamental to his success. He attributed the high success rate of his study to detailed surgical planning. Bahat[65] also reported that site preparation is guided by the objective of minimizing ostectomy while maintaining an optimum implant direction.

It should be remembered that shorter surgical burs and drill stoppers are needed for short-implant surgery. The main goal, even more than for longer implants, is to achieve optimal primary stability, avoiding micromovement and ensuring a favorable osseointegration environment, and trying to avoid crestal bone resorption.[65]

Bone quality seems to play a decisive role in determining implant prognosis. The implant surface directly affects implant survival/success rate, obtaining significantly higher percentages with treated surfaces.[44]

Planning is critical when using short implants in severely atrophied cases. Anatomical landmarks (eg nerve, sinus) must be identified and avoided.

2.7 Complications encountered with short implants

2.7.1 Treatment of complications

In short implants, the complications are the same as those occurring with standard or long implants. However, if implant failure occurs, advanced surgery is needed to recover the lost bone so that new implants can be placed.

Short implant failure cannot be attributed to a single factor. It has been associated with poor bone quality (usually in the posterior maxilla where type IV bone is predominately found), lack of primary stability, jaw type, number of implants, smoking, parafunction, gender, infection, and implant diameter.[18] Overheating of the implant reception site during surgical preparation is another important complication associated with more frequent bone loss and implant failure.[47] If one or more of these factors is present when placing short implants, there is a higher risk of implant failure.

To reduce this complication it is important to use a novel low-speed drilling procedure that avoids overheating of the surgical site but allows recovery of large quantities of living bone particles,[47] or drill with copious irrigation at 600 to 800 rpm. The greatest complications arise when two or more of the complications mentioned above occur at the same time.[18]

From a biomechanical point of view, the rationale for the use of short implants is well documented.[47] When an implant is loaded, the majority of the shear forces are distributed at the level of the first few threads to the crestal cortical bone; therefore, once the minimum implant height is osseointegrated, implant width is more important than additional length.[48] Some risk factors, such as increased crown height and bite forces, may increase stress when using short implants. Eliminating or minimizing the lateral force on the prosthesis and force distribution by splinting multiple implants can significantly reduce stress on implants and therefore increase survival rates. Excessive stress may be problematic for the bone tissue, leading to a hypertrophic response and local overload that can provoke bone loss in the locations of the acting force.[47]

Fracture or loosening of mechanical and prosthetic components, soft tissue inflammation, fistula formation, pain or infection, marginal bone loss, and peri-implantitis can occur. There is a tendency toward the implant failure happening before prosthesis placement (54.9%), as reported in a literature review by Goodacre et al.[30] However, higher numbers of failures after prosthesis placement have also been reported.[30] Despite this, a common finding in all of these studies was the tendency of failures to occur in the first year of function. Occlusal overload was found to be an important risk factor, even in cases with reported bruxism.[25,65] The most distal position usually involves greater masticatory load than the anterior one.

2.7.2 Prevention of failures and complications

Care should be taken with short-implant patients in terms of maintenance, performance of controls, and strict reviewing of the peri-implant bone and soft tissue health. In short implants, peri-implantitis will be more catastrophic than in longer implants, and the implant will probably be lost.

Short-implant placement should be avoided in situations with compromised esthetics, in patients with poor oral hygiene, in bruxists with unfavorable occlusion, when there is sufficient bone length to place longer implants, or in type IV bones with reduced height and associated with other risk factors.

2.8 Clinical cases

All the cases presented in this chapter have in common insufficient height and/or proximity to anatomical landmarks, such as the IAN or the mental nerve, to allow placement of standard implants.

Case 1 (Figs 2-4 to 2-12)

Courtesy of Dr J Ortega

Case 1 shows a patient requiring tooth replacement in the mandibular posterior quadrants with dental implants, but with insufficient space for standard dimension dental implants. Bone augmentation procedures and short implants were suggested to the patient, who after eval-

Figs 2-4 to 2-12 Case 1

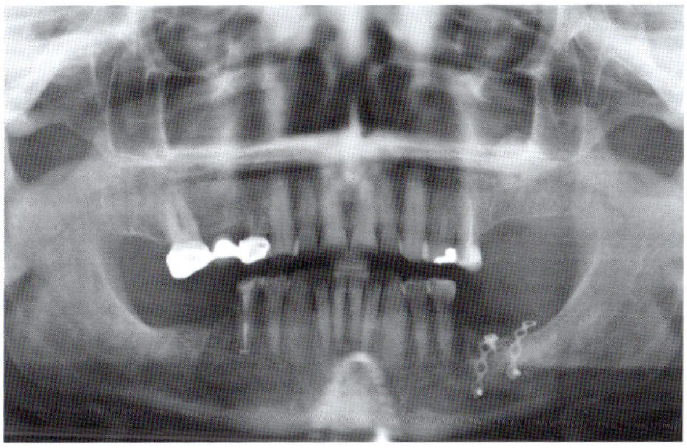

Fig 2-4 Initial panoramic radiograph.

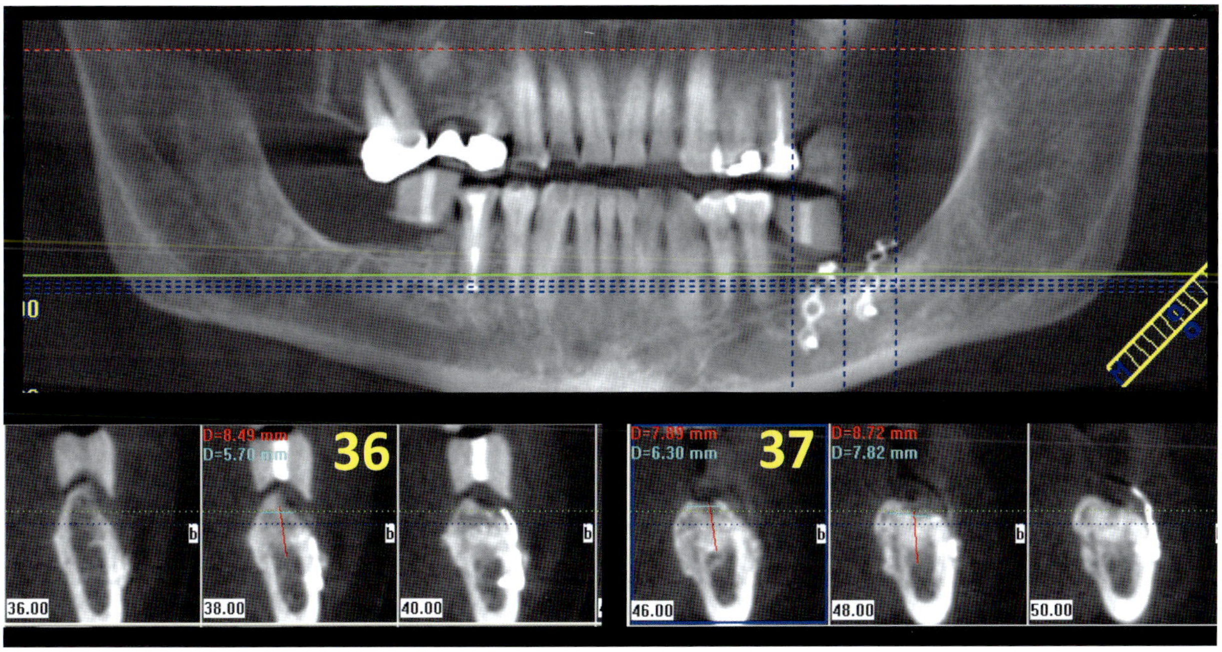

Fig 2-5 CBVT (cone beam volumetric tomography) images of Case 1. Implant in position 36: width 5.70 mm, height 8.49 mm. Implant in position 37: width 6.30 mm, height 7.83 mm.

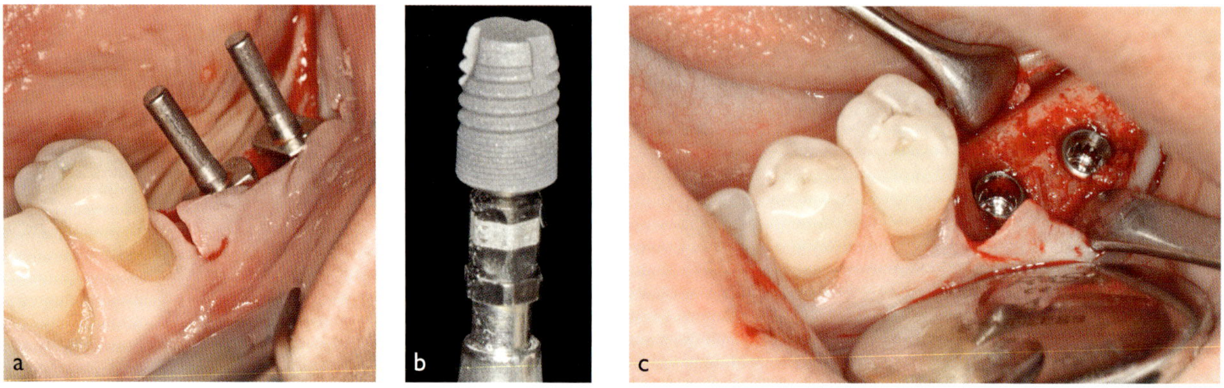

Figs 2-6a to c Implant surgery of the third quadrant. (a) Direction indicators in positions 36 and 37. (b) Astra Tech® (Mölndal, Sweden) implant, 4 × 6 mm. (c) Implants placed.

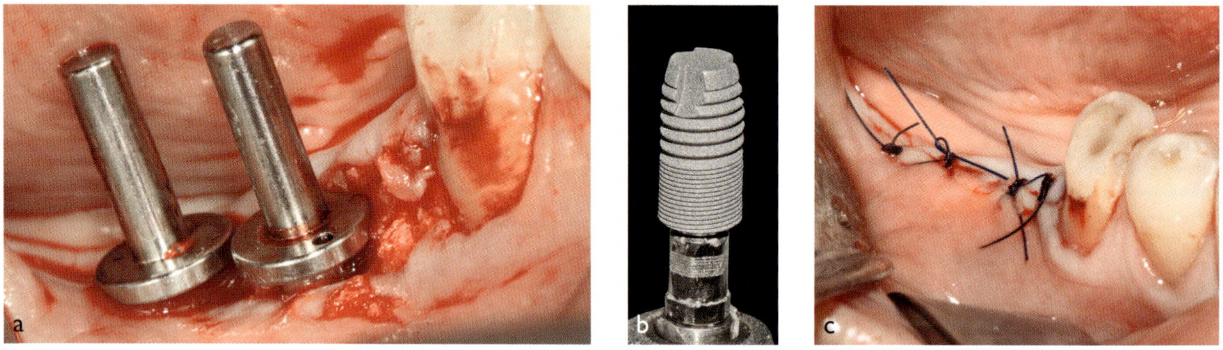

Figs 2-7a to c Implant surgery of the fourth quadrant. (a) Direction indicators in positions 46 and 47. (b) Astra Tech® (Mölndal, Sweden) implant, 4 × 8 mm. (c) Implants placed and suture of the flap.

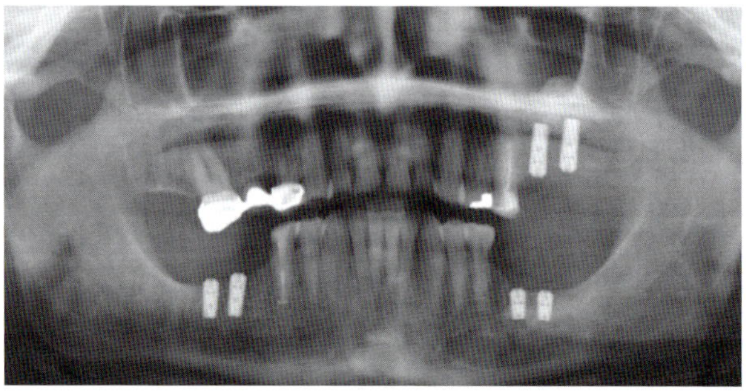

Fig 2-8 Postsurgical panoramic radiograph.

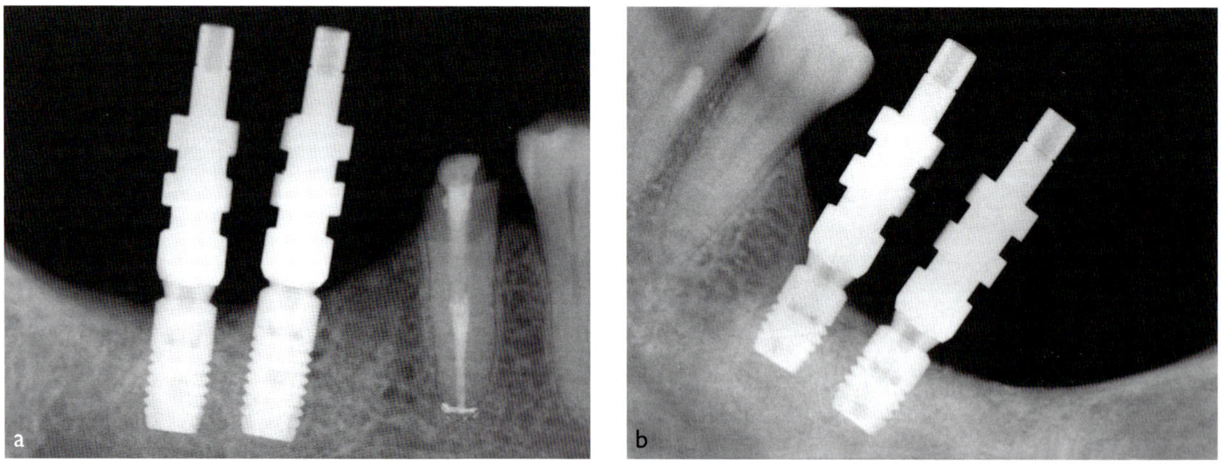

Figs 2-9a and b Periapical radiographs of the impression copings inserted. (a) Fourth quadrant. (b) Third quadrant.

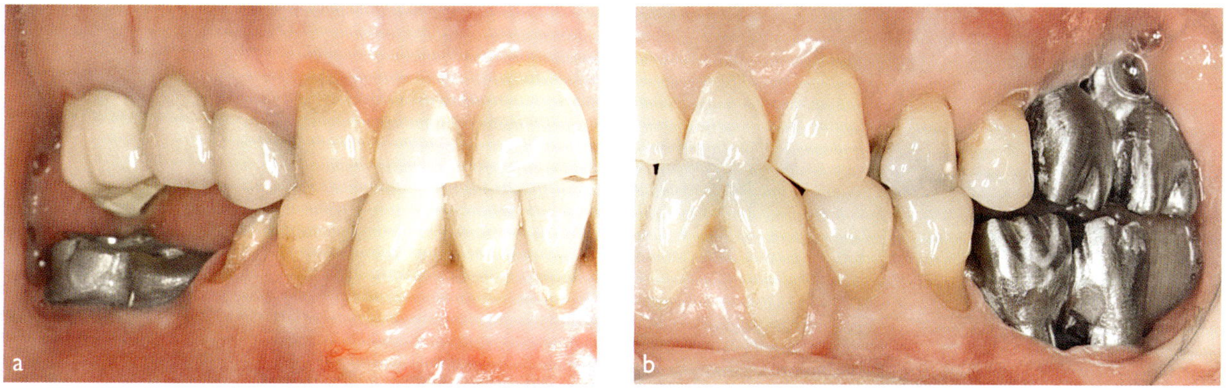

Figs 2-10a and b Metal try-in. (a) Fourth quadrant. (b) Third quadrant.

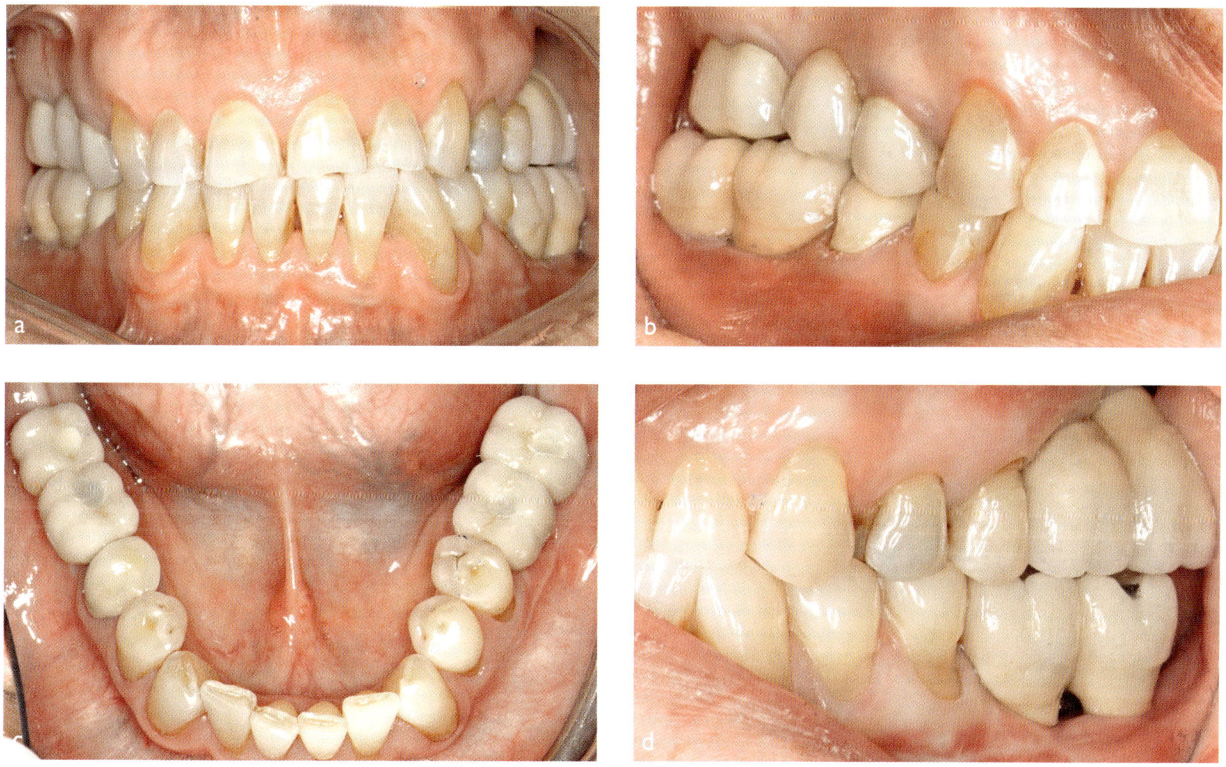

Figs 2-11a to d Final insertion of the crowns. (a) Anterior view. (b) Fourth quadrant. (c) Occlusal view. (d) Third quadrant.

uating the advantages and disadvantages declined the surgical procedures for bone augmentation. According to the space available, two implants with the same diameter of 4 mm and lengths of 6 and 8 mm (Fig 2-7) were chosen for the right mandibular quadrant. In the left mandibular quadrant bone availability was even less, leaving extra-short implants the only option (4 × 6 mm implants) (Fig 2-6). Implants were placed with a standard two-phase protocol and were left buried during the healing process, which took 3 months. After the second healing phase, healing abutments were left for an additional 1-month period. Impressions were taken and the rehabilitation phase was then completed. Crowns were splinted in order to distribute the load and to prevent overloading of the C/I interface. The final situation is shown in Figs 2-11 and 2-12.

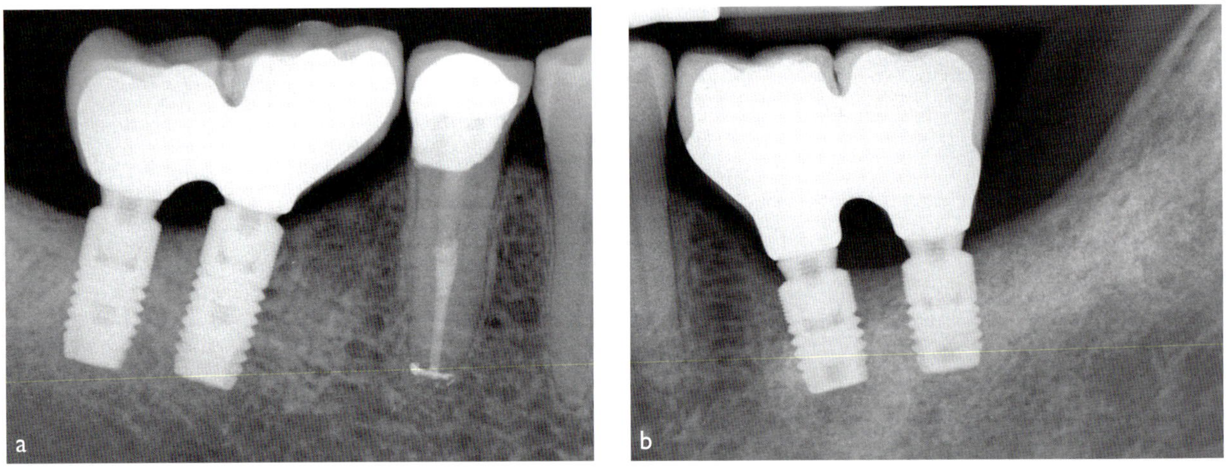

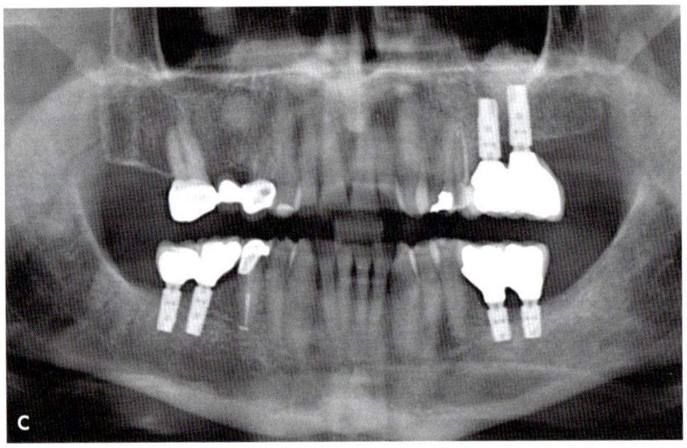

Figs 2-12a to c Final radiographs. (a) Fourth quadrant periapical radiograph. (b) Third quadrant periapical radiograph. (c) Final panoramic radiograph.

Figs 2-13 to 2-20 Case 2

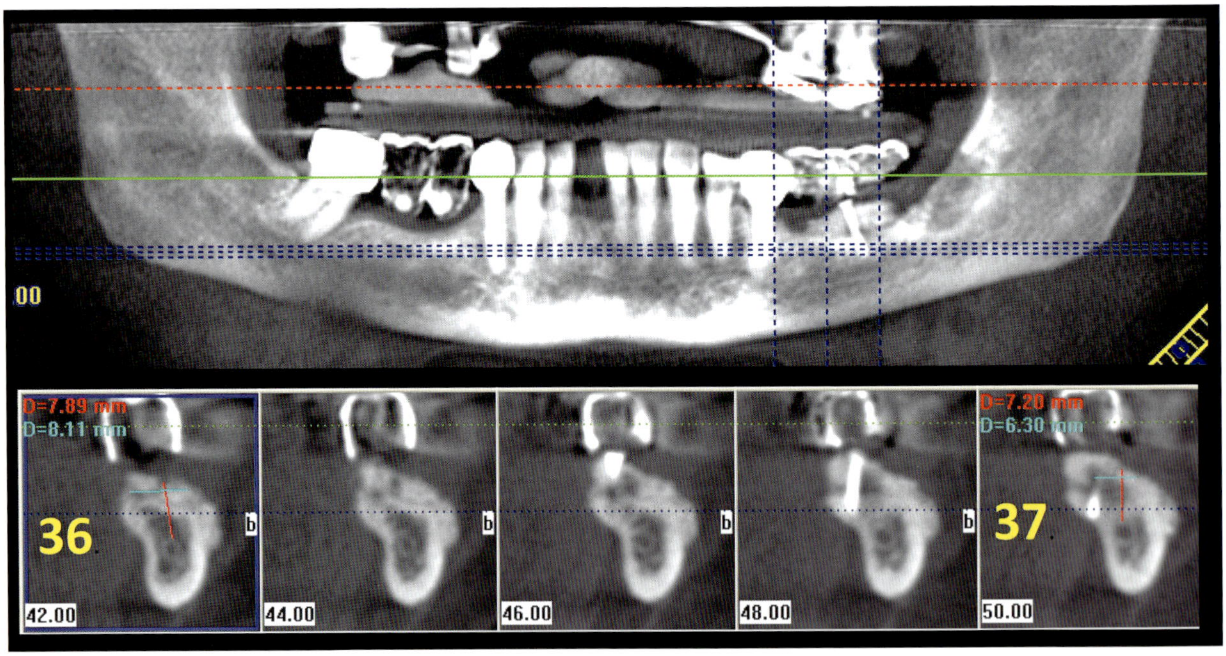

Fig 2-13 Initial panoramic view of the CBVT (cone beam volumetric tomography) and sectional images of the area 36 and 37.

Case 2 (Figs 2-13 to 2-20)

Courtesy of Dr J Ortega

In this patient, extreme resorption of the mandible made the task of placing implants in this area almost impossible. Vertical augmentation by means of a bone block was performed, and after a 6-month healing period two short implants ware placed over the bone block. Noteworthy is the fact that even with 4-mm vertical augmentation, 6-mm-long implants were the maximum possible in this case.

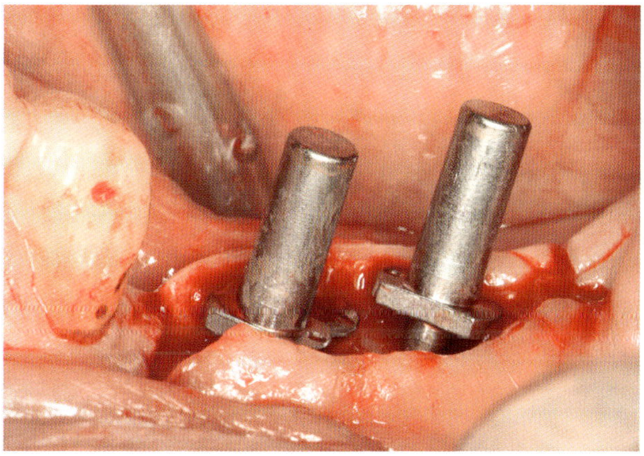

Fig 2-14 Direction pins inserted in implant positions 36 and 37.

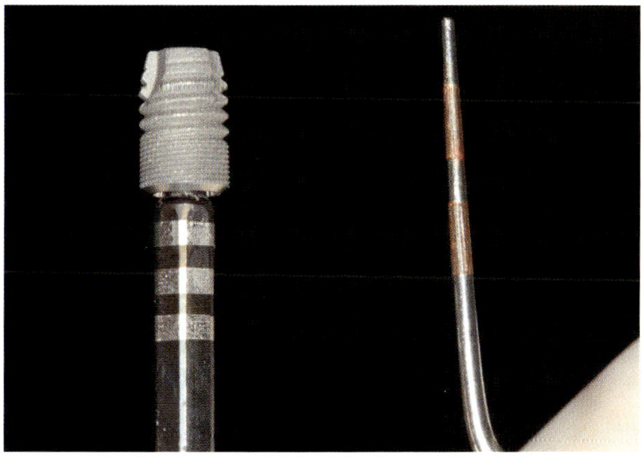

Fig 2-15 Insertion of Astra Tech® implant of 4 × 6 mm.

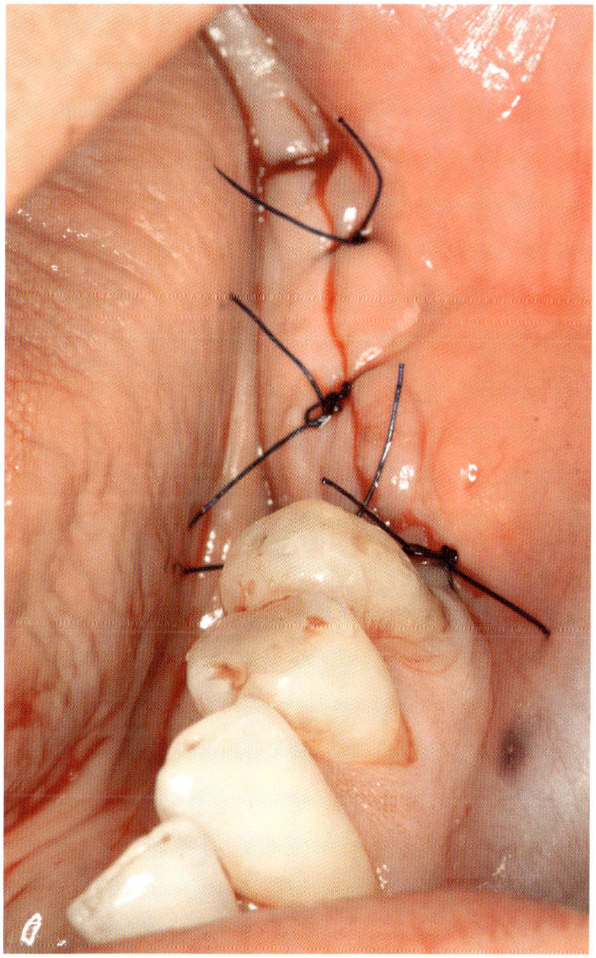

Fig 2-16 Suture of the surgical flap.

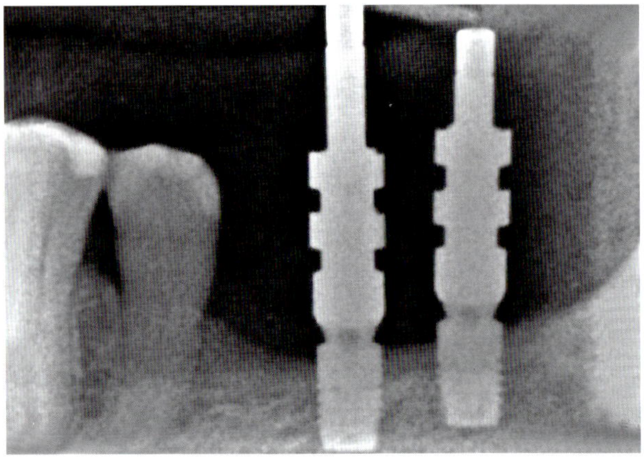

Fig 2-17 Periapical radiograph of the inserted impression copings.

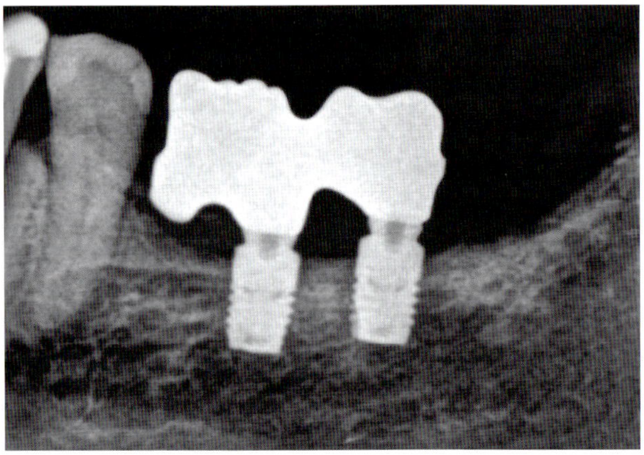

Fig 2-18 Metal try-in on implants 36 and 37.

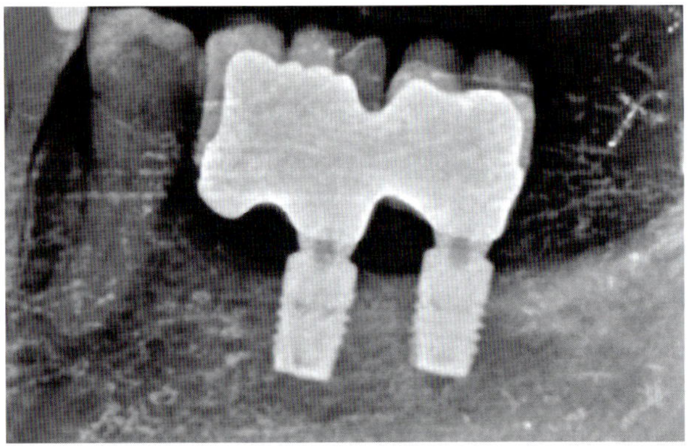

Fig 2-19 Periapical radiograph of the final insertion of the prosthetic crowns.

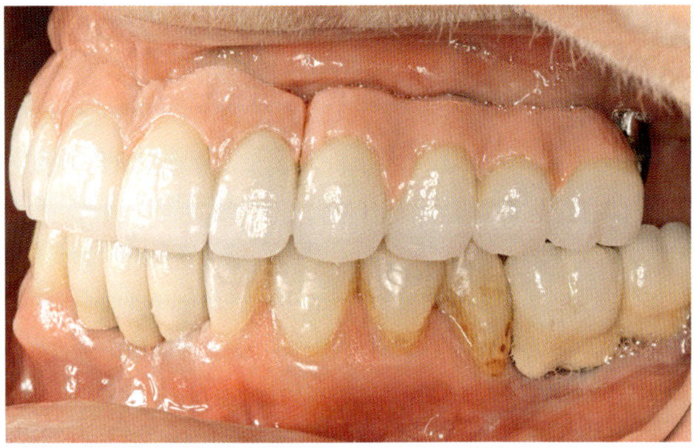

Fig 2-20 Final insertion of the crowns.

Case 3 (Figs 2-21 to 2-27)

Courtesy of Drs M Quevedo and M Molins

A severe atrophy of the mandible was present in this patient in both quadrants. Bone block grafting was refused by the patient. Due to a very limited residual bone over the mental foramens and alveolar nerves, surgery was planned using computer software (Figs 2-23 and 2-24). Finally, short implants of 4 × 6 mm were placed in the posterior regions of the mandible using partially guided surgery. The case was finished by splinting short with longer implants in the third and fourth quadrants (Fig 2-27).

Figs 2-21 to 2-27 Case 3

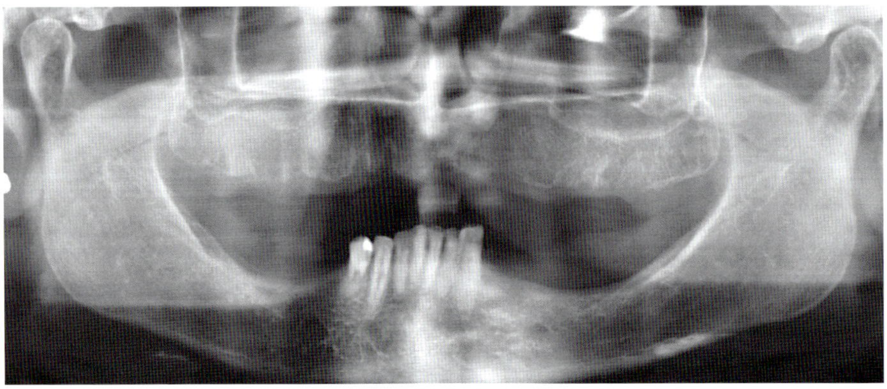

Fig 2-21 Initial panoramic radiograph. Notice the advanced resorption of the posterior mandible.

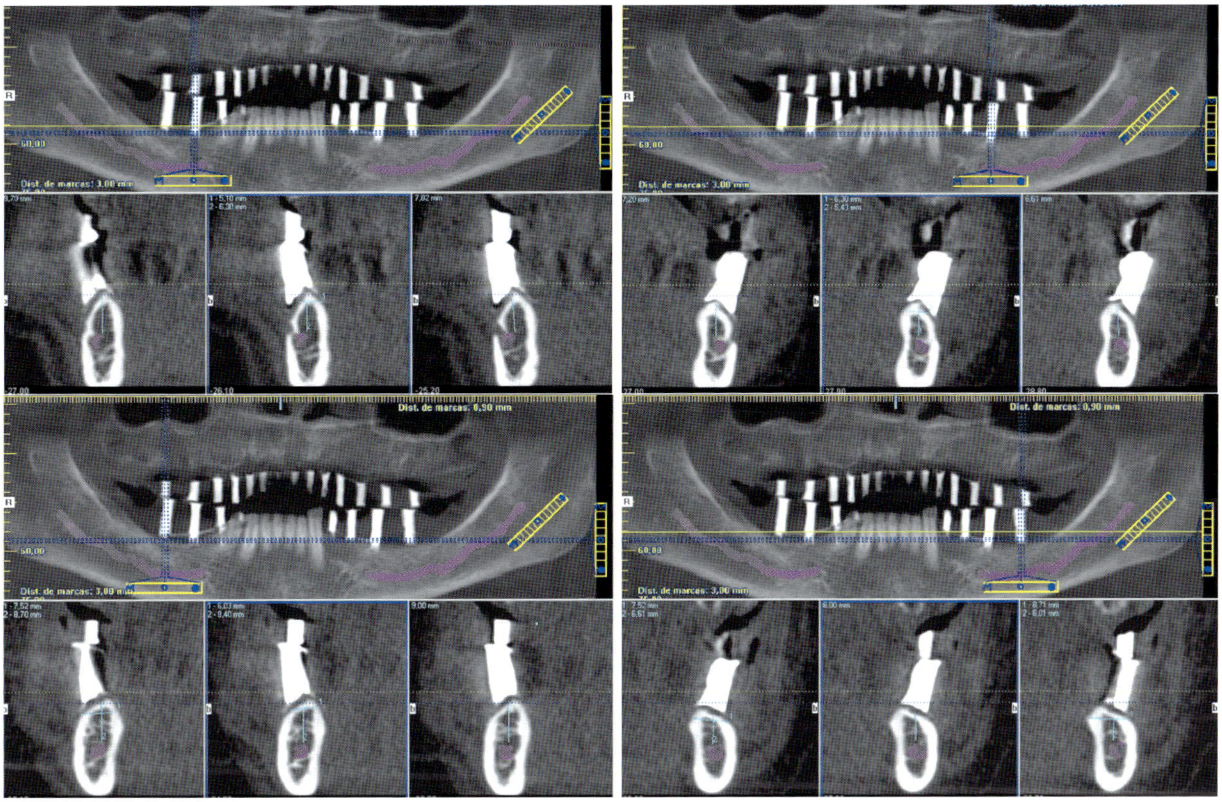

Fig 2-22 CBVT (cone beam volumetric tomography) exploration of both quadrants (third and fourth).

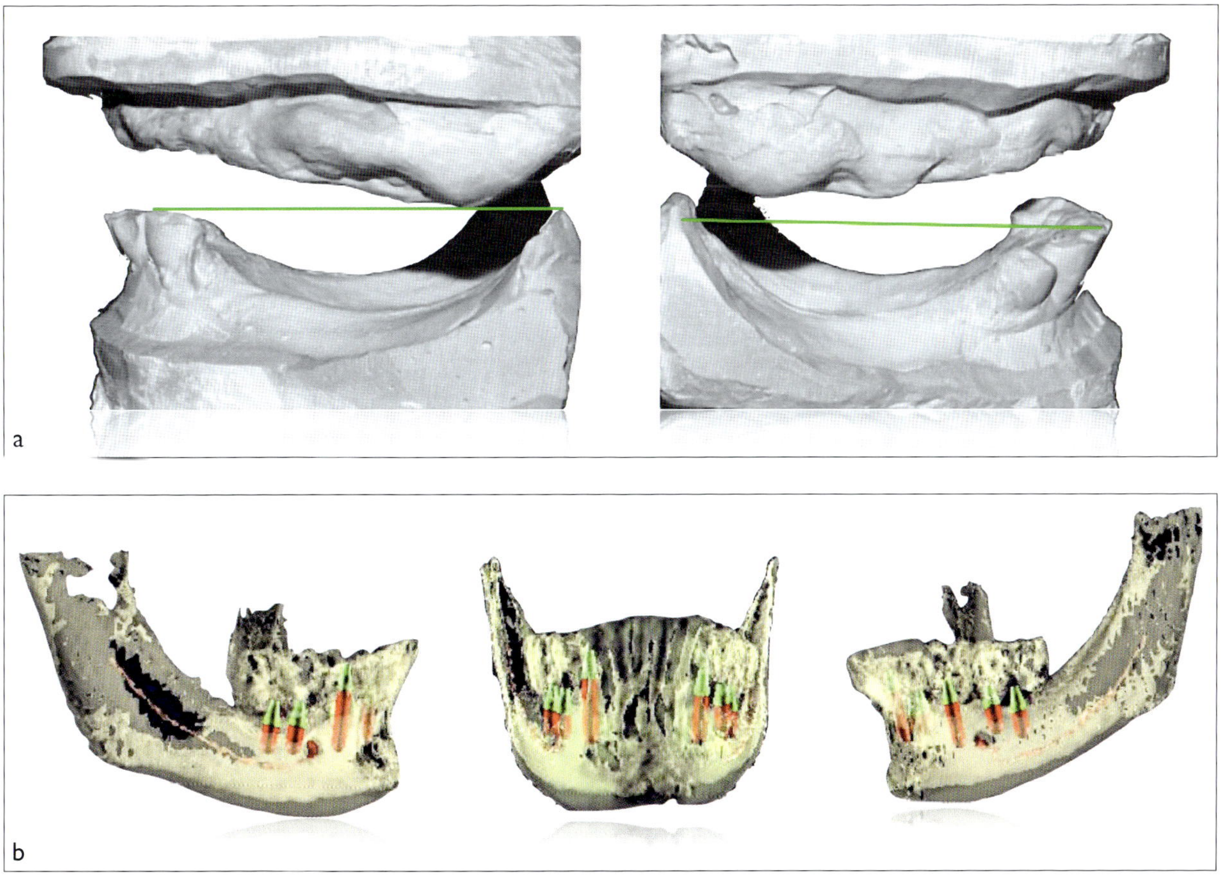

Figs 2-23a and b (a) Study models. (b) Planned implant surgery with computer software.

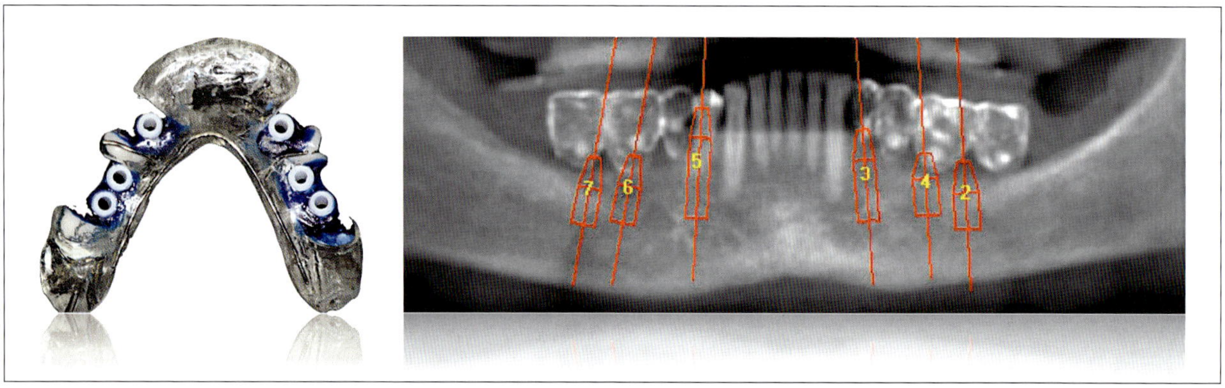

Fig 2-24 A partially guided surgical stent was fabricated for the implant surgery.

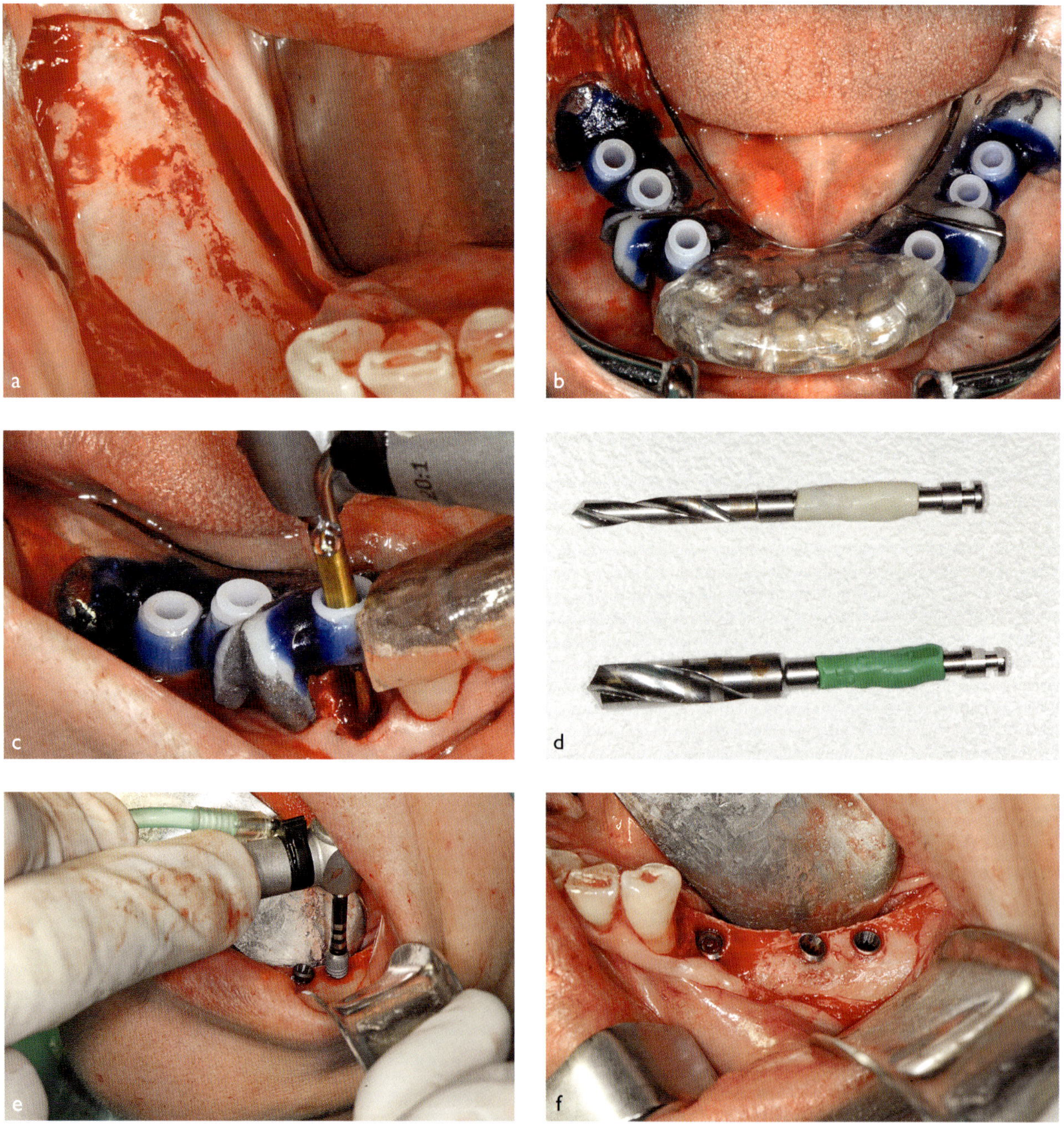

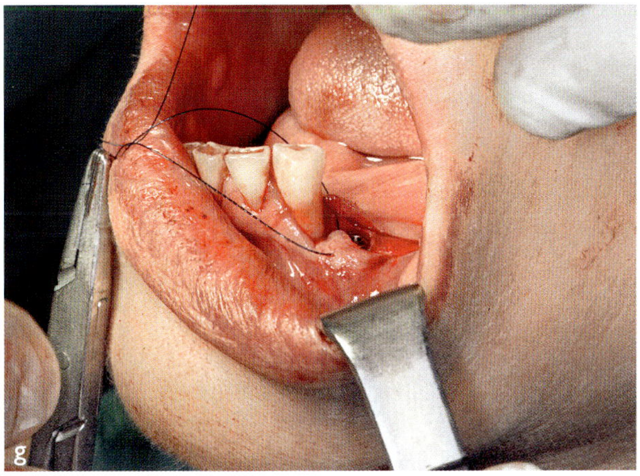

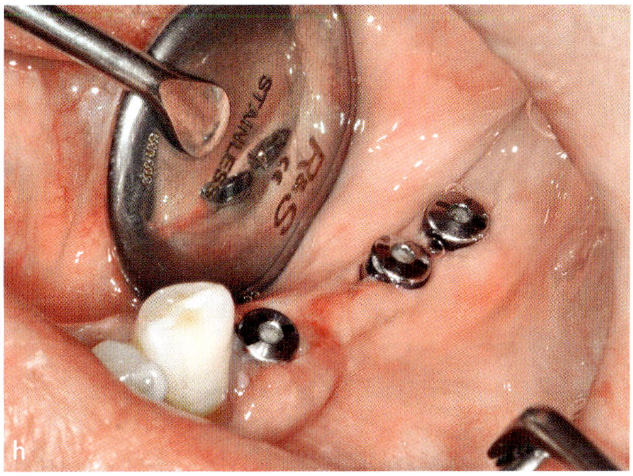

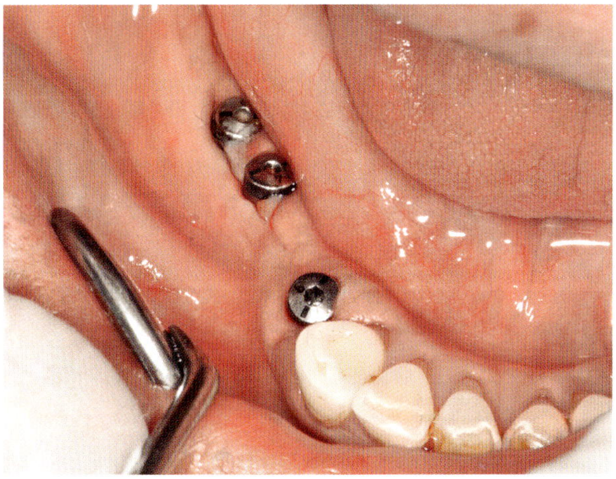

Fig 2-25a to i Implant surgery sequence of the fourth and third quadrant. (a) Full thickness flap elevation. (b) Insertion of the surgical stent. (c) Guided drilling of the implant bed. (d) Surgical drills used for short implants. (e) Placement of the short implants. (f) Implants in their final position. (g) Suturing of the flap. (h) Healing abutments, third quadrant. (i) Healing abutments, fourth quadrant.

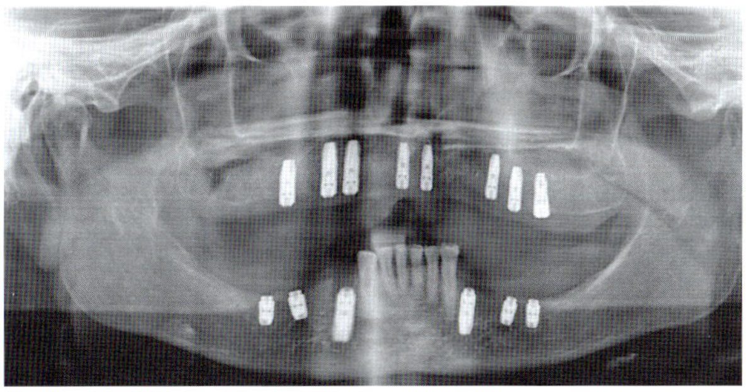

Fig 2-26 Postsurgical panoramic radiograph showing the implants placed.

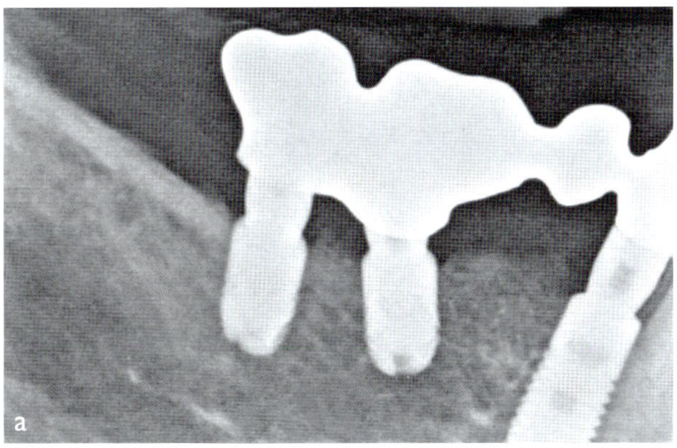

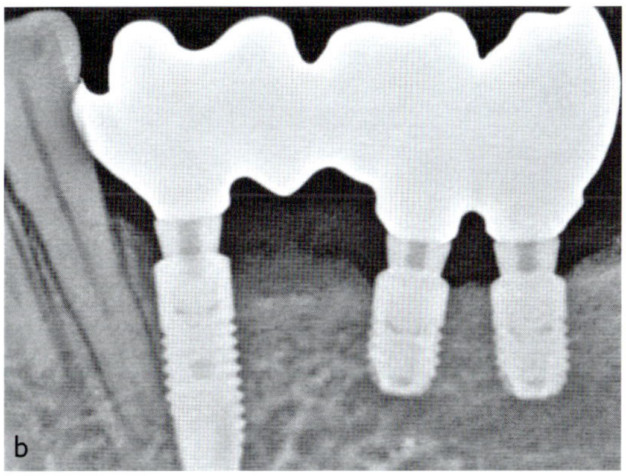

Figs 2-27a and b Periapical radiographs showing the final crowns in (a) the fourth and (b) the third quadrant to check the adjustment.

Case 4 (Figs 2-28 to 2-30)

Courtesy of Drs N Ginebreda and F Bibiloni

In this case, right mandibular resorption was present in the position of the first and second molars. The distance over the mandibular canal was less than 8 mm. Two short implants were planned to replace the missing molars. Finally, a fixed partial denture was placed, splinting the implants (Fig 2-30).

Figs 2-28 to 2-30 Case 4

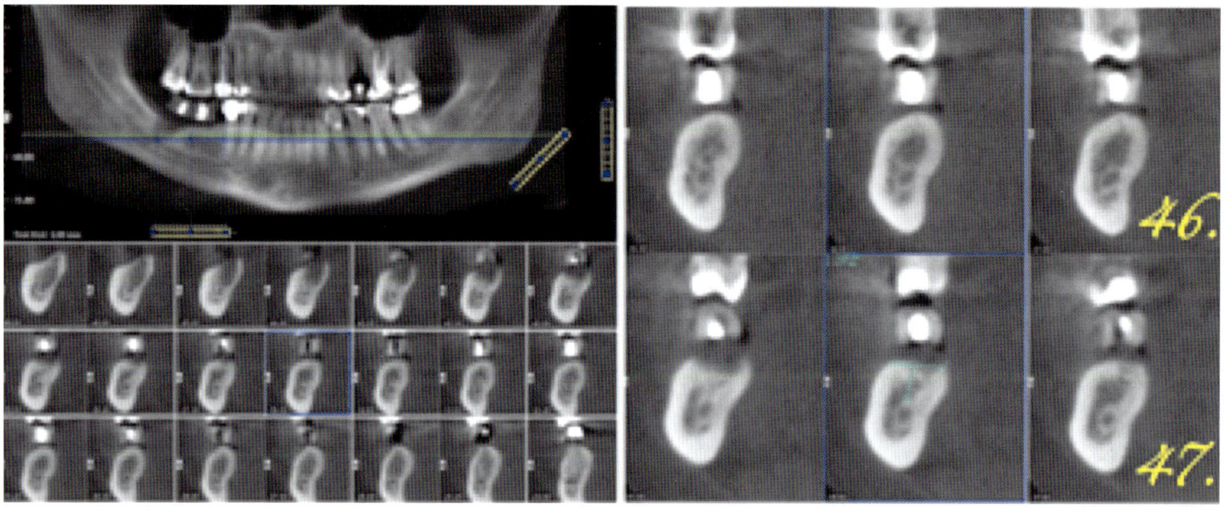

Fig 2-28 Initial CBVT (cone beam volumetric tomography) exploration of the fourth quadrant.

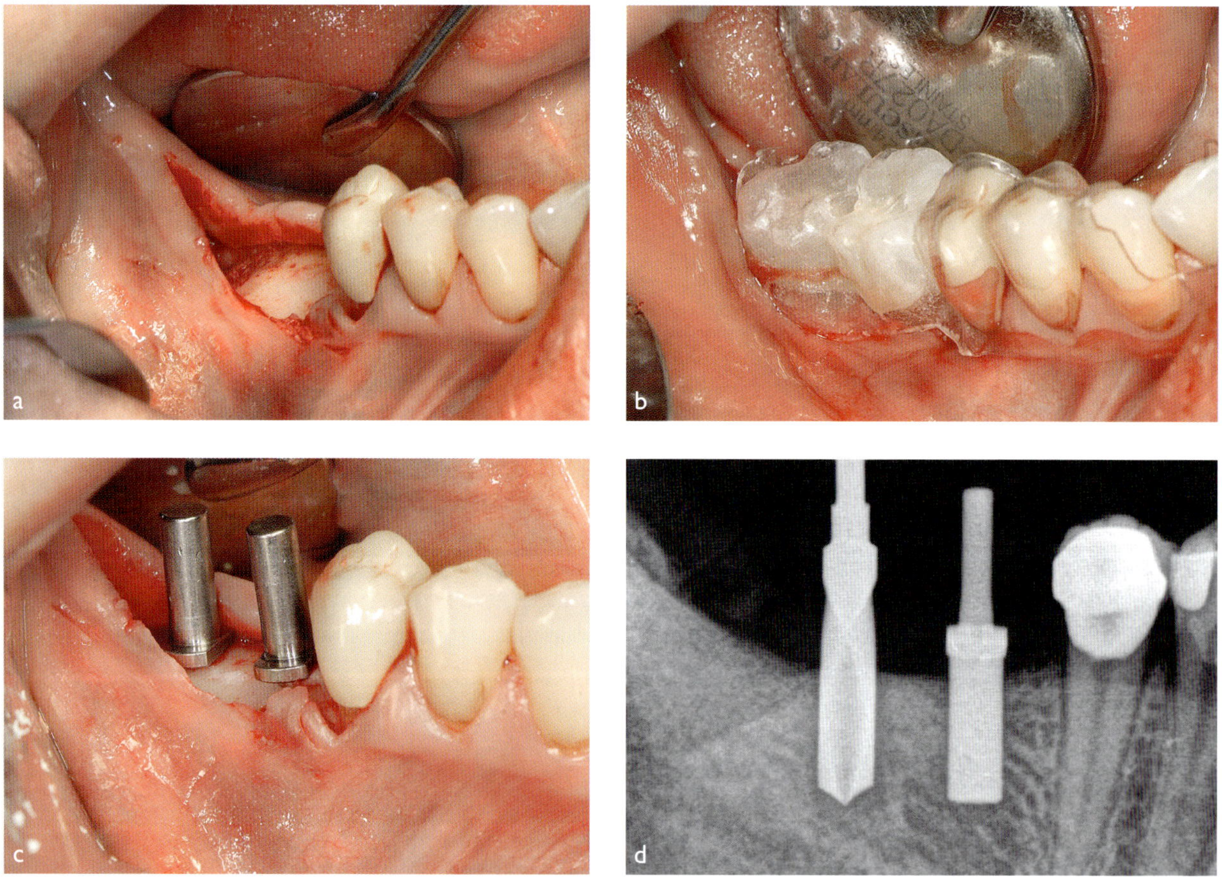

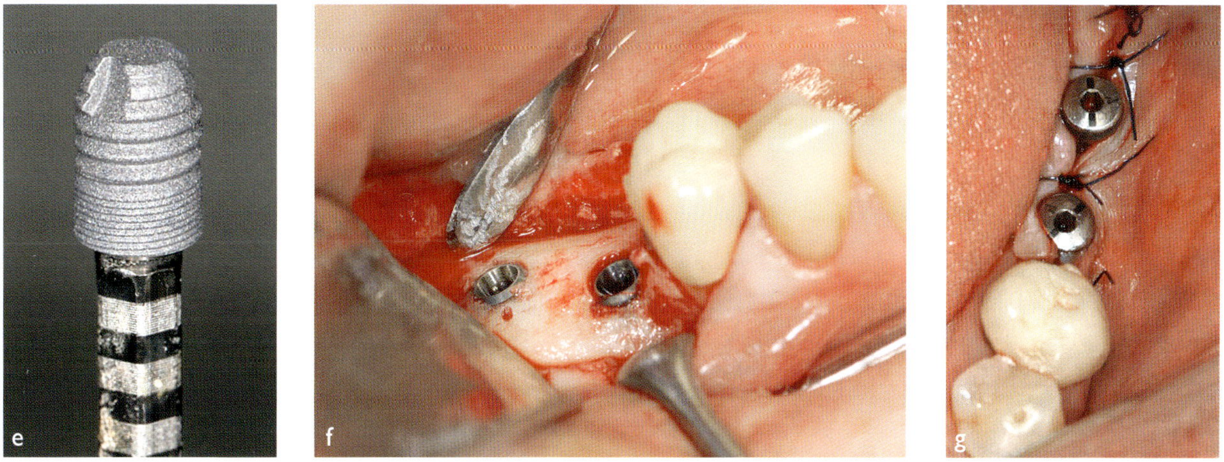

Figs 2-29a to g Implant surgery sequence. (a) Flap incision. (b) Surgical stent. (c) Direction pins inserted. (d) Periapical radiograph to check depth and proximity to neighboring teeth. (e) Placement of two Astra Tech® implants 4 × 6 mm. (f) Implants inserted into the osteotomies. (g) Flap suture around healing abutments.

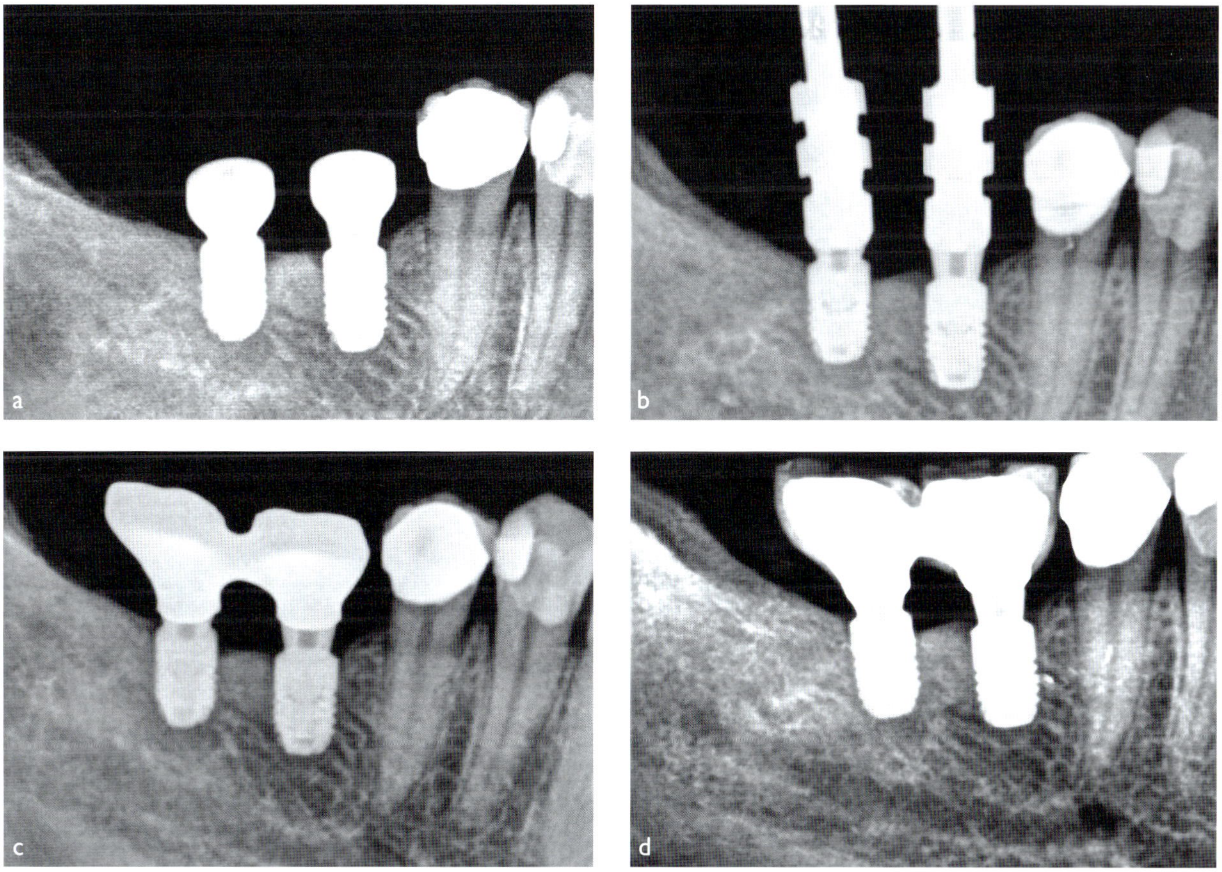

Figs 2-30a to d Periapical radiographs 2 months after implant surgery. (a) Implants with healing abutments. (b) Impression copings inserted. (c) Metal try-in for cement retained restoration. (d) Final insertion of the prosthetic crowns.

Figs 2-31 to 2-35 Case 5

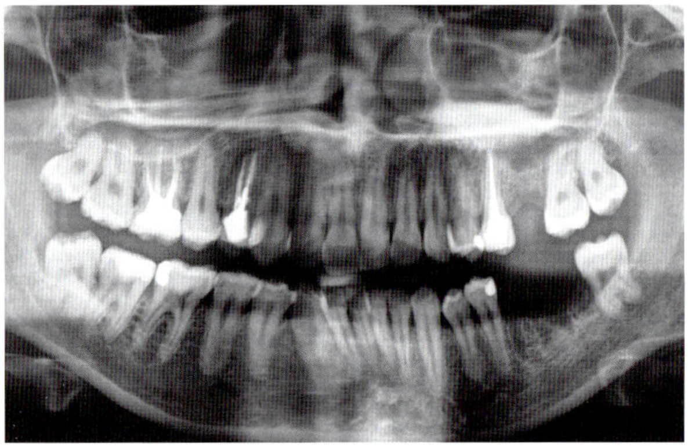

Fig 2-31 Initial panoramic radiograph, showing absence of teeth 25, 36, and 37.

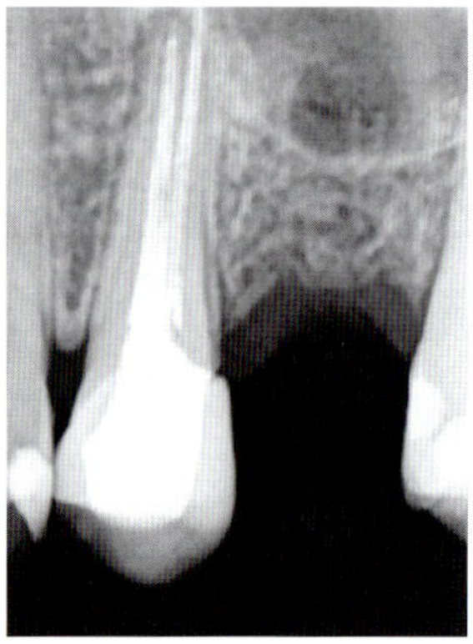

Fig 2-32 Initial periapical radiograph showing reduced bone height.

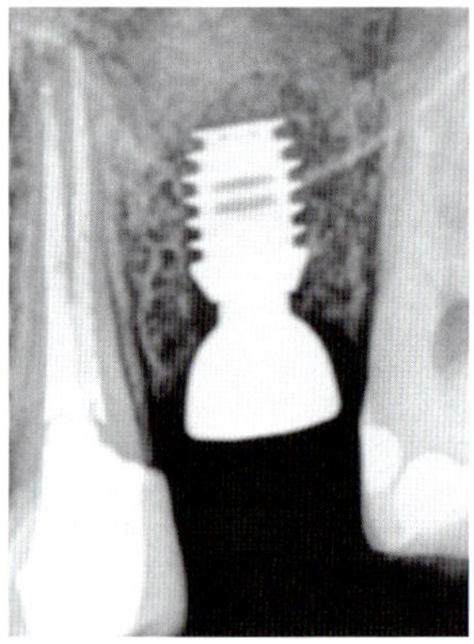

Fig 2-33 Implant placed with simultaneous sinus lift with osteotomes. Notice the radiopacity of the biomaterial around the apical part of the implant.

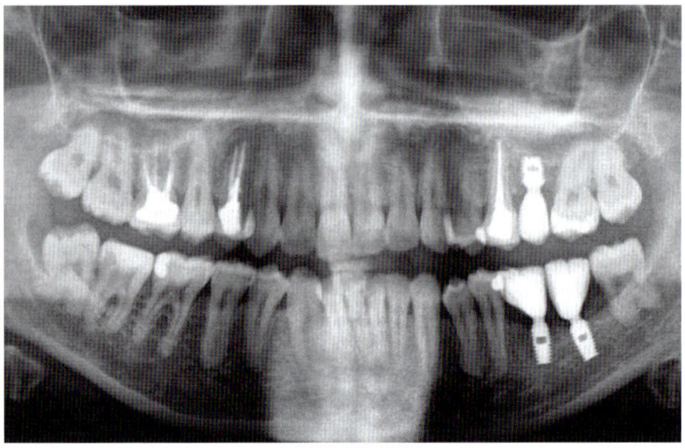

Fig 2-34 Final restorations placed.

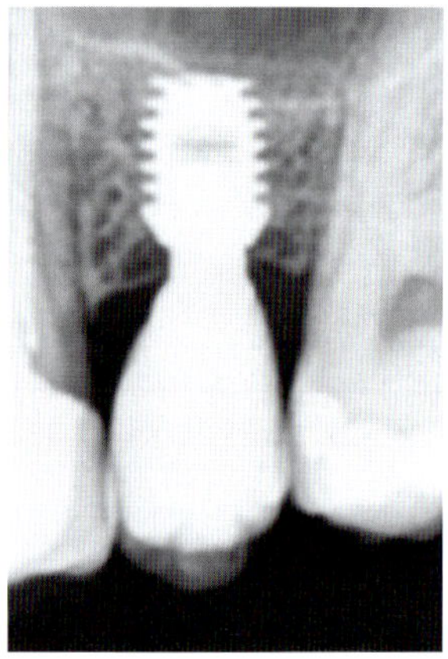

Fig 2-35 Periapical radiograph showing the placement of the cement retained restoration.

Case 5 (Figs 2-31 to 2-35)

Courtesy of Dr A Barroso

This case demonstrates a situation where both the mandible and the maxilla were rehabilitated using short implants. In the mandible, extractions without ridge preservation led to a situation with inadequate bone height. In the maxilla the aim was to avoid a lateral sinus lift procedure. A 6 mm-long implant was chosen to replace the first maxillary molar, with a simultaneous atraumatic crestal sinus lift, and two 7 mm-long implants were used to replace the mandibular molars. The procedure was performed using a two-phase protocol and rehabilitation took place 4 months after implant placement.

Case 6 (Figs 2-36 and 2-37)

Courtesy of Dr A Barroso

This case was an edentulous left mandibular restored using unsplinted short implants. Single crowns were placed in the second premolar, first molar, and second molar (Fig 2-36).

Figs 2-36 and 2-37 Case 6

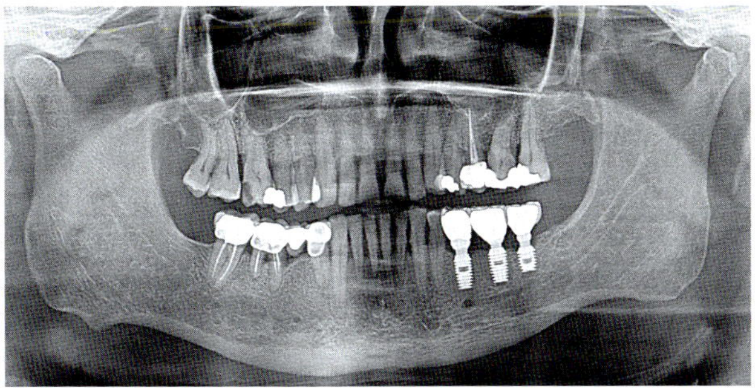

Fig 2-36 Panoramic radiograph showing the unsplinted implant-supported restorations on implants numbers 35, 36, and 37.

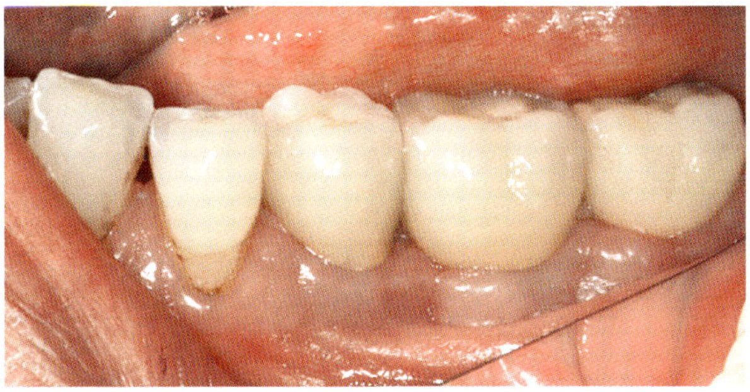

Fig 2-37 Clinical picture showing soft tissue adaptation of the cement-retained restorations.

2.9 Conclusions

- Short implants are especially intended for posterior atrophic mandibles/maxillas. They can often replace complex reconstructive surgery, being an alternative therapy in atrophic cases.
- The ideal short implant should be an implant with a rough surface, a diameter of ≥4 mm, an internal connection and platform modification, and no shorter than 6 mm.
- "More is more" when deciding the number of short implants to be placed.
- Careful selection and radiological 3D evaluation of the patient is crucial. An occlusal analysis should be made.
- Periodical occlusal/hygiene controls should be made.
- Peri-implantitis is equal to failure when dealing with short implants.

References

1. Driskell TD. Clinical use of aluminum oxide endosseous implants. J Oral Implantol 1977;7:53-76.
2. Chess JT. Restoration of lost dentition using aluminum oxide endosteal implants. Dent Clin North Am 1980;24:521-533.
3. Niznick GA. The Core-Vent implant system. J Oral Implantol 1982;10:379-418.
4. Hahn J. Clinical experience with the Titanodont subcortical implant system. J Oral Implantol 1983;11:72-88.
5. Kirsch A. The IMZ osteointegrated implant system. Dent Clin North Am 1989;33:733-791. Review.
6. Becker W, Berg L, Becker BE. Untreated periodontal disease: a longitudinal study. J Periodontol 1979;50:234-244.
7. Kotsovilis S, Fourmousis I, Karoussis IK, Bamia C. A systematic review and meta-analysis on the effect of implant length on the survival of rough-surface dental implants. J Periodontol 2009;80:1700-1718.
8. Lee JH, Frias V, Lee KW, Wright RF. Effect of implant size and shape on implant success rates: a literature review. J Prosthet Dent 2005;94:377-381.
9. Renouard F, Nisand D. Short implants in the severely resorbed maxilla: a 2-year retrospective clinical study. Clin Implant Dent Relat Res 2005;7(Suppl 1):S104-110.
10. Dori S, Peleg M, Barnea E. Alveolar ridge augmentation with hip corticocancellous allogenic block graft prior to implant placement. Refuat Hapeh Vehashinayim 2008;25:28-38,54.
11. Fugazzotto PA. Shorter implants in clinical practice: rationale and treatment results. Int J Oral Maxillofac Implants 2008;23:487-496.
12. Tawil G, Aboujaoude N, Younan R. Influence of prosthetic parameters on the survival and complication rates of short implants. Int J Oral Maxillofac Implants 2006;21:275-282.
13. Feldman S, Boitel N, Weng D, Kohles SS, Stach RM. Five-year survival distributions of short-length (10 mm or less) machined-surfaced and Osseotite implants. Clin Implant Dent Relat Res 2004;6:16-23.
14. Ten Bruggenkate CM, Asikainen P, Foitzik C, Krekeler G, Sutter F. Short (6-mm) nonsubmerged dental implants: results of a multicenter clinical trial of 1 to 7 years. Int J Oral Maxillofac Implants 1998;13:791-798.
15. Chung DM, Oh TJ, Lee J, Misch CE, Wang HL. Factors affecting late implant bone loss: a retrospective analysis. Int J Oral Maxillofac Implants 2007;22:117-126.
16. Griffin TJ, Cheung WS. The use of short, wide implants in posterior areas with reduced bone height: a retrospective investigation. J Prosthet Dent 2004;92:139-144.
17. Renouard F, Nisand D. Impact of implant length and diameter on survival rates. Clin Oral Implants Res 2006;17 (Suppl 2):35-51.
18. Das Neves FD, Fones D, Bernardes SR, do Prado CJ, Neto AJ. Short implants: an analysis of longitudinal studies. Int J Oral Maxillofac Implants 2006;21:86-93.
19. Tinti C, Parma-Benfenati S. Clinical classification of bone defects concerning the placement of dental implants. Int J Periodontics Restorative Dent 2003;23:147-155.
20. Esposito M, Grusovin MG, Coulthard P, Worthington HV. The efficacy of various bone augmentation procedures for dental implants: a Cochrane systematic review of randomized controlled clinical trials. Int J Oral Maxillofac Implants 2006;21:696-710.
21. Aghaloo T, Moy P. Which hard tissue augmentation techniques are the most successful in furnishing bony support for implant placement? Int J Oral Maxillofac Implants 2007;22(Suppl):49-70.
22. Morand M, Irinakis T. The challenge of implant therapy in the posterior maxilla: providing a rationale for the use of short implants. J Oral Implantol 2007;33:257-266.
23. Misch CE, Steignga J, Barboza E, Misch-Dietsh F, Cianciola LJ, Kazor C. Short dental implants in posterior partial edentulism: a multicenter retrospective 6-year case series study. J Periodontol 2006;77:1340-1347.

24. Toffler M. Treating the atrophic posterior maxilla by combining short implants with minimally invasive osteotome procedures. Pract Proced Aesthet Dent 2006;18:301-308.
25. Triplett RG, Mason ME, Alfonso WF, McAnear JT. Endosseous cylinder implants in severely atrophic mandibles. Int J Oral Maxillofac Implants 1991;6:264-269.
26. Adell R, Lekholm U, Gröndahl K, Branemark PI, Lindström J, Jacobsson M. Reconstruction of severely resorbed edentulous maxillae using osseointegrated fixtures in immediate autogenous bone grafts. Int J Oral Maxillofac Implants 1990;5:233-246.
27. Johns RB, Jemt T, Heath MR, et al. A multicenter study of overdentures supported by Branemark implants. Int J Oral Maxillofac Implants 1992;7:513-522.
28. Friberg B, Gröndahl K, Lekholm U, Branemark PI. Long-term follow-up of severely atrophic edentulous mandibles reconstructed with short Branemark implants. Clin Implant Dent Relat Res 2000;2:184-189.
29. Jemt T, Lekholm U. Implant treatment in edentulous maxillae: a 5-year follow-up report on patients with different degrees of jaw resorption. Int J Oral Maxillofac Implants 1995;10:303-311.
30. Goodacre CJ, Bernal G, Rungcharassaeng K, Kan JY. Clinical complications with implants and implant prostheses. J Prosthet Dent 2003;90:121-132.
31. Testori T, Wiseman L, Woolfe S, Porter SS. A prospective multicenter clinical study of the Osseotite implant: four-year interim report. Int J Oral Maxillofac Implants 2001;16:193-200.
32. Tawil G, Younan R. Clinical evaluation of short, machined-surface implants followed for 12 to 92 months. Int J Oral Maxillofac Implants 2003;18:894-901.
33. Cochran DI. A comparison of endosseous dental implant surfaces. J Periodontol 1999;70:1523-1539.
34. Deporter DA, Watson PA, Pillar RM, et al. A retrospective clinical study in human of endosseous dental implant partially covered with a powder-sintered porous coating: 3-to-4 year results. Int J Oral Maxillofac Implants 1996;11:87-95.
35. Pilliar RM. Processing and properties of endosseous dental implant surfaces: design for increased osseointegration potential. Oral Health 2000;8:51-58.
36. Albrektsson T, Zarb G, Worthington PMD, Eriksson AR. The long term efficacy of currently used dental implants: a review and proposed criteria of success. Int J Oral Maxillofac Implants 1986;1:11-25.
37. Lekholm U, van Steenberghe D, Herrmann I, et al. Osseointegrated implants in the treatment of partially edentulous jaws: a prospective 5-year multicenter study. Int J Oral Maxillofac Implants 1994;9:627-635.
38. Bahat O. Treatment planning and placement of implants in the posterior maxillae: report of 732 consecutive Nobelpharma implants. Int J Oral Maxillofac Implants 1993;8:151-161.
39. Misch CE. Prótesis dental sobre implantes. Barcelona: Elsevier Mosby, 2006.
40. Weng D, Jacobson Z, Tarnow D, et al. A prospective multicenter clinical trial of 3i machined-surface implants: results after 6 years of follow-up. Int J Oral Maxillofac Implants 2003;18:417-423.
41. Gentile MA, Chuang SK, Dodson TB. Survival estimates and risk factors for failure with 6 x 5.7-mm implants. Int J Oral Maxillofac Implants 2005;20:930-937.
42. Venuleo C, Chuang S-K, Weed M, Dibart S. Long term bone level stability on short implants: a radiographic follow-up study. J Maxillofac Oral Surg 2008;7:340-345.
43. Romeo E, Ghisolfi M, Rozza R, Chiapasco M, Lops D. Short (8-mm) dental implants in the rehabilitation of partial and complete edentulism: a 3- to 14-year longitudinal study. Int J Prosthodont 2006;19:586-592.
44. Goene R, Bianchesi C, Hüerzeler M, et al. Performance of short implants in partial restorations: 3-year follow-up of Osseotite implants. Implant Dent 2005;14:274-280.
45. Corrente G, Abundo R, des Ambrois AB, Savio L, Perelli M. Short porous implants in the posterior maxilla: a 3-year report of a prospective study. Int J Periodontics Restorative Dent 2009;29:23-29.
46. Malo P, de Araujo Nobre M, Rangert B. Short implants placed one-stage in maxillae and mandibles: a retrospective clinical study with 1 to 9 years of follow-up. Clin Implant Dent Relat Res 2007;9:15-21.
47. Anitua E, Orive G, Aguirre JJ, Andía I. Five-year clinical evaluation of short dental implants placed in posterior areas: a retrospective study. J Periodontol 2008;79:42-48.
48. Deporter DA, Caudry S, Kermalli J, Adegbembo A. Further data on the predictability of the indirect sinus elevation procedure used with short, sintered, porous-surfaced dental implants. Int J Periodontics Restorative Dent 2005;25:585-593.
49. Nedir R, Bischof M, Briaux JM, Beyer S, Szmukler-Moncler S, Bernard JP. A 7-year life table analysis from a prospective study on ITI implants with special emphasis on the use of short implants. Results from a private practice. Clin Oral Implants Res 2004;15:150-157.
50. Deporter D, Pilliar RM, Todescan R, Watson P, Pharoah M. Managing the posterior mandible of partially edentulous patients with short, porous-surfaced dental implants: early data from a clinical trial. Int J Oral Maxillofac Implants 2001;16:653-658.
51. Misch CE, Judy KW. Classification of partially edentulous arches for implant dentistry. Int J Oral Implantol 1987;4:7-13.
52. Lekholm U, Zarb G. Patient selection. In: Branemark PI, Zarb G, Albrektsson T (eds). Tissue Integrated Prosthesis: Osseointegration in Clinical Dentistry. Chicago: Quintessence, 1985:109-209.
53. Deporter DA, Todescan R, Dominguez Campelo L, Pilliar RM. Implantes de superficie porosa sinterizada: aprovechamiento de ventajas clínicas únicas. Periodoncia 2002:6:369-382.
54. Pilliar RM. Overview of surface variability of metallic endosseous dental implants: textured and porous surface-structured designs. Implant Dent 1998;7:305-314.
55. Hagi D, Deporter DA, Pilliar RM, Arenovich T. A targeted review of study outcomes with short (7 mm) endosseous dental implants placed in partially edentulous patients. J Periodontol 2004;75:798-804.
56. Jemt T, Lekholm U. Oral implant treatment in posterior partially endetulous jaws: a 5-year follow-up report. Int J Oral Maxillofac Implants 1993;8:635-640.
57. Reiger MR, Mayberry M, Brose MO. Finite element analysis of six endosseous implants. J Prosthet Dent 1990;63:671-676.
58. Van Oosterwyck. The influence of bone mechanical properties and implant fixation upon bone loading around oral implants. Clin Oral Implants Res 1998;9:407-418.
59. Birdi H, Schulte J, Kovacs A, Weed M, Chuang SK. Crown-to-implant ratios of short length implants. J Oral Implantol 2010;36:425-433.
60. Blanes RJ. Crown–implant ratio and dental implant complications. Clin Oral Impl Res 2009;20(Suppl 4):67-72.
61. Lun LB. A biomechanical rationale for the use of short implants. J Oral Implantol 1991;17:126-131.
62. Akca K. Finite element stress analysis of the effect of short implant usage in place of cantilever extensions in mandibular posterior edentulism. J Oral Rehabil 2002;29:350-356.
63. Degidi M, Piattelli A, Iezzi G, Carinci F. Wide-diameter implants: analysis of clinical outcome of 304 fixtures. J Periodontol 2007;78:52-58.
64. Davarpanah M, Martínez H, Etienne D, Wide diameter implants: new concepts. Int J Periodontics Restorative Dent 2001;21:149-159.
65. Bahat O. Branemark system implants in the posterior maxilla: clinical study of 660 implants followed for 5 to 12 years. Int J Oral Maxillofac Implants 2000;15:646-653.

Chapter 3

Is socket preservation possible?

Vanessa Ruiz Magaz, Estafania Solans, Tania Perez

3.1 Introduction

Loss of alveolar bone may be attributed to a variety of factors, such as endodontic pathology, periodontitis, facial trauma, and aggressive maneuvers during extraction. The consequence is usually the loss of the ridge contours, leading to esthetic problems or impairing ideal implant placement.

It is possible to minimize such problems by performing ridge preservation procedures in extraction sockets using grafting materials with or without barrier membranes.[1] According to the American Academy of Periodontology (AAP), an alveolus is the socket in the bone into which a tooth is attached by means of the periodontal ligament. Therefore the terms alveolus or socket can be used indistinctly.

The change of the buccal wall will be more pronounced than that of its lingual/palatal counterpart.[2] Schropp et al.[3] measured dimensional changes in 46 healing sockets in 16 patients and it was found that a reduction in buccolingual width of approximately 50% (from 12.0 mm to 5.9 mm) took place over a 12-month period, with two-thirds of this change occurring in the first 3 months after extraction (Table 3-1).

Table 3-1 Average width and height reduction in the alveolar crest

Authors	Width and height reduction	Healing time
Bartee[4]	Width: 60% Height: 40%	6 months
Schropp et al.[3]	Width: 50% (12.0 mm to 5.9 mm)	12 months
Chen et al.[5]	Width: 50% (5 mm to 7 mm) Height: 2.0 mm to 4.5 mm	6–12 months

Amler[6] in 1960 described five stages in the healing of a post-extraction alveolar bone (Fig 3-1):

- First stage: The coagulation occurs almost immediately with the formation of a "blood clot" of red and white cells, initiating hemolysis.

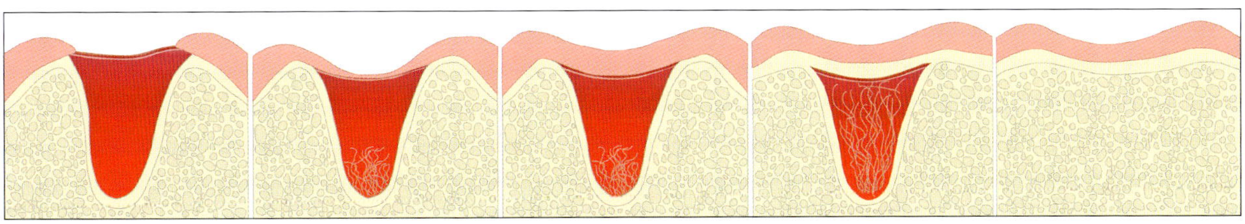

Fig 3-1 Amler's five stages in the healing of post-extraction sockets in alveolar bone.[6] Stage 1: coagulation, formation of a "blood clot", initiating hemolysis. Stage 2: granulation tissue replaces the clot. Stage 3: connective tissue replaces granulation tissue; the epithelium lining the wound is complete. Stage 4: calcification of osteoid tissue. Stage 5: closure of the alveolar epithelium and bone fill.

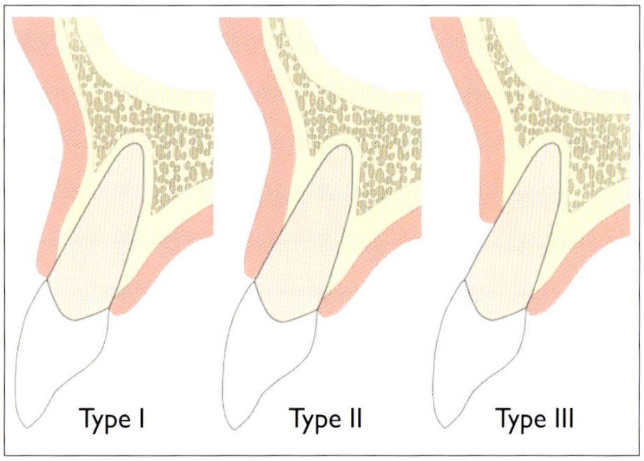

Fig 3-2 Elian's classification of post-extraction defects.[7] Type I socket: the facial soft tissue and buccal plate of bone are at normal levels in relation to the cementoenamel junction of the pre-extracted tooth and remain intact post-extraction. Type II socket: facial soft tissue is present but the buccal plate is partially missing following extraction of the tooth. Type III: the facial soft tissue and the buccal plate are both markedly reduced after tooth extraction.

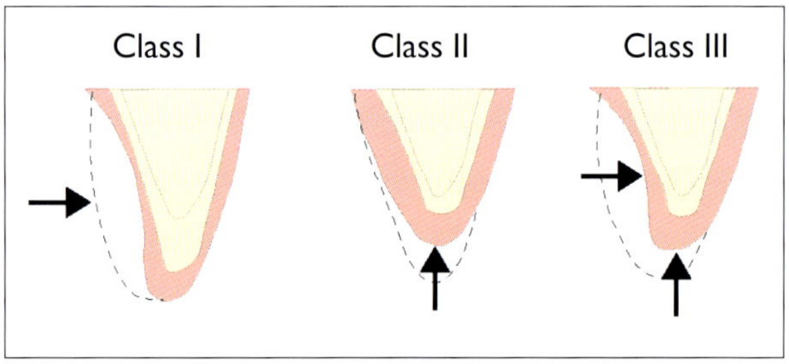

Fig 3-3 Seibert's classification of ridge defects.[8] Class I: defects have tissue loss in a buccolingual dimension with normal apicocoronal dimension. Class II: defects have tissue loss in an apicocoronal dimension with normal buccolingual dimension. Class III: defects present a combination of both deficiencies in width and height.

- Second stage: The granulation tissue replaces the clot on the fourth or fifth day. The angiogenesis is initiated through the chain of endothelial cells and capillary formation.
- Third stage: The connective tissues (collagen fibers, fibroblasts) gradually replace the granulation tissue over a period of 14 to 16 days. The epithelium lining the wound is complete.
- Fourth stage: The calcification of osteoid tissue begins, starting at the base and periphery of the socket over a period of 7 to 10 days. The trabecular bone almost completely fills the socket at 6 weeks. Activity of osteoblasts reaches a maximum, and there is a proliferation of cellular elements of connective tissue and osteoblasts (osteoid tissue) beneath gaps around immature bone, between the 4th and 6th week after extraction. After the 8th week, the osteogenic process appears to descend.
- Fifth stage: The complete closure of the alveolar epithelium occurs after 4 or 5 weeks. Substantial bone fill occurs between the 5th and 10th week. And at 16 weeks, bone fill has been completed, with little evidence of osteogenic activity during this period, although bone fill will continue for some months without reaching the neighboring tooth bone level.[1]

In socket preservation, the goal is to maintain both hard and soft tissue levels. However, the placement of an intrasocket osseous graft minimizes, but does not eliminate, loss of horizontal and vertical ridge dimensions.[1,6]

There have been a number of proposed systems to classify extraction sockets. After years of socket research, it has become obvious that although there are multiple variables related to each extraction socket, the key factor that determines the kind of socket present following extraction is the presence or absence of the buccal hard and soft tissue. Therefore, Elian[7] proposed a simplified classification of extraction sockets (Fig 3-2):

- Type I socket: the facial soft tissue and buccal plate of bone are at normal levels in relation to the cementoenamel junction of the pre-extracted tooth and remain intact post-extraction.
- Type II socket: facial soft tissue is present but the buccal plate is partially missing following extraction of the tooth.
- Type III: the facial soft tissue and the buccal plate are both markedly reduced after tooth extraction.

Ridge defects could also be classified. In 1983, Seibert[8] proposed a simple classification system (Fig 3-3):

- Class I: defects have tissue loss in a buccolingual dimension with normal apicocoronal dimension.
- Class II: defects have tissue loss in an apicocoronal dimension with normal buccolingual dimension.
- Class III: defects present a combination of both deficiencies in width and height.[9]

Regarding socket preservation, many techniques have been proposed. These include using flaps or flapless surgery, the use of different types of bony grafts or replacement materials, and several kinds of membranes ranging from absorbable to non-absorbable.[7] Moreover, although

Table 3-2 Advantages and disadvantages of non-resorbable and resorbable membranes

Type of membrane	Advantages	Disadvantages	Examples
Non-resorbable	• Numerous studies demonstrate their success • May be titanium-reinforced • Remain intact until removal • Easily attached with titanium or resorbable tacks • Greater bone fill if membrane not exposed • Minimal tissue response if membrane not exposed	• Require a second surgery for removal • Increase patient morbidity • If exposed, must be removed • Can be technique-sensitive	• ePTFE membranes, eg Gore-Tex (Gore Medical, Flagstaff, AZ, USA) • Titanium-reinforced Gore-Tex
Resorbable	• Numerous studies demonstrate their success • Do not require surgical removal • Decreased patient morbidity • Improved soft-tissue healing • Tissue-friendly reaction to membrane exposure • Cost effective; one surgery only • Does not have to be removed if exposed	• Uncertain duration of barrier membrane function • Difficult to track down • Slightly less bone fill than non-resorbable membranes • Inflammatory response from tissues may interfere with healing and GBR • Can be technique-sensitive	• Neomem (bovine collagen matrix; Citagenix, Laval, Quebec, Canada) • Bio-Gide (porcine collagen matrix; Geistlich, Wolhusen, Switzerland) • Ossix (cross-linked collagen barrier; Implant Innovations, Palm Beach Gardens, FL, USA)

there are tangible benefits of using alveolar preservation techniques, there is no available literature to show which procedure is the best is terms of predictability. Alveolar bone resorption and socket remodeling involve a complex cascade of events that can include multiple modes of action, such as biomechanical stimulation, wound closure, and scaffolding effects.

Various graft materials including autogenous, allogenous, xenogenic, and alloplastic bone grafts have been used to preserve the alveolar ridge following tooth extraction.[1] These bone filling materials should ideally possess the following characteristics:[10]

- Easy to use and manage.
- Not prone to infection or migration.
- Able to attract precursor bone cells.
- Hydrophilic.
- Easily accessible.
- Unable to transmit infectious diseases to the patient.

Regarding the use of membranes, a wide range of barrier membranes has been reported in numerous studies. There are two major categories: non-resorbable membranes and resorbable membranes, and they include expanded polytetrafluoroethylene (e-PTFE), collagen, acellular dermal matrix (ADM), polyglycolic acid, and polyglactin.[11,12] Table 3-2 lists their advantages and disadvantages.

Unfortunately, it seems that ridge preservation has not become routine clinical practice although studies have demonstrated that it is a predictable technique that has many advantages. However, further studies are needed to evaluate the long-term effects of ridge preservation materials and to develop standardized protocols for their use.

This chapter will review the current scientific literature on socket preservation and will try to define the best technique. In order to do so, the following topics will be addressed:

- 3.2 Ridge preservation topics
  - 3.2.1 Is there a significant difference between performing ridge preservation and the healing of the socket by clot alone?
  - 3.2.2 Which grafting material can be used?
  - 3.2.3 Is bone formed in preserved sockets?
  - 3.2.4 Does the type, position, or reason for extraction of the tooth affect ridge preservation?
  - 3.2.5 Does ridge preservation affect the success rate of implants?

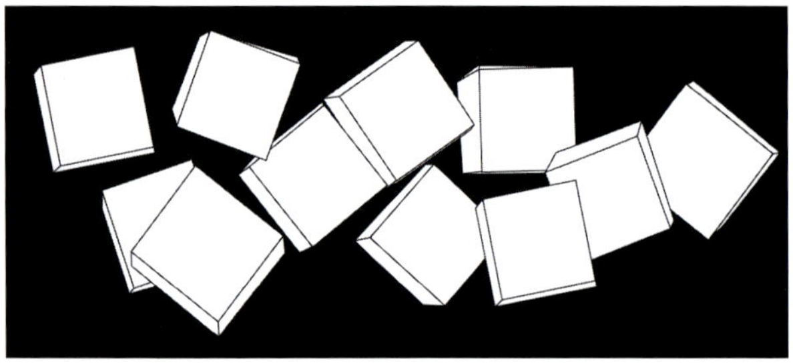

Fig 3-4 Polylactic-polyglycolic sponges for alveolar preservation.

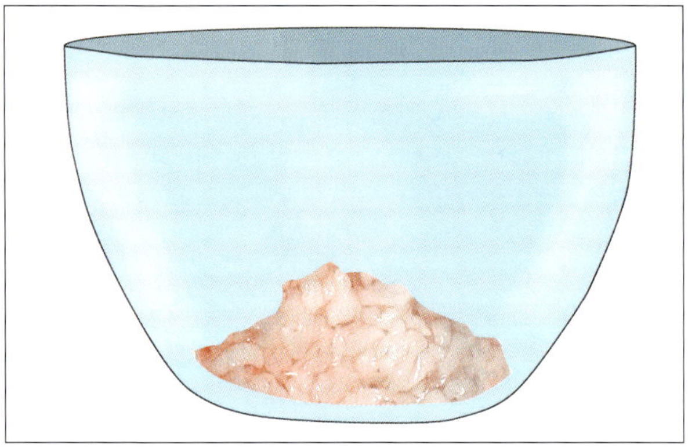

Fig 3-5a Xenograft (bovine deproteinized bone).

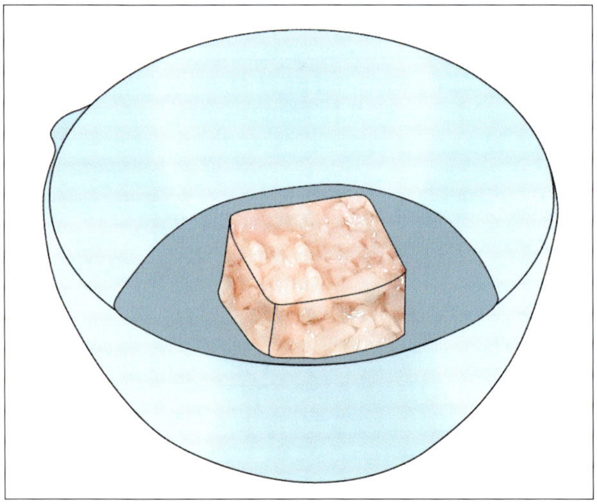

Fig 3-5b Composite bovine derived xenograft (Bio-Oss Collagen®; Geistlich, Wolhusen, Switzerland) consisting of approximately 90% deproteinized cancellous bone particles embedded in a biodegradable collagen matrix of porcine origin (10%). The collagen facilitates the handling of the graft particles and holds the graft at the desired place with a good adaptation to the defect's shape.

- 3.3 Socket preservation materials
  - 3.3.1 What are the available bone substitutes?
  - 3.3.2 Should a membrane be placed after an extraction?
  - 3.3.3 Is it necessary to achieve primary wound closure to cover the membranes and biomaterials?
  - 3.3.4 Complications encountered while dealing with biomaterials in socket preservation
- 3.4 Socket preservation techniques
  - 3.4.1 Bartee's technique
  - 3.4.2 Peñarrocha's technique
  - 3.4.3 Elian's technique
  - 3.4.4 Hernández Alfaro's technique
- 3.5 Conclusions

3.2 Ridge preservation topics

3.2.1 Is there a significant difference between performing ridge preservation and the healing of the socket by clot alone?

Several studies compare post-extraction sockets in which socket preservation was performed with post-extraction sockets without a socket preservation technique.

Several biomaterials were compared with clot healing alone, assessed by clinical parameters in height and width dimensions:

- Mineralized freeze-dried bone allograft (FDBA).[13]
- Aloplastic materials, like bioactive glass (BG) combined with calcium sulfate[14] or polylactide–polyglycolide sponges[11] (Fig 3-4).
- Autologous bone.[12]
- Xenograft (Fig 3-5).[11,15]

The observation period ranged from 4 to 9 months. Most of the studies included sockets with a four-wall configuration. Regarding the clinical outcomes, ridge preservation procedures were effective in limiting horizontal and vertical ridge alterations in post-extraction sites. However, the extraction method was the most important factor to preserve the alveolar bone loss regardless of how the socket was treated after extraction (Table 3-3).[16]

Recommendations

- Alveolar preservation should be performed in areas eligible to receive a delayed implant.
- Socket preservation should be performed in areas supporting a pontic or where an implant could be placed in the future.
- In the esthetic area, bone architecture should be maintained for optimal results.

3.2.2 Which grafting material should be used?

Comparisons of grafting materials have been reported, and present clinical measurements.

There is evidence that ridge preservation maintains significantly more ridge width and height, with most grafting materials being effective, and only slight differences between them. According to the current literature, when a socket preservation technique is performed by covering the alveolus using a membrane barrier, such as ADM or a bioabsorbable collagen wound dressing material, the horizontal and vertical dimensions are better preserved if the membrane is combined with a biomaterial placed inside the socket,[12,19] regardless of the barrier membrane that has been used.[20]

When comparing a xenograft with a synthetic bone substitute or a xenograft with an allograft, it was observed that ridge width and height dimensions were similarly preserved with both graft materials.[21,22]

Hydroxyapatite shows better preservation of vertical bone level than calcium sulfate, and this probably can be explained by the faster resorption of this biomaterial compared with hydroxyapatite (Table 3-4).[23]

Recommendations

Given the low number of publications and the different healing times, it is not possible to conclude that one biomaterial is better than another.

3.2.3 Is bone formed in preserved sockets?

With normal healing, an untreated extraction socket will become filled with vital bone. When a socket is filled with any type of biomaterial, whether a xenograft, allograft, or alloplastic material, the retention of non-vital bone graft particles results.[13,29] The amount and type of bone formed has been the main focus of histologic ridge preservation studies.

Table 3-3 Clinical studies comparing ridge preservation techniques versus healing of the sockets by a blood clot

Authors	Study type	Patients	Number of sockets	Position/ reason for extraction	Test/control	Observation period	Socket wall configuration	Results	Outcome
Camargo et al.[17]	Prospective	16	16/16	2 anterior or premolar teeth/ND	Bioactive glass combined with calcium sulfate/ clot	6 months	ND	Height; test: .38 ± 3.18 mm; control: 1.00 ± 2.25 mm Width; test: 3.48 ± 2.68 mm; control: 3.06 ± 2.41 mm	
Iasella et al.[3]	RCT	24	12/12	Non-molar teeth extractions/ND	Mineralized FDBA and collagen membrane/ clot	4–6 months	4-wall configuration	Width; test: -1.2 ± 0.9 mm; control: -2.6 ± 2.3 mm. Height; test had significantly less loss than control	Most predictable maintenance of ridge width and height by ridge preservation
Serino et al.[18]	CCT	45	26 test, 13 control	Mixed/ND	PL-PG sponge/ clot	6 months	ND	Mid-buccal dimensions; test: +1.3 mm; control: -0.8 mm	Overall less resorption in test group
Nevins et al.[15]	RCT	9	9 test, 17 control	Maxillary anterior teeth/ periodontally compromised teeth	Bio-Oss/clot	1–3 months	4-wall configuration	Height; test: -2.42 ± 2.58 mm; control: -5.24 ± 3.72 mm	The difference between the groups was statistically significant

CCT, controlled clinical trial; ND, not described; PL-PG, polylactide–polyglycolide; RCT, randomized controlled trial

Table 3-4 Clinical studies comparing different grafting materials

Authors	Study type	Patients	Number of sockets	Position/ reason for extraction	Test/control	Observation period	Socket wall configuration	Results	Outcome
Vance et al.[21]	RCT	24	12/12	Nonmolar/ND	Test: CMC/CaS with DFDBA and CaS barrier. Control: Bio-Oss and collagen membrane	4 months	ND	Width: both groups lost 0.5 ± 0.8 mm. Height; vertical midbuccal; test: -0.3 ± 0.7 mm; control: +0.7 ± 1.2 mm	Ridge width and height dimensions were similarly preserved with both graft materials
Neiva et al.[24]	RCT	24	12/12	Maxillary premolar teeth/ND	Test: putty & P15 + bioabsorbable collagen wound dressing. Control: clot + bioabsorbable collagen	4 months	ND	Width; test: -1.31 ± 0.96 mm; control: -1.43 ± 1.05 mm. Height; test: -0.15 ± 1.76 mm; control: -0.56 ± 1.04 mm	Significant differences in height between the groups
Fotek et al.[25]	RCT	20	9 test, 11 control	Maxillary incisor, canine, or premolar/tooth fracture with an endodontic failure	Test: mineralized bone allograft + ADM. Control: mineralized bone allograft + PTFE	4 months	ND	Loss of buccal plate width; test: -0.44 mm; control: 0.30 mm. Height; test: -1.11 mm; control: -0.25 mm	No statistically significant difference was found between the two treatment modalities
Crespi et al.[26]	RCT	15	15 test, 15 test, 15 control	Molar or premolar regions/ ND	Test 1: MHA in granule form + collagen sheet. Test 2: CaS + collagen sheet. Control: unfilled sockets	3 months	Three bone walls and loss of the buccal plate	Height; MHA group: -0.48 ± 0.21 mm; CaS group: -2.48 ± 0.65 mm; control group: -3.75 ± 0.63 mm	The MHA group showed significantly better preservation of vertical bone level than the other two groups
Fernandes et al.[27]	RCT	18	18 test, 18 control	Maxillary anterior teeth/ hopeless teeth	Test: AMB/P-15 + ADM. Control: blood clot + ADM	6 months	ND	External vertical buccal measurement; test: -1.20 ± 2.02 mm; control:-1.50 ± 1.15 mm. Width; test: -2.53 ± 1.81 mm; control: -3.40 ± 1.39 mm	In the horizontal measurement, there was a statistical difference between the groups
Mardas et al.[28]	RCT	26	ND	Mandibular or maxillary incisor, canine or premolar/ hopeless teeth	Test: SBC. Control: DBBM. In both groups collagen barrier	8 months	In case a bony wall was severely damaged or completely lost, the patient was excluded	Width; test: -1.1 ± 1 mm; control: -2.1 ± 1 mm	Both materials preserved the mesiodistal bone height of the ridge

ADM, acellular dermal matrix; AMB/P-15, anorganic bovine bone matrix with a synthetic cell-binding peptide P-15; CCT, controlled clinical trial; CaS, calcium sulfate; CMC/CaS, carboxymethyl cellulose and calcium sulfate; DBBM, deproteinized bone bovine mineral; DFDBA, demineralized freeze-dried bone allograft; MHA, magnesium-enriched hydroxyapatite; ND, not described; RCT, randomized controlled trial; SBC, Straumann® bone ceramic.

The amount of bone formed depends on the time point when the socket content is examined during the healing process.[11]

Bone histomorphometry is the mean by which bone remodeling, modeling, and structure may be quantitatively assessed. It provides information that is not currently available from other approaches, such as bone densitometry and biochemical markers of bone turnover.

Bone histomorphometry is the only procedure that allows the assessment of:

- Bone turnover.
- Static and dynamic tissue and cell activities of modeling and remodeling.
- Bone quality (microarchitecture, texture of bone matrix – lamellar or woven bone, microdamage, and presence of mineralization defects).
- Mechanisms underlying bone mass changes at the tissue and cellular levels.

There is a lack of homogeneity in the published studies regarding the healing time of preserved sockets. The different healing times make it difficult to obtain comparable results between studies, so there is no clear evidence that one material is superior to another in terms of new bone formation. Healing times vary from 3 to 12 months. The degree of bone maturation is intimately linked to this time.

The biomaterial healing times may also vary. For example, for sockets preserved with polylactide–polyglycolide sponges it is necessary to wait only 3 months, while studies with deproteinized bovine bone mineral (DBBM) or demineralized freeze-dried bone allograft (DFDBA) showed a healing time of at least 6 to 9 months.[14,21,30,31]

Regarding the amount of newly formed bone in preserved sockets, no biomaterial appears to be superior. All the biomaterials have biocompatible properties. Biomaterials such as carboxymethyl cellulose and calcium sulfate may favor more rapid vascular and cellular ingrowth, which would facilitate vital bone formation and resorption of DFDBA particles.[9]

BG-treated sockets demonstrate more vital bone than DFDBA-treated or untreated sockets. This finding may be attributed to the osteoconductive nature of the BG particles. BG particles contain a calcium phosphate layer, which is similar to the mineral phase of bone and is responsible for the osteoconductive properties.[32] DBBM is the most common grafting material and has been shown to be a biocompatible bone filler with good osteoconductive properties (Table 3-5).[14,38]

The residual graft particles have been distinguished in different histomorphometric studies regardless of the material used, with the exception of those alveoli preserved with sponges and calcium sulfate.

In summary, ridge preservation procedures are accompanied by varying degrees of new bone formation and residual graft materials in the extraction socket. The use of grafting material allows new bone formation in extraction sockets. However, the use of different grafting materials and their different healing periods make comparisons difficult. The long-term effect of residual grafting material on implant survival and success has not been reported. The material chosen may reflect operator preference, the length of time before the implant is to be placed, and commercial availability.[13]

Recommendations

- There is mixed evidence that one grafting material is better than another or better than the clot alone in terms of the amount of newly formed bone.
- The clinician may choose the biomaterial depending on his/her preference.

3.2.4 Does the type, position, or reason for extraction of the tooth affect ridge preservation?

It is not known whether tooth type or position in the oral cavity has any effect on ridge preservation. The majority of studies investigated anterior maxillary single-rooted teeth, probably because in the esthetic zone bone architecture is mandatory for a good treatment result.

In the posterior regions, resorption following tooth extraction occurs in the same way as in the anterior regions. However, the vestibular wall is thicker so implant placement is easier compared with in the anterior regions. This does not mean alveolar preservation is not indicated or not important in posterior regions.

It should also be taken into account that maxillary sites demonstrated a greater loss of ridge width than mandibular sites and most ridge resorption occurred on the buccal aspects of the ridge.[13]

Table 3-5 Clinical studies showing degrees of new bone formation and residual graft materials in the extraction sockets

Author	Study type	Patients	Number of sockets	Position/reason for extraction	Test/control	Healing time	Socket wall configuration	Results	Outcome
Artzi et al.[12]	CCT	15	15	Maxilla, single-root teeth/ND	DBBM	9 months	3–4 walls	VB: 46.3%; CT: 22.9%; DBBM: 30.8%	The resorbability of DBBM is not recognized at 9 months
Artzi et al.[19]	CCT	15	15	Maxilla, single-root teeth/ND	DBBM	9 months	3–4 walls	VB respective socket depth; coronal:17.1%; mid: 48.3%; apical: 63.9%	DBBM is a biocompatible filler. Graft particles were not resorbed at 9 months
Froum et al.[33]	CCT	19	30	All teeth. Periodontal or prosthetic reason	BG/DFDBA/ blood clot	6–8 months	4 walls	BG: VB 22–88%; CT 35.3%; RG 5.5% DFDBA: VB 23–48.1%; CT 51.6%; RG 13.5% Control: VB 17–53.1%; CT 67%	BG sockets had more VB than DFDBA and control ones. VB was not statistically significant among the 3 groups
Serino et al.[18]	CCT	45	26 test, 20 control	All teeth/ND	PL-PG sponge/ blood clot	6 months	ND	PL-PG: VB 67%; control: VB 56%	At 6 months new bone was mineralized. No presence of graft particles
Carmagnola et al.[34]	CCT	21	31	All teeth. Periodontal or endodontic reason, or root fracture	G1: DBBM + collagen membrane. G2: collagen membrane. G3: blood clot.	G1: 7 months G2: 4 months G3: 1-15 years	ND	G1: LB 26 ± 23.7%; WB 8.4 ± 8%; BM 26.2 ± 15.9%; CT 18.1 ± 17%; RG 21.1 ± 20% G2: LB 40.1 ± 15.9%; WB 12.9 ± 15.7%; MB 46 ± 16.7% G3: LB 56.1 ± 18.1%; WB 0.5 ± 1%; BM 43 ± 18%	G1 were comprised of connective tissue and small amounts of newly formed bone surrounding the graft particles
Iasella et al.[13]	RCT	24	12 test, 12 control	Non-molar teeth extraction/ND	Mineralized FDBA + collagen membrane/ blood clot	4-6 months	4 walls		
Vance et al.[21]	RCT	24	12 G1, 12 G2	Non-molar tooth extraction/ND	G1: DFDBA + putty + CaS. G2: DBBM + collagen membrane.	4 months	ND	G1; VB: 61 ± 9% G2; VB: 26 ± 20%	More vital bone in G1
Guarnieri et al.[35]	CCT	10	10 test, 5 control	Maxilla and mandible non-molar teeth/ND	CaS	3 months	ND	Test group: VB 58%; CT not found and RG not found	Calcium sulfate it is almost completely resorbable and allows bone formation at 3 months

Serino et al.[16]	CCT	20	7 test, 9 control, 4 dropouts	Monoradicular teeth. Periodontal reason	Test: PL-PG acid sponge. Control: blood clot	3 months	At least 8 mm of alveolar bone height	Test group: VB 59.9%; CT ND; RG not found Control group: VB 48.8%; CT ND	PL-PG acid did not interfere with bone formation and it is a suitable material
Neiva et al.[24]	RCT	24	12 test, 12 control	Maxillary premolars/ ND	Test: HA + peptide 15 and a collagen dressing Control: collagen dressing	4 months	<80% of bone loss	Test group: VB 29.9 ± 8.46%; CT 65.2 ± 6.4%; RG 6.25% Control group: VB 36.5 ± 7.7%; CT 62.6 ± 7.41%	A favorable response was observed when putty P15 was applied to extraction sockets
Hoffmann et al.[36]	Retrospective	276	276. Only 0 biopsies analyzed	All teeth/periodontal reason	dPTFE membrane	12 months	Buccal and lingual plate present	A significant newly formed tissue was mainly bone	
Molly et al.[22]	CCT	8	36	All teeth/periodontal reason	G1: DBBM + ePTFE. G2: PL-PG sponge + ePTFE. G3: Calcium carbonate ceramic + ePTFE. Control: covered PTFE	6 months	ND	G1: VB 20.7 ± 15.8%; RG 20.2 ± 17% G2: VB 27.9 ± 20.6%; RG 5.6 ± 8.9% G3: VB 24 ± 22%; RG 12 ± 16.4% Control: 29.4 ± 17.1%	A relatively high amount of DBBM and calcium carbonate remained after 6 months
Mangano et al.[23]	CC	1	3 test	Mandibular canine and premolars/periodontal reason	HA	20 years	ND	VB: 25.4 ± 3.2%; RG: 38.1 ± 4.1%; Marrow spaces: 41.3 ± 5.2%	Intimate binding between bone and HA particles was present and were surrounded closely by bone
Heberer et al.[20]	CCT	16	18 test	12 maxillary molars; 2 mandibular molars; 2 premolars; 1 anterior maxilla/endodontic reason	DBBM with collagen	6 weeks	4 walls	VB: 28%; CT:54%; RG: 11%	Sockets presenting bone formation rates similar to those found after a 3-month healing period
Beck et al.[37]	CCT	33	38 test	Single-root teeth/ fracture, endodontic reason and no restorable caries	DFDBA	Group 1: early healing 14 weeks Group 2: delayed healing 27 weeks	10 mm bony support	G1: VB 45.8%; CT 39.6%; RG 14.6% G2: VB 45%; CT 41.3%; RG 13.5%	Waiting 6 months after using DFDBA does not provide a greater amount of new bone formation or less residual bone particles compared to that after only 3 months

BM, bone marrow; CaS, calcium sulfate; CC, clinical case; CCT, controlled clinical trial; CT, connective tissue; dPTFE, dense polytetrafluoroethylene, G1, group 1; HA, hydroxyapatite; LB, lamellar bone; ND, not described; PL-PG, polylactide–polyglycolide; RCT, randomized controlled trial; RG, remaining graft; VB, vital bone; WB, woven bone.

Recommendations

- Perform alveolar preservation in the anterior teeth after tooth loss, regardless of subsequent treatment to follow.
- Always perform alveolar preservation in multiple extractions.
- Rate socket preservation in posterior regions.

3.2.5 Does ridge preservation affect the success rate of implants?

The requirements for successful osseointegration of dental implants are a sufficient quantity and quality of osseous tissue to ensure the stabilization of the implant, and to allow bone-to-implant contact of the entire surface intended for osseointegration (as reported by Albrektsson and Linder[38] and Adell[39]).

Tissue integrated prostheses in clinical dentistry were statistically analysed after observation times of 5 to 12 years by Adell in 1985.[39] The masticatory function of the patients was restored to the same level as that of patients with natural dentitions of corresponding extent. Psychosocially the patients were almost entirely relieved of their previous severe handicaps related to edentulousness. In all mandibles and in 90% of maxillae the bridges were continuously stable. The marginal soft tissue reactions were mild and the marginal bone loss less than 1.0 mm during the first year and then only 0.05 to 0.07 mm annually. After the first year, hardly any implants were lost and almost no marginal bone. The implant survival rates were 84% and 93% for those in maxillae and mandibles respectively. These results allow a very predictable prognosis to be given for tissue integrated prostheses.

The criteria for successful implants described by Albrektsson et al.[40] reported the following: absence of mobility, pain, peri-implant infection or suppuration, as well as radiographic peri-implant bone loss of <1 mm during the first year, followed by 0.2 mm for each successive year. The criterion for implant survival was that the implants remained in function at the time of evaluation, not necessarily meeting all the success criteria.

There is a lack of long-term information on the longevity of preserved ridges and the survival/success of implants placed. There is almost no information on which technique or material provides a more stable long-term result.[11]

Success rates are also satisfactory when placing implants in previously grafted bone. In a retrospective study of 607 titanium plasma-sprayed implants placed in regenerated bone (with DFDBA), 97.2% of maxillary implants and 97.4% of mandibular implants were successful for an average of 11 years.[41] Even higher success rates in augmented bone have been reported by Simion et al.[42] These numbers are similar to the success rates for implants placed in mature bone.

The waiting time for the placement of implants after alveolar preservation does not seem to affect implant success. A study where the healing time ranged from 3 to 11 months produced similar results in terms of implant survival. It has been shown that earlier placement of implants into preserved sockets does not negatively impact upon the clinical outcome with respect to implant success.[29]

Regarding implants placed in native bone, no differences in the long-term survival rate are observed between those implants placed in preserved sockets. Implants placed at post-extraction sockets augmented with any kind of biomaterial exhibited minimal marginal bone loss, similar to implants placed in native bone (Table 3-6).[14,30]

Recommendations

Implants placed in preserved ridges have survival and predictability similar to implants placed in native bone. Therefore alveolar preservation does not affect the success rate of implants.

3.3 Socket preservation materials

3.3.1 What are the available bone substitutes?

In order to prevent bone resorption after tooth extraction, numerous animal and clinical studies validate the concept of ridge preservation by the placement of biomaterials into fresh extraction sockets. Several studies have proposed various ridge preservation techniques including the placement of graft materials and/or the use of occlusive membranes, with success rates of implants placed in regenerated bone comparable to the success rates of implants placed in native bone. There are three primary goals of ridge preservation:

- Modulation of early-stage ridge resorption.
- Increased bone density.
- Facilitation of future dental implant surgery.

Autologous grafts have long been considered to be the gold standard material for bone-grafting procedures. However, the need for a donor site can increase pain and morbidity. Hence, bone substitutes have gained increasing acceptance as an alternative to autologous bone for patients requiring bone augmentation, in an effort to decrease the morbidity associated with autologous graft harvesting. Allografts, xenografts, and alloplasts come in many forms (Table 3-7), and data support their safety, clinical applicability, and low antigenicity.[9]

Generally, materials available for placement into extraction sites can be considered either non-resorbable or resorbable. In fact, even the non-resorbable materials undergo some physiochemical dissolution. The most important feature of these materials is that they allow placement of endosseous implants into the grafted site, even in the presence of some unresorbed particles. Another group of materials may be considered short-term resorbable materials because they are readily resorbed and replaced by host tissue over the typical healing period. Similar in use to the transitional materials, they may increase bone density, prevent early ridge resorption, and facilitate the placement of dental implants. Due to the more rapid turnover of these materials, they should be selected when implant placement will be performed within 3 to 6 months, before significant ridge resorption takes place.[4]

Table 3-6 Clinical studies showing survival rate of implants placed in preserved sockets an in native bone

Author	Study type	Patients	Number of sockets	Position/ reason for extraction	Test/control	Healing time	Socket wall configuration	Results	Outcome
Norton and Wilson[29]	CCT	17	40 and 40 implants	ND, periodontal/ endodontal reason, or trauma	Bioactive glass	3 to 11 months	4 walls	SR: 88.6%. 2 drop-outs (96.8%) BL at 36 months: M 0.5 mm; D 0.4 mm	Implants will survive for up to 3 years in sockets grafted with bioactive glass, even when such grafts appear to only slowly conduct new bone growth
Molly et al.[22]	CCT	8	36	All teeth/periodontal reason	Group 1: DBBM + ePTFE. Group 2: PL-PG sponge + ePTFE. Group 3: Calcium carbonate ceramic + ePTFE. Control: covered PTFE	6 months	ND	A good primary stability was found at the moment of implant insertion and also at abutment connection	Prognosis of early implant osseointegration was not influenced by the insertion of the bone biomaterials
Crespi et al.[26]	CCT	15	Test 45, 15 sockets in each group	All teeth/ND	Group 1: Calcium sulfate. Group2: DBBM. Group3: HA	3 months	3 walls	At 24 months 100% survival rate	Implant survival of such treatment modality was not negatively influenced by grafting materials of different composition
Koutouzis and Lundgren[30]	Retrospective	60	Test 30, control 30	All teeth/ND	Test: DFDBA. Control: native bone	4 months	ND	At 12 months survival rate was 100% for both groups. Mean marginal bone loss: 0.15 mm at 12 months for both	Implants placed at post-extraction sockets augmented with DFDBA exhibited minimal marginal bone loss and is similar to implants placed in native bone

BL, bone loss; CCT, controlled clinical trial; D, distal; HA, hydroxyapatite; M, mesial; PL-PG, polylactide–polyglycolide; SR, success rate

Table 3-7 Sources of grafting material for guided bone regeneration

Graft material	Definition	Examples
Autogenous graft	Material that is transferred from one position to another within the same individual	Graft may be intraoral or extraoral depending on the harvesting site
Allograft	Material that is transferred from a donor of the same species	The most common graft is freeze-dried bone graft, which may be mineralized or demineralized (FDBA or DFDBA) and free frozen bone (FFB)
Xenograft	Material that is transferred from a donor of another species, processed appropriately	Bovine hydroxyapatite, porcine hydroxyapatite, coralline hydroxyapatite, and equine hydroxyapatite
Alloplastic material	Synthetic material, usually inert, used as a substitute for bone grafts	Bioactive glass, beta-tricalcium phosphate, hydroxyapatite, collagen hydroxyapatite, and calcium sulfate

The characteristics of various bone substitutes are described in Chapter 8.

Synthetic resorbable materials, also known as alloplastic biomaterials, are available in several forms. Among them are microporous resorbable hydroxyapatite (HA), microcrystalline, nonceramic resorbable HA and beta-tricalcium phosphate (β-TCP). While they are chemically similar to bone, they differ from anorganic bovine bone in crystalline structure, carbonate content, and porosity. The use of any of these materials alone will require from 4 to 12 months for significant graft turnover and bone formation to occur. In large defects, even longer periods may be required for mature bone formation. Due to the eventual resorption and replacement of these materials by host bone, the duration of ridge preservation cannot be accurately predicted. A reasonable time frame for most sites, in the author's experience, would be from 3 to 5 years. After that time, physiologic bone remodeling may ultimately cause the grafted ridge to assume its natural state.

In some situations when dental implant placement is going to occur after 3 to 6 months post-extraction, the use of rapid turnover biomaterials is indicated. Typically, DFDBA or autogenous bone is combined with a low-density HA, TCP, or anorganic bone matrix (ABM) product in a 50:50 or 75:25 ratio. The function of this composite graft is to provide a synergistic scaffold for new bone formation. The DFDBA or autogenous bone used alone has not been shown to significantly increase bone density in extraction sites probably due to its rapid turnover time. Autologous grafts are considered to be the ideal material for bone grafting procedures because their osteogenic, osteoinductive, and osteoconductive properties. Transplantation of living cells increases the possibility of retained cell viability and graft revascularization. In addition, autologous grafts do not present a risk of disease transmission because donor and recipient are the same individual. However, they do increase the risk of additional pain, infection, and donor site morbidity because an additional surgical procedure is necessary for harvesting.[9]

3.3.2 Should a membrane be placed after an extraction?

Historically, achieving primary closure and prevention of graft particle loss and infection has been a major problem associated with primary (immediate) grafting of extraction sockets. Clinicians are often confronted with grafting a socket in which primary closure cannot be obtained. Placement of a barrier material can accomplish two clinical goals for the clinician. The first is that it allows primary surgical closure over the socket and graft material while remaining intact as a guided bone regenerative barrier for at least 4 months. The second is that it increases the amount of bound-down keratinized connective tissue at that site.

The concept of using synthetic membranes in the socket preservation technique has gained wide acceptance. The use of an occlusive membrane eliminates the problem of particle migration while simultaneously preventing soft tissue and epithelial migration into the healing socket.

Despite the reported benefits of using a membrane there has not been a membrane material designed for extraction site grafting. Non-resorbable membranes such as e-PTFE (Fig 3-6) have a common complication, the exposure of the membrane and subsequent graft infection. It seems that they are not suitable for post-extraction

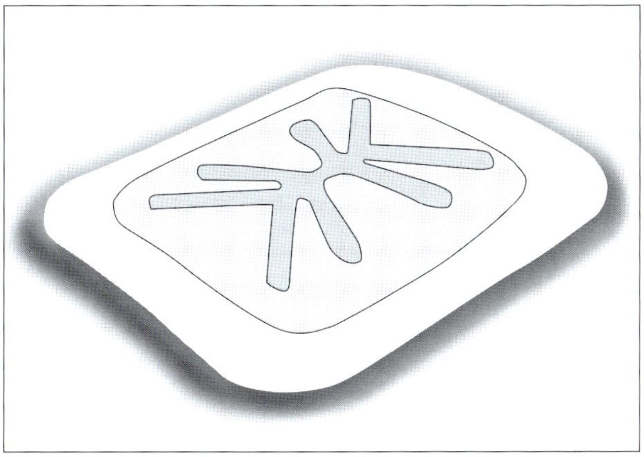

Fig 3-6 PTFE membrane.

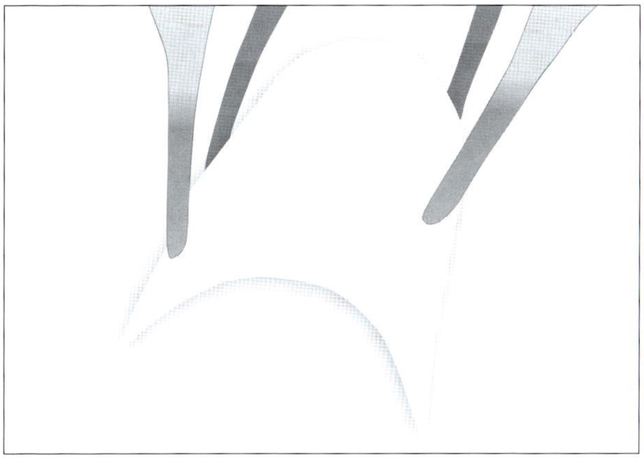

Fig 3-7 Collagen membrane.

sites. Despite these complications, it has been suggested that, in some cases, it may be esthetically advantageous to intentionally leave membranes exposed in order to preserve the architecture of the keratinized mucosa.

Another type of membrane is resorbable membranes, that may be effective for extraction site reconstruction, but primary closure is required to prevent premature membrane dissolution. Collagen membranes may be preferable because of their physiological absorption process and high biocompatibility with oral tissues (Fig 3-7). In addition, collagen is a hemostatic agent and possesses the ability to stimulate platelet aggregation and to enhance fibrin linkage, which may lead to initial clot formation, stability, and maturation. Furthermore, collagen has been demonstrated to be chemotactic for fibroblasts *in vitro*.[43] This property could enhance cell migration and promote primary wound coverage, which is fundamental for bone growth (Fig 3-7 collagen membrane).[9]

The acellular dermal matrix graft (ADMG) has been used in periodontal plastic surgery for increasing the amount of keratinized tissue. The ADMG is obtained from tissue donor banks, and is processed in order to remove all cells that are the components necessary for survival and transmission of viruses. The ADMG is able to act as a bioactive scaffold for migration of fibroblasts, epithelial cells, and endothelial cells (Fig 3-8).[32]

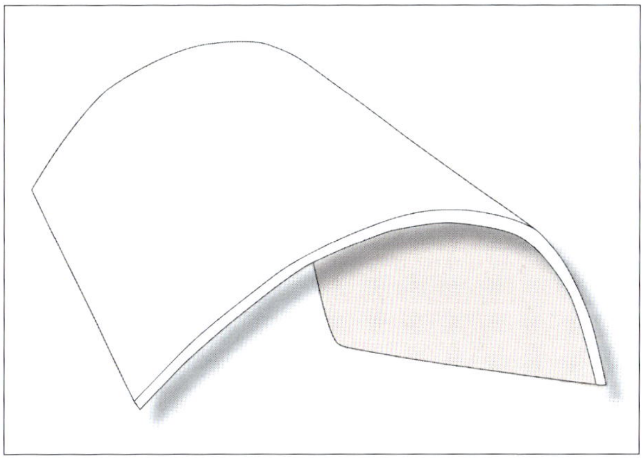

Fig 3-8 Acellular dermal matrix.

3.3.3 Is it necessary to achieve primary wound closure to cover the membranes and biomaterials?

The majority of the published studies report primary closure. Primary closure can be achieved either by a coronally advanced flap covering the graft, the socket alone or the membrane, or by a pedicled palatal flap.[11] However, in some publications, flaps were replaced without obtaining complete socket coverage (Fig 3-9).

Achieving partial closure of the wound but covering the exposed socket/graft with a collagen membrane has also been documented. With the aim of reducing bacterial colonization, all patients were instructed to use chlorhexidine 0.12% twice daily until soft tissue closure.[13] On the other hand, if a non-resorbable membrane like e-PTFE is used it is mandatory to get primary wound closure. If exposed they present more problems than collagen membranes, as they become highly contaminated. Exposure of membranes may lead to compromised results.[11] Not all studies mention exposure rates, but the average is around 25%.[21]

Titanium membranes are not as flexible as other membranes, and this could favor their increased exposure.

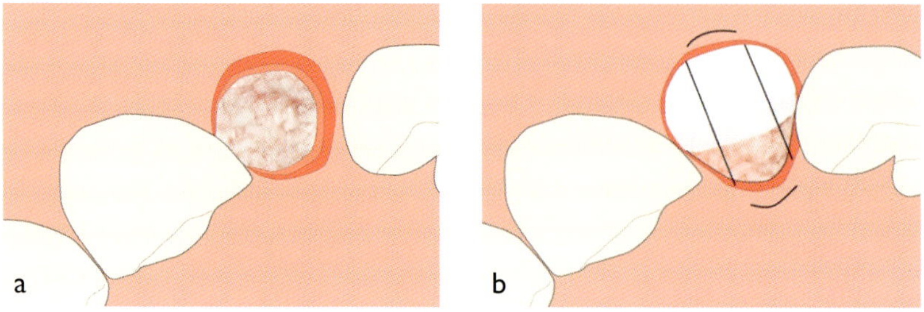

Fig 3-9a and b Socket preservation with biomaterial without (a) and with (b) coverage with a resorbable membrane.

Another factor that could contribute to the exposure is the suturing technique used to get a free tension flap.[44]

An alveolar reconstruction site can be covered using a number of techniques, including different types of membranes, autogenous tissue grafts, or with a vestibular advancement flap, although the latter can compromise the mucogingival architecture. Pedicled flaps generally have a better prognosis than free grafts. They are autogenous, easy to tailor, vascularized, and have the capacity to generate keratinized mucosa at the crest, thus maintaining the mucogingival border in the proper place. The palatal connective tissue flap compares favorably with membranes and free grafts.[45]

Recommendations

- Given the diversity of soft tissue closure and concomitant procedures, an assessment of whether primary wound closure is necessary for successful outcome is difficult. It would appear that ridge preservation can be successful irrespective of closure technique.
- When using a non-resorbable membrane, it is necessary to obtain primary wound closure for predictable results.

3.3.4 Complications encountered while dealing with biomaterials in socket preservation

The most common complication when a socket preservation technique is performed is membrane exposure. Depending on its size it can be related to the partial/total loss or infection of the bone graft. The exposure rate can range from 25% to 45%.[31,44] Postoperative membrane exposure may occur due to the presence of tension in the flaps when suturing or the use of provisional dentures that impinged on the regenerated areas during the primary stages of healing.

Membrane exposure may be detrimental to bone regeneration because blood supply is affected, the healing of the graft is compromised and the socket is prone to possible bacterial infection.[42] Collagen membranes also may be exposed, showing an exposure rate of 31%, but the complication is much easier to control than in a non-resorbable membrane.[11]

In the event that the membrane is exposed in the first 6 to 8 weeks of healing, the site can be rinsed out daily with 12% chlorhexidine. If it exposes 8 weeks later, a partial thickness flap should be made adjacent to the augmented site and the barrier should be removed, then the flap margins should be resutured. Attention should be paid not to disturb the granulation tissue beneath the membrane.[46]

The use of barrier membranes in socket augmentation procedures has been shown to have clinical effectiveness in preserving alveolar ridges after tooth extraction. Results show that membrane-covered sites present with significantly less ridge atrophy than control sites.[47] Some minor complications or difficulties associated with barrier membrane use during socket augmentation procedures include the potential reduction of keratinized gingiva, alterations of gingival contours, and migration of the mucogingival junction, as a result of coronal displacement of the flap to achieve soft tissue closure over the membrane.

Recommendations

- If a non-resorbable membrane is used, it is important to obtain a tension-free flap to ensure primary wound closure for avoiding exposure complications.
- If a resorbable membrane is used it better to close the wound, but if this is not possible socket preservation can be successful.
- The use of chlorhexidine 0.12% is recommended in small doses to control contamination of the membrane and promote soft tissue closure.

3.4 Socket preservation techniques

In a review by Darby et al.[11] in which the aim was to evaluate the techniques and outcomes of post-extraction socket preservation and the efficacy of these procedures in relation to subsequence implant placement, nine different methods for socket preservation were identified. The techniques range from simply placing the graft in the extraction socket to raising and replacing a flap in the original position, with or without a membrane exposed to the oral cavity.

The most commonly used method was a graft that was placed in the extraction socket, covered by a membrane, and followed by flap advancement to achieve complete or partial primary closure. The second most commonly employed technique was covering a graft by coronal advancement or rotation of the flap, but without a membrane. The third most common surgical technique was the placement of membrane alone over the extraction socket, with full or partial cover by the soft tissue. Other methods investigated included placement of the graft alone, covering the graft socket with a membrane alone, ridge preservation solely by coverage with a membrane, placing a graft and covering with a collagen bone dressing, placing a sponge in the socket without any coverage, and placing a sponge with soft tissue coverage.[11]

In socket preservation procedures, the first rule is to perform atraumatic extraction of teeth with maximal preservation of the buccal and lingual cortical plate. This may be accomplished through careful luxation and judicious use of burs to section ankylosed or curved roots. Following root removal, sharp curettage should be carried out to remove remnants of periodontal ligament as well as any soft tissues such as periradicular cysts. These tissues may harbor pathogenic bacteria that can lead to postoperative complications. Active infection is the only absolute contraindication. The presence of purulent drainage, swelling, or pain indicates active infection, which may cause graft failure. If infection is suspected, preoperative antibiotics should be given and continued for 7 to 14 days. If symptoms resolve, the site may be considered safe for extraction and grafting.[48] Moreover, excessive tension on the flaps with sutures should be avoided to maximize blood flow within the flap and avoid necrosis of the flap margins.

Some of these techniques are described step by step in the following sections.

3.4.1 Bartee's technique

Barry K Bartee described a socket preservation technique using a dense polytetrafluoroethylene (dPTFE) membrane as a barrier to contain the graft particles and to facilitate bone regeneration in extraction sites (Fig 3-10).[48]

Following tooth removal, sharp curettage should be carried out to remove remnants of periodontal ligament as well as any soft tissue.

Perforation of the socket cortical plate (decortication) is optional but may be helpful in establishing blood supply to the graft from the adjacent bone. This may be accomplished with a slow-speed round bur. Caution is advised to avoid damage to vital structures such as adjacent tooth roots or neurovascular structures.

After tooth extraction the graft material is moistened with sterile saline in a sterile dish to form a cohesive paste that can be delivered to the extraction site. Using a periosteal elevator or syringe technique, the material is delivered to the extraction site and packed gently to the apex of the site. Over-packing must be avoided because this only hinders revascularization of the site. A section of membrane material is then cut to fit over the site(s), extending 3 to 4 mm beyond the socket margins onto host bone. The membrane should be trimmed to maintain a 1.0-mm margin from adjacent tooth roots to facilitate reattachment of the papilla to the interdental bone. A paper or foil template may be used to avoid wasting membrane material during trimming. If needed, the membrane may be stretched slightly and molded over the fingertips to form a convex dome over the alveolar ridge. The membrane should fit over the site(s) and under the mucoperiosteal flap without wrinkling or buckling. If necessary, the membrane should be further trimmed or the subperiosteal dissection of the flap should be extended to achieve a passive and stable fit of the membrane directly over the bone. Do not overlap two or more pieces of membrane at any time.

Finally, suturing is accomplished with interrupted sutures at the interdental papillae and a single or horizontal mattress suture across the socket opening. Primary closure is not required for extraction-site grafting and will only make membrane removal more difficult; so this membrane is left partially exposed in the oral cavity. The recommended suture material is 3-0 polyglycolide or PTFE monofilament.

Fig 3-10a to f Bartee's socket preservation technique.

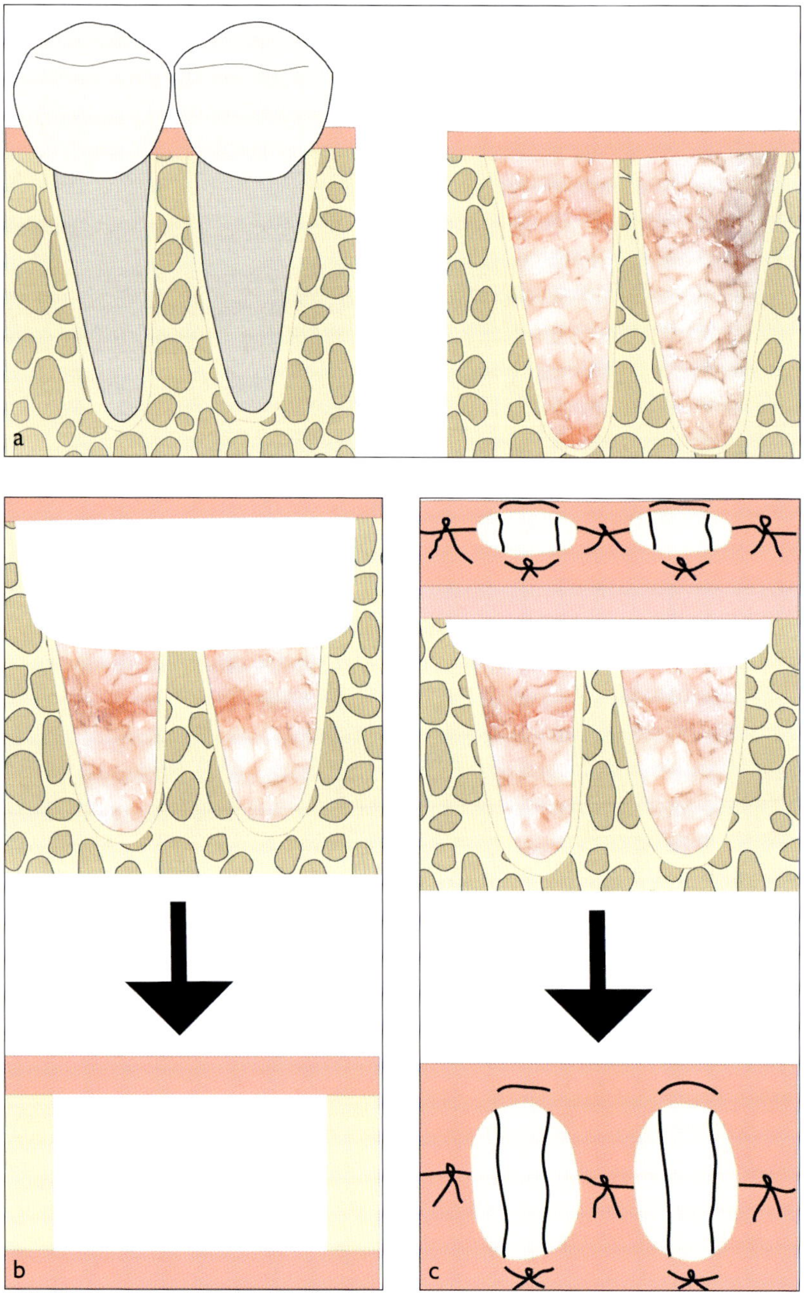

Fig 3-10a After tooth extraction the graft material is delivered to the extraction site and packed gently to the apex of the site.

Fig 3-10b The dPTFE membrane should fit over the site and under the mucoperiosteal flap without wrinkling or buckling.

Fig 3-10c Suturing is accomplished with interrupted sutures. Primary closure is not required.

Thorough irrigation of the site is performed to remove all remaining graft particles, especially those between the flap edges or between the flap and the underlying membrane. These particles would provide a conduit for oral bacteria to infiltrate the graft. Temporary bridges or dentures may be placed immediately over the graft–membrane complex. Postoperatively, the patient should be observed at 1 week. The patient should be instructed to gently clean around the site with a cotton swab or cotton gauze to prevent plaque accumulation on the membrane. At 2 weeks, sutures should be removed and the membrane cleaned if there is significant bacterial accumulation (Fig 3-10).

Membrane removal is performed at 3 or 4 weeks postoperatively, depending on the size of the defect and the condition of the socket walls. Defects that are large or have one or more walls missing may benefit from

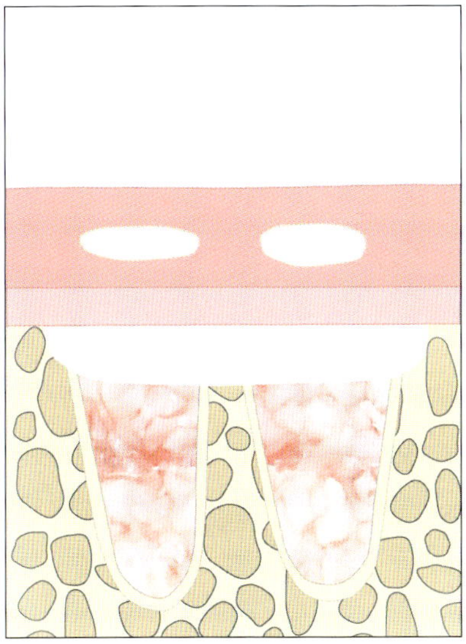

Fig 3-10d At 2 weeks, sutures should be removed and the membrane should be cleaned if there is significant bacterial accumulation.

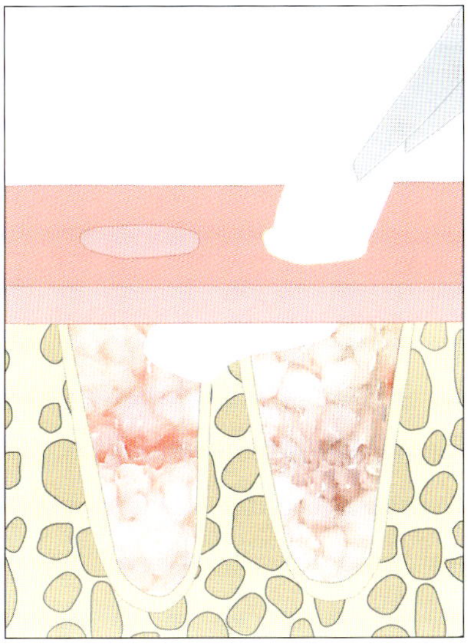

Fig 3-10e Membrane removal is performed at 3 or 4 weeks postoperatively. Removal is accomplished by grasping the membrane with forceps and gently removing it from the tissue bed.

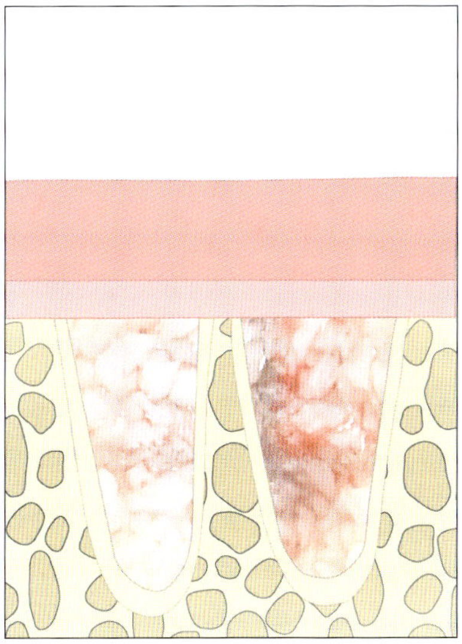

Fig 3-10f Re-epithelialization of the underlying tissue will occur over the next 7 to 10 days.

the longer healing period. Removal is accomplished by grasping the membrane with forceps and gently removing it from the tissue bed. No infiltrative anesthesia is required for this procedure; however, topical anesthetic may be used. In the context of extraction site grafting, is it not necessary to leave the membrane in place for longer than 4 weeks. Upon removal, the graft material can usually be visualized, well consolidated in the osteoid matrix underlying the membrane. Re-epithelialization of the underlying tissue will occur over the next 7 to 10 days. Depending on the graft material placed, 12 to 16 weeks is required for mineralization of the socket to occur. Large defects or those with missing walls may require up to 6 months for maturation.

3.4.2 Peñarrocha's technique

Peñarrocha et al.[49] describe a socket preservation technique of the anterior maxillary process using a trephine core and covering it with soft tissue rotated palatal flap (Fig 3-11).

The surgery is performed under local anesthesia, using a trapezoidal full-thickness flap with vertical incisions. Teeth are extracted atraumatically and curettage is subsequently performed (Fig 3-11a). A bone core is grafted from the neighboring buccal vestibular region (canine in the case report) using a 6-mm trephine bur under abundant sterile saline irrigation (Fig 3-11b). The bone cores are stabilized by tapping them against the sockets (Fig 3-11c). Since primary soft tissue sealing is not possible, rotated soft palatal flaps are raised.

The vestibular bone cavities must be filled with collagen sponges, while surgical cement is applied to the palatal zone. Suturing is performed with 3/0 silk (Fig 3-11d), and amoxicillin (500 mg 3 times a day for 7 days) is prescribed, along with 0.12% chlorhexidine mouthwash. Special care should be taken to prevent the provisional prosthesis, which is placed over the central incisors, from applying pressure to the surgical gingival site.

3.4.3 Elian's technique

A new socket preservation technique was presented by Elian et al.[7] in 2007. The socket repair technique proposed is for type II sockets, where a significant amount of the buccal plate is missing following extraction (Fig 3-12a).

Once the tooth is diagnosed as hopeless, it is removed atraumatically, utilizing flapless extraction with care not to disturb the interproximal papillae and labial soft tissue (Fig 3-12b). The socket is then debrided with surgical curettes, and any infected tissue is removed. A finger should be placed over the buccal tissue when curetting the buccal part of the socket to prevent perforation of the soft tissue.

Fig 3-11a to e Peñarrocha's technique. Trapezoidal full-thickness flap with vertical incisions is raised.

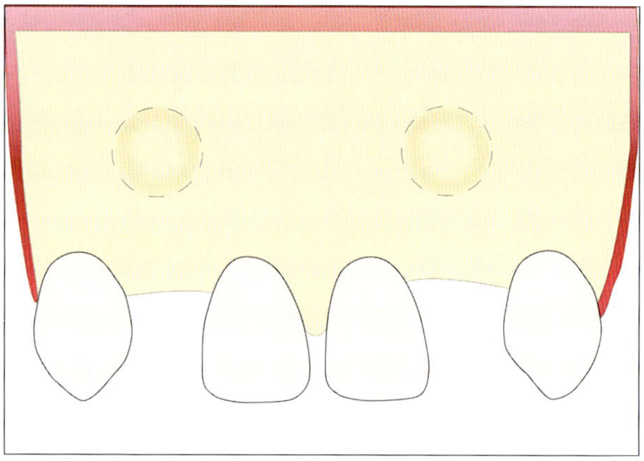

Fig 3-11a Teeth are extracted. A trephine bur is used to mark the vestibular bone core.

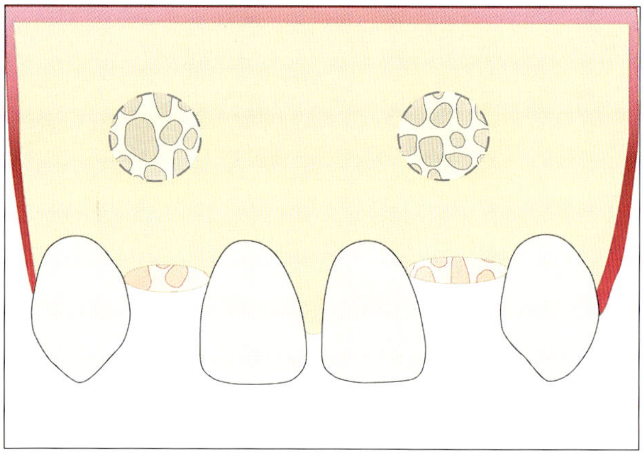

Fig 3-11b A bone core is grafted from the neighboring buccal vestibular regions.

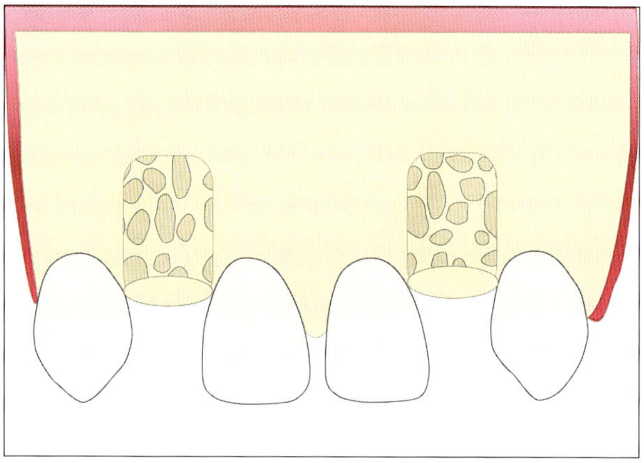

Fig 3-11c The bone cores are placed into the socket.

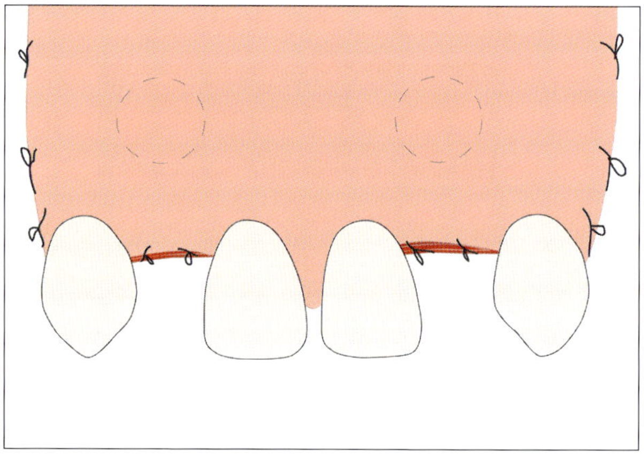

Fig 3-11d The vestibular flap is sutured with 3/0 silk to the palatal side.

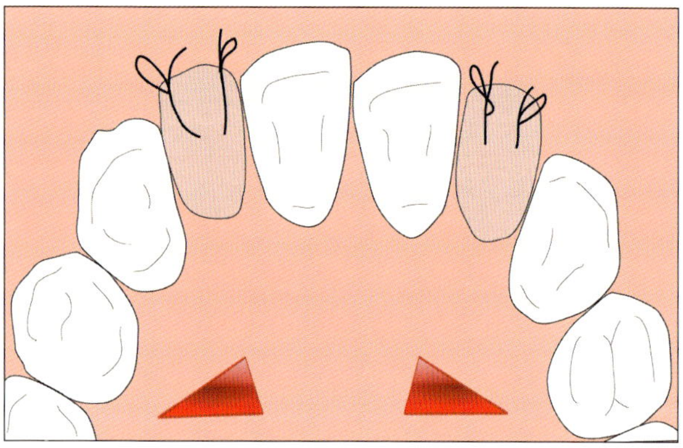

Fig 3-11e Rotated pedicle flaps with interposition of connective tissue harvested from the palate is used in order to achieve and maintain passive primary closure over the grafted area.

A collagen membrane is contoured into a modified V-shape (Fig 3-12c). The membrane should be strong so that it can be sutured and maintain a long absorption time to allow for guided bone regeneration. The membrane must also be firm enough to allow insertion into the socket without collapsing. The barrier used in this technique is an absorbable collagen membrane. The narrow part of the trimmed membrane is placed into the socket and should be wide enough to extend laterally past the defect in the buccal wall. Placing the membrane on the external aspect of the buccal wall could compromise its blood supply and cause an increased chance of resorption. The wider part of the membrane should be trimmed and be able to cover the opening of the socket following graft placement.

Following final shaping, the membrane is positioned into the socket lining the buccal tissues. The socket is then filled with a bone graft; pressure from the graft against the membrane will help keep it in place and push out the contour of the buccal tissue (Fig 3-12c). Ideally, the graft material should be compressed into the socket

Fig 3-12a to d Elian's technique.

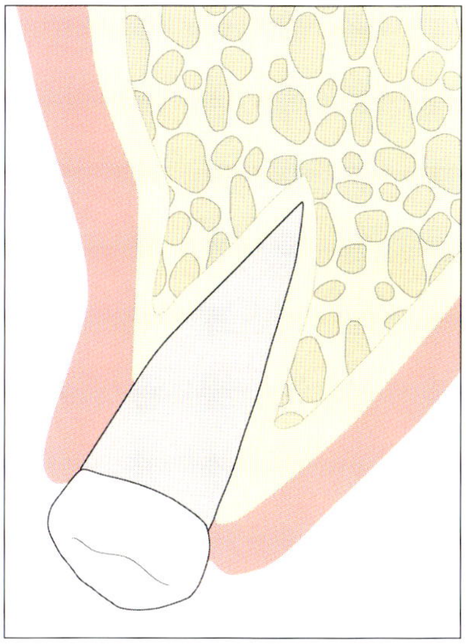

Fig 3-12a Indication for Type II sockets: a significant amount of the buccal plate is missing.

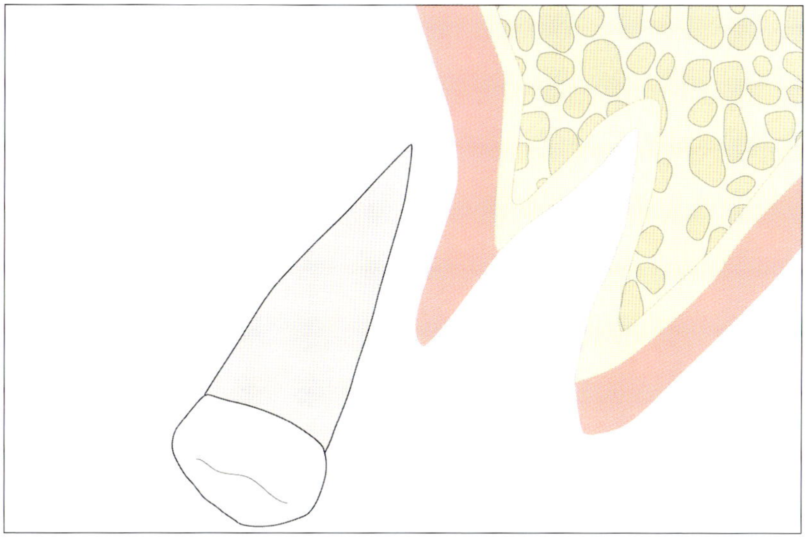

Fig 3-12b Flapless extraction and tooth removed atraumatically.

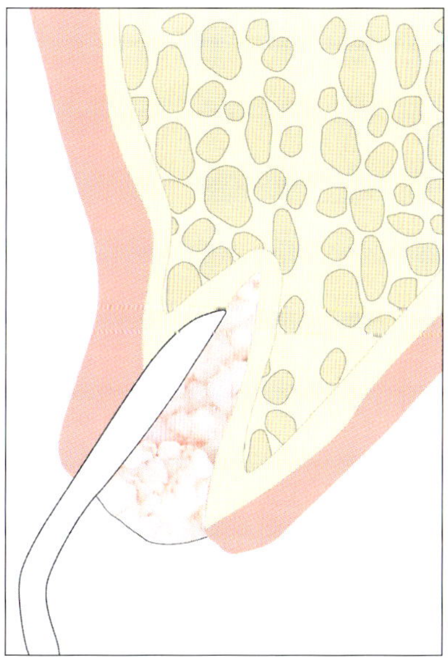

Fig 3-12c Once the membrane is shaped, it is positioned into the socket lining the buccal tissues. The socket is then filled with a bone graft.

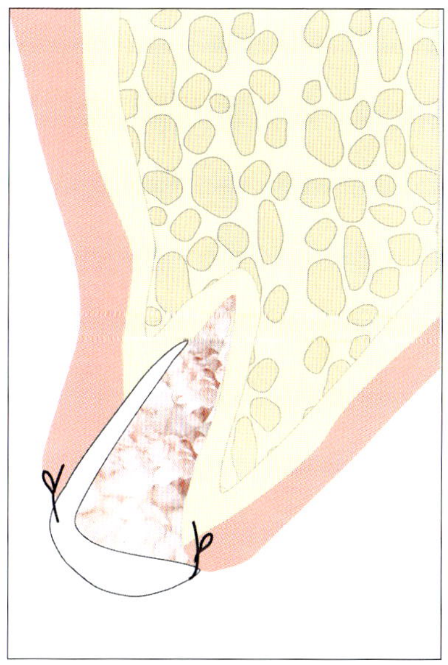

Fig 3-12d The membrane is sutured to the palatal tissue.

and remain in place. The graft material recommended for this technique is a small particle, mineralized cancellous freeze-dried bone allograft. This graft material should be hydrated for 5 minutes and retain enough moisture for the particles to aggregate when inserted. This allograft material allows good compression and its mineralized component permits slow resorption. It also helps keep the shape of the socket while new bone fills the socket during healing. After the graft is compressed, the top part of the membrane is extended over the opening of the socket. The membrane is then sutured with two or three 5-0 absorbable sutures to the palatal tissue (Fig 3-12d).

3.4.4 Hernández Alfaro's technique

A ridge-preservation technique was described by Hernández Alfaro et al.[45] in 2005. The authors describe this technique as simple and with minimal donor site morbidity and time consumption. This technique is described

Fig 3-13 Hernández-Alfaro's technique.

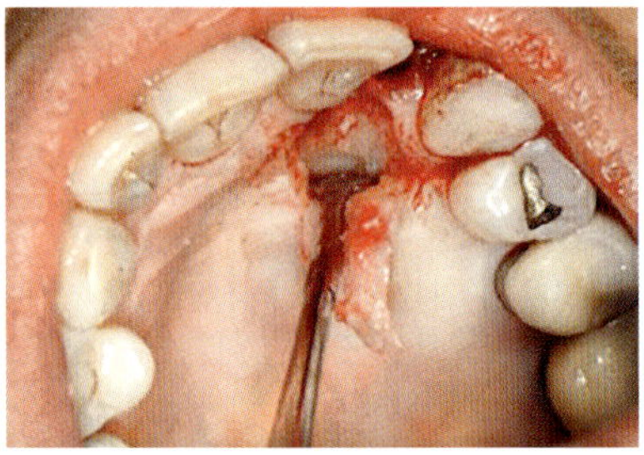

Fig 3-13a A palatal para-marginal incision is made from one tooth posterior to one tooth anterior to the planned area that will be reconstructed.

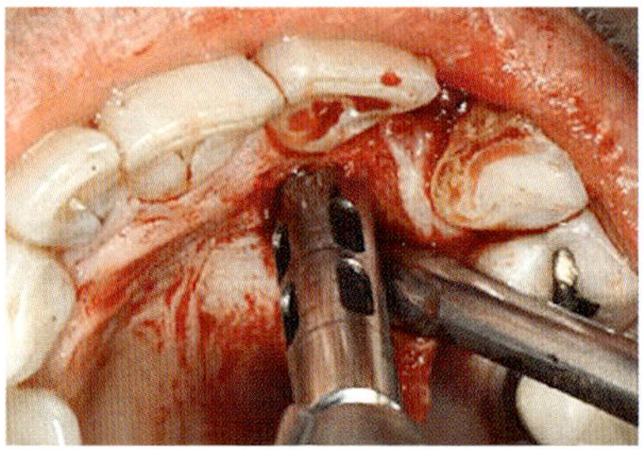

Fig 3-13b The trephine is placed perpendicular to the vault until the cortical plate is engaged. It is then angled to reach a direction parallel to the neighboring roots.

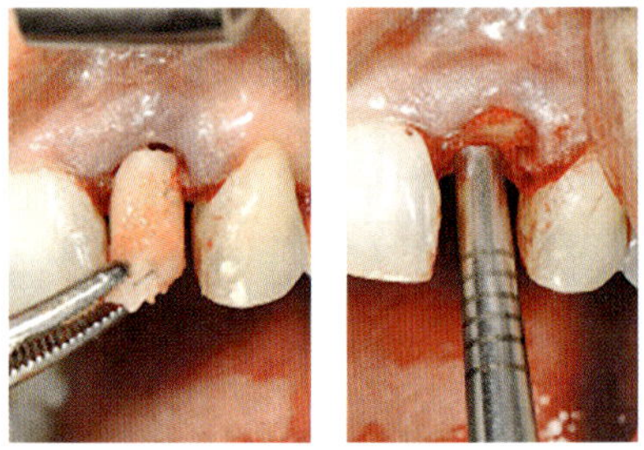

Fig 3-13c The autogenous bone graft is transferred to the socket (*left*) and can then be tapered with a flat-ended osteotome (*right*).

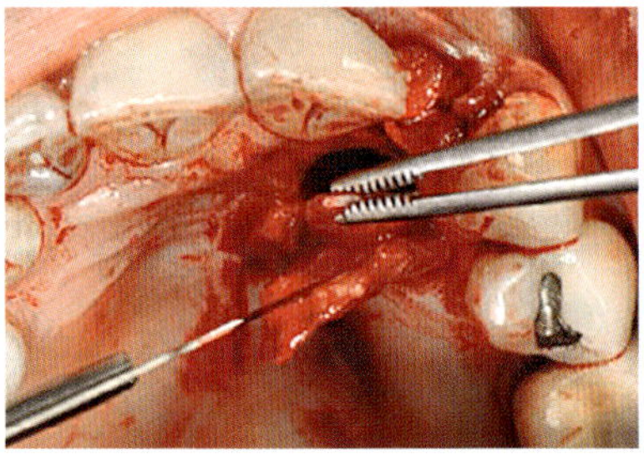

Fig 3-13d Soft tissue coverage is provided by a partial thickness subepithelial palatal pedicle flap.

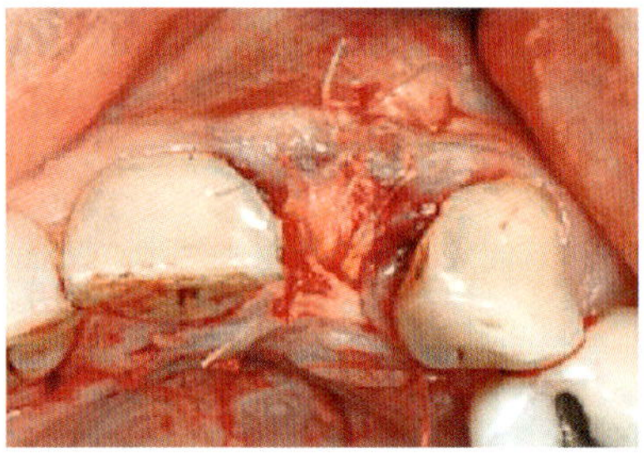

Fig 3-13e The connective palatal tissue flap is sutured over the reconstructed area and afterwards the flap is resutured to its original place.

for alveolar reconstructions in cases where bone resorption has already occurred.[36] Autologous palatal bone is used as a bone grafting material.

In this technique the soft tissue surrounding the alveolus is not modified. A palatal para-marginal incision is made from one tooth posterior to one anterior to the planned reconstruction. An anterior relieving incision allows uncovering of the palatal vault in this area (Fig 3-13a). A bone trephine is used to harvest a bone core from the palatal vault in the vicinity of the defect. The trephine diameter is determined by adding 1 mm to the defect size. A safety margin of 3 mm of bone is left between the planned osteotomy defect area. The trephine is then placed perpendicular to the vault until engaged in the cortical plate. It is then angled to reach a direction parallel to the neighboring roots (Fig 3-13b).

The depth of the osteotomy varies depending on the reconstructive needs and the precalculated height of the vault.

The graft is transferred to the defect site. Because of the vault shape, grafts can have a wedge shape at the end. This end edge is placed inside the alveolus to be reconstructed. The graft can then be tapered inside the defect with a flat-ended osteotome (Fig 3-13c). The flat coronal side of the graft is left at the desired vertical level in relation to the neighboring teeth. Since the size of the graft is predetermined according to the defect to be reconstructed, a tight relation with the remaining alveolar walls is achieved.

Soft tissue coverage is then provided by a partial thickness subepithelial pedicled flap isolated from the main flap (Fig 3-13d). The connective tissue flap is sutured in place with 5-0 monofilament sutures. The epithelial part of the flap is resutured to its original place with resorbable sutures, thus covering the donor area (Fig 3-13e).

3.5 Conclusions

- Socket preservation procedures are effective in limiting horizontal and vertical ridge resorption post-extraction sites.

- Ridge preservation techniques are accompanied by varying degrees of bone formation and residual graft material in the extraction socket. This depends on the material and techniques used.
- It seems that there is insufficient scientific evidence to support the superiority of one technique over another.
- The material chosen may reflect operator preference, the substitution rate and the length of time before the implant is to be placed.
- Preserving extraction sockets improves our ability to provide esthetic restorations to our patients without decreasing the predictability and function of those prostheses.

References

1. Irinakis T. Rationale for socket preservation after extraction of a single-rooted tooth when planning for future implant placement. J Can Dent Assoc 2006;72:917-922.
2. Araujo MG, Lindhe J. Ridge preservation with the use of Bio-Oss collagen: a 6-month study in the dog. Clin Oral Implants Res 2009;20:433-440.
3. Schropp L, Kostopoulos L, Wenzel A. Bone healing following immediate versus delayed placement of titanium implants into extraction sockets: a prospective clinical study. Int J Oral Maxillofac Implants 2003;18:189-199.
4. Bartee BK. Extraction site reconstruction for alveolar ridge preservation. Part 1: rationale and materials selection. J Oral Implantol 2001;27:187-193.
5. Chen ST, Wilson TG Jr, Hammerle CH. Immediate or early placement of implants following tooth extraction: review of biologic basis, clinical procedures, and outcomes. Int J Oral Maxillofac Implants 2004;19(Suppl):12-25.
6. Amler MH, Johnson PL, Salman I. Histological and histochemical investigation of human alveolar socket healing in undisturbed extraction wounds. J Am Dent Assoc 1960;61:32-44.
7. Elian N, Cho SC, Froum S, Smith RB, Tarnow DP. A simplified socket classification and repair technique. Pract Proced Aesthet Dent 2007;19:99-104; quiz 6.
8. Seibert JS. Reconstruction of deformed, partially edentulous ridges, using full thickness onlay grafts. Part II. Prosthetic/periodontal interrelationships. Compend Contin Educ Dent 1983;4: 549-562.
9. Wang HL, Kiyonobu K, Neiva RF. Socket augmentation: rationale and technique. Implant Dent 2004;13:286-296.
10. Yukna RA, Castellon P, Saenz-Nasr AM, et al. Evaluation of hard tissue replacement composite graft material as a ridge preservation/augmentation material in conjunction with immediate hydroxyapatite-coated dental implants. J Periodontol 2003;74: 679-686.
11. Darby I, Chen ST, Buser D. Ridge preservation techniques for implant therapy. Int J Oral Maxillofac Implants 2009;24(Suppl):260-271.
12. Artzi Z, Tal H, Dayan D. Porous bovine bone mineral in healing of human extraction sockets. Part 1: histomorphometric evaluations at 9 months. J Periodontol 2000;71:1015-1023.
13. Iasella JM, Greenwell H, Miller RL et al. Ridge preservation with freeze-dried bone allograft and a collagen membrane compared to extraction alone for implant site development: a clinical and histologic study in humans. J Periodontol 2003;74:990-999.
14. Fiorellini JP, Nevins ML. Localized ridge augmentation/preservation. A systematic review. Ann Periodontol 2003;8:321-327.
15. Nevins M, Camelo M, De Paoli S et al. A study of the fate of the buccal wall of extraction sockets of teeth with prominent roots. Int J Periodontics Restorative Dent 2006;26:19-29.
16. Serino G, Rao W, Iezzi G, Piattelli A. Polylactide and polyglycolide sponge used in human extraction sockets: bone formation following 3 months after its application. Clin Oral Implants Res 2008;19:26-31.
17. Camargo PM, Lekovic V, Carnio J, Kenney EB. Alveolar bone preservation following tooth extraction: a perspective of clinical trials utilizing osseous grafting and guided bone regenera Oral Maxillofac Surg Clin North Am 2004;16:9-18.
18. Serino G, Biancu S, Iezzi G, Piattelli A. Ridge preservation following tooth extraction using a polylactide and polyglycolide sponge as space filler: a clinical and histological study in humans. Clin Oral Implants Res 2003;14:651-658.
19. Artzi Z, Tal H, Dayan D. Porous bovine bone mineral in healing of human extraction sockets: 2. Histochemical observations at 9 months. J Periodontol 2001;72:152-159.
20. Heberer S, Al-Chawaf B, Hildebrand D, Nelson JJ, Nelson K. Histomorphometric analysis of extraction sockets augmented with Bio-Oss Collagen after a 6-week healing period: a prospective study. Clin Oral Implants Res 2008;19:1219-1225.
21. Vance GS, Greenwell H, Miller RL, Hill M, Johnston H, Scheetz JP. Comparison of an allograft in an experimental putty carrier and a bovine-derived xenograft used in ridge preservation: a clinical and histologic study in humans. Int J Oral Maxillofac Implants 2004;19:491-497.
22. Molly L, Vandromme H, Quirynen M, Schepers E, Adams JL, van Steenberghe D. Bone formation following implantation of bone biomaterials into extraction sites. J Periodontol 2008;79: 1108-1115.
23. Mangano C, Piattelli A, Perrotti V, Iezzi G. Dense hydroxyapatite inserted into postextraction sockets: a histologic and histomorphometric 20-year case report. J Periodontol 2008;79:929-933.
24. Neiva RF, Tsao YP, Eber R, Shotwell J, Billy E, Wang HL. Effects of a putty-form hydroxyapatite matrix combined with the synthetic cell-binding peptide P-15 on alveolar ridge preservation. J Periodontol 2008;79:291-299.
25. Fotek PD, Neiva RF, Wang HL. Comparison of dermal matrix and polytetrafluoroethylene membrane for socket bone augmentation: a clinical and histologic study. J Periodontol 2009;80:776-785.
26. Crespi R, Capparè P, Gherlone E. Dental implants placed in extraction sites grafted with different bone substitutes: radiographic evaluation at 24 months. J Periodontol 2009;80:1616-1621.
27. Fernandes PG, Novaes AB Jr, de Queiroz AC, de Souza SL, Taba M Jr, Palioto DB, Grisi MF. Ridge preservation with acellular dermal matrix and anorganic bone matrix cell-binding peptide P-15 after tooth extraction in humans. J Periodontol 2011;82;72-79.
28. Mardas N, Chadha V, Donos N. Alveolar ridge preservation with guided bone regeneration and a synthetic bone substitute or a bovine-derived xenograft: a randomized, controlled clinical trial. Clin Oral Implants Res 2010;21:688-698.
29. Norton MR, Wilson J. Dental implants placed in extraction sites implanted with bioactive glass: human histology and clinical outcome. Int J Oral Maxillofac Implants 2002;17:249-257.
30. Koutouzis T, Lundgren T. Crestal bone-level changes around implants placed in post-extraction sockets augmented with demineralized freeze-dried bone allograft: a retrospective radiographic study. J Periodontol 2010;81:1441-1448.

31. Zubillaga G, Von Hagen S, Simon BI, Deasy MJ. Changes in alveolar bone height and width following post-extraction ridge augmentation using a fixed bioabsorbable membrane and demineralized freeze-dried bone osteoinductive graft. J Periodontol 2003;74: 965-975.
32. Luczyszyn SM, Papalexiou V, Novaes AB Jr, Grisi MF, Souza SL, Taba M Jr. Acellular dermal matrix and hydroxyapatite in prevention of ridge deformities after tooth extraction. Implant Dent 2005;14:176-184.
33. Froum S, Cho SC, Rosenberg E, Rohrer M, Tarnow D. Histological comparison of healing extraction sockets implanted with bioactive glass or demineralized freeze-dried bone allograft: a pilot study. J Periodontol 2002;73:94-102.
34. Carmagnola D, Adriaens P, Berglunch T. Healing of human extraction sockets filled with Bio-Oss. Clin Oral Impants Res 2003;14: 137-143.
35. Guarnieri R, Pecora G, Fini M et al. Medical grade calcium sulfate hemihydrate in healing of human extraction sockets: clinical and histological observations at 3 months. J Periodontol 2004;75: 902-908.
36. Hoffmann O, Bartee BK, Beaumont C, Kasaj A, Deli G, Zafiropoulos GG. Alveolar bone preservation in extraction sockets using non-resorbable dPTFE membranes: a retrospective non-randomized study. J Periodontol 2008;79:1355-1369.
37. Beck TM, Mealey BL. Histologic analysis of healing after tooth extraction with ridge preservation using mineralized human bone allograft. J Periodontol 2010;81:1765-1772.
38. Albrektsson T, Linder L. Intravital, long-term follow-up of autologous experimental bone grafts. Arch Orthop Trauma Surg 1981;98:189-193.
39. Adell R. Tissue integrated prostheses in clinical dentistry. Int Dent J 1985;35:259-265.
40. Albrektsson T, Zarb G, Worthington P, Eriksson AR. The long-term efficacy of currently used dental implants: a review and proposed criteria of success. Int J Oral Maxillofac Implants 1986;1:11-25.
41. Fugazzotto PA. Success and failure rates of osseointegrated implants in function in regenerated bone for 72 to 133 months. Int J Oral Maxillofac Implants 2005;20:77-83.
42. Simion M, Maglione M, Iamoni F, Scarano A, Piattelli A, Salvato A. Bacterial penetration through Resolut resorbable membrane in vitro. An histological and scanning electron microscopic study. Clin Oral Implants Res 1997;8:23-31.
43. Postlethwaite AE, Seyer JM, Kang AH. Chemotactic attraction of human fibroblasts to type I, II, and III collagens and collagen-derived peptides. Proc Natl Acad Sci U S A. 1978;75:871-875.
44. Pinho MN, Roriz VL, Novaes AB Jr et al. Titanium membranes in prevention of alveolar collapse after tooth extraction. Implant Dent 2006;15:53-61.
45. Hernandez Alfaro F, Pages CM, Garcia E, Corchero G, Arranz C. Palatal core graft for alveolar reconstruction: a new donor site. Int J Oral Maxillofac Implants 2005;20:777-783.
46. El Helow K, El Askary Ael S. Regenerative barriers in immediate implant placement: a literature review. Implant Dent 2008;17: 360-371.
47. Camelo M, Nevins ML, Schenk RK, Simion M, Rasperini G, Lynch SE, Nevins M. Clinical, radiographic, and histologic evaluation of human periodontal defects treated with Bio-Oss and Bio-Guide. Int J Periodontics Restorative Dent 1998;18:321-331.
48. Bartee BK. Extraction site reconstruction for alveolar ridge preservation. Part 2: membrane-assisted surgical technique. J Oral Implantol 2001;27:194-197.
49. Penarrocha M, Garcia-Mira B, Martinez O. Localized vertical maxillary ridge preservation using bone cores and a rotated palatal flap. Int J Oral Maxillofac Implants 2005;20:131-134.

Chapter 4

Immediate implants: are they safe?

Jordi Ortega Martinez, Natália Oliveira, Federico Hernández Alfaro

4.1 Introduction

Since the first appearance and popularization of dental implants, different techniques and materials have been developed, leading to a great variety of treatment options. Treatment times have been one of the issues most influenced by such development.

Constant pressure and increased demands from patients led dentists to shorten the "standard protocol" times, instead placing and restoring dental implants immediately. What may have started as an experiment soon proved to have the same effectiveness and survival when compared with the conventional protocol previously described by Bränemark.[1] Further studies have shown that even with these high survival rates, the final result may be unsuccessful, since in some cases the esthetic outcome may be compromised, and will not fulfill patient expectations.[2]

To begin with, this procedure was considered unpredictable, but with the development of new protocols and improved diagnosis it now has similar final results to other loading protocols, in some cases even better.

Being technique-sensitive and dependent on proper diagnosis and clinical skills, this procedure should only be carried out when indicated. Therefore it is important to understand the advantages and precise indications of placing immediate implants.

The objective of this chapter is to explain when and how to place immediate implants, as well as to demystify controversies related to this type of procedure.

4.2 Background

The traditional surgical protocol of implant placement used to be followed by a period of several months' healing after the dental extraction.[1] This is referred to as a delayed approach.[3] However, recent evidence suggests that implants placed using the immediate placement technique have similar survival rates to implants placed using the delayed approach in healed sites.[2,4,5]

Due to a physiologic resorption of the socket after extraction and without the use of any preventive methods, socket bone loss is of approximately 50%, especially in the maxilla.[2,5-7] Two methods are described to reduce this resorption:

- Graft the socket with an osteoconductive material (allograft or xenograft) or autologous bone (see Chapter 3 on socket preservation).
- Perform immediate implant placement after tooth extraction.

Immediate placement of a dental implant was described for the first time more than 30 years ago, by Schulte and Heimke,[8] consisting in positioning the implant in the same surgical procedure as the tooth extraction. Since then, different placement and loading protocols have evolved from the first protocols in order to achieve quicker and easier surgical treatment (Fig 4-1). Nowadays, immediate implant placement after tooth extraction is a widely acceptable procedure with high survival rates ranging from 93.9% to 100%.[9-17]

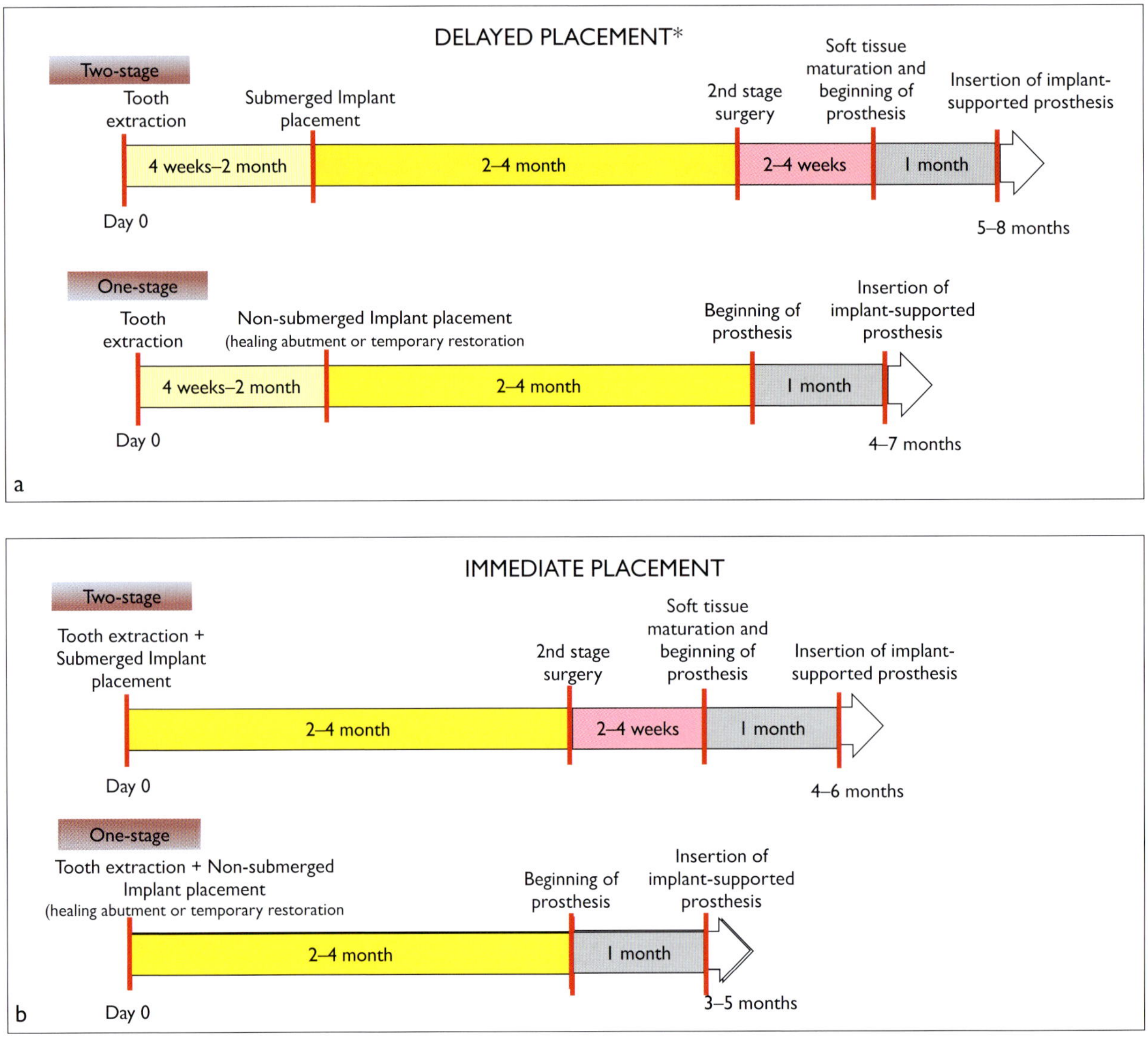

Figs 4-1a and b Treatment sequence diagrams recommended for standard surgical delayed and immediate implant placement procedures (soft and hard tissue regeneration are not contemplated, therefore variable timings may be applicable). *Considered after soft tissue and/or partial bone tissue healing (4–16 weeks).

4.3 Socket physiology

In order to comprehend the concept of immediate implant placement and consequent advantages and disadvantages, it is important to understand the healing process that the socket undergoes after a tooth extraction. Although this timing varies according to the author and the patient, the following indicative timeline illustrates the socket healing process.[18]

- Day 0: Day of tooth extraction, after a few minutes the hemorrhage stops, a blood clot is formed, and an inflammatory process is established.
- Day 2–3: The blood clot is established, leading to the formation of granulation tissue.
- Day 7: Granulation tissue is established and some connective tissue osteoid and epithelium begins to form.
- Day 20: Connective tissue replaces the previously present granulation tissue and osteoid tissue starts to mineralize at the socket periphery. Complete epithelium closure occurs after approximately 25 to 35 days.
- Day 40: The socket is filled with connective tissue, immature bone and epithelium.
- Day 60: Soft tissue is healed and mature bone is present.

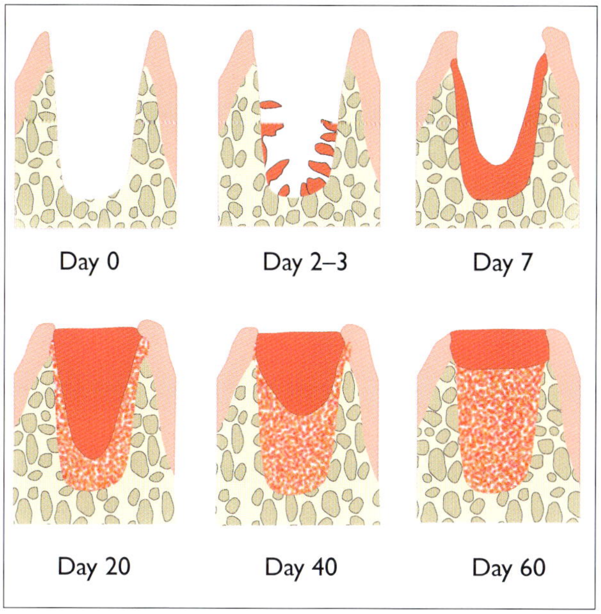

Fig 4-2 Schematic representation of socket healing process (modified from Amler[18] with permission).

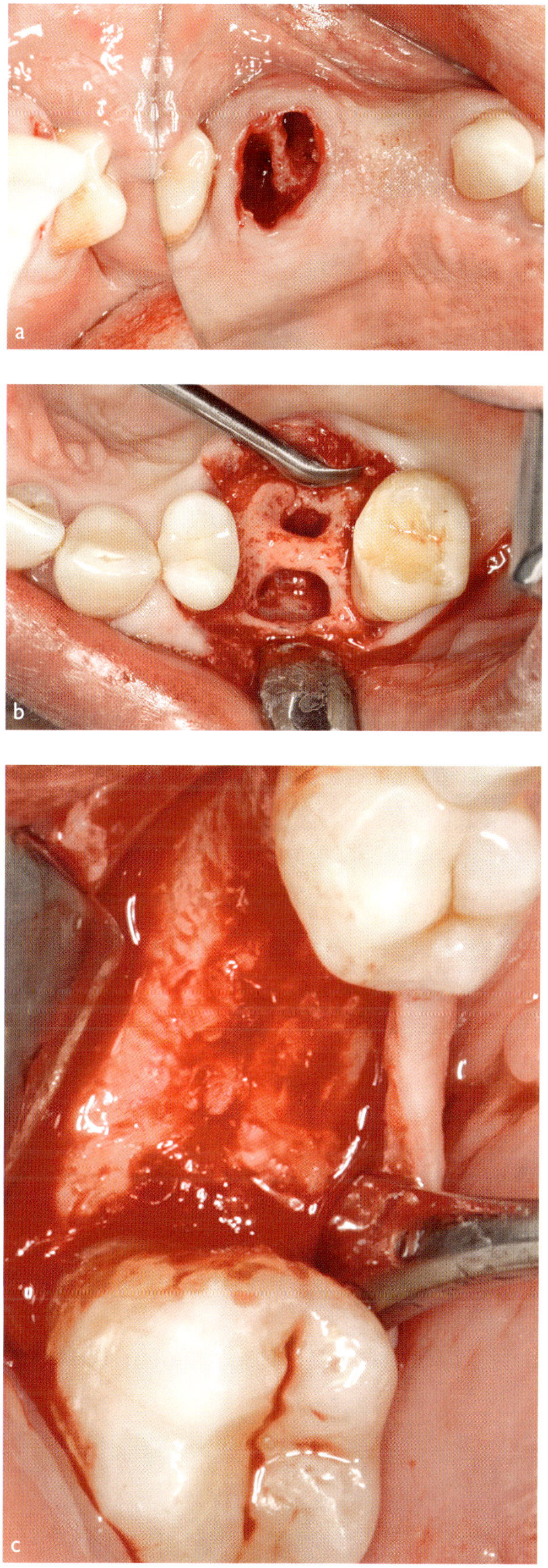

Figs 4-3a to c Socket healing phases. (*a*) Post-extraction socket. (*b*) Partial socket healing. (*c*) Total socket healing.

Despite the presence of mature bone after 2 months, bone remodeling may continue even 1 year after extraction until there is normalization with the adjacent edentulous bone level. However, despite the variance between individuals, the majority of bone alterations occur during these first months (Figs 4-2 and 4-3).[19-21]

Several studies analyzed the different external and internal modifications in vertical and horizontal level after tooth extraction (Table 4-1).[22-26] These changes are more pronounced in molars than premolars, and in the mandible than the maxilla. Nevertheless, other factors, such as the presence of bone dehiscence, buccal bone thickness, and periodontal biotype should be considered in order to predict the degree of future soft tissue recession, which is usually accompanied by bone alterations.[25-28]

Caplanis et al.[29] described an extraction defect sounding (EDS) classification according to hard and soft tissue alterations immediately following tooth removal, as well as providing basic treatment guidelines. Extraction defects were separated into type 1 (EDS-1), type 2 (EDS-2), type 3 (EDS-3), and type 4 (EDS-4) (Table 4-2 and Fig 4-4).

Elian et al.[28] reported a simplified classification of extraction sockets and recommended repair techniques

Table 4-1 Socket dimensional changes during healing

Reference	Healing time (months)	Vertical change (mean ± SD) (mm)	Buccolingual change (mean ± SD) (mm)
Lekovic et al.[22]	6	-0.86 ± 0.14	-
Lekovic et al.[23]	6	-1.50 ± 0.26	-
Camargo et al.[24]	6	1.00 ± 2.25	3.06 ± 2.41
Iasella et al.[25]	4 to 6	-0.90 ± 1.60	-2.63 ± 2.29
Schropp et al.[26]	12	-0.7	-5.9

Table 4-2 Descriptive table of EDS defects (reproduced with permission from Caplanis et al.[29]

Defect type	General assessment	No. socket walls affected	Biotype	Hard tissue (mm)	Distance to reference (mm)	Ideal soft tissue	Treatment recommendations
EDS-1	Pristine	0	Thick	0	0–3	Predictable	Immediate implant (one-stage
EDS-2	Pristine to slight damage	0–1	Thin or thick	0–2	3–5	Achievable but not predictable	Site preservation or immediate implant (one- or two-stage)
EDS-3	Moderate damage	1–2	Thin or thick	3–5	6–8	Slight compromise	Site preservation then implant placement (two-stage)
EDS-4	Severe	2–3	Thin or thick	≥6	≥9	Compromised	Site preservation then site development then implant placement (three-stage)

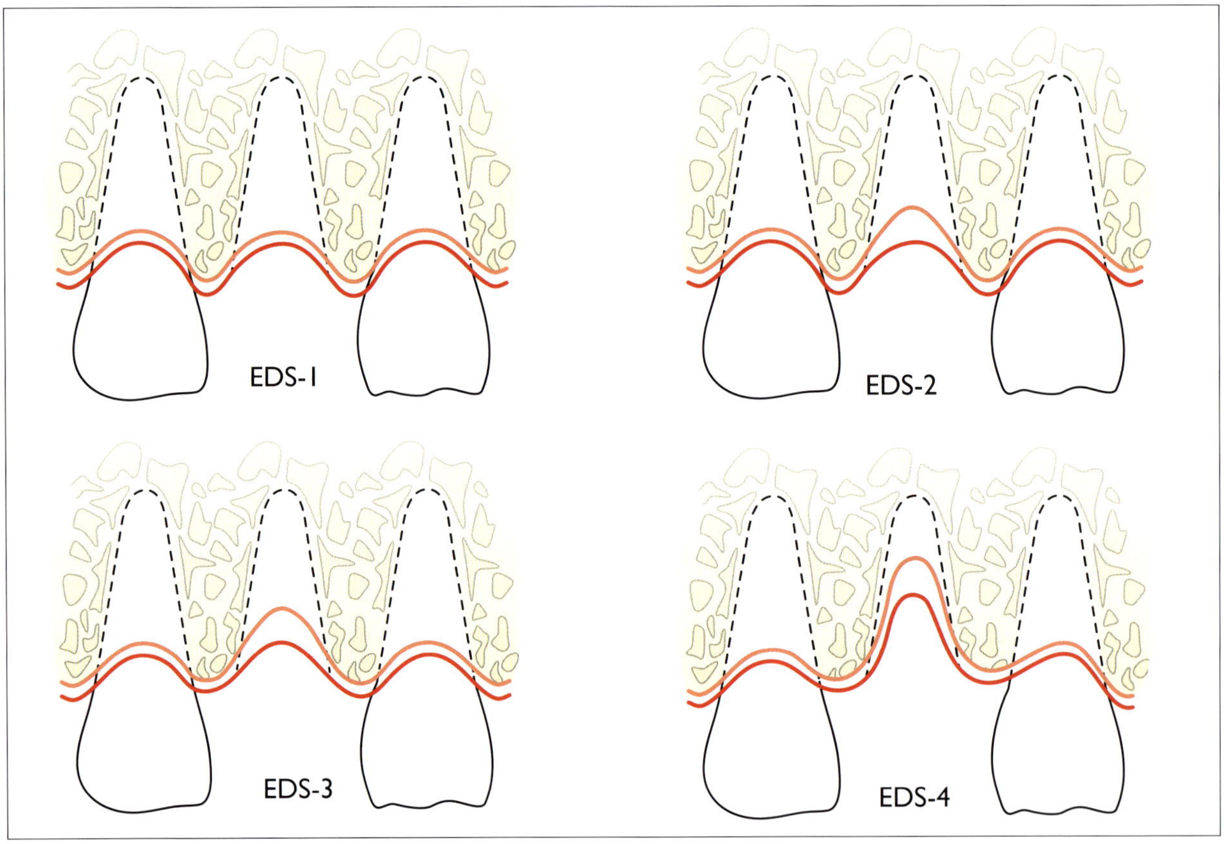

Fig 4-4 Illustration of EDS defects (reproduced with permission from Caplanis et al.[29]).

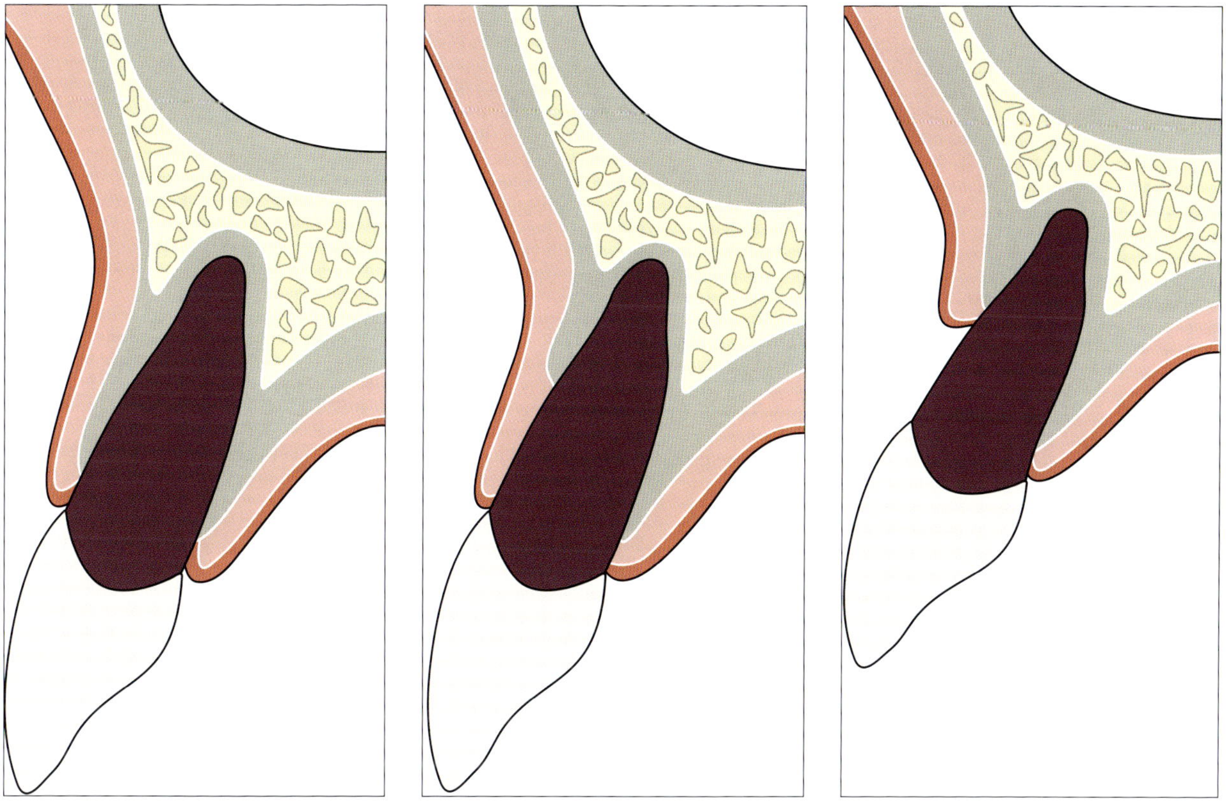

Fig 4-5 Illustration of the three types of extraction socket (reproduced with permission from Elian et al.[28]).

in the esthetic zone, dividing the sockets into three types according to the facial soft tissue and bone buccal plate present (Fig 4-5). In type I sockets, according to Elian's classification (see Chapter 3), the facial soft tissue and buccal plate bone are intact and at normal levels in relation to the cementoenamel junction (CEJ) of the pre-extracted tooth, and immediate implant placement may be applied without compromising the esthetic outcome. In types II or III, a staged placement is recommended although additional soft and hard tissue surgery may be necessary.[28]

As previously mentioned, after tooth extraction, socket alterations are usually more pronounced at the buccal plate than at the palatal or lingual portion of the extraction site.[30-32] Bundle bone is a "tooth-related" tissue that delineates the alveolar socket, and has a thickness of approximately 0.8 mm.[33] Since the bundle bone blood supply is provided by the periodontal ligament vessel, once the tooth is extracted it will remodel and eventually disappear.[34] As a consequence, 2–3 mm of the coronal bone wall may resorb during the healing process.

Ridge alterations that occur following tooth removal are mainly the result of tooth loss and its consequent function.[33] This concept has to be taken into account prior to immediate implant placement. In order to reduce possible complications that may result from this physiologic process, implants should be positioned slightly more palatally/lingually and apically than the existent socket wall and/or regeneration should be considered.

4.4 Classification

The first classification that described implant placement timing as mature, recent, delayed, or immediate, was reported by Wilson and Weber,[35] based on soft tissue healing and predictability of guided bone regeneration (GBR) procedures. Further classifications based on hard and soft tissue healing and treatment time were subsequently described, as shown in Table 4-3.[36-38]

In order to clarify every aspect of immediate implants, the following topics will be discussed:

- 4.5 Immediate implants
  - 4.5.1 Advantages of immediate implants
  - 4.5.2 Indications for placement of immediate implants

Table 4-3 Timing of implant placement

Reference	Classification	Implant placement
Hämmerle et al.[36]	Type I	In fresh extraction sockets
	Type II	After soft tissue coverage (4–8 weeks)
	Type III	Radiographic bone fill (12–16 weeks)
	Type IV	Healed socket (>16 weeks)
Esposito et al.[37]	Immediate	In fresh extraction sockets
	Immediate-delayed	<8 weeks post extraction
	Delayed	>8 weeks post extraction
Chen and Buser[38]	Immediate	Same day
	Early	Soft tissue healing (4–8 weeks)
		Partial bone healing (12–16 weeks)
	Late	Complete bone healing (>6 months)

- 4.5.3 Does the surgical technique differ from delayed implant placement?
- 4.5.4 Where can immediate implants be placed?
- 4.6 Considerations before placement of an immediate implant
- 4.6.1 Are there significant differences in crestal bone resorption between immediate and delayed implants?
- 4.6.2 Do immediate implants have a significant effect on soft tissue recession outcomes?
- 4.6.3 Does the presence of periapical infection affect immediate implant success or survival rate?
- 4.7 Gap treatment
- 4.7.1 Is it necessary to graft the gap?
- 4.7.2 When grafting, which is the best biomaterial? Is a membrane necessary? Is it necessary to obtain primary wound closure?
- 4.8 Implant primary stability
- 4.8.1 Are there significant differences in implant stability between immediate and delayed implants?
- 4.9 Compromised situations
- 4.9.1 Immediate implants versus delayed implants: survival and success rates in molar sites
- 4.9.2 Immediate implants in periodontally affected sites
- 4.9.3 Immediate implants versus delayed implants: survival rates and bone loss in periodontal patients
- 4.10 Conclusions
- 4.11 Clinical cases

4.5 Immediate implants

4.5.1 Advantages of immediate implants

At the fourth ITI (International Team for Implantology) Consensus Conference (November 2009), the advantages and disadvantages for implant placement at various points in time after tooth extraction were reported.[2] They concluded that immediate implant placement is technically more difficult than delayed implant placement when attempting to obtain primary stability and adequate prosthetic positioning. They also identified an increased risk of mucosal recession with time, despite the satisfactory esthetic outcome shown in 80% of cases, according to their esthetic index. The survival rates of post-extraction implants are high and comparable with those of implants placed in healing sites.[2] Various clinical considerations have been suggested in order to decide whether an immediate implant placement approach may be the treatment choice, and Table 4-4 lists the relative advantages and disadvantages.[27,39,40]

Based on clinical experience and scientific data, the criteria for immediate implant success are considered to be atraumatic tooth extraction, minimally invasive surgical approach, and implant primary stability.[41,42]

Table 4-4 Advantages and disadvantages of immediate implant placement

Advantages	Disadvantages
Fewer surgical interventions required	The morphology of the site, leading to increased surgical difficulty
Shorter treatment time	The presence of periapical pathology
Ideal three-dimensional implant positioning references	The absence/reduction of keratinized tissue
The presumptive preservation of alveolar bone at the side of the tooth extraction	Esthetic compromise with thin tissue biotypes
Soft tissue esthetics and maintenance	Lack of complete soft tissue closure over the extraction socket

Table 4-5 Indications and contraindications for immediate implant treatment

Indications	Contraindications
All tooth extraction without active infection (caries, crown or root fractures, endodontic problems)	Absence of bone walls surrounding dental implant
Traumatic tooth avulsion with bone walls preserved	Insufficient apical bone to achieve primary stability
Temporary tooth root resorption with permanent tooth agenesis	Presence of anatomic limitation (inferior dental nerve or sinus)
Post-orthodontic root resorption	Acute periapical infection

Figs 4-6a to c Ideal 3D implant positioning.

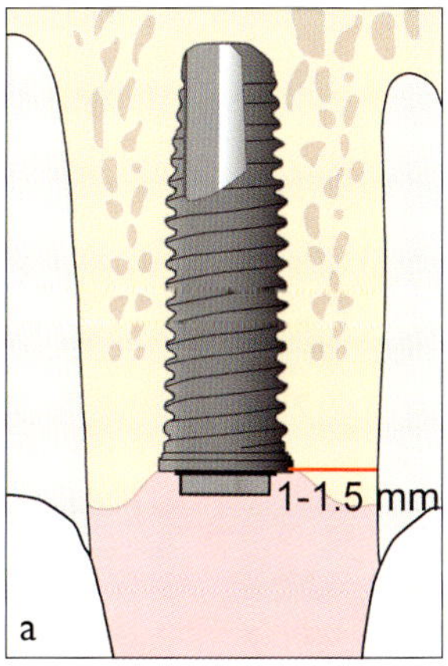

Fig 4-6a Mesiodistal position: minimal distance 1.0–1.5 mm from the adjacent teeth.

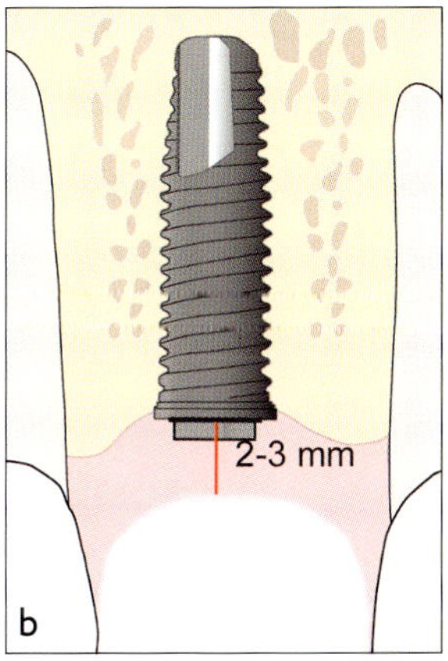

Fig 4-6b Apicocoronal position: apical from CEJ of adjacent teeth (tissue level implants 2 mm, bone level implants 3 mm, from the gingival level of the future restoration).

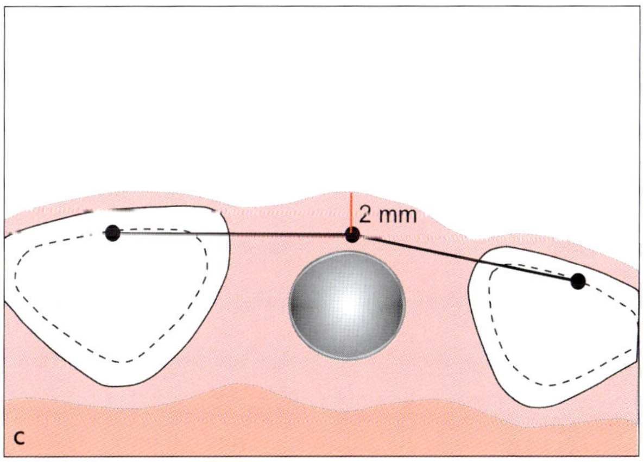

Fig 4-6c Buccopalatal position: 1.5–2 mm towards the palatal, maintaining minimally 2 mm of buccal wall.

4.5.2 Indications for placement of immediate implants

There are no specific indications or contraindications for immediate implant therapy other than those for any implant surgery (Table 4-5). Immediate implants are normally selected for esthetic reasons or to reduce treatment time.[6,43,44]

4.5.3 Does the surgical technique differ from delayed implant placement?

The procedure for immediate implant placement must be considered different regardless of whether the esthetics is compromised. Nevertheless, ideal three-dimensional (3D) implant positioning (Fig 4-6) must be assessed, as well as appropriate implant diameter according to the socket morphology.[5,6,41,45,46]

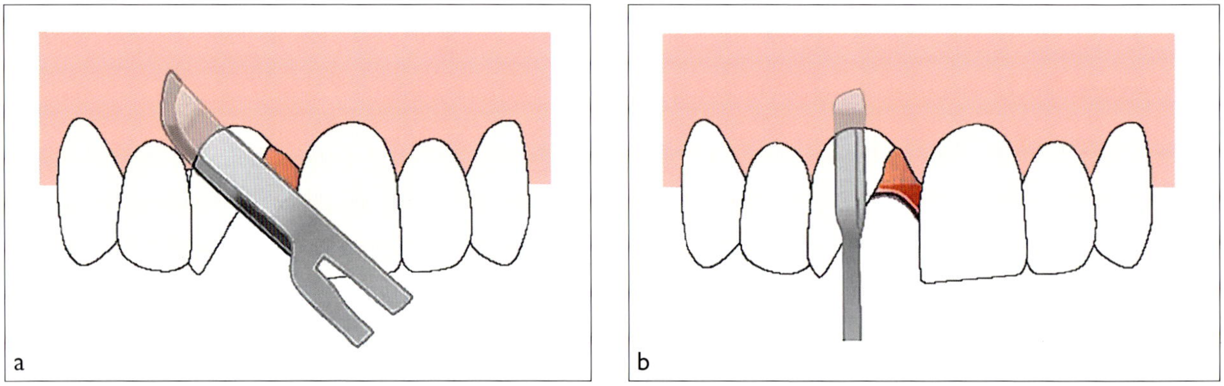

Figs 4-7a and b Atraumatic dental extraction with (a) microsurgical scalpel or (b) periotomes.

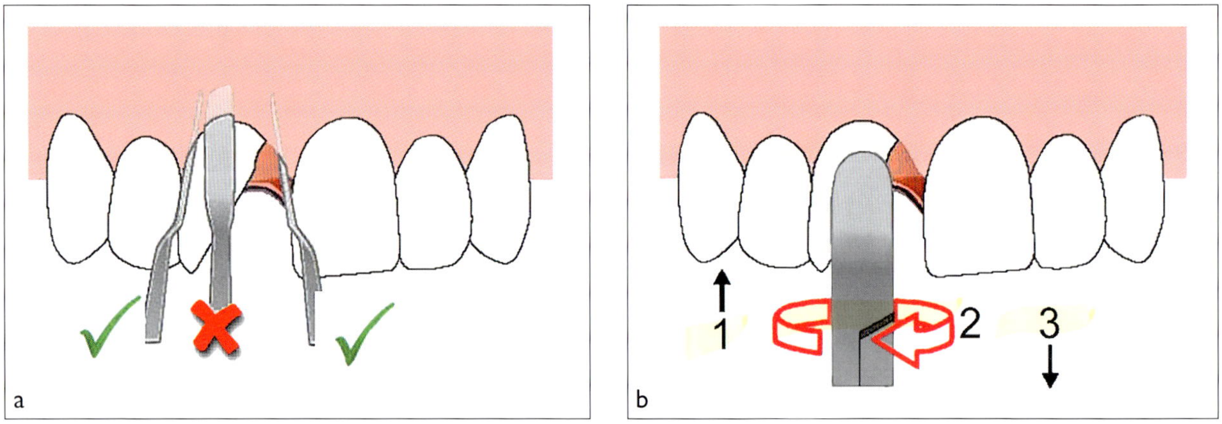

Figs 4-8a and b Atraumatic extraction with application of peritomes and forceps. (a) Periotomes should be applied along the socket, with the exception of the vestibular wall. (b) Application of apical pressure (1 – press) and rotation movements along the axis of the tooth (2 – turn) to shear the PDL fibers (3 – pull).

- Atraumatic dental extraction to preserve the integrity of alveolar bone walls: dental extraction should be performed with no bone fractures. Periodontal ligament (PDL) should be broken with a microsurgical scalpel or periotomes (Fig 4-7).
- Mesiodistal or buccolingual movements should be avoided to prevent breakage of thin bone walls (Fig 4-8).
- Buccal wall must be kept to prevent bone loss in this area, which is the most susceptible to resorption (Fig 4-9).
- Complete debridement of all the alveolar walls with curettes, which should also be used to assess socket morphology and integrity (Fig 4-9).
- Implant drilling should be performed towards the palatolingual area and the implant head should not emerge too buccally, achieving primary stability from the apical area of the socket (at least 3 to 5 mm of intimate bone-to-implant contact [BIC]), maintaining at least 2 mm from the external buccal wall, 3 mm in between implants, and 1.5 mm from a natural tooth (Fig 4-6). The use of a surgical stent is recommended, to orientate implant placement (Figs 4-10).
- If the gap distance is significant, grafting may be necessary to avoid soft tissue growth and allow the implant to osseointegrate (Fig 4-11).
- Primary closure of the wound should be achieved by soft tissue (pedicled flap, connective tissue graft or coronal reposition of the flap) or covered by a resorbable membrane to protect the surgical area. A non-submerged technique is also reported in the literature with predictable outcomes with the use of a provisional restoration or a healing abutment.[7]

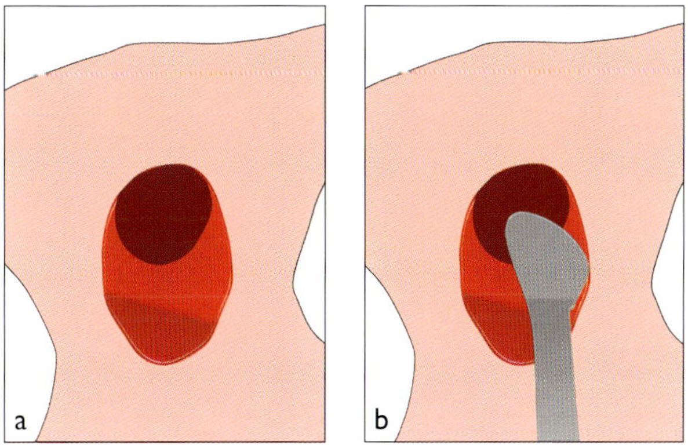

Figs 4-9a and b Socket integrity. (a) Visual and tactile determination of the integrity of the socket wall with the absence of dehiscences. (b) Debridement of the alveolar wall with a curette.

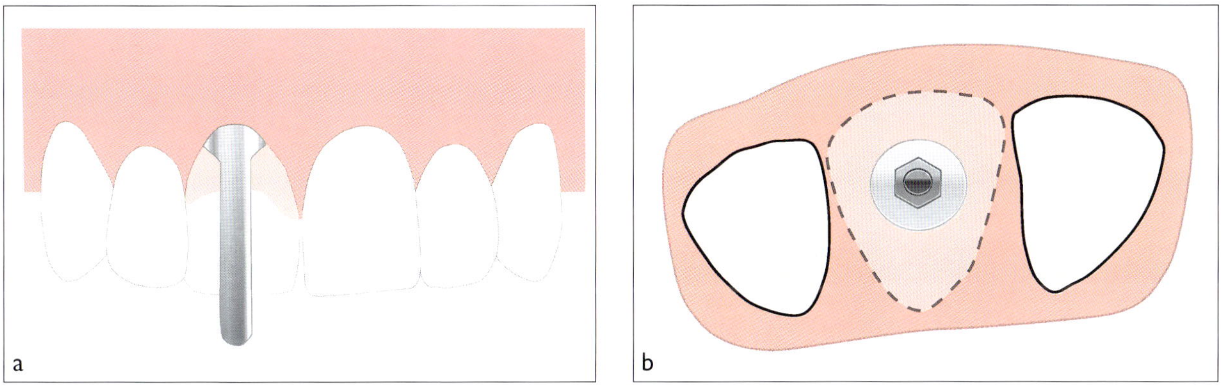

Figs 4-10a and b Positioning of the try-in pin through the surgical stent, to confirm correct implant drilling.

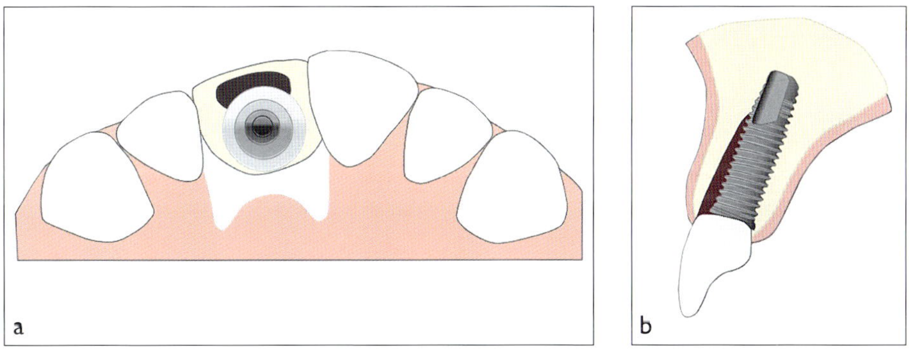

Figs 4-11a and b Immediate implant positioning in the anterior esthetic area, with placement of biomaterial in the gap.

4.5.4 Where can immediate implants be placed?

Uniradicular teeth (anterior area)

The first bur (marking drill) should be placed at an angle to the palatal wall, to create a slight indentation for anchorage and reduce slippage of the drill into the socket. During the osteotomy, once anchorage is obtained, the bur is straightened in order to obtain a parallel trajectory to the palatal or lingual wall. The head of the implant should be positioned at least 2 mm from the external buccal bone and 3 mm apical from the imaginary CEJ of the future tooth. Drilling must be performed palatally, not along the socket morphology, for the implant head to emerge correctly and not too bucally. An implant buccal position will limit prosthetic solutions and lead to esthetic and biological complications (Fig 4-12).[39,47,48]

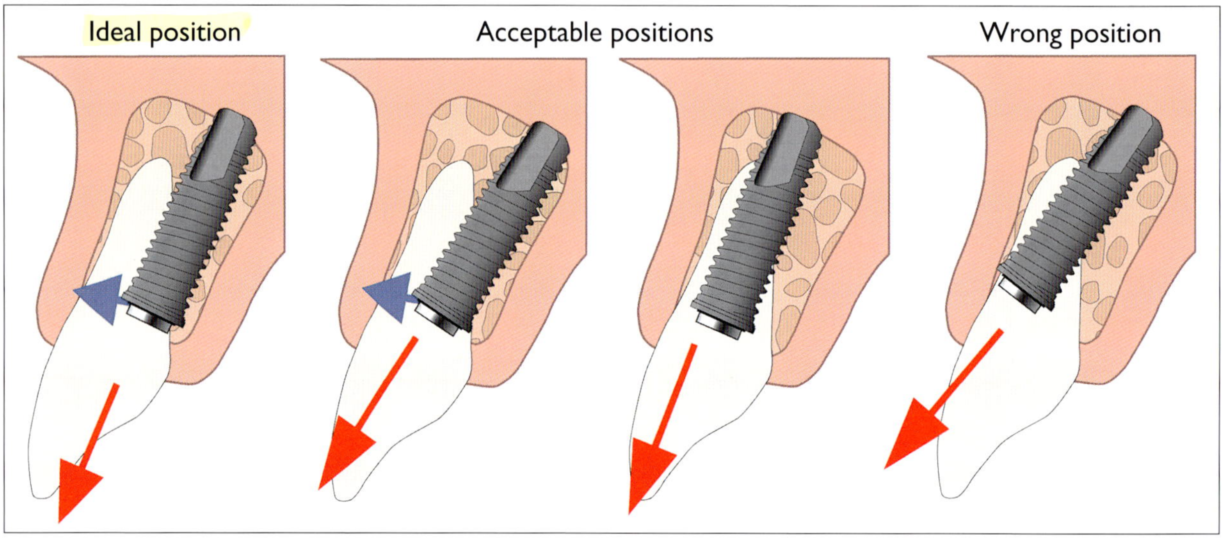

Fig 4-12 Immediate implant positioning in the anterior esthetic area (reproduced with permission from Funato et al.[47]).

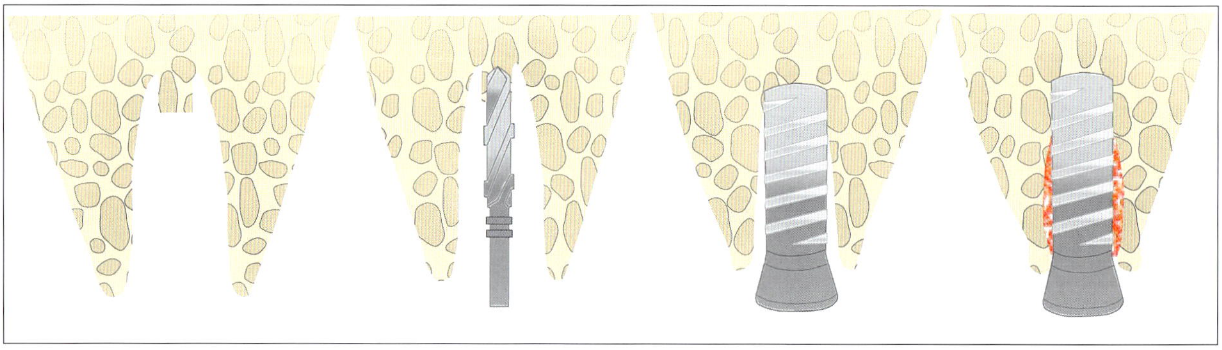

Fig 4-13 Immediate implant positioning for the maxillary premolars (reproduced with permission from Fugazzotto et al.[49]).

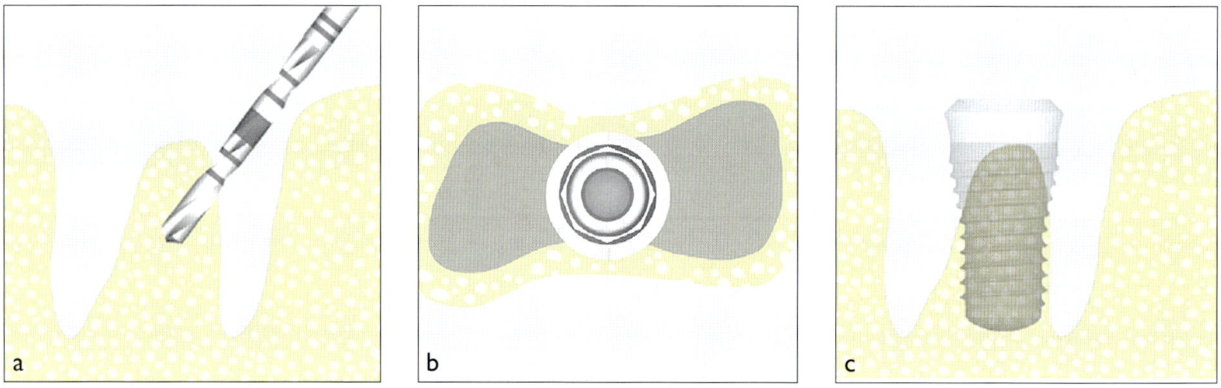

Figs 4-14a to c Immediate implant positioning for mandibular molars. (a) Initial drill angulations in relation to the septa to obtain anchorage. (b) Occlusal view. (c) Saggital view. (Reproduced with permission from Fugazzotto[52].)

Uniradicular teeth (posterior area)

Primary stability is easily achieved and esthetic considerations are lower than in the anterior zone. However, the ideal 3D positioning is the same as in the esthetic anterior area, slightly palatal or lingual.

Biradicular premolars and canines

Placed preferentially in the center of the socket (anchoring to the interradicular septum) or in the palatal root, rather than the vestibular root. Usually a gap is created and the clinician must decide whether or not to fill it (Fig 4-13).[49]

Maxillary molars

Palatal root or center of the socket (septa) placements are preferable. Owing to the presence of three roots, primary stability is often challenging and delayed implant placement has to be considered.[50,51]

Mandibular molars

The interradicular septum is usually wide enough to receive a wide diameter implant and esthetic demands are not crucial. The bur should enter angled in relation to the septa and during osteotomy, and once anchorage is obtained this angle should be straightened, to obtain an ideal 3D positioning mesiodistally and buccolingually. However, the gap should always be filled because of the mesial and distal root anatomy (Fig 4-14).[52]

4.6 Considerations before placement of an immediate implant

4.6.1 Are there significant differences in crestal bone resorption between immediate and delayed implants?

Crestal bone loss is predictable when an implant is placed in a healed crest, but when a dental implant is placed inside a fresh socket, there is no exact control over where the implant head is placed related to the marginal bone. Moreover, there is a tendency to submerge further the immediate implants to reduce adverse effects of the resorption process.[53]

Interproximal bone level changes are well recorded, but few of them show differences between immediate and delayed protocols. Although many articles describe limited marginal bone loss or gain in immediate implant therapy, caution is needed when interpreting the results since few of these studies report radiographic outcomes.[37,54-57]

Even more important is the preservation of the buccal bone level because of esthetic considerations. However, only two studies register buccal bone resorption, with slightly increased bone loss when compared with interproximal changes.[58,59]

Table 4-6 Mucosal recession with immediate implants

Reference	Frequency (%)	Remarks
Lindeboom et al.[64]	8.7	Recession 1–2mm
	30.0	Recession <1mm
Chen et al.[7]	33.3	Recession at 6 months
Kan et al.[65]	34.8	Recession ≥ 1.5 mm
	8.3	V-shape defects
	42.8	U-shape defects
	100.0	UU-shape defects
Evans and Chen[66]	45.2	Total of recessions ≥ 0.5 mm
	26.2	Recession 0.5–1.0 mm
	9.5	Recession 1.0–1.5mm
	9.5	Recession >1.5mm

Lately, implants with platform switching have been considered, to prevent bone resorption and allow soft tissue to seal the abutment connection far from the bone-to-implant interface.[60] It is accepted that this design will reduce apical migration of hard and soft tissues, obtaining optimal peri-implant stability.[41,61-63]

Recommendations

- There are no significant differences in interproximal bone loss between immediate and delayed implant placement protocols.
- Immediate implant placement does not prevent bone loss.
- Caution must be taken during post-extraction implant placement in relation to the apicocoronal position, and the CEJ of adjacent teeth should be used as a measurement reference. The implant head should be placed 3 mm apical to the CEJ of adjacent teeth.

4.6.2 Do immediate implants have a significant effect on soft tissue recession outcomes?

Most studies do not find statistical or clinical differences between immediate implants compared with the delayed protocol, and soft tissues are no better preserved in the immediate protocol (Table 4-6).[7,20,64-68] However, studies do not focus on the buccal keratinized tissue (such as crestal bone), although this should be considered because of the esthetic concerns. Susceptibility to recession in the anterior area may lead to exposure of the implant metal margin, resulting in a grey, unnatural coloration of the gingiva.[67]

To preserve the buccal bone and reduce the risk of recession, normally a flapless surgical approach is recommended when placing immediate implants. When there is a high risk of fenestration or a submerged approach is performed, a mucoperiosteal flap may be used, permitting primary closure of the wound.[17,69] Reports indicate that when a flap is released and the periosteum detached, the bone is more prone to resorption, especially in the presence of thin buccal walls (see Case 5).[69,70] This may be caused by the reduction in vascularization. This flap advancement may alter the mucogingival line, and when the keratinized tissue is scarce it can cause a mucogingival problem that may require further surgical intervention, with poor esthetic prognosis.[7]

Platform-switching implant shoulder design and the distance from the crestal bone to the contact point of the restoration are also current considerations described in the literature as criteria to obtain/maintain interproximal papillae.[42,71] Nevertheless, careful case selection is advised in the esthetic area since certain indicators such as thin tissue biotype, thin facial bone, dehiscence of facial bone, and implant malposition may increase the risk or a poor esthetic outcome.

4.6.3 Does the presence of periapical infection affect immediate implant success or survival rate?

The survival rate of implants placed when periapical pathology is present is still controversial, since the results of most recent studies are contradictory and unclear.

In most of the studies when a periapical infection was present the implant was not placed immediately, and instead a delayed placement protocol was performed or patients were excluded.[7,20,41,42,58,67,71-74] However, in recent studies, implants placed immediately after the extraction of teeth with chronic periapical lesions appear to present similar results to those without.[57,64,75,76]

Regardless, with chronic periapical infection immediate implant placement should be considered and caution is recommended. Even after correct debridement, there may be remains of scar or granulomatous tissue, which can endanger treatment outcome,[13,77] and in some compromised cases, the necessary primary stability may not be achieved.[57]

Care should be taken for patients with a medical history of allergies to penicillin, in which case alternative antibiotics are prescribed. Despite the lack of unequivocal scientific evidence relating systemic antibiotics to lower implant survival rates directly, the same reports show a higher failure rate in patients who are allergic to penicillin when alternative antibiotics are prescribed.[78]

Recommendations

- Immediate implant placement with active periapical infection is not recommended and may be considered a contraindication, especially in patients allergic to penicillin.
- Socket debridement must always be performed previous to immediate implant placement, especially when a chronic periapical infection is present.
- Chronic periapical infection may make the surgical procedure more difficult, but immediate implants can be placed.

4.7 Gap treatment

Socket morphology, especially in the molar area and canines, is wider than implant diameter; therefore the gap left from the socket wall and the implant surface should be considered to be treated in order to avoid soft tissue invasion and crestal bone loss. Gap treatment is a controversial matter, in various aspects, as described below.

4.7.1 Is it necessary to graft the gap?

In accordance with several reviews, immediate implant gap treatment using autogenous bone grafts, xenografts, or allografts may improve the process of bone formation between the implant and the surrounding socket walls, increase survival rates, and reduce socket resorption.[5,13,27,54,79] Horizontal reduction can be controlled with grafting better than vertical, and it will be greater in the presence of a dehiscence or any buccal defect.[2,54] However, when small gaps are present, grafting procedures may or may not be applied. It has been reported with immediate or early implant placement that peri-implant gaps of 2 mm or less healed spontaneously.[37,54]

Table 4-7 Gap treatment procedures

Reference	Gap dimension treated	Gap regeneration	Survival rate (%)
Block et al.[20]	Not specified	Allograft	-
Canullo et al.[41]	> 1mm	Bovine bone matrix	100
Siciliano et al.[74]	Not specified	Bio-Oss® and Bio-Gide®	100
Del Fabbro et al.[81]	> 1mm	PRGF + autogenous bone chips	98.4
Cafiero et al.[72]	> 1mm	Bio-Oss® and Bio-Gide®	100
Crespi et al.[67]	> 2 mm	Autogenous chips	100
Siegenthaler et al.[57]	All gaps	Bio-Oss® and Bio-Gide®	100
Chen et al.[7]	Not specified	Bio-Oss®, Bio-Oss® and Bio-Gide®, no regeneration	100
Lang et al.[71]	> 1mm	Bio-Oss® and Bio-Gide®	-
Lindeboom et al.[64]	Not specified	Autogenous corticocancellous bone and membrane	92
Vila and Rangert[80]	> 1mm	Small gaps: autogenous bone + film celluloses Large gaps: Bio-Oss®	100
Vanden Bogaerde et al.[82]	Not specified	No defect: no regeneration Closed defect: autologous bone graft Open defect: bone graft + resorbable membrane	100
Schropp et al.[56]	< 2mm	Spontaneous healing	91

4.7.2 When grafting, which is the best biomaterial? Is a membrane necessary? Is it necessary to obtain primary wound closure?

Bovine bone matrix and resorbable collagen membranes are the most common grafting materials applied, when the distance between the implant and the bone wall needs to be filled in order to reduce crestal bone resorption.[7,41,57,71,72,74,80] Most studies report the use of Bio-Oss® and Bio-Gide® (Geistlich, Wolhusen, Switzerland) when the gap exceeds 1 mm.[41,71,72] Nonetheless, other materials like mineralized bone allograft and autogenous bone graft with and without plasma rich in growth factors (PRGF), have also been used successfully in order to treat these gaps (Table 4-7).[7,20,41,56,57,64,67,71,72,74,80-82] In a prospective randomized study evaluating healing of marginal defects in immediate transmucosal implants grafted, the three groups (receiving Bio-Oss®, Bio-Oss® and resorbable collagen membrane, and no graft as a control group) presented no significant differences regarding vertical defects.[7] Although horizontal resorption was significantly greater in the control group, the survival rate was 100%.[7]

When grafting of the gap is performed, in order to prevent soft tissue migration, it is still unclear if it is necessary to place a membrane or if placement of a provisional restoration is sufficient.[52,83] In the case of placing a resorbable membrane, it is preferable to obtain primary closure, either by coronally positioning the flap or with pedicle flap techniques, in order to reduce membrane exposure and have a more predictable grafting outcome.[7,17,51,52,72,84,85]

Recommendations

Gap distance:

- Gap ≥ 2 mm: grafting is recommended.
- Gap 1–2 mm: unclear if grafting is necessary, spontaneous healing has been described.

Gap grafting material:

- Best grafting material is controversial; various materials (autograft, xenograft, or allograft) may be used with favorable results.

Gap primary closure:

- It is unclear if primary closure is necessary when grafting the gap.

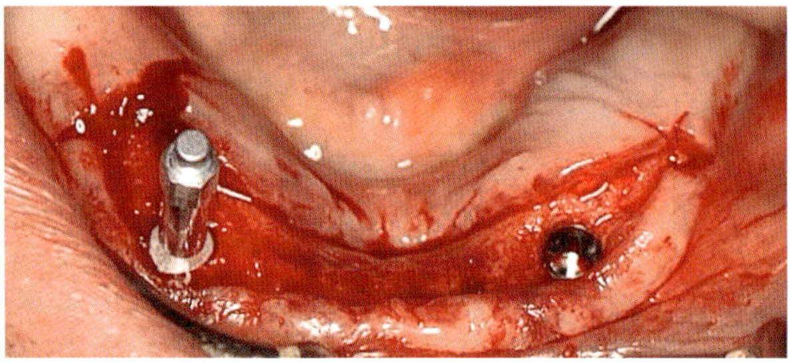

Fig 4-15a Smart peg placed in a NobelActive® implant (Nobel Biocare, Zurich, Switzerland).

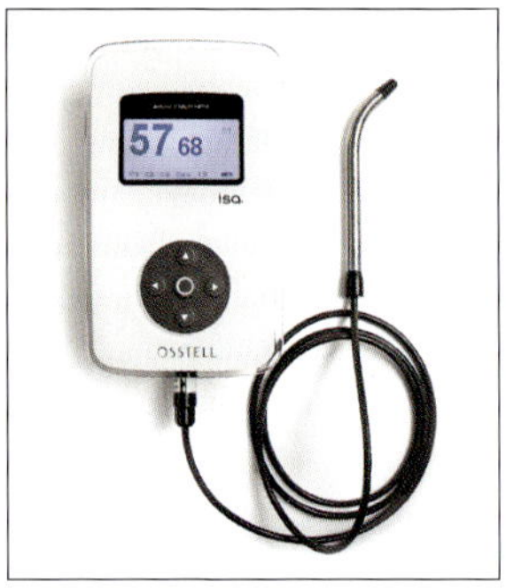

Fig 4-15b Osstell ISQ® device for resonance frequency analysis (RFA).

Table 4-8 Primary stability measurements according to the literature

Reference	Insertion torque (N/cm)	ISQ
Calvo-Guirado et al.[62]	-	> 60 (mean 71.1 ± 6.2)
Palattella et al.[59]	-	Test group: 65 ± 5 / 72 ± 3 Control group: 65 ± 5/ 73 ± 2
Lindeboom et al.[64]	-	6 months Immediate: 64.5 ± 3.9 Delayed: 64.5 ± 4.4
Canullo et al.[41]	Initial insertion 32–45	-
Ribeiro et al.[42]	40	-
Crespi et al.[67]	40	60

4.8 Implant primary stability

An important clinical factor to ensure osseointegration is primary implant stability; in the case of immediate implants this is mandatory. There are several methods described to measure this parameter. The most common are insertion torque (N/cm) and resonance frequency analysis (RFA), which can be measured using the Osstell Mentor® device (Osstell, Gothenburg, Sweden; Fig 4-15).[20,63,68,72,74,82] These measurements may be used as references to determine implant stability, using the implant stability quotient (ISQ). However, the only precise methods to determine BIC are histology and histomorphometric analysis.[3,86]

4.8.1 Are there significant differences in implant stability between immediate and delayed implants?

Studies comparing implant stability between delayed and immediately placed implants seem to indicate lower ISQ values in immediately placed implants compared with implants placed in pristine bone (Table 4-8).[41,42,59,62,64,67] Although these differences tend to disappear over time, ISQ values seem to increase progressively during healing over the first few months in immediate implants.[63,68,72]

Implant design may also have an effect in the primary stability obtained during implant placement. Many authors consider that it is easier to obtain primary stability with rough surfaces, aggressive thread design, and tapered implants.[53,71]

Recommendations

- Primary stability must be obtained during immediate implant placement.
- Tapered implants with aggressive threads may be beneficial.

4.9 Compromised situations

4.9.1 Immediate implants versus delayed implants: survival and success rates in molar sites

Most studies present comparable survival rates when comparing immediate and delayed implant placement in molar sites (Table 4-9).[50-52,72,78,87-91] However, there seems to be a slightly lower survival rate for implants placed in the maxilla, partly because most of them were associated with atraumatic sinus procedures and also as consequence of lower bone density, which makes obtain-

Table 4-9 Immediate implant placement in molar sites according to the literature

Reference	No. implants	Follow-up (months)	Survival rate (%)	Gap grafting	Technique
Schwartz-Arad et al.[91]	50 (16 maxilla, 35 mandible)	15	Maxilla: 82.3 Mandible: 92.3	Autogenous bone + resorbable and non-resorbable membranes	Submerged
Artzi et al.[90]	12 maxilla	9–90	88.6	β-TCP	Non-submerged
Bianchi and Sanfilippo[87]	42 maxilla, mandible	72–108	100	Autogenous connective tissue graft or without grafting	96 submerged 20 non-submerged
Fugazzotto[50]	83 maxilla	12.4	100	DFDBA + resorbable and non-resorbable membranes	Submerged
Wagenberg and Froum[78]	202 maxilla, 261 mandible	12–193	Maxilla: 93.56 Mandible: 95.02	FDBA + Vicryl membrane	Submerged
Levin et al.[88]	21 maxilla, mandible	6–125	100	Deproteinized bovine bone	Submerged
Penarrocha-Diago et al.[89]	32 maxilla, mandible	12	100	Autogenous bone	Non-submerged
Cafiero et al.[72]	82	12	100	Deproteinized bovine bone and resorbable membrane	Non-submerged
Fugazzotto[51]	391 maxilla	40.3	99.5	DFDBA + resorbable and non-resorbable membranes	Submerged
Fugazzotto[52]	341 mandible	30.8	99.1	Demineralized bovine bone with and without bone chips and covered resorbable and non-resorbable membranes; 9 implants were not grafted	Submerged except 9 implants

β-TCP, beta-Tricalcium phosphate; DFDBA, demineralized freeze-dried bone allograft; FDBA, freeze-dried bone allograft.

ing primary stability more difficult.[51,90] In molar sites the majority of implants were placed simultaneously with a grafting material. After this procedure most authors preferred to submerge the implant and obtain primary wound closure.[50-52,78,91] When a non-submerged approach was used the authors applied a healing abutment and displaced the soft tissue, adapting it as much as possible.[72,90] A few articles that analyze bone loss indicate similar results for implants placed in post-extraction and healed molar sites.[51,52,89,91]

Recommendations

- Immediate implants in molar sites seem to have similar survival rates to delayed implants; however, there is lack of information in relation to long-term success.
- Immediate implant placement in molar sites is technically challenging in terms of obtaining correct 3D positioning and soft tissue manipulation.

4.9.2 Immediate implants in periodontally affected sites

Immediate implants are indicated in the esthetic zone and in patients without periodontal affection. However, in recent years this concept has slightly altered. As a result of increased patient demands and the demonstrable results of immediate implant loading, one of the treatment options for periodontal patients with unsalvageable teeth is tooth extraction with immediate implant placement and loading.

It is clear that prior to immediate implant placement, periodontal patients must receive treatment including oral hygiene instructions, and scaling and root planing, to control the inflammation and minimize the effect on healing. After periodontal treatment, evidence suggests that if correct debridement is performed prior to placement, an immediate implant may be placed.[2,76,92]

Table 4-10 Immediate implant placement in patients with previous periodontal disease according to the literature

Reference	No. immediate implants	Follow-up	Mean bone loss (mm)	Cumulative survival rate (%)
Evian et al.[93]	43	943 days	-	P: 78.18
Wagenberg and Froum[78]	1925	1–16 years	-	P : 96.3 H: 91.8
Maló et al.[92]	433	5 years	1.7	P: 91
Horwitz et al.[95]	41	1 year	-0.71 to -0.99	P: 84
Deng et al.[96]	84 (50 maxilla, 34 mandible)	1 year	-1.12 ± 0.18	P: 95 (maxilla 92, mandible 100)
Alves et al.[97]	108 (74 maxilla, 85 mandible)	3 years	-	P: 98.74 (maxilla 98.65, mandible 98.82)

H, non-periodontal patients; P, periodontal history

4.9.3 Immediate implants versus delayed implants: survival rates and bone loss in periodontal patients

Some studies report immediate implant placement in patients with periodontal history, indicating comparable survival rates to delayed implant placement (Table 4-10).[70,78,92-97] However, there are few comparative studies with well-designed clinical protocols evaluating the effect of different timing of placement in periodontal patients and the relation with implant survival, as well as bone loss.[93,94]

Previous periodontal history should be considered a risk factor for immediate implant placement. More studies are necessary in order to give rigorous clinical long-term guidelines according to a patient's periodontal diagnosis.

Recommendations

- Patients with periodontal history have acceptable survival rates, but may present lower success rates, since reports suggest higher incidence of bone loss, increased probing depths, and peri-implantitis.
- There is limited evidence in periodontal patients to indicate similar survival rates for immediate and delayed implant placement.

4.10 Conclusions

- Interproximal bone level and soft tissue recession: crestal bone as well as soft tissue preservation could be achieved with either by immediate implant placement following tooth extraction or by a delayed protocol. No statistically significant differences were found in medium and long-term follow-up studies.
- Treatment of the gap between implant and bone wall: there is no consensus as to whether bone augmentation with GBR for immediate implants placed into fresh extraction sites is necessary, and which is the most predictable procedure. However Bio-Oss® and membrane therapy seem to show a higher buccal position of the gingival margin in the anterior area.
- Presence of periapical infection: chronic periapical infection is a risk factor but not an absolute contraindication for immediate implant placement. However, debridement of the alveolus should be performed. The presence of a periapical infection should be carefully considered.
- Implant primary stability: primary implant stability is an important factor in achieving osseointegration. Several methods have been used to quantify this parameter, such as insertion torque values and RFA. However, few scientific studies reveal comparative data between immediate and delayed implant placement. It seems that there are no significant differences between primary stability of immediate and delayed implants, and in both cases implant stability increases during the healing process.
- Immediate implants in molar sites: immediate implants in molar sites seem to have similar survival rates to delayed implants. However, each case has to be analyzed, weighing the potential benefits and disadvantages.

Figs 4-16 to 4-28 Case 1.

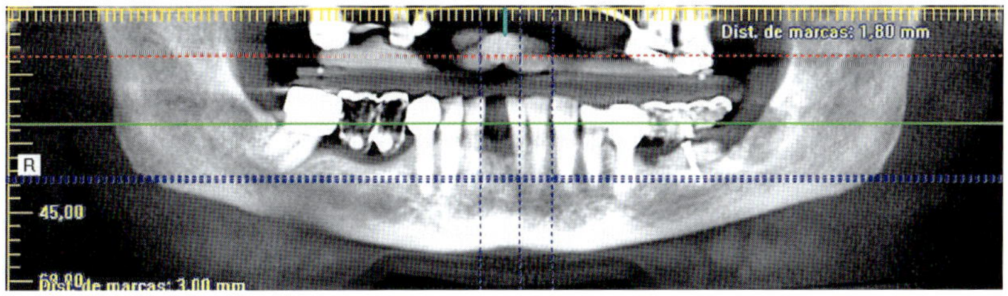

Fig 4-16 Pretreatment panoramic radiograph.

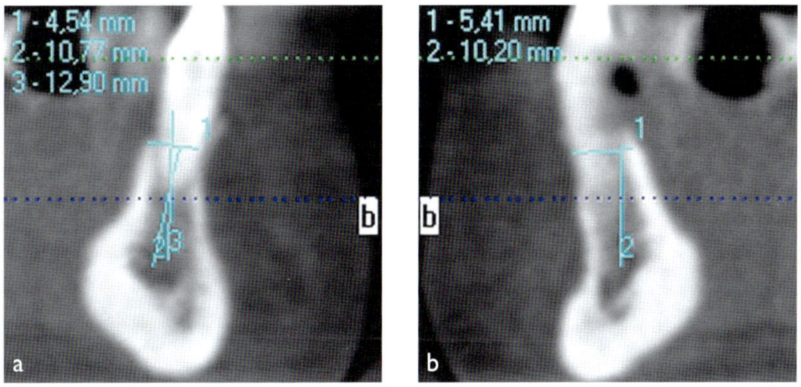

Figs 4-17a and b Measurement of available apical bone on CT (computerized tomography) scan.

- Periodontal disease: there is limited evidence indicating similar survival rates with immediate or delayed implant placement in periodontal patients. Nevertheless, periodontal history should be considered a risk factor for implant placement and the patient should be informed.
- Based on the literature discussed in this chapter, immediate implant placement following tooth extraction may be a viable alternative to delayed placement. However, it requires careful case selection and a specific treatment protocol because it is a very sensitive technique and more difficult to execute than a conventional protocol.

4.11 Clinical cases

Case 1 (Figs 4-16 to 4-28)

Presented is an example of two immediate implants placed in the anterior mandible. A 64-year-old patient attended the University Dental Clinic (Clínica Universitaria Odontológica [CUO]) at the International University of Catalonia (Universitat Internacional de Catalunya [UIC]).

The patient suffered a stroke 5 years previously and a postoperative pulmonary embolism. She also presented with hypertension. The patient was referred to the current specialist for any necessary preventive measures prior to oral surgery treatment.

To plan the treatment, a full prosthetic and radiological study was performed (Fig 4-16).

The available apical bone was detected for stabilization of immediate implants following tooth extraction (as teeth were periodontally hopeless) (Fig 4-17).

Careful debridement was undertaken and an atraumatic dental extraction was performed, keeping all bone walls available (Figs 4-18 to 4-20).

Implant placement was performed according to commercial brand protocol (Figs 4-21 and 4-22). Ideally implants should be finally inserted with a torque wrench to ensure optimal primary stability (Fig 4-23).

The jumping distance left between the implant surface and the bone wall was less than 2 mm; therefore, it healed spontaneously (Fig 4-24). The flap did not involve buccal bone wall to minimize bone loss in this critical area. Sutures were made to approximate the wound (Fig 4-25).

Postoperative radiographs were taken (Figs 4-26) to control implant placement. Wound healing 1 week after implant surgery is shown in Fig 4-27.

Radiologic control 3 months post-surgery is shown in Fig 4-28. The bundle bone had been resorbed although the implants were osseointegrated. The implants did not present dehiscence, but had a very thin buccal bone wall.

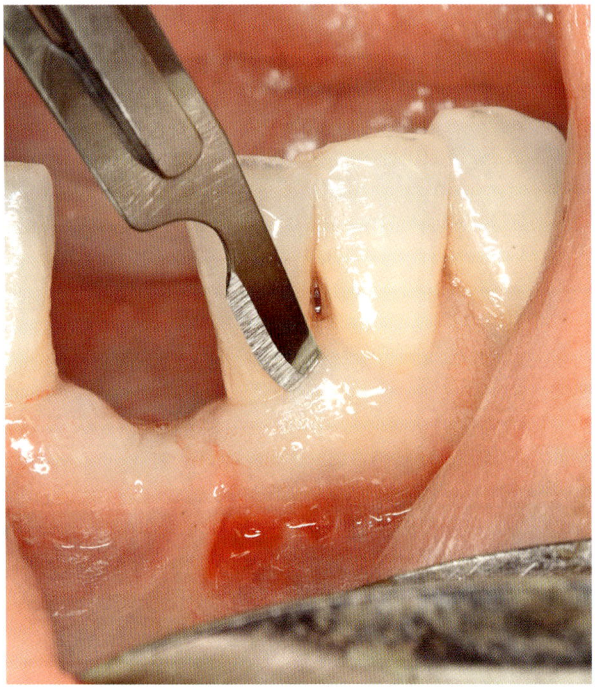

Fig 4-18 Debridement.

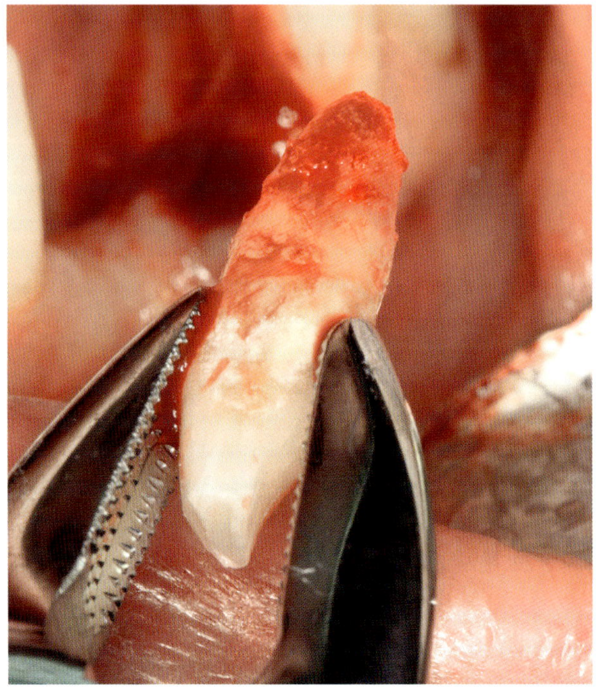

Fig 4-19 Extraction.

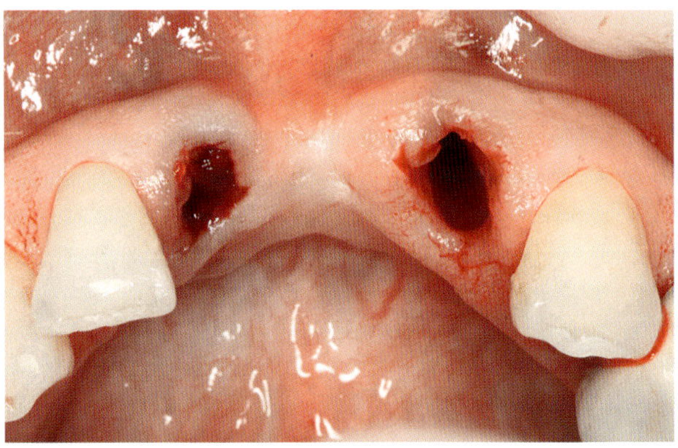

Fig 4-20 Atraumatic dental extraction, keeping all bone walls available.

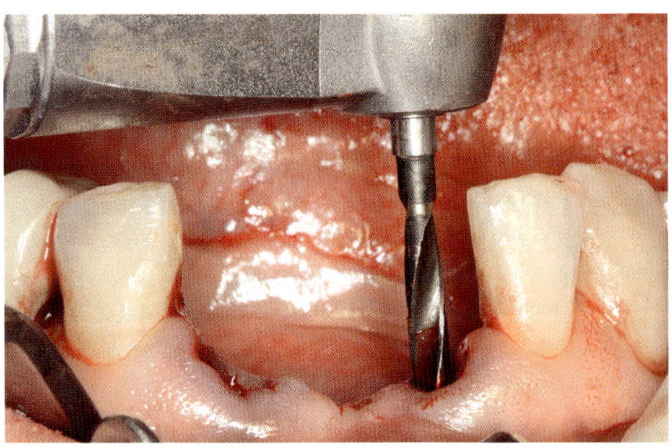

Fig 4-21 Implants were placed according to commercial brand protocol.

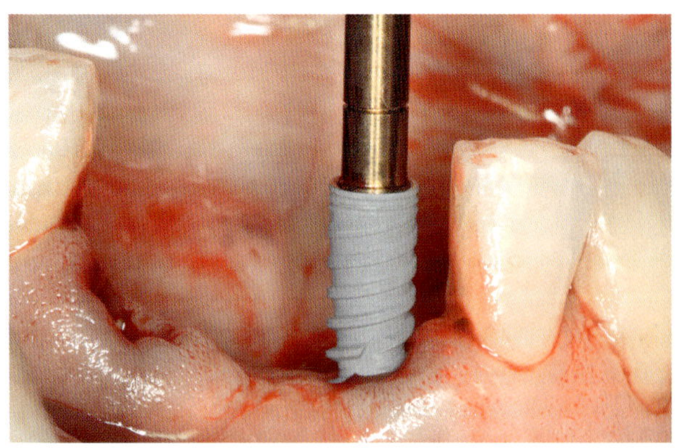

Fig 4-22 Implant placement.

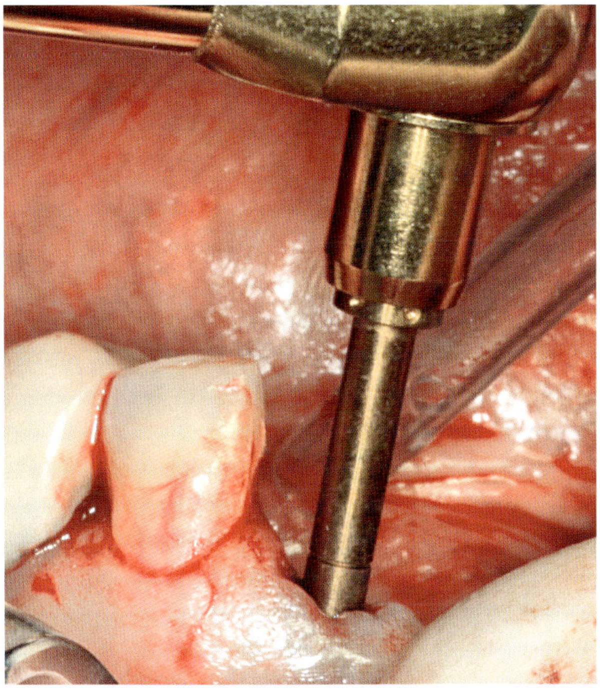

Fig 4-23 Ideally implant should be finally inserted with torque wrench to ensure optimal primary stability.

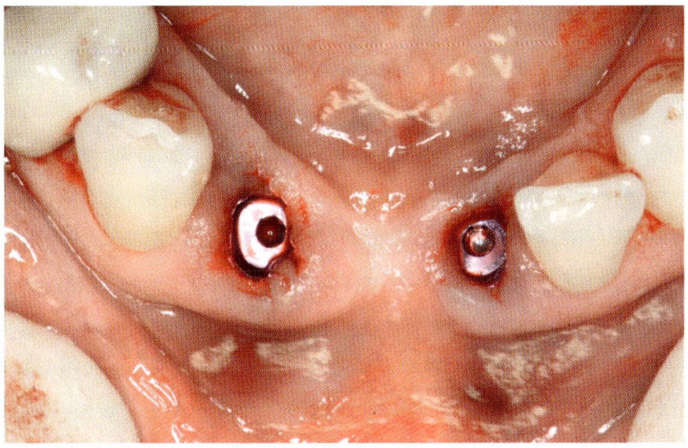

Fig 4-24 Occlusal view. Note implants are placed slightly palatally.

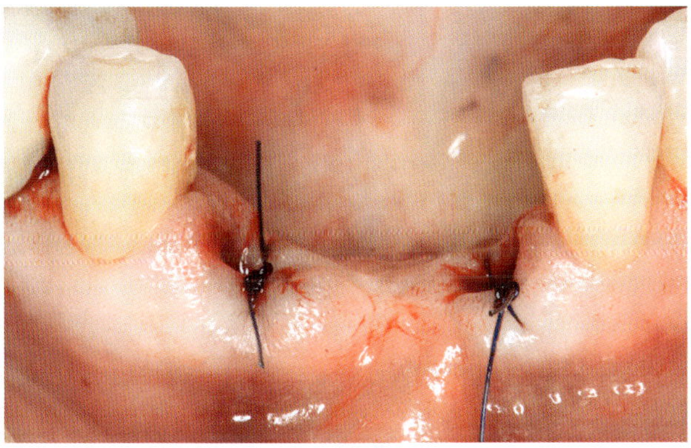

Fig 4-25 The wounds are sutures tension-free.

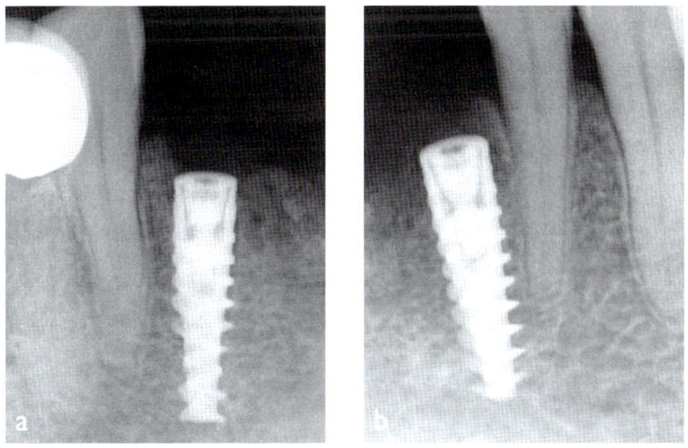

Figs 4-26a and b Postoperative radiograph to control implant placement.

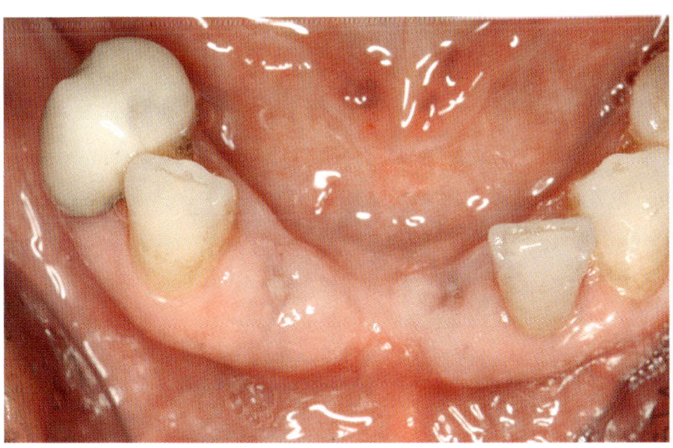

Fig 4-27 Wound healing 1 week postoperatively.

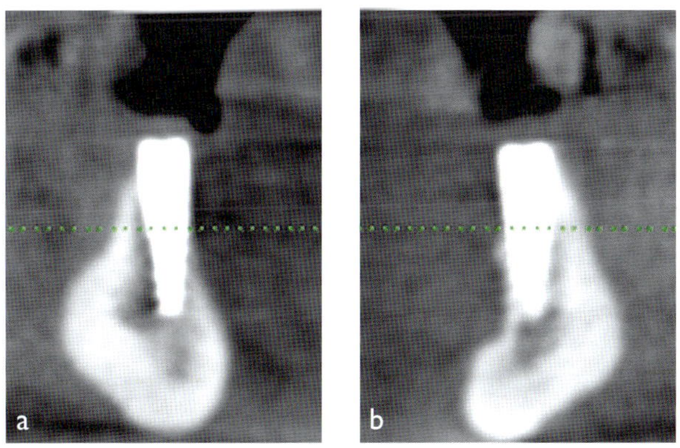

Figs 4-28a and b Radiographs taken 3 months after surgery.

Case 2 (Figs 4-29 to 4-47)

A 45-year-old patient attended the CUO at the IUC to rehabilitate teeth 24 to 26. The patient had no medical concerns; however, he smoked up to 10 cigarettes a day.

A radiological study was performed (Figs 4-29 to 4-32). There was a retained root in the area of tooth 24. Sufficient apical bone was present to ensure primary stability of both dental implants. The clinical preoperative situation is shown in Fig 4-33. Careful debridement was performed before dental extraction (Fig 4-34). A 15C surgical blade is commonly used for ultrafine precision of an atraumatic debridement before dental extraction (Fig 4-35).

Special care was taken to preserve all socket walls (Fig 4-36). The flap did not involve buccal bone wall to minimize bone loss in this critical area (Fig 4-37).

Implant placement is shown in Figs 4-38 to 4-40. The insertion torque was 35 Ncm and the ISQ was over 60, as measured using RFA.

As the gap was over 2 mm, this was filled with a biomaterial and covered with a collagen membrane (Fig 4-40). Resorbable membrane was left exposed and sutured tension-free (Fig 4-41). Figures 4-42 and 4-43 show the healing 1 week post-operatively. Soft tissue healing was by second intention as the wound progress was not ideal (Figs 4-42 and 4-43).

The occlusal view before prosthetic rehabilitation is shown in Fig 4-44. Prosthetic abutments were created (Fig 4-45). The cemented final restoration is shown in Fig 4-46, and Fig 4-47 shows the buccal view of the final restoration.

Figs 4-29 to 4-47 Case 2.

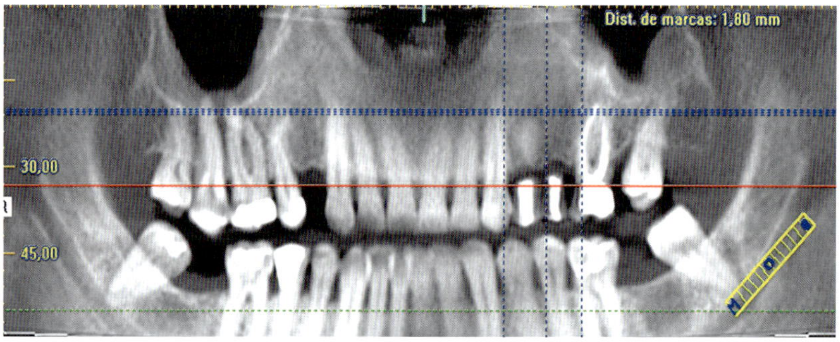

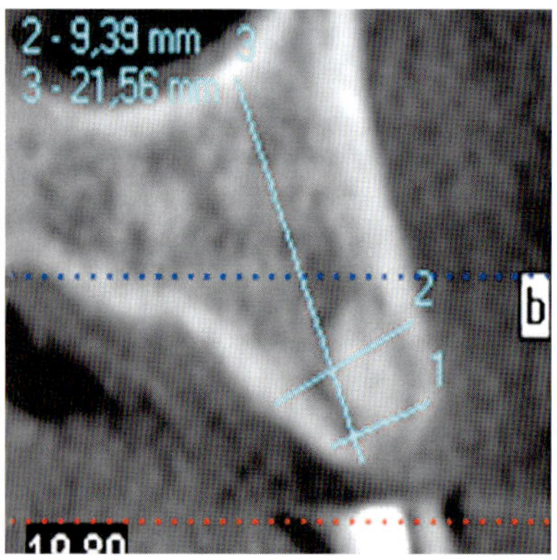

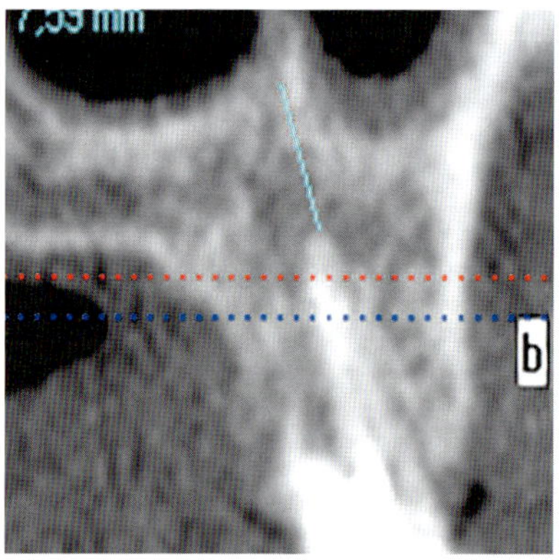

Figs 4-29 to 4-31 Preoperative CT (computerized tomography) scans.

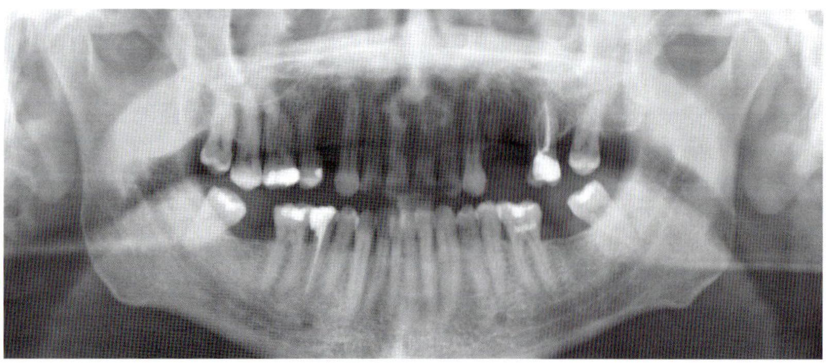

Fig 4-32 Preoperative panoramic radiograph.

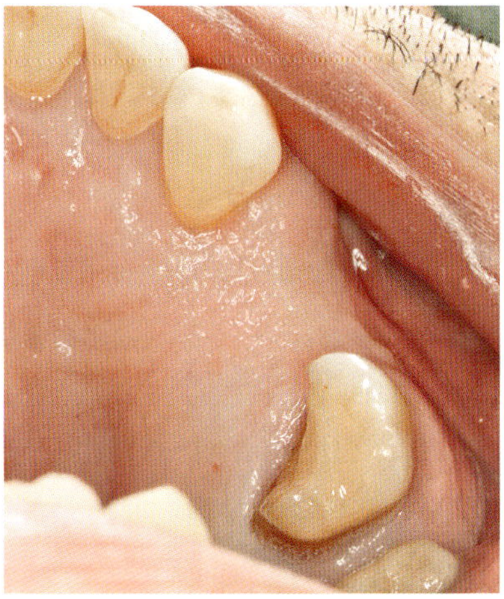

Fig 4-33 Clinical preoperative situation.

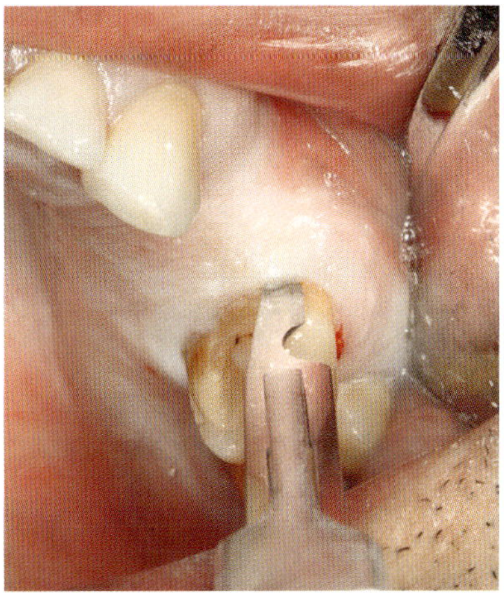

Fig 4-34 Debridement.

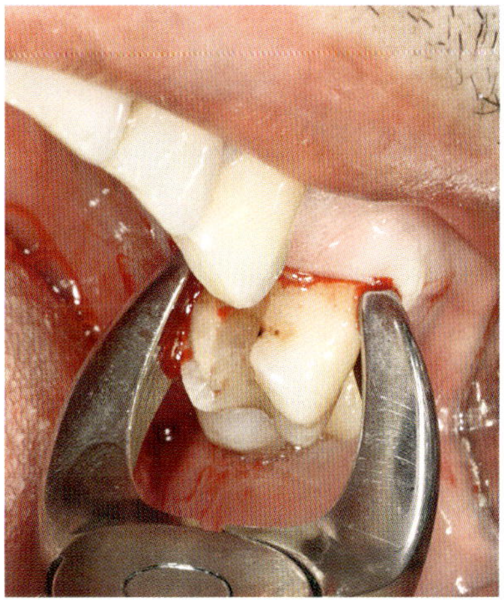

Fig 4-35 Extraction.

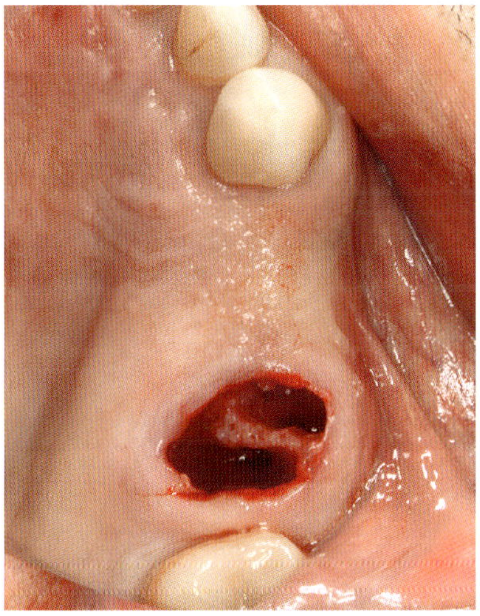

Fig 4-36 Care was taken to preserve socket walls.

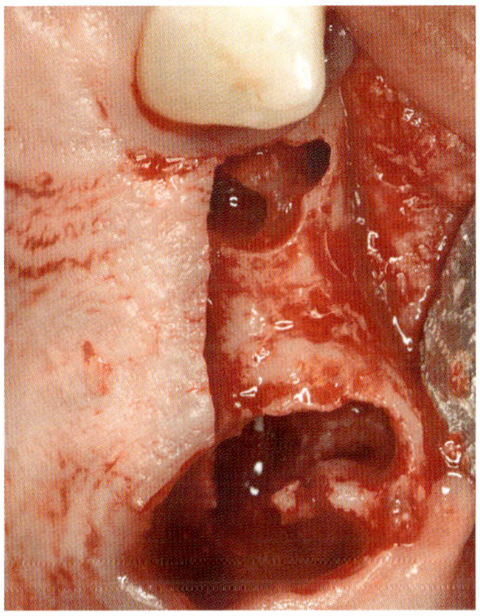

Fig 4-37 The flap did not involve buccal bone wall to minimize bone loss in this critical area.

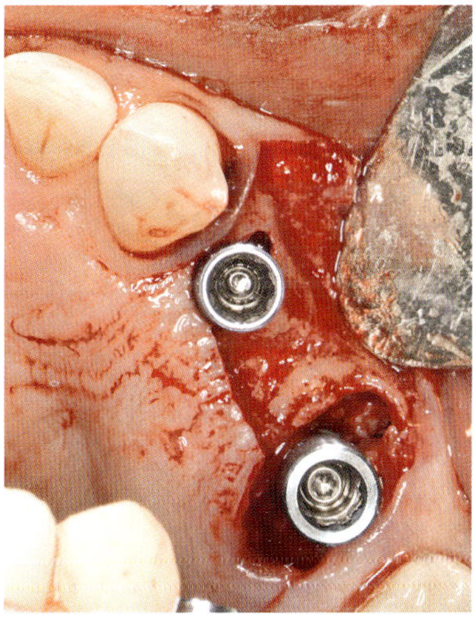

Fig 4-38 Implant placement.

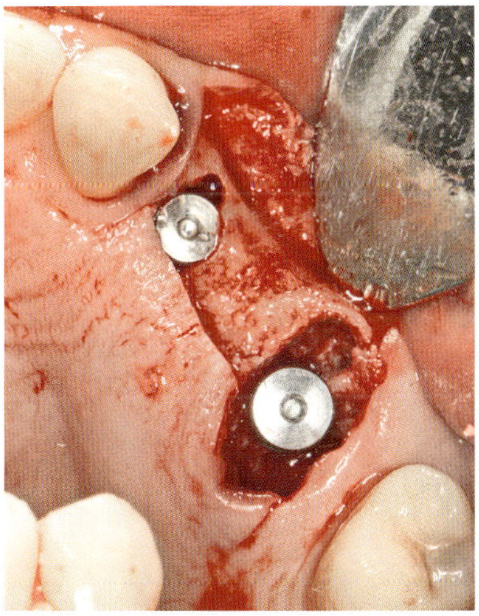

Fig 4-39 Implant placement.

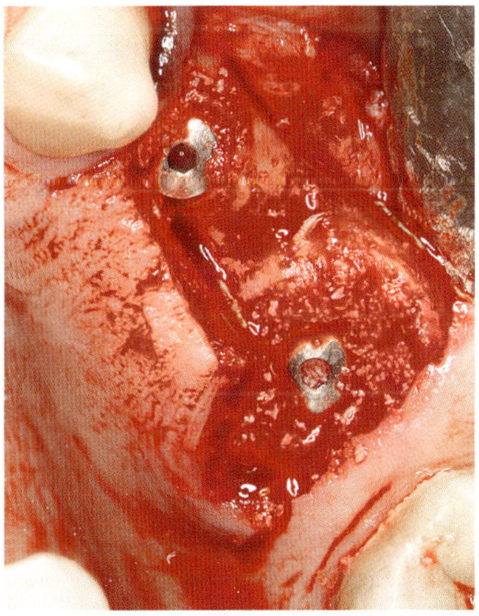

Fig 4-40 The gap was filled with a biomaterial and covered with a collagen membrane.

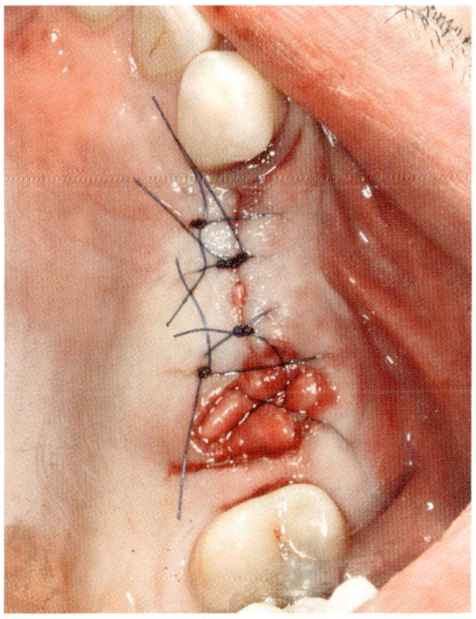

Fig 4-41 Resorbable membrane was left exposed and sutured tension-free.

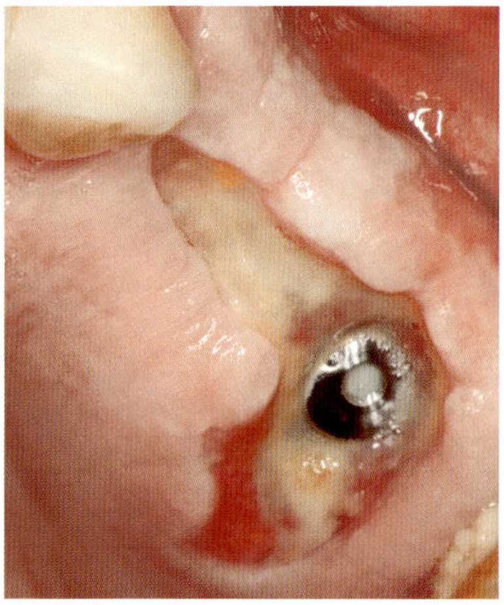

Fig 4-42 Healing 1 week postoperatively.

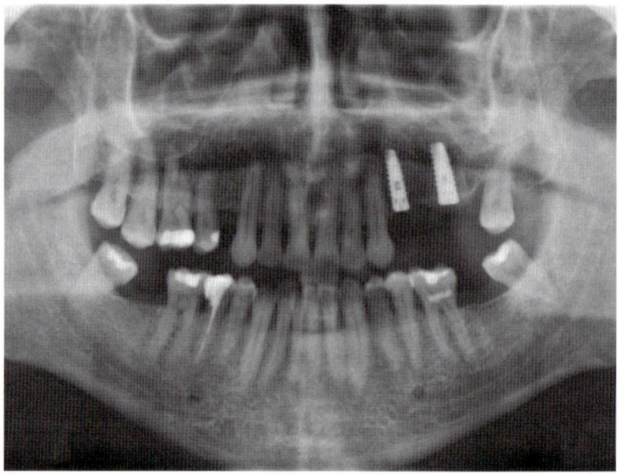

Fig 4-43 Panoramic radiograph taken 1 week postoperatively to control placement of implants.

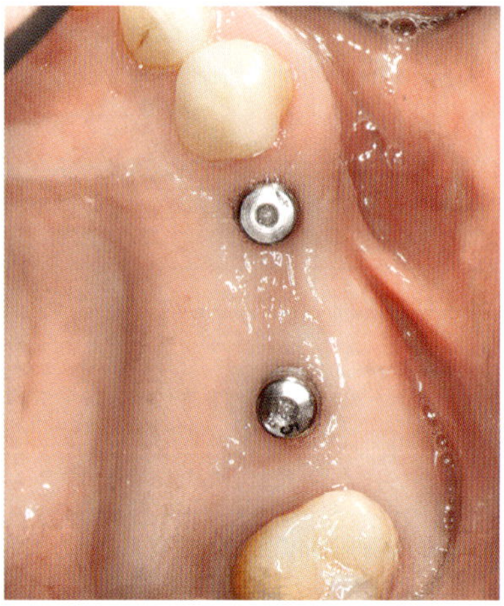

Fig 4-44 Occlusal view before prosthetic restoration.

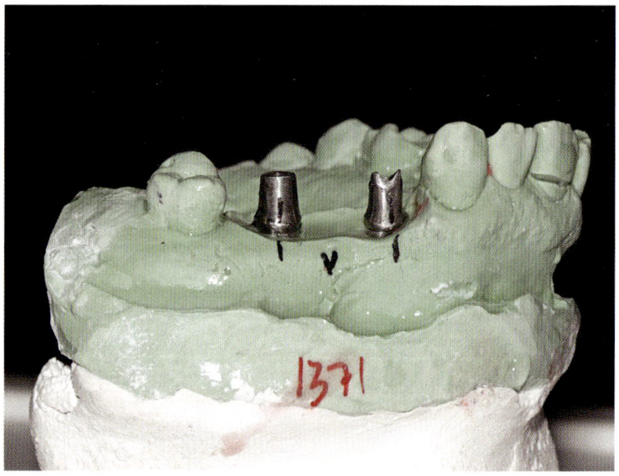

Fig 4-45 Creation of prosthetic abutments.

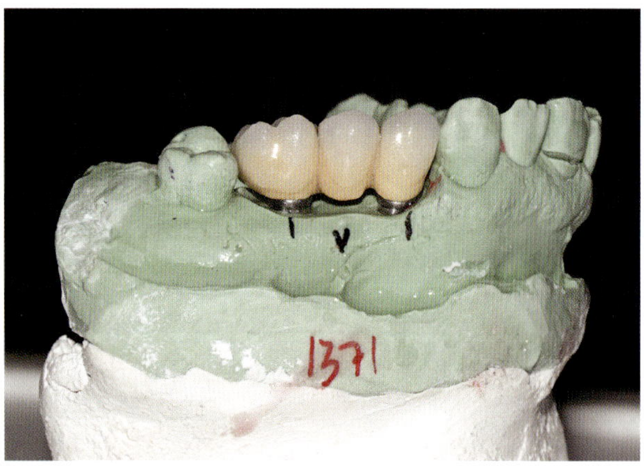

Fig 4-46 The cemented final restoration.

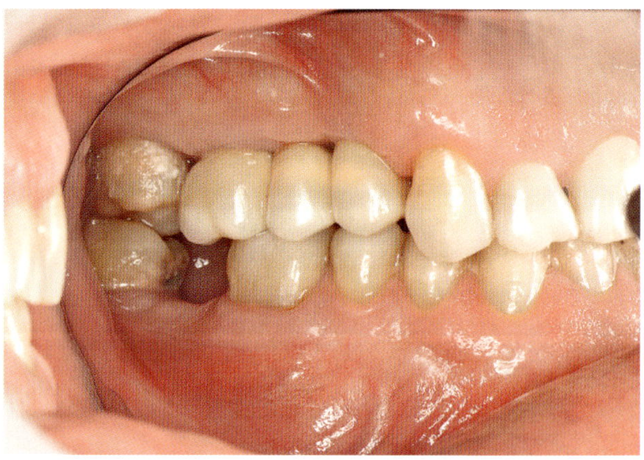

Fig 4-47 Buccal view of final restoration.

Case 3 (Figs 4-48 to 4-59)

A 62-year-old patient attended the CUO at UIC to rehabilitate her oral cavity with a full maxillary and mandibular prosthodontic–implant rehabilitation.

She did not present with any medical concerns, and was a non-smoker.

Debonding of the fixed partial denture (FPD) positioned at 23 left an unrestorable canine root with no ferrule (Figs 4-48 and 4-49). Atraumatic dental extraction (Fig 4-50) was performed. Immediate postextraction implants were drilled on the palatal bone wall (Fig 4-51). The final implant position is shown in Figs 4-52 and 4-53.

There was early implant head exposure after 1 week of healing (Fig 4-54). Second-stage surgery was performed and there was an optimal amount of keratinized tissue surrounding the position 23 dental implant (Fig 4-55). Figures 4-56 to 4-59 show the final treatment outcome.

Figs 4-48 to 4-59 Case 3.

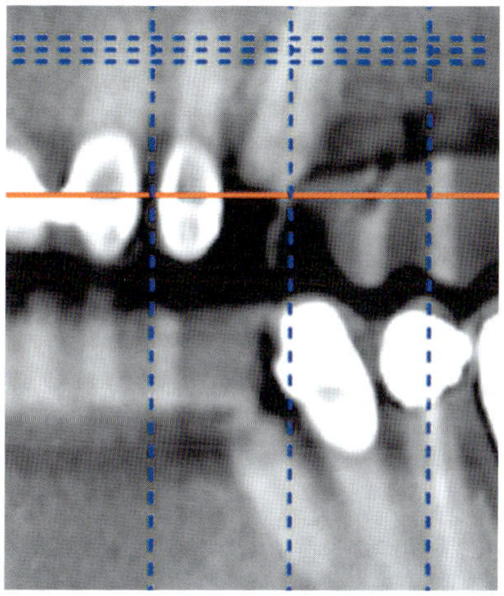

Fig 4-48 Pretreatment computerized tomography (CT) scan.

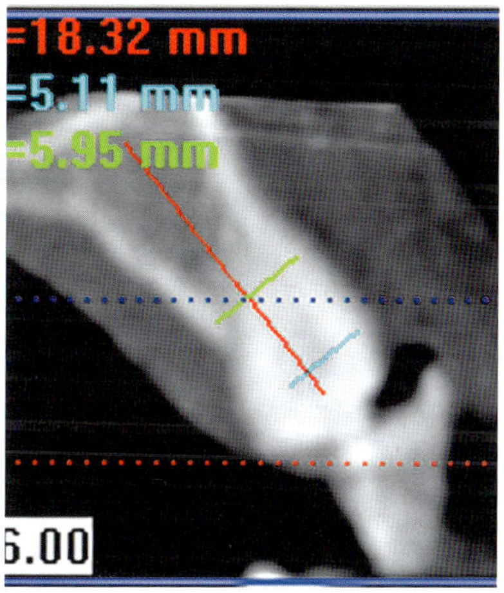

Fig 4-49 CT scan shows unrestorable canine root with no ferrule.

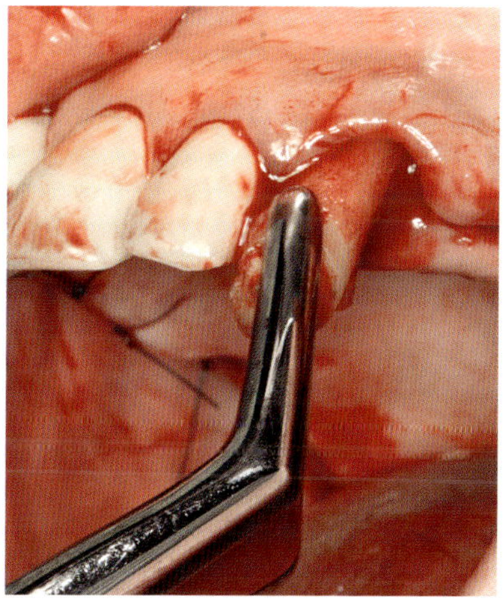

Fig 4-50 Atraumatic dental extraction.

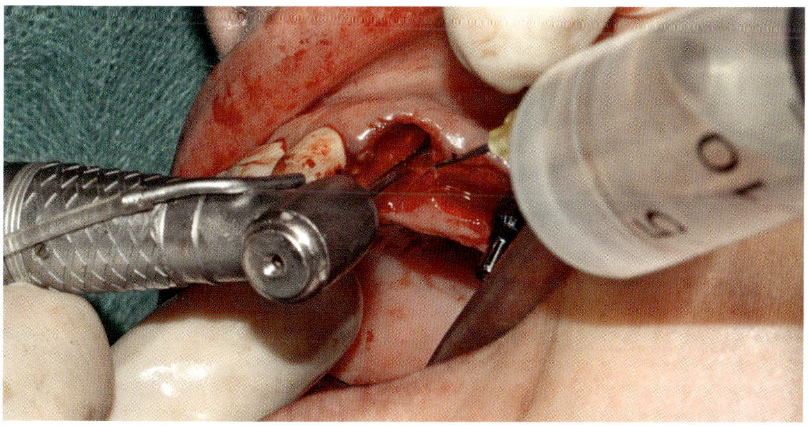

Fig 4-51 Postextraction implants were drilled on the palatal bone wall.

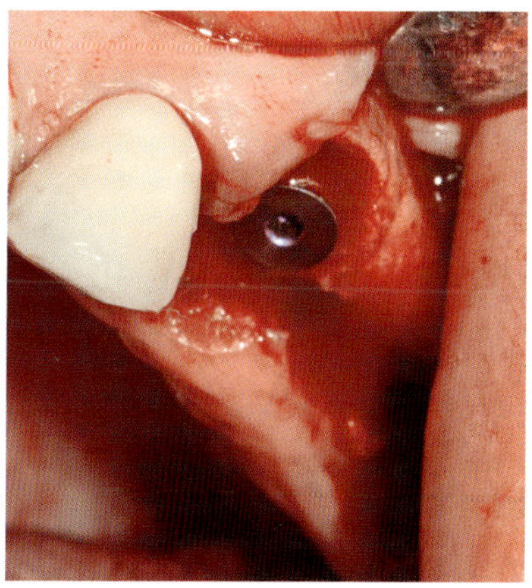

Fig 4-52 Immediate implant placement.

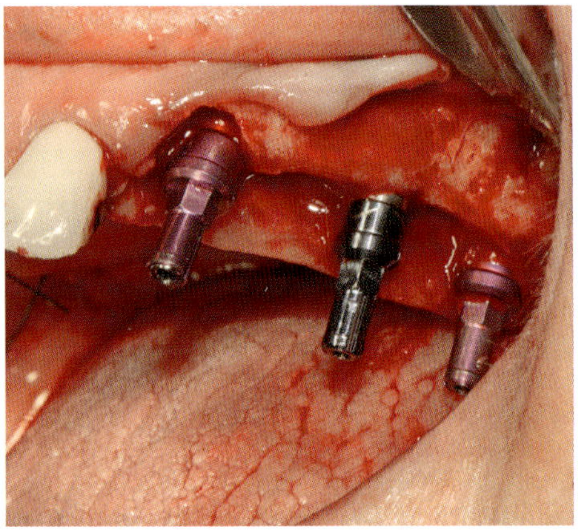

Fig 4-53 Final implant position.

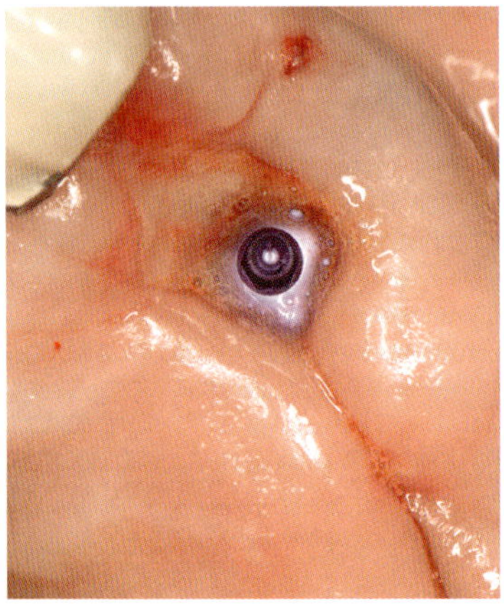

Fig 4-54 Early implant head exposure after 1 week of healing.

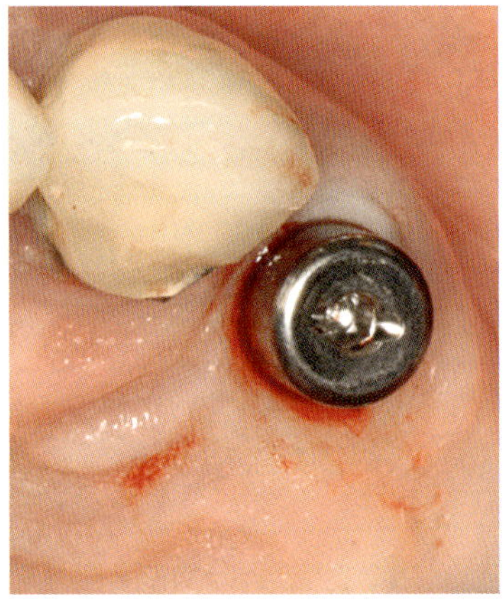

Fig 4-55 Second-stage surgery.

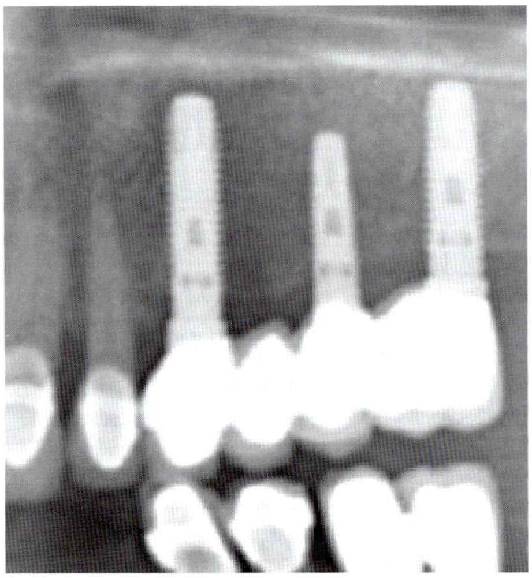

Fig 4-56 Radiograph showing final treatment outcome.

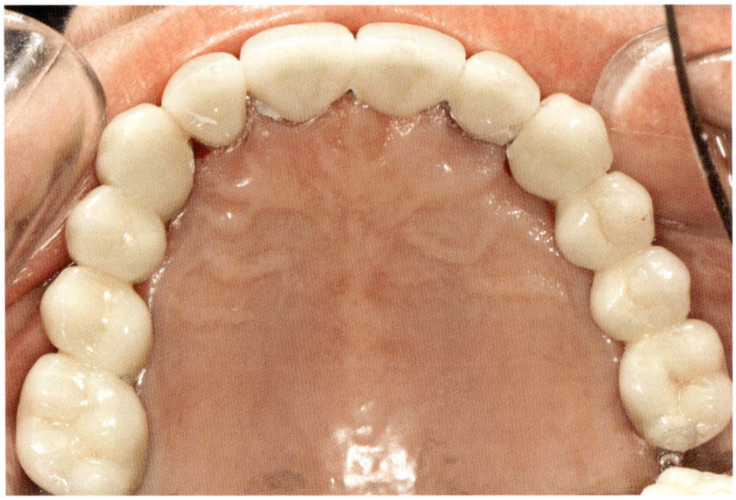

Fig 4-57 Final occlusal view.

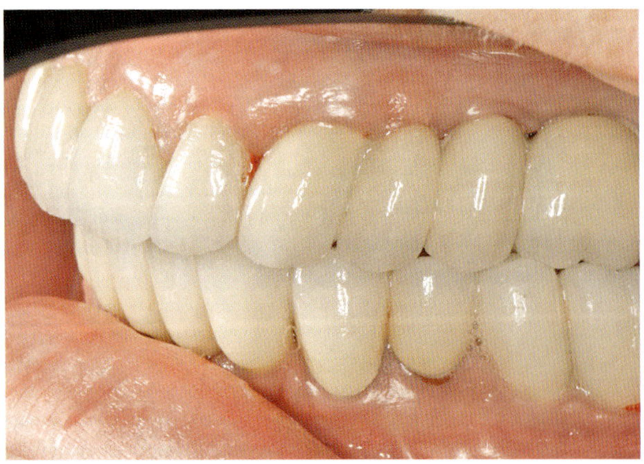

Fig 4-58 Final lateral view.

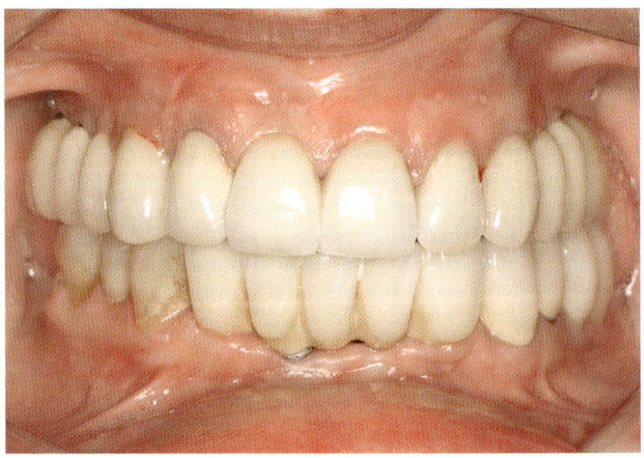

Fig 4-59 Final anterior view.

Case 4 (Figs 4-60 to 4-78)

A 61-year-old patient (Fig 4-60) attended the CUO at the UIC to rehabilitate tooth 43 due to fracture of the crown and lack of ferrule.

The patient presented no medical concerns and did not smoke. Intraoral photographs were taken (Figs 4-61 and 4-62). The radiological study (Figs 4-63 and 4-64) revealed the fractured root of tooth 43. There was sufficient apical bone to ensure primary stability.

Atraumatic extraction of the dental root was performed, maintaining the integrity of all socket walls (Fig 4-65). After careful debridement of the socket, the implant was placed in the interradicular septum (Figs 4-66), as the mandibular canine presented two roots. Since the gap was over 2 mm (Fig 4-67), a mucoperiosteal flap was elevated and biomaterial was placed (Bio-Oss®; Fig 4-68). A collagen membrane was placed over the regeneration (Bio-Gide®) (Fig 4-69).

For primary soft tissue closure, periosteal incisions were performed with coronal positioning of the flap (Fig 4-70). Postoperative radiographs were taken to check implant placement (Fig 4-71 and 4-72). Healing after implant placement is shown in Figs 4-73 and 4-74. The final crown is shown in Fig 4-75. Healing and final rehabilitation are shown in Figs 4-76 to 4-78.

Figs 4-60 to 4-78 Case 4.

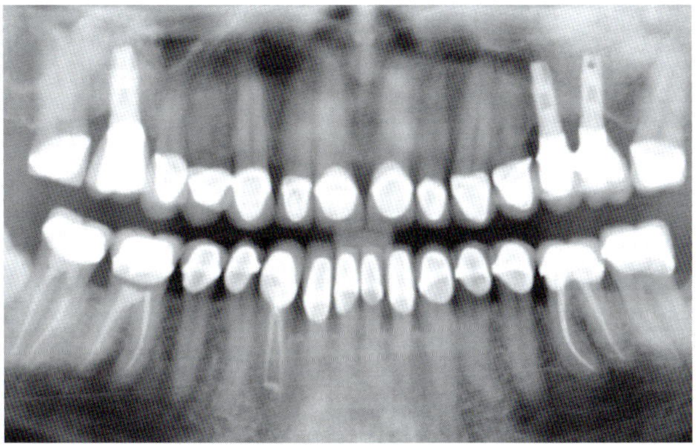

Fig 4-60 Panoramic radiograph taken prior to the tooth fracture.

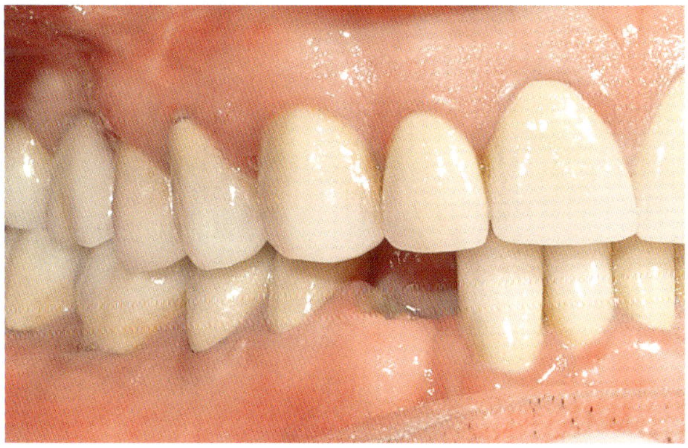

Fig 4-61 Initial lateral view of fractured tooth 43.

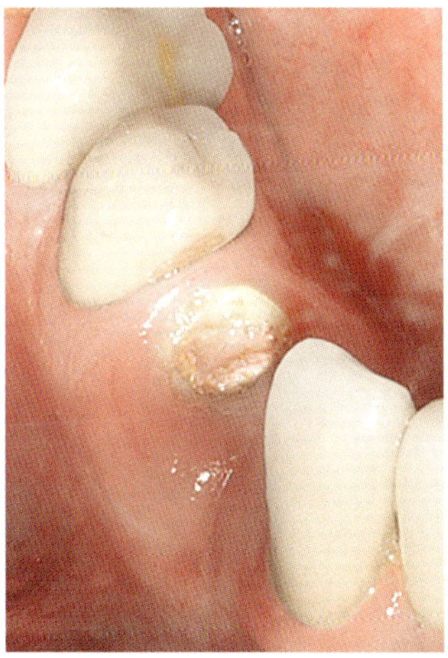

Fig 4-62 Initial occlusal view of fractured tooth 43.

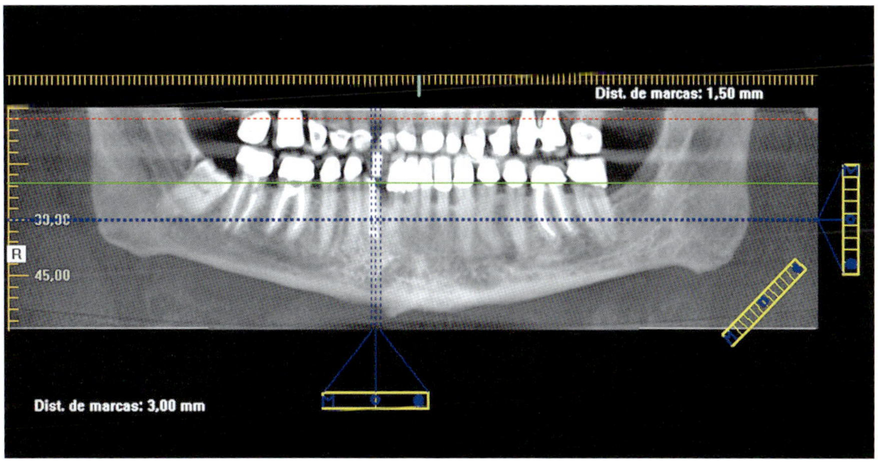

Fig 4-63 CT scan prior to immediate implant placement.

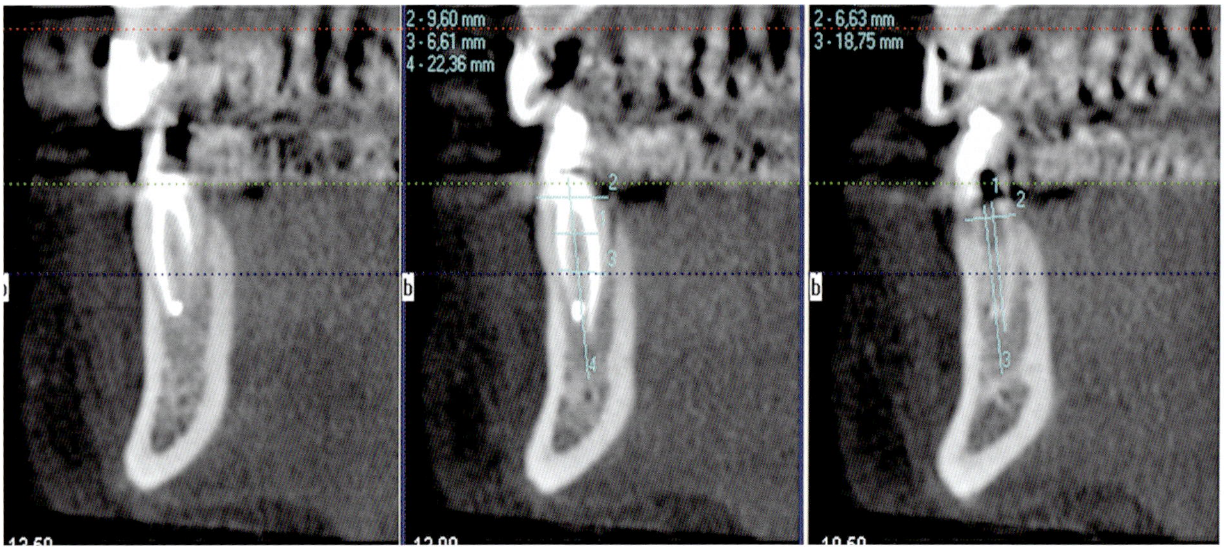

Fig 4-64 Details from CT axial scan showing measurements prior to immediate implant placement.

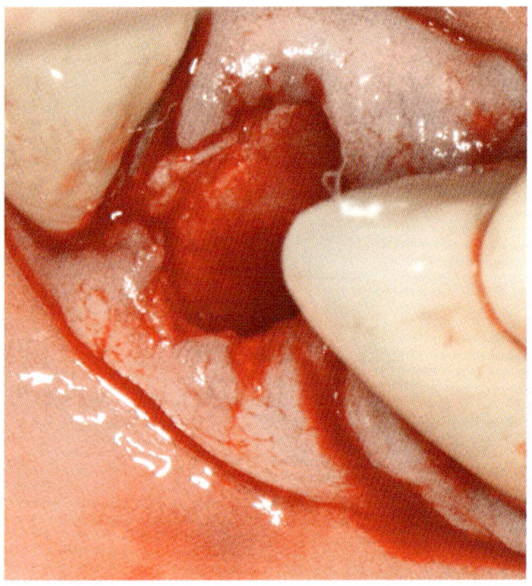

Fig 4-65 The socket after extraction.

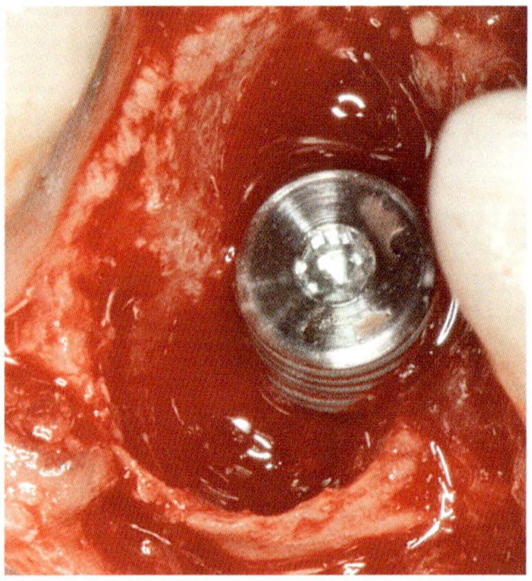

Fig 4-66 Immediate implant placement anchored to the interradicular septum.

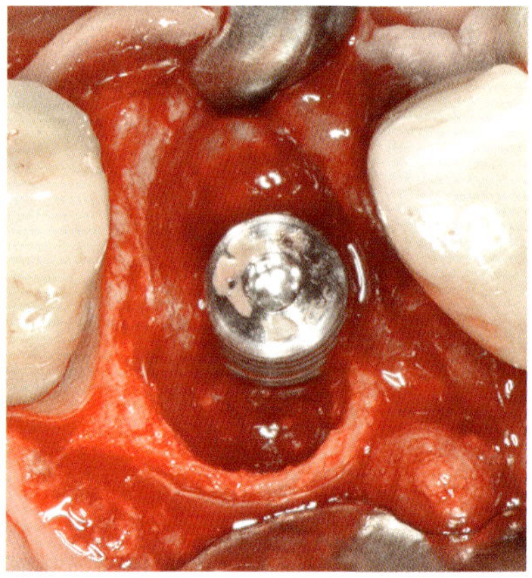

Fig 4-67 The gap distance over 2 mm.

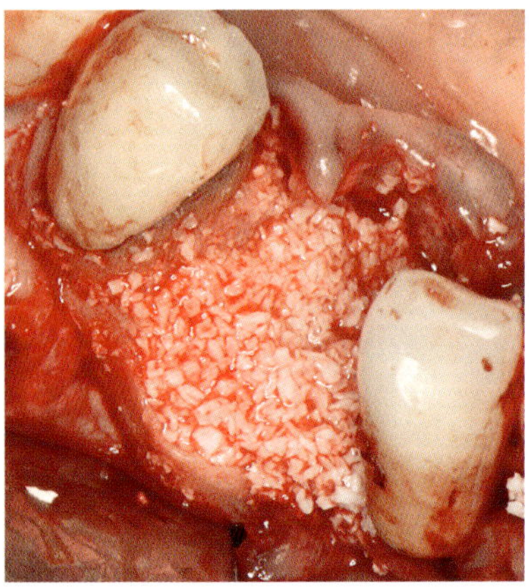

Fig 4-68 Mucoperisoteal flap and regeneration of the gap with biomaterial (Bio-Oss®).

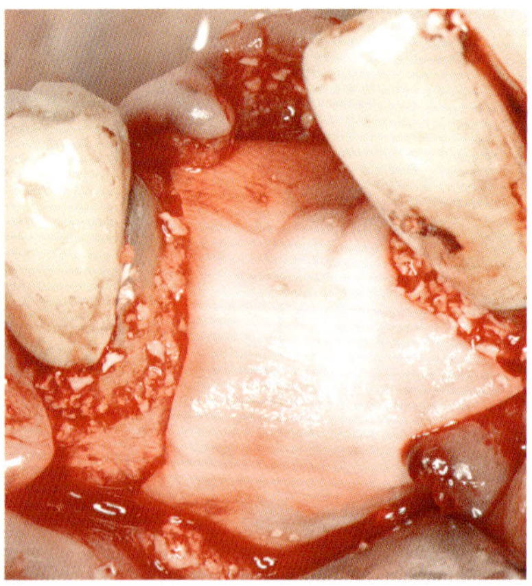

Fig 4-69 Placement of collagen membrane over the regeneration (Bio-Gide®).

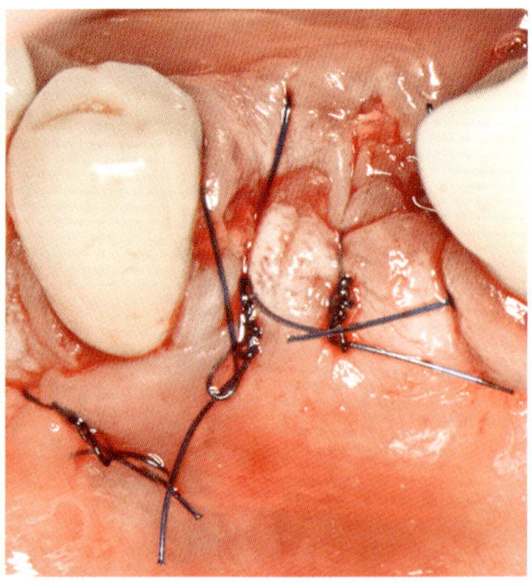

Fig 4-70 Primary soft tissue closure without tension.

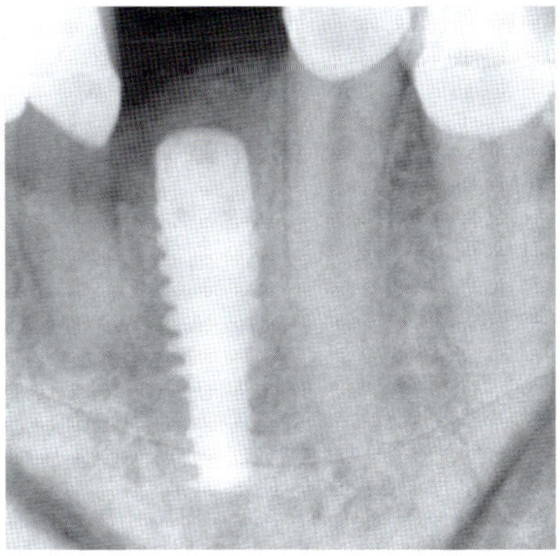

Fig 4-71 Periapical radiograph after immediate implant placement and regeneration.

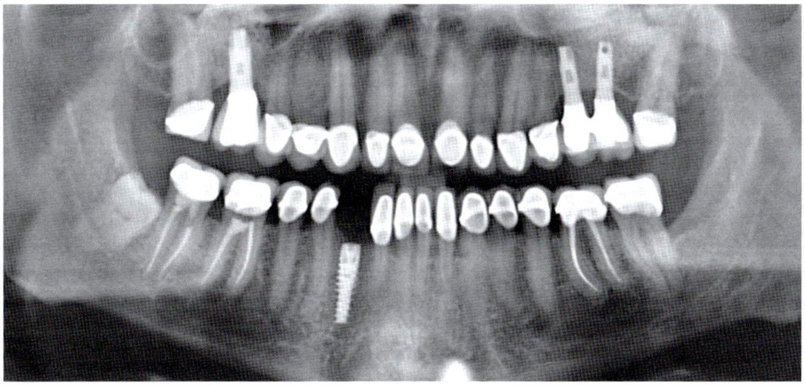

Fig 4-72 Panoramic radiograph after immediate implant placement.

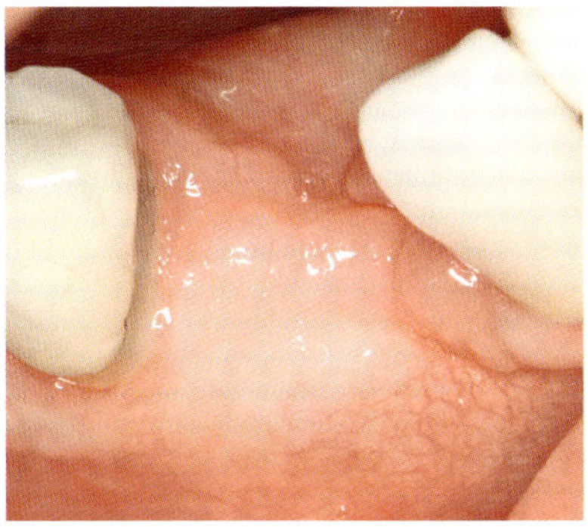

Fig 4-73 Situation 15 days postsurgery.

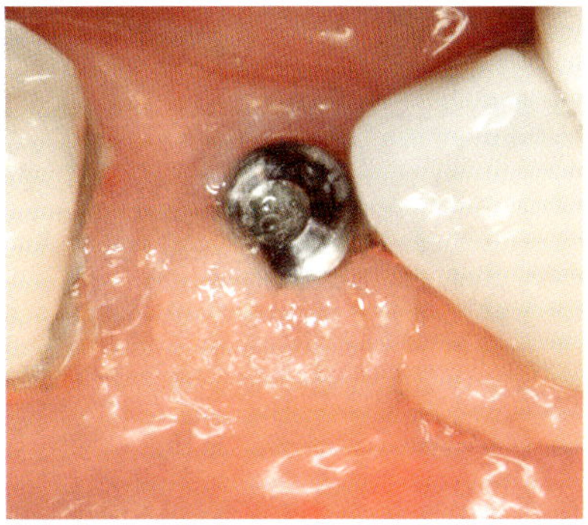

Fig 4-74 Healing after second-stage surgery.

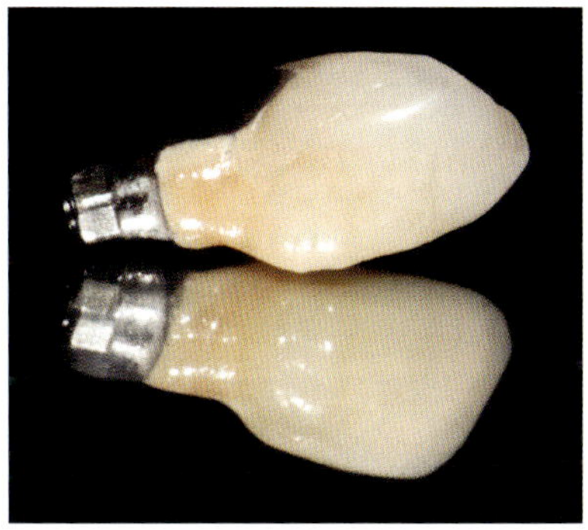

Fig 4-75 Final crown.

Fig 4-76 Final anterior view.

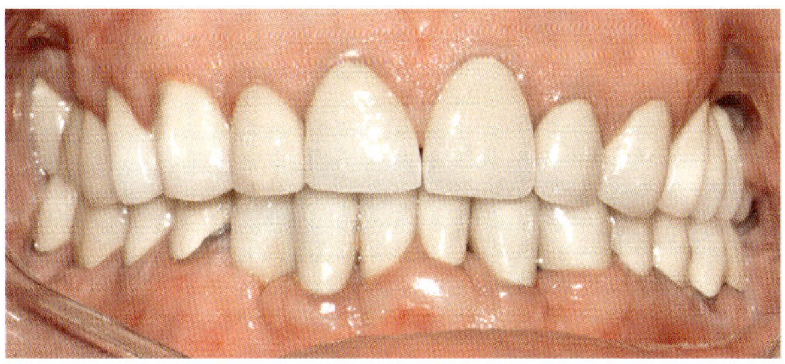

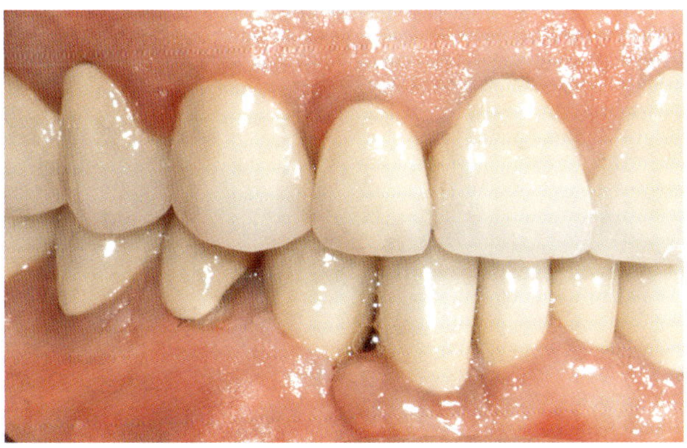

Fig 4-77 Final lateral view.

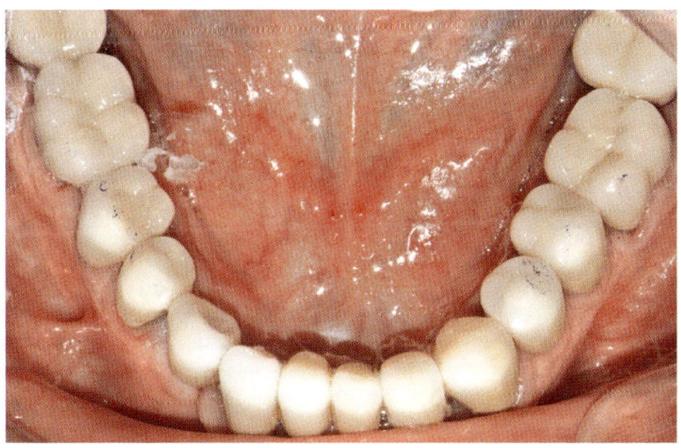

Fig 4-78 Final occlusal view.

Case 5 (Figs 4-79 to 4-91)

The patient attended the CUO at the UIC. The initial situation is shown in Figs 4-79 to 4-82. Two canine roots were extracted (Figs 4-83 and 4-85). In the first quadrant an implant was placed with a flapless approach, and since the gap was less than 2 mm it was not filled with biomaterial (Fig 4-84). In the second quadrant there was a fenestration during implant placement. A mucoperiosteal flap was raised (Fig 4-86) and regenerated with biomaterial and a membrane in the apical portion (Figs 4-87 and 4-88). One-week postoperatively it can be seen that the simple act of raising a flap led to increased bone resorption (Figs 4-89 to 4-91).

Figs 4-79 to 4-91 Case 5.

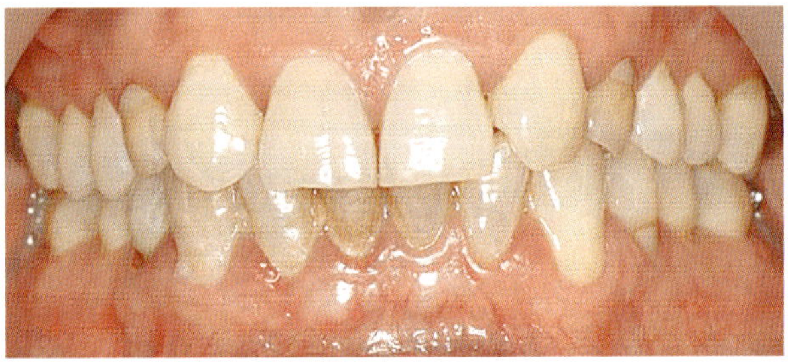

Fig 4-79 Initial anterior view.

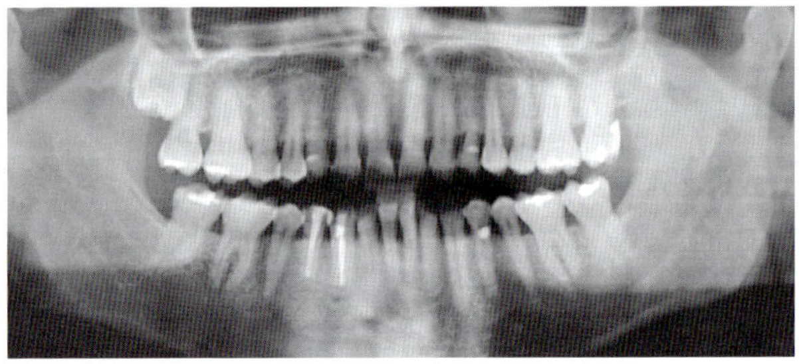

Fig 4-80 Initial panoramic radiograph.

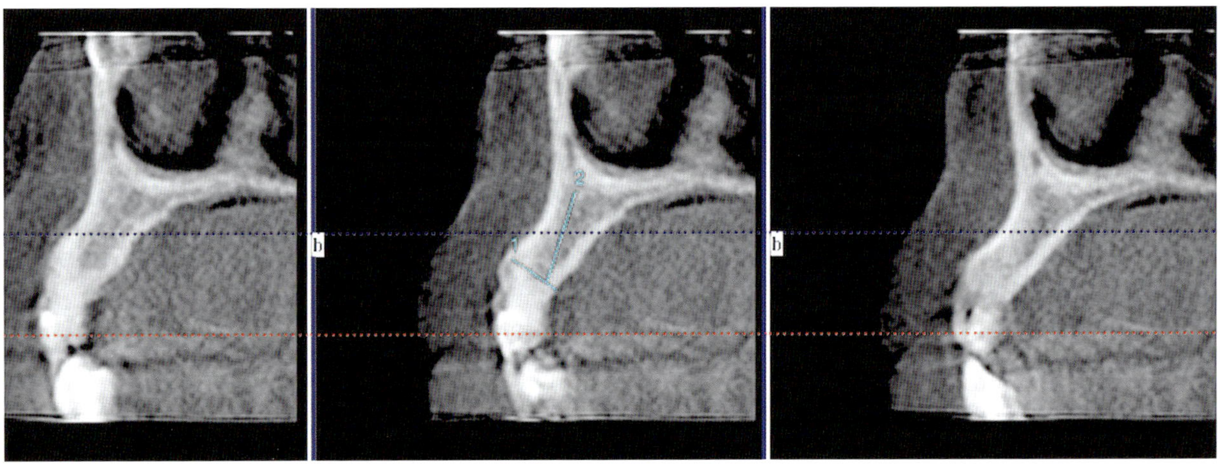

Fig 4-81 First quadrant CT scan.

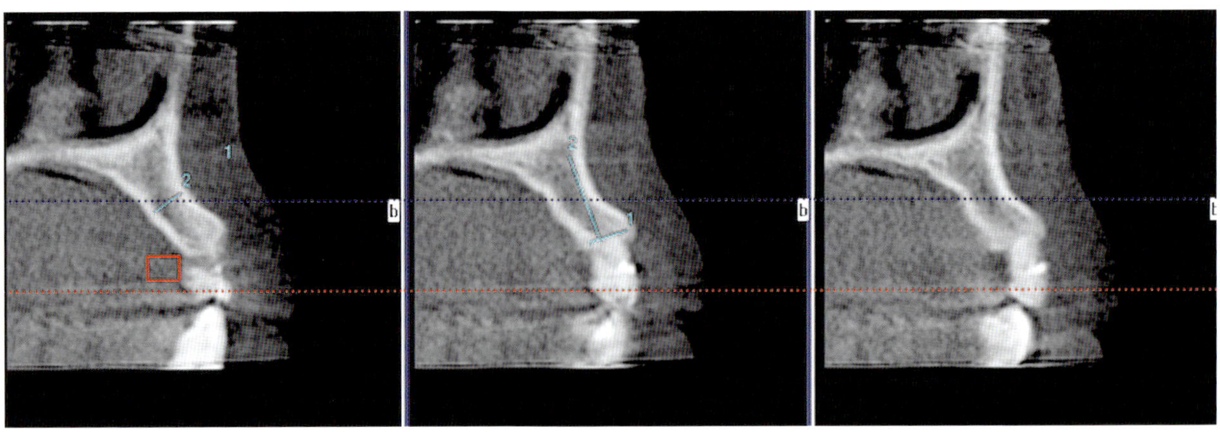

Fig 4-82 Second quadrant CT scan.

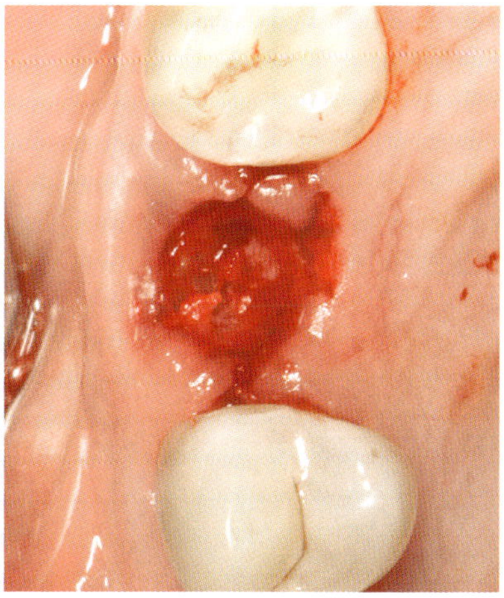

Fig 4-83 First quadrant: extraction socket.

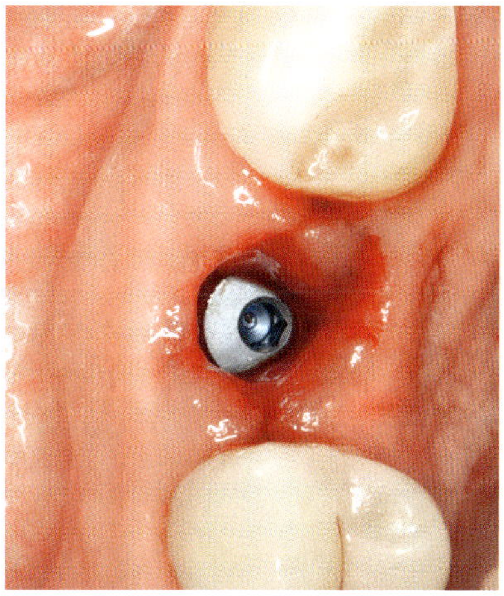

Fig 4-84 First quadrant: flapless implant placement without regeneration (gap less than 2 mm).

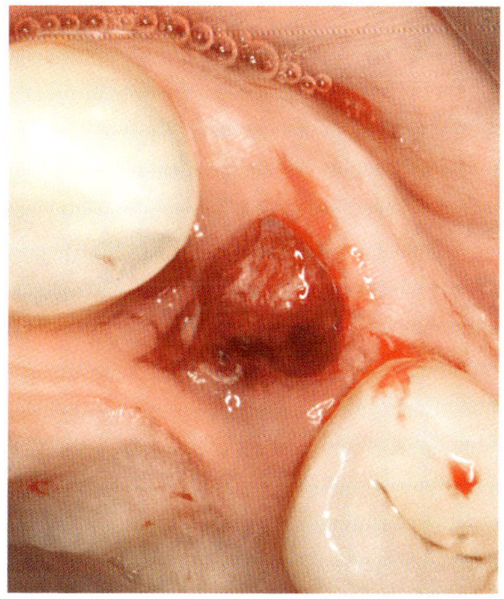

Fig 4-85 Second quadrant: extraction socket.

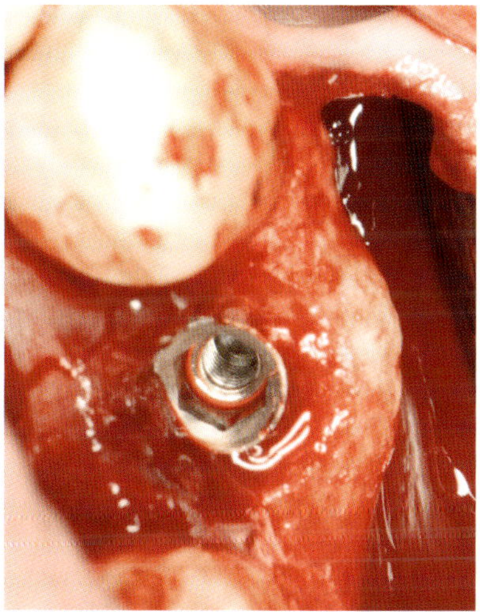

Fig 4-86 Second quadrant: immediate implant placement. Owing to fenestration during implant placement, a mucoperiosteal flap was raised.

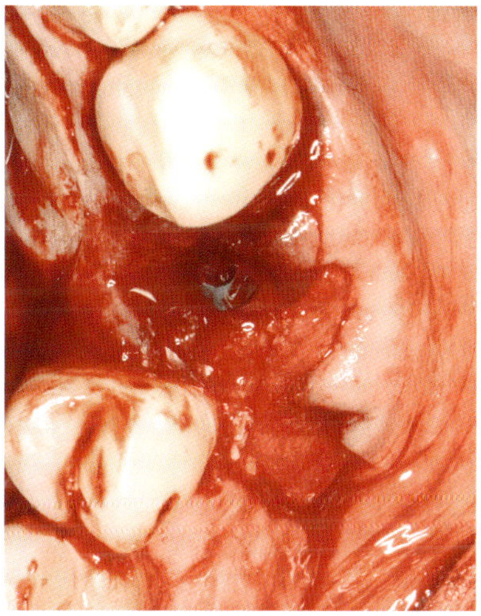

Fig 4-87 Second quadrant: apical regeneration with biomaterial (Bio-Oss®) and a collagen membrane (Bio-Gide®).

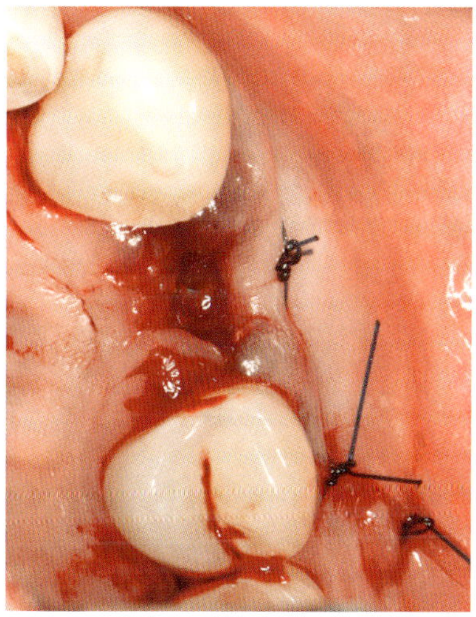

Fig 4-88 Second quadrant: suture.

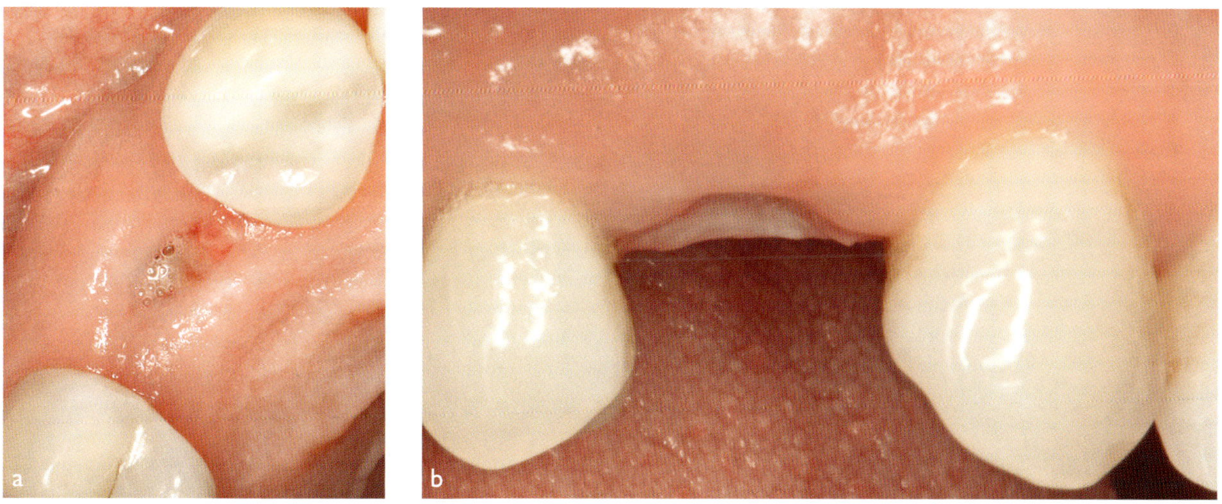

Figs 4-89a and b First quadrant, situation 1 week postoperatively: (a) occlusal view; (b) lateral view.

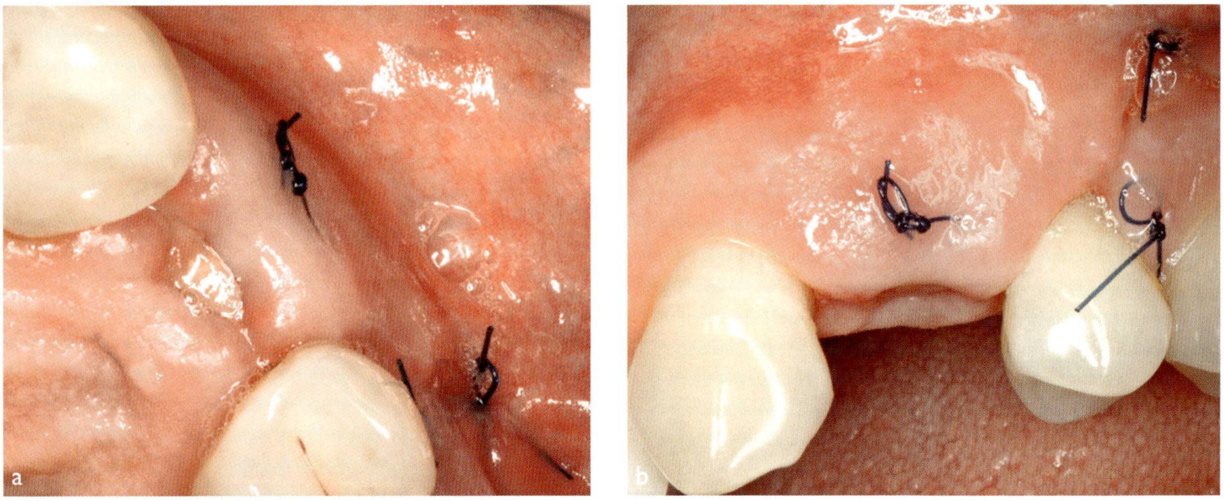

Figs 4-90a and b Second quadrant, situation 1 week postoperatively: (a) occlusal view; (b) lateral view

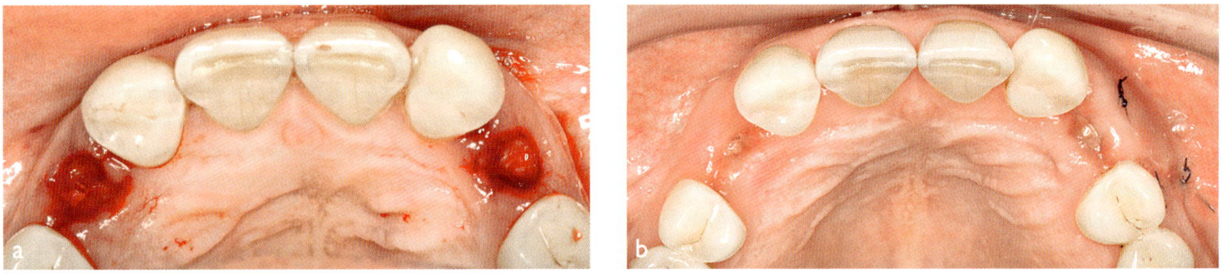

Figs 4-91a and b Occlusal views of extraction sockets: (a) after extraction; (b) situation 1 week postoperatively (immediate flapless implant placement in the first quadrant, and immediate implant placement with a mucoperiosteal flap in the second quadrant).

References

1. Branemark PI, Hansson BO, Adell R, Breine U, Lindstrom J, Hallen O, et al. Osseointegrated implants in the treatment of the edentulous jaw. Experience from a 10-year period. Scand J Plast Reconstr Surg Suppl 1977;16:1-132.
2. Chen ST, Beagle J, Jensen SS, Chiapasco M, Darby I. Consensus statements and recommended clinical procedures regarding surgical techniques. Int J Oral Maxillofac Implants 2009;24 (Suppl):272-278.
3. Albrektsson T, Zarb G, Worthington P, Eriksson AR. The long-term efficacy of currently used dental implants: a review and proposed criteria of success. Int J Oral Maxillofac Implants 1986;1:11-25.
4. Atieh MA, Payne AG, Duncan WJ, de Silva RK, Cullinan MP. Immediate placement or immediate restoration/loading of single implants for molar tooth replacement: a systematic review and meta-analysis. Int J Oral Maxillofac Implants 2010;25:401-415.
5. Fugazzotto PA. Treatment options following single-rooted tooth removal: a literature review and proposed hierarchy of treatment selection. J Periodontol 2005;76:821-831.
6. Davarpanah M, Szmukler-Moncler S. Immediate Loading of Dental Implants: theory and clinical practice. Chicago: Quintessence Books, 2008.
7. Chen ST, Darby IB, Reynolds EC. A prospective clinical study of non-submerged immediate implants: clinical outcomes and esthetic results. Clin Oral Implants Res 2007;18:552-562.
8. Schulte W, Heimke G. The Tubinger immediate implant. Quintessenz 1976;27:17-23.
9. Kan JY, Rungcharassaeng K, Lozada J. Immediate placement and provisionalization of maxillary anterior single implants: 1-year prospective study. Int J Oral Maxillofac Implants 2003;18:31-39.
10. Esposito M, Grusovin MG, Willings M, Coulthard P, Worthington HV. The effectiveness of immediate, early, and conventional loading of dental implants: a Cochrane systematic review of randomized controlled clinical trials. Int J Oral Maxillofac Implants 2007;22:893-904.
11. De Rouck T, Collys K, Cosyn J. Immediate single-tooth implants in the anterior maxilla: a 1-year case cohort study on hard and soft tissue response. J Clin Periodontol 2008;35:649-657.
12. Greenstein G, Cavallaro J Jr, Tarnow D. Dental implants in the periodontal patient. Dent Clin North Am 2010;54:113-128.
13. Schropp L, Isidor F. Timing of implant placement relative to tooth extraction. J Oral Rehabil 2008;35(Suppl 1):33-43.
14. Ferrara A, Galli C, Mauro G, Macaluso GM. Immediate provisional restoration of postextraction implants for maxillary single-tooth replacement. Int J Periodontics Restora tive Dent 2006;26:371-377.
15. den Hartog L, Slater JJ, Vissink A, Meijer HJ, Raghoebar GM. Treatment outcome of immediate, early and conventional single-tooth implants in the aesthetic zone: a systematic review to survival, bone level, soft-tissue, aesthetics and patient satisfaction. J Clin Periodontol 2008;35:1073-1086.
16. Buser D, Belser U, Wismeijer D. ITI Treatment Guide: Implant Placement in Post-Extraction Sites – Treatment Options. Chicago: Quintessence Publishing, 2008.

17. Schwartz-Arad D, Chaushu G. Placement of implants into fresh extraction sites: 4 to 7 years retrospective evaluation of 95 immediate implants. J Periodontol 1997;68:1110-1116.
18. Amler MH. The time sequence of tissue regeneration in human extraction wounds. Oral Surg Oral Med Oral Pathol 1969;27: 309-318.
19. Atwood DA. Reduction of residual ridges: a major oral disease entity. J Prosthet Dent 1971;26:266-279.
20. Block MS, Mercante DE, Lirette D, Mohamed W, Ryser M, Castellon P. Prospective evaluation of immediate and delayed provisional single tooth restorations. J Oral Maxillofac Surg 2009;67(Suppl 11):89-107.
21. Andreasen JO, Petersen JK, Laskin DM. Textbook and color atlas of tooth impactions, diagnosis, treatment. Copenhagen: Munksgaard, 1997.
22. Lekovic V, Kenney EB, Weinlaender M, Han T, Klokkevold P, Nedic M, et al. A bone regenerative approach to alveolar ridge maintenance following tooth extraction. Report of 10 cases. J Periodontol 1997;68:563-570.
23. Lekovic V, Camargo PM, Klokkevold PR, Weinlaender M, Kenney EB, Dimitrijevic B, et al. Preservation of alveolar bone in extraction sockets using bioabsorbable membranes. J Periodontol 1998;69:1044-1049.
24. Camargo PM, Lekovic V, Weinlaender M, Klokkevold PR, Kenney EB, Dimitrijevic B, et al. Influence of bioactive glass on changes in alveolar process dimensions after exodontia. Oral Surg Oral Med Oral Pathol Oral Radiol Endod 2000;90:581-586.
25. Iasella JM, Greenwell H, Miller RL, Hill M, Drisko C, Bohra AA, et al. Ridge preservation with freeze-dried bone allograft and a collagen membrane compared to extraction alone for implant site development: a clinical and histologic study in humans. J Periodontol 2003;74:990-999.
26. Schropp L, Kostopoulos L, Wenzel A. Bone healing following immediate versus delayed placement of titanium implants into extraction sockets: a prospective clinical study. Int J Oral Maxillofac Implants 2003;18:189-199.
27. Chen ST, Wilson TG Jr, Hammerle CH. Immediate or early placement of implants following tooth extraction: review of biologic basis, clinical procedures, and outcomes. Int J Oral Maxillofac Implants 2004;19(Suppl):12-25.
28. Elian N, Cho SC, Froum S, Smith RB, Tarnow DP. A simplified socket classification and repair technique. Pract Proced Aesthet Dent 2007;19:99-104; quiz 6.
29. Caplanis N, Lozada JL, Kan JY. Extraction defect assessment, classification, and management. J Calif Dent Assoc 2005;33:853-863.
30. Botticelli D, Berglundh T, Lindhe J. Hard-tissue alterations following immediate implant placement in extraction sites. J Clin Periodontol 2004;31:820-828.
31. Araujo MG, Lindhe J. Dimensional ridge alterations following tooth extraction. An experimental study in the dog. J Clin Periodontol 2005;32:212-218.
32. Araujo MG, Sukekava F, Wennstrom JL, Lindhe J. Ridge alterations following implant placement in fresh extraction sockets: an experimental study in the dog. J Clin Periodontol 2005;32:645-652.
33. Araujo MG, Sukekava F, Wennstrom JL, Lindhe J. Tissue modeling following implant placement in fresh extraction sockets. Clin Oral Implants Res 2006;17:615-624.
34. Araujo MG, Lindhe J. Ridge alterations following tooth extraction with and without flap elevation: an experimental study in the dog. Clin Oral Implants Res 2009;20:545-549.
35. Wilson TG, Weber HP. Classification of a therapy for areas of deficient bony housing prior to dental implant placement. Int J Periodontics Restorative Dent 1993;13:451-459.
36. Hammerle CH, Chen ST, Wilson TG Jr. Consensus statements and recommended clinical procedures regarding the placement of implants in extraction sockets. Int J Oral Maxillofac Implants 2004;19(Suppl):26-28.
37. Esposito M, Grusovin MG, Coulthard P, Worthington HV. The efficacy of various bone augmentation procedures for dental implants: a Cochrane systematic review of randomized controlled clinical trials. Int J Oral Maxillofac Implants 2006;21:696-710.
38. Chen S, Buser D. Implants in post-extraction sites: A literature update. In: Buser D, Belser U, Wismeijer D (eds). ITI Treatment Guide. Berlin: Quintessence Publishing, 2008:9-15.
39. Bhola M, Neely AL, Kolhatkar S. Immediate implant placement: clinical decisions, advantages, and disadvantages. J Prosthodont 2008;17:576-581.
40. Barzilay I. Immediate implants: their current status. Int J Prosthodont 1993;6:169-175.
41. Canullo L, Iurlaro G, Iannello G. Double-blind randomized controlled trial study on post-extraction immediately restored implants using the switching platform concept: soft tissue response. Preliminary report. Clin Oral Implants Res 2009;20:414-420.
42. Ribeiro FS, Pontes AE, Marcantonio E, Piattelli A, Neto RJ, Marcantonio E Jr. Success rate of immediate nonfunctional loaded single-tooth implants: immediate versus delayed implantation. Implant Dent 2008;17:109-117.
43. Davarpanah M, Martinez H, Kebir M, Tecucianu J-F. Clinical Manual of Implant Dentristy, 1st ed. London: Quintessence Publishing, 2003.
44. Misch CE. Contemporary Implant Dentistry, 3rd ed. St Louis: Elsevier Mosby, 2009.
45. Block M. Color Atlas of Dental Implant Surgery, 1st ed. Philadelphia: WB Saunders, 2001.
46. Douglass GL, Merin RL. The immediate dental implant. J Calif Dent Assoc 2002;30:362-365, 8-74.
47. Funato A, Salama MA, Ishikawa T, Garber DA, Salama H. Timing, positioning, and sequential staging in esthetic implant therapy: a four-dimensional perspective. Int J Periodontics Restorative Dent 2007;27:313-323.
48. Becker W, Goldstein M. Immediate implant placement: treatment planning and surgical steps for successful outcome. Periodontol 2000 2008;47:79-89.
49. Fugazzotto PA. Implant placement in maxillary first premolar fresh extraction sockets: description of technique and report of preliminary results. J Periodontol 2002;73:669-674.
50. Fugazzotto PA. Implant placement at the time of maxillary molar extraction: technique and report of preliminary results of 83 sites. J Periodontol 2006;77:302-309.
51. Fugazzotto PA. Implant placement at the time of maxillary molar extraction: treatment protocols and report of results. J Periodontol 2008;79:216-223.
52. Fugazzotto PA. Implant placement at the time of mandibular molar extraction: description of technique and preliminary results of 341 cases. J Periodontol 2008;79:737-747.
53. Sanz M, Cecchinato D, Ferrus J, Pjetursson EB, Lang NP, Lindhe J. A prospective, randomized-controlled clinical trial to evaluate bone preservation using implants with different geometry placed into extraction sockets in the maxilla. Clin Oral Implants Res 2010;21:13-21.
54. Atieh MA, Payne AG, Duncan WJ, Cullinan MP. Immediate restoration/loading of immediately placed single implants: is it an effective bimodal approach? Clin Oral Implants Res 2009;20:645-659.
55. Kupershmidt I, Levin L, Schwartz-Arad D. Inter-implant bone height changes in anterior maxillary immediate and non-immediate adjacent dental implants. J Periodontol 2007;78:991-996.
56. Schropp L, Kostopoulos L, Wenzel A, Isidor F. Clinical and radiographic performance of delayed-immediate single-tooth implant placement associated with peri-implant bone defects. A 2-year prospective, controlled, randomized follow-up report. J Clin Periodontol 2005;32:480-487.

57. Siegenthaler DW, Jung RE, Holderegger C, Roos M, Hammerle CH. Replacement of teeth exhibiting periapical pathology by immediate implants: a prospective, controlled clinical trial. Clin Oral Implants Res 2007;18:727-737.
58. Crespi R, Cappare P, Gherlone E, Romanos GE. Immediate versus delayed loading of dental implants placed in fresh extraction sockets in the maxillary esthetic zone: a clinical comparative study. Int J Oral Maxillofac Implants 2008;23:753-758.
59. Palattella P, Torsello F, Cordaro L. Two-year prospective clinical comparison of immediate replacement vs. immediate restoration of single tooth in the esthetic zone. Clin Oral Implants Res 2008;19:1148-1153.
60. Atieh MA, Ibrahim HM, Atieh AH. Platform switching for marginal bone preservation around dental implants: a systematic review and meta-analysis. J Periodontol 2010;81:1350-1366.
61. Canullo L, Rasperini G. Preservation of peri-implant soft and hard tissues using platform switching of implants placed in immediate extraction sockets: a proof-of-concept study with 12- to 36-month follow-up. Int J Oral Maxillofac Implants 2007;22:995-1000.
62. Calvo-Guirado JL, Ortiz-Ruiz AJ, Lopez-Mari L, Delgado-Ruiz R, Mate-Sanchez J, Bravo Gonzalez LA. Immediate maxillary restoration of single-tooth implants using platform switching for crestal bone preservation: a 12-month study. Int J Oral Maxillofac Implants 2009;24:275-281.
63. Rodriguez-Ciurana X, Vela-Nebot X, Segala-Torres M, Calvo-Guirado JL, Cambra J, Mendez-Blanco V, et al. The effect of interimplant distance on the height of the interimplant bone crest when using platform-switched implants. Int J Periodontics Restorative Dent 2009;29:141-151.
64. Lindeboom JA, Tjiook Y, Kroon FH. Immediate placement of implants in periapical infected sites: a prospective randomized study in 50 patients. Oral Surg Oral Med Oral Pathol Oral Radiol Endod 2006;101:705-710.
65. Kan JY, Rungcharassaeng K, Liddelow G, Henry P, Goodacre CJ. Periimplant tissue response following immediate provisional restoration of scalloped implants in the esthetic zone: a one-year pilot prospective multicenter study. J Prosthet Dent 2007;97(Suppl 6):S109-118.
66. Evans CD, Chen ST. Esthetic outcomes of immediate implant placements. Clin Oral Implants Res 2008;19:73-80.
67. Crespi R, Cappare P, Gherlone E, Romanos GE. Immediate occlusal loading of implants placed in fresh sockets after tooth extraction. Int J Oral Maxillofac Implants 2007;22:955-962.
68. Lops D, Chiapasco M, Rossi A, Bressan E, Romeo E. Incidence of inter-proximal papilla between a tooth and an adjacent immediate implant placed into a fresh extraction socket: 1-year prospective study. Clin Oral Implants Res 2008;19:1135-1140.
69. Malo P, Nobre M. Flap vs. flapless surgical techniques at immediate implant function in predominantly soft bone for rehabilitation of partial edentulism: a prospective cohort study with follow-up of 1 year. Eur J Oral Implantol 2008;1:293-304.
70. Schwartz-Arad D, Chaushu G. Immediate implant placement: a procedure without incisions. J Periodontol 1998;69:743-750.
71. Lang NP, Tonetti MS, Suvan JE, Pierre Bernard J, Botticelli D, Fourmousis I, et al. Immediate implant placement with transmucosal healing in areas of aesthetic priority. A multicentre randomized-controlled clinical trial I. Surgical outcomes. Clin Oral Implants Res 2007;18:188-196.
72. Cafiero C, Annibali S, Gherlone E, et al. Immediate transmucosal implant placement in molar extraction sites: a 12-month prospective multicenter cohort study. Clin Oral Implants Res 2008;19:476-482.
73. Cornelini R, Cangini F, Covani U, Wilson TG Jr. Immediate restoration of implants placed into fresh extraction sockets for single-tooth replacement: a prospective clinical study. Int J Periodontics Restorative Dent 2005;25:439-447.
74. Siciliano VI, Salvi GE, Matarasso S, Cafiero C, Blasi A, Lang NP. Soft tissues healing at immediate transmucosal implants placed into molar extraction sites with buccal self-contained dehiscences. A 12-month controlled clinical trial. Clin Oral Implants Res 2009;20:482-488.
75. Truninger TC, Philipp AO, Siegenthaler DW, Roos M, Hämmerle CH, Jung RE. A prospective, controlled clinical trial evaluating the clinical and radiological outcome after 3 years of immediately placed implants in sockets exhibiting periapical pathology. Clin Oral Implants Res 2011;22:20-27.
76. Waasdorp JA, Evian CI, Mandracchia M. Immediate placement of implants into infected sites: a systematic review of the literature. J Periodontol 2010;81:801-808.
77. Quirynen M, Vogels R, Alsaadi G, Naert I, Jacobs R, van Steenberghe D. Predisposing conditions for retrograde peri-implantitis, and treatment suggestions. Clin Oral Implants Res 2005;16:599-608.
78. Wagenberg B, Froum SJ. A retrospective study of 1925 consecutively placed immediate implants from 1988 to 2004. Int J Oral Maxillofac Implants 2006;21:71-80.
79. Becker W. Immediate implant placement: treatment planning and surgical steps for successful outcomes. Br Dent J 2006;201:199-205.
80. Villa R, Rangert B. Early loading of interforaminal implants immediately installed after extraction of teeth presenting endodontic and periodontal lesions. Clin Implant Dent Relat Res 2005;7(Suppl 1):S28-35.
81. Del Fabbro M, Boggian C, Taschieri S. Immediate implant placement into fresh extraction sites with chronic periapical pathologic features combined with plasma rich in growth factors: preliminary results of single-cohort study. J Oral Maxillofac Surg 2009;67:2476-2484.
82. Vanden Bogaerde L, Rangert B, Wendelhag I. Immediate/early function of Branemark System TiUnite implants in fresh extraction sockets in maxillae and posterior mandibles: an 18-month prospective clinical study. Clin Implant Dent Relat Res 2005;7(Suppl 1):S121-30.
83. Smith RB, Tarnow DP, Brown M, Chu S, Zamzok J. Placement of immediate implants and a fixed provisional restoration to replace the four mandibular incisors. Compend Contin Educ Dent 2009;30:408-410, 13-5; quiz 16,18.
84. Chen ST, Darby IB, Adams GG, Reynolds EC. A prospective clinical study of bone augmentation techniques at immediate implants. Clin Oral Implants Res 2005;16:176-184.
85. Esposito M, Grusovin MG, Achille H, Coulthard P, Worthington HV. Interventions for replacing missing teeth: different times for loading dental implants. Cochrane Database Syst Rev 2009:CD003878.
86. Jun SH, Chang BM, Weber HP, Kwon JJ. Comparison of initial stability parameters and histomorphometric analysis of implants inserted into extraction sockets: human fresh cadaver study. Int J Oral Maxillofac Implants 2011;25:985-990.
87. Bianchi AE, Sanfilippo F. Single-tooth replacement by immediate implant and connective tissue graft: a 1-9-year clinical evaluation. Clin Oral Implants Res 2004;15:269-277.
88. Levin L, Laviv A, Schwartz-Arad D. Long-term success of implants replacing a single molar. J Periodontol 2006;77:1528-1532.
89. Penarrocha-Diago M, Carrillo-Garcia C, Boronat-Lopez A, Garcia-Mira B. Comparative study of wide-diameter implants placed after dental extraction and implants positioned in mature bone for molar replacement. Int J Oral Maxillofac Implants 2008;23:497-501.
90. Artzi Z, Parson A, Nemcovsky CE. Wide-diameter implant placement and internal sinus membrane elevation in the immediate postextraction phase: clinical and radiographic observations in 12 consecutive molar sites. Int J Oral Maxillofac Implants 2003;18:242-249.

91. Schwartz-Arad D, Grossman Y, Chaushu G. The clinical effectiveness of implants placed immediately into fresh extraction sites of molar teeth. J Periodontol 2000;71.839-844.
92. Malo P, de Araujo Nobre M, Rangert B. Implants placed in immediate function in periodontally compromised sites: a five-year retrospective and one-year prospective study. J Prosthet Dent 2007;97(Suppl 6):S86-95.
93. Evian CI, Emling R, Rosenberg ES, Waasdorp JA, Halpern W, Shah S, et al. Retrospective analysis of implant survival and the influence of periodontal disease and immediate placement on long-term results. Int J Oral Maxillofac Implants. 2004;19:393-398.
94. Shibly O, Kutkut A, Patel N, Albandar JM. Immediate implants with immediate loading vs. conventional loading: 1-year randomized clinical trial. Clin Implant Dent Relat Res 2010;14:663-671.
95. Horwitz J, Zuabi O, Machtei E. Radiographic changes around immediately restored dental implants in periodontally susceptible patients: 1-year results. Int J Oral Maxillofac Implants 2008;23: 531-538.
96. Deng F, Zhang H, Shao H, He Q, Zhang P. A comparison of clinical outcomes for implants placed in fresh extraction sockets versus healed sites in periodontally compromised patients: a 1-year follow-up report. Int J Oral Maxillofac Implants 2010;25: 1036-1040.
97. Alves CC, Correia AR, Neves M. Immediate implants and immediate loading in periodontally compromised patients-a 3-year prospective clinical study. Int J Periodontics Restorative Dent 2010;30:447-455.

Chapter 5

Can I rely on software-guided surgery?

Alberto Sicilia, Alberto Rodríguez, Isabel Cuesta

5.1 Introduction

Traditionally, preoperative diagnosis in implantology was based on two-dimensional (2D) interpretation of radiographic information, obtained basically from panoramic and/or periapical radiographs. In the 1990s, evolution in this field led to more generalized use of computerized tomography (CT),[1] together with the elaboration of radiographic and surgical templates.[2,3] However, despite the availability of CT technology, during these early stages clinicians would only receive 2D information and had to go through a mental process of "limited three-dimensionalization" (Fig 5-1) in order to approach realistic surgical readiness and to adequately plan the placement of fixtures, which carried significant limitations.[4]

This need for more elaborate and trustworthy 3D information led to the design, at the turn of the century,[5] of specific implant design programs based on 3D handling (Fig 5-2) of information obtained by CT or cone beam computerized tomography (CBCT), creating the new concept of computer-aided implant surgery (CAIS).[4]

There is a certain terminological confusion in this field, so for the purpose of clarity, we will use in this chapter the term CAIS to refer globally to all procedures where information is obtained by scanning jaws (CT or CBCT), and then processed by a specific type of software that allows for the virtual 3D planning of dental implants, and which finally assists the surgeon during implant placement in the patient's mouth. The term aided, while somewhat ambiguous, is also conveniently generic, as it encompasses all procedures based on the use of surgical templates and navigation systems, as well as other surgical uses of the 3D information obtained, which we will discuss at the end of this section.

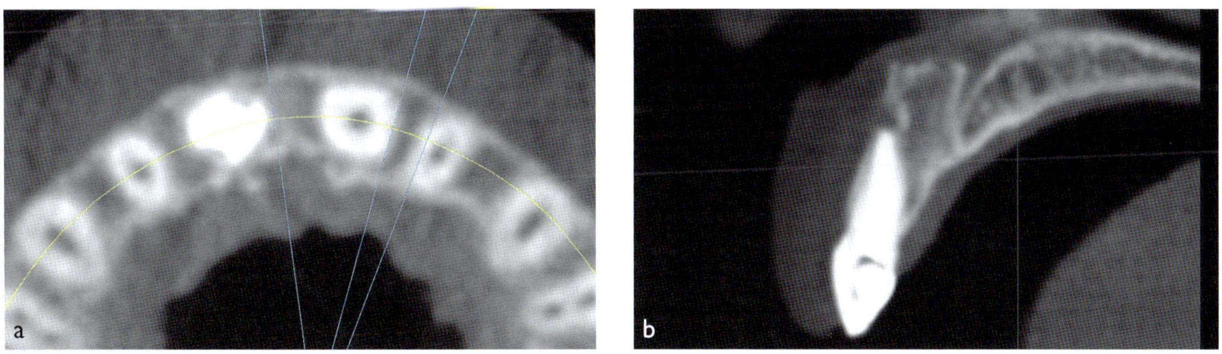

Figs 5-1a and b Computerized tomography (CT) displayed with a traditional approach. The analysis was based on the clinician's evaluation of 2D images from different perspectives: occlusal view, perpendicular section of the ridge, and pantographic reconstruction. The clinician had to undergo a "limited 3D mental reconstruction" to carry out the planning.

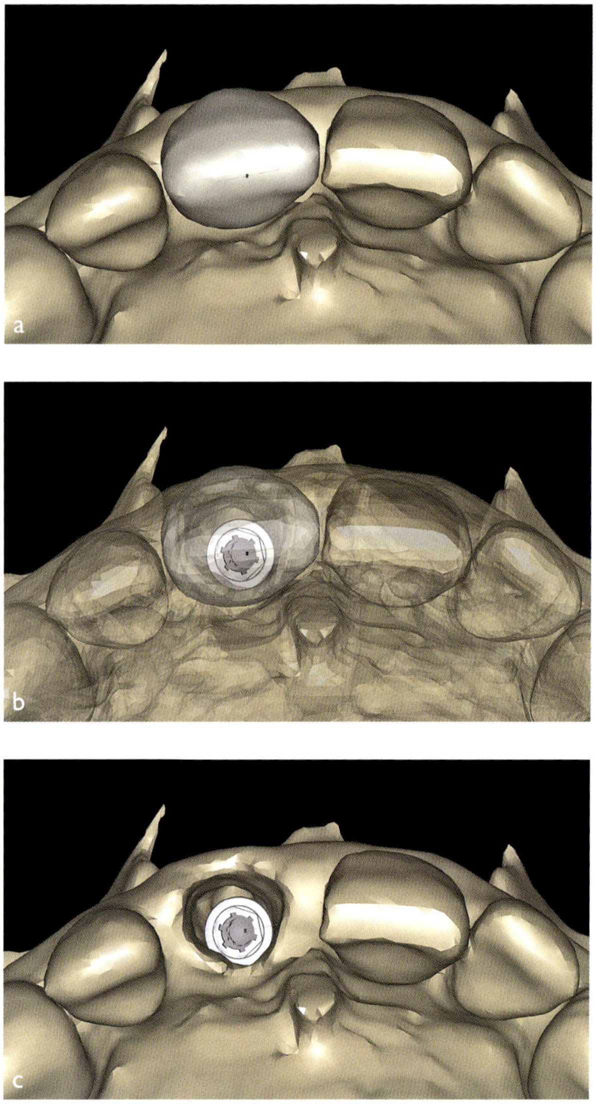

Figs 5-2a to c The production of 3D models allows us to draw up a plan based on virtual surgery. This case, for example, involved the extraction of a central incisor (a), the virtual placement of an immediate implant (b), and the assessment of the resulting residual bone defect (c).

The following topics will be assessed:

- 5.2 What types of CAIS procedures are available for clinical use?
  - 5.2.1 Template-based or static procedures
  - 5.2.2 Navigation system or dynamic procedures
  - 5.2.3 Conclusions
- 5.3 How reliable are CAIS systems?
  - 5.3.1 Conclusions
- 5.4 Is bone density useful as a planning tool?
  - 5.4.1 Conclusions
- 5.5 What are the benefits and drawbacks of each type of system?
  - 5.5.1 Conclusions
- 5.6 What are the limitations of CAIS?
  - 5.6.1 Acceptable reliability, occasional deviations
  - 5.6.2 A need to combine different systems
  - 5.6.3 Lack of information on soft tissue
- 5.7 Computer-oriented surgery: a new dynamic concept

5.2 What types of CAIS procedures are available for clinical use?

5.2.1 Template-based or static procedures

The most commonly used and widely documented approach is based on the creation of a surgical template using digital information. This is known as static computer-assisted surgery, or computer-guided surgery.[6] With this procedure, information obtained through 3D planning is used to produce a surgical template by means of computer-aided design/computer-aided manufacturing (CAD/CAM) procedures, which allows implants to be placed on the patient's jaws in a way that duplicates precisely the virtual design. This begins with the laboratory production of a radiographic template designed to hold a prosthetic base, teeth and/or markers, which could be radiopaque. This radiographic template is placed into the patient's mouth during the CT/CBCT scan, for which its precise positioning and stability are paramount. Information from the scanned jaws and from the radiographic template used is processed to build a 3D model from which the clinician creates the virtual plan (Fig 5-3). Finally, a surgical template is made, which will act as a link between the virtual world (3D planning) and the real world (the patient), as well as the immediate provisional prosthesis (Fig 5-4).[7]

There are two types of guided surgery, which differ essentially by the method used to build the surgical template: those that use stereolithographic templates and those that use mechanical templates.[6]

Stereolithographic templates

Stereolithography is a rapid prototyping procedure, patented by Chuck Hull in 1986. It is based on a digital

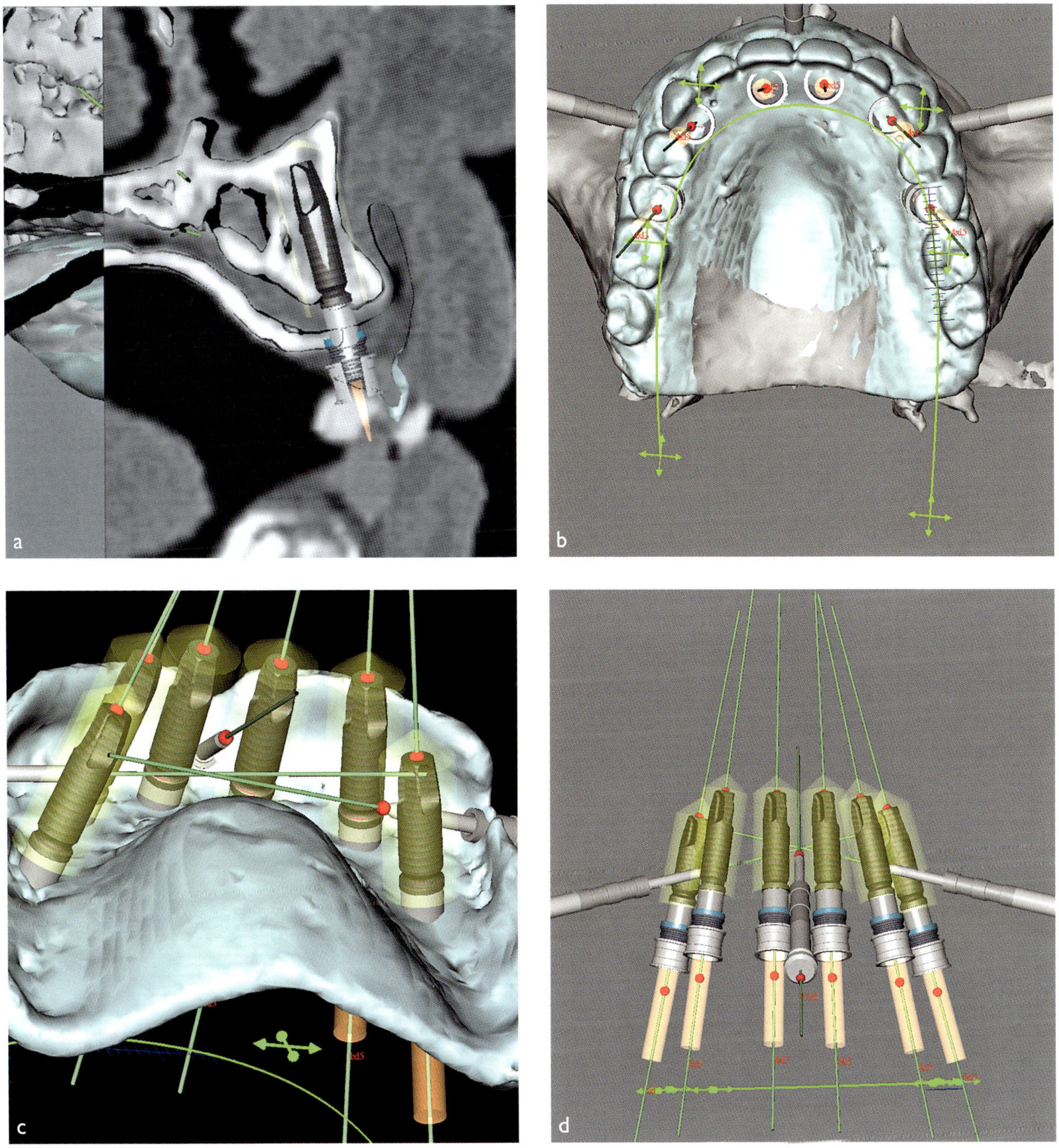

Figs 5-3a to d Following a full esthetic and functional examination, a radiographic template is produced, containing all the necessary information on the spatial positioning of the teeth and reference (fiducial) marks for patient indexing. This enables the virtual planning of the implants and provides digital information for creating the drilling template.

model of the element to be copied (in this case the surgical template), which is previously broken down by the design program into sections or layers, representing parallel planes perpendicular to a specific axis. The surgical template is built layer by layer. Stereolithographic production machinery, which is limited to industrial use, consists of a container filled with photopolymerizable resin set on a platform that can be moved vertically (Fig 5-5). When template construction begins, the platform is at its highest position, slightly below the surface of the resin. The information from the first layer is copied by means of laser-activated polymerization of the supernatant resin, and the laser draws onto it the information from that first layer. Once this process is

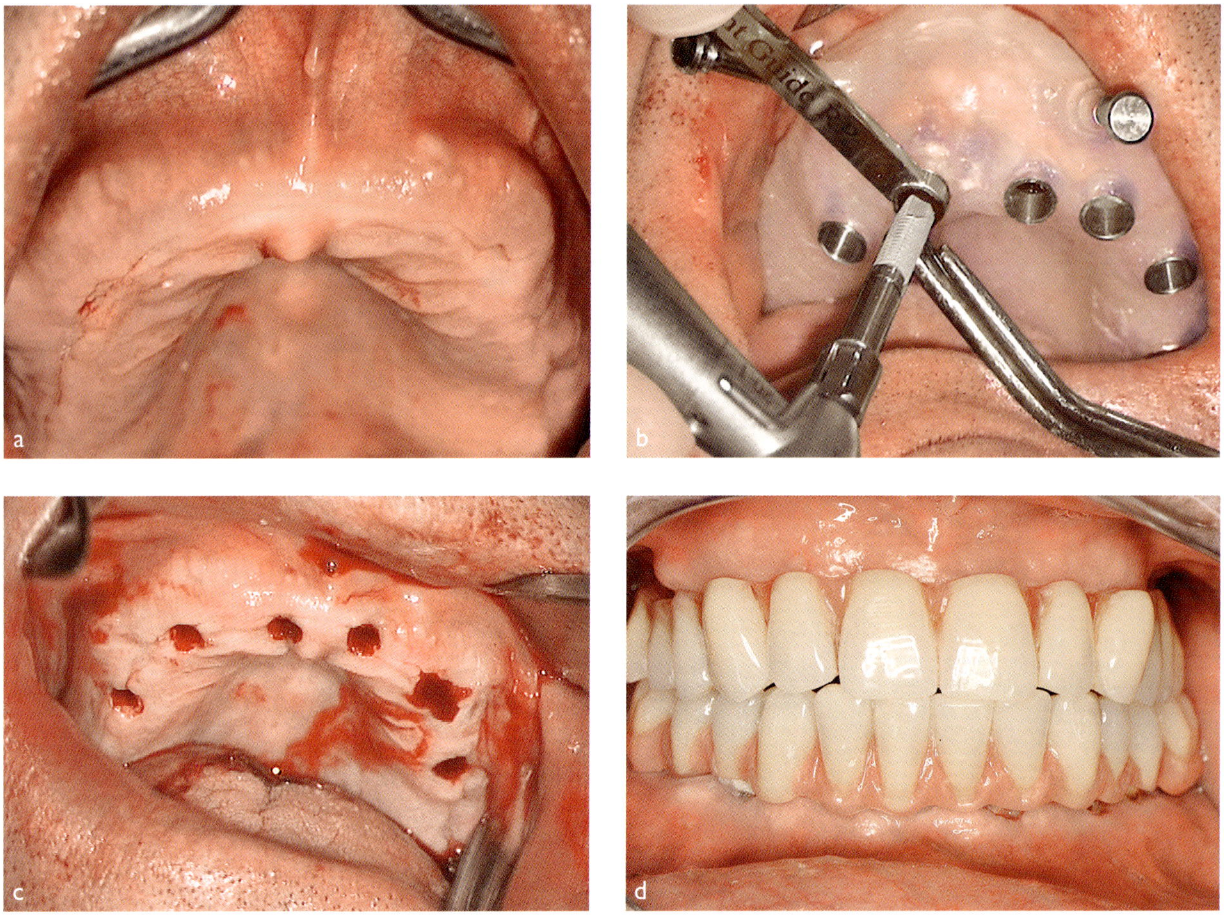

Figs 5-4a to d Aided by the stereolithographic template, implants can be placed by making small, circular incisions by means of a minimally invasive technique, which requires neither flap raising nor suturing. Surgery finishes with the immediate placement of an implant-supported provisional prosthesis.

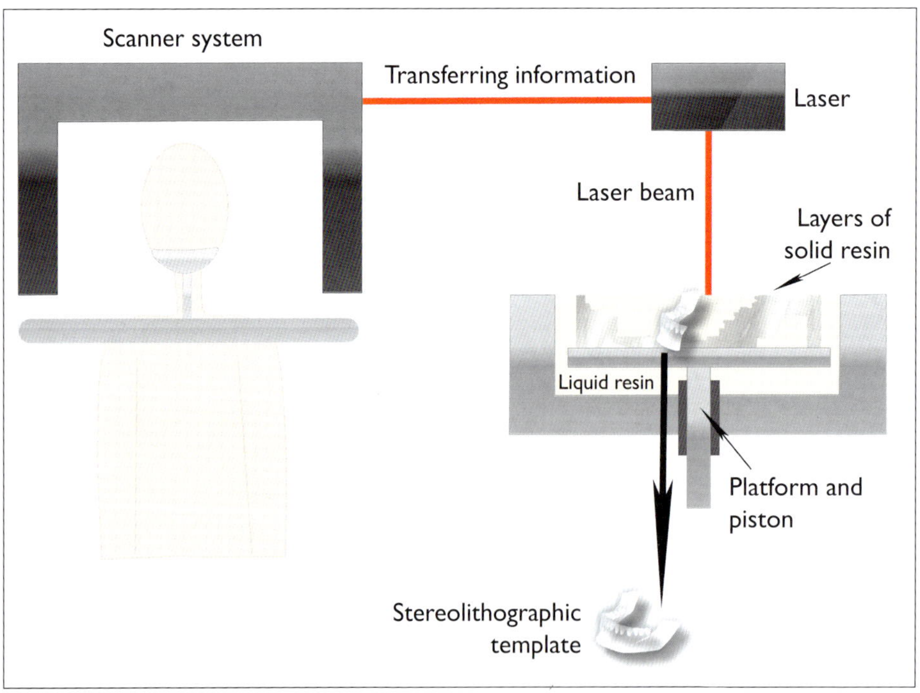

Fig 5-5 Diagram showing fabrication of a stereolithographic template.

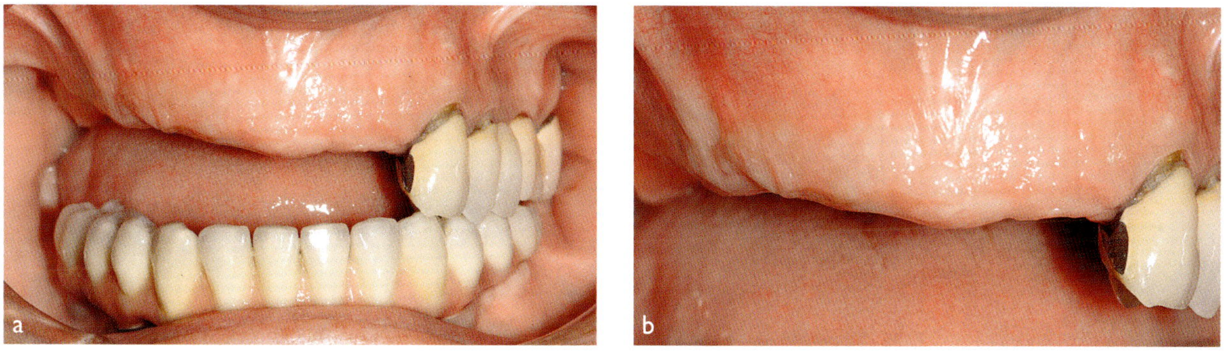

Figs 5-6a and b A 45-year-old woman who, 6 months previously, underwent examination of the right maxillary sinus followed by extensive reconstructive surgery with horizontal ridge augmentation in the anterior section and maxillary right molar region. She shows good keratinized tissue and an adequately sized ridge. Transmucosal implant placement in 11, 21, 13, 15 and 16 (Med3D®) is scheduled.

complete, the platform moves downwards slightly and the laser beam draws the next layer onto the new supernatant resin, photopolymerizing an additional layer, which adheres to the previous one. Once this process is complete and the final prototype is cleaned, its photopolymerization is finalized in an ultraviolet oven and the titanium cylinders are manually fitted in the prototype, so that the clinician can use the instruments and components necessary to drill the alveoli and place the implants.

There are various systems that use this procedure, perhaps the most noteworthy being the SAFE® method based on the SimPlant® software program (Materialise Dental, Leuven, Belgium) (Fig 5-2) and the NobelGuide® method (Nobel Biocare, Gothenburg, Sweden) (Figs 5-3 and 5-4).

Mechanical templates

Mechanical template production is a simpler process, which may be carried out in a conventional dental laboratory or in the clinic itself. It is based on the initial manufacturing of an acrylic radiographic template, which features fiducial markers for indexing the patient. Once the planning stage is complete, using precision computer-guided mechanical devices, the template is perforated at the point in which the implants are to be placed and the titanium guide cylinders are set in place in the exact position and direction. Systems that utilize this procedure include Med3D® (med3D, Heidelberg, Germany) (Figs 5-6 to 5-8) and Straumann® CARES® Guided Surgery protocols (Straumann, Basel, Switzerland).

5.2.2 Navigation system or dynamic procedures

Conversely, in the so-called dynamic or navigation procedures, a communication system generally based on an infrared camera allows for the drilling and placement of the implant to be continuously monitored. The 3D planning and the patient are indexed by means of a template holding a bow with radiopaque markers. In this type of procedure, a "physical surgical template" has not been previously manufactured; instead, orientation is based on combined images transmitted by the navigation system (Figs 5-9 to 5-11). These can range from the display of the drills or of the implant superimposed over the 3D planning for the patient in real time, to the merging of information in symbol format, such as a target and a depth gauge for adjusting the drilling site, axis, and depth.[4,6] One of the most widespread navigation systems used in implant surgery is RoboDent® (RoboDent, Ismaning, Germany) (Figs 5-9 to 5-11).

5.2.3 Conclusion

Types of computer-assisted surgery include static systems, which use a surgical template, or dynamic systems that use navigation technology. Templates may be manufactured industrially (stereolithographic) or in a dental laboratory, or in the clinic itself using less complex computer-guided tools, known as mechanical systems.

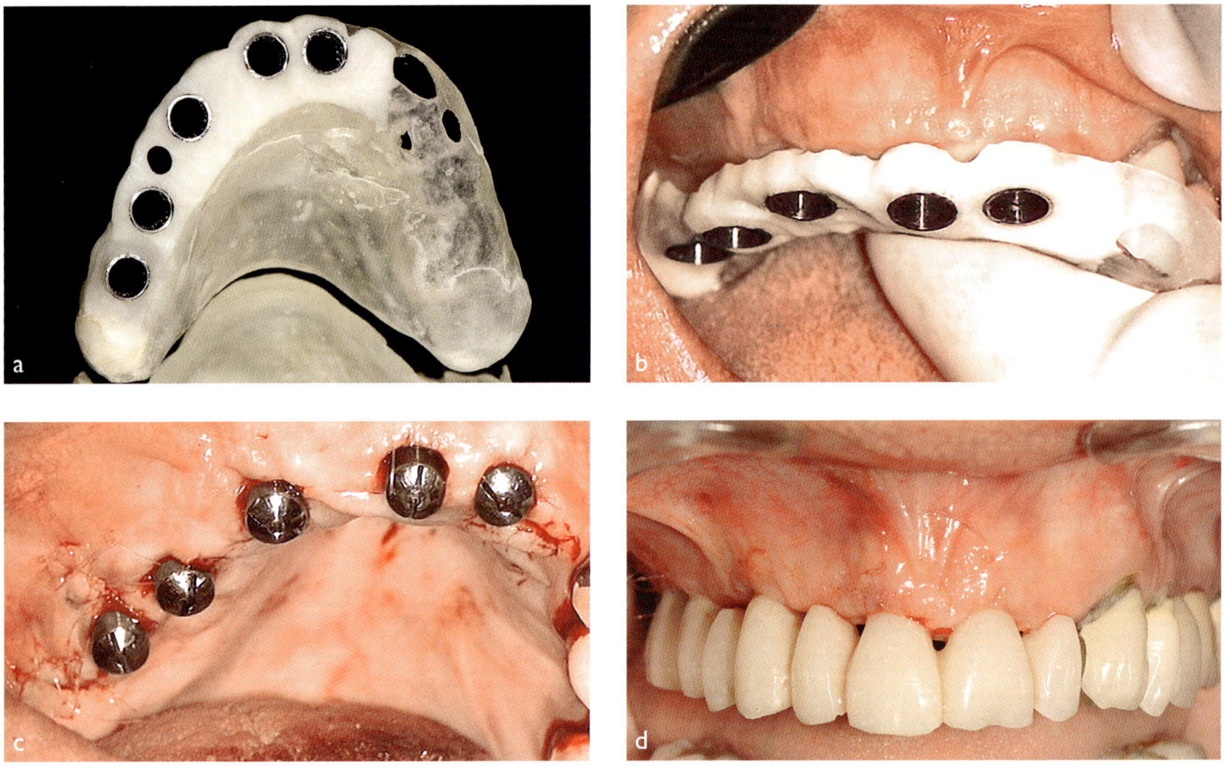

Figs 5-7a to d (Same patient as in Fig 5-6) A mechanical surgical template is fabricated, followed by the performance of combined techniques of minimally invasive surgery, transmucosal surgery, and mini-flaps for implant placement with the least possible trauma. The connective tissue obtained after creating the access hole for implant placement is grafted to a cul-de-sac created on the vestibular side of each implant site, to improve the contour shape and increase the size of the keratinized buccal tissue. An immediate provisional metal-free acrylic prosthesis is placed.

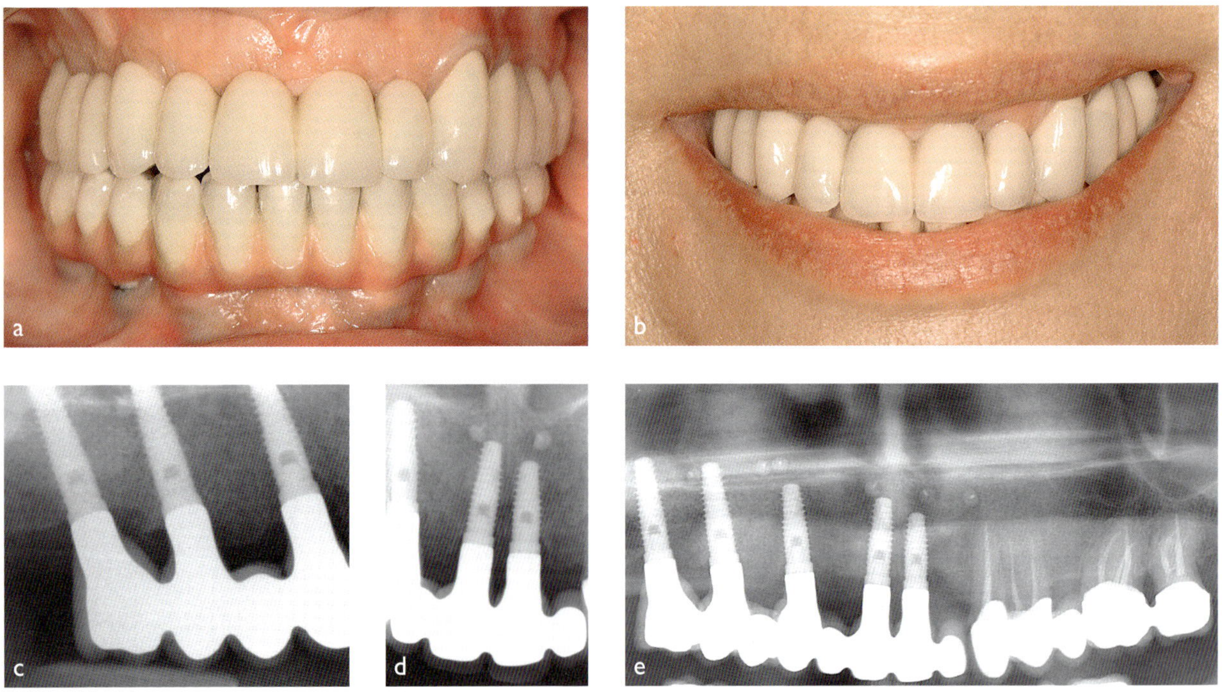

Figs 5-8a to e (Same patient as in Fig 5-6) Final restoration with a non-segmented dental implant-supported prosthesis (teeth 17 to 12) and conventional prosthesis on the left side.

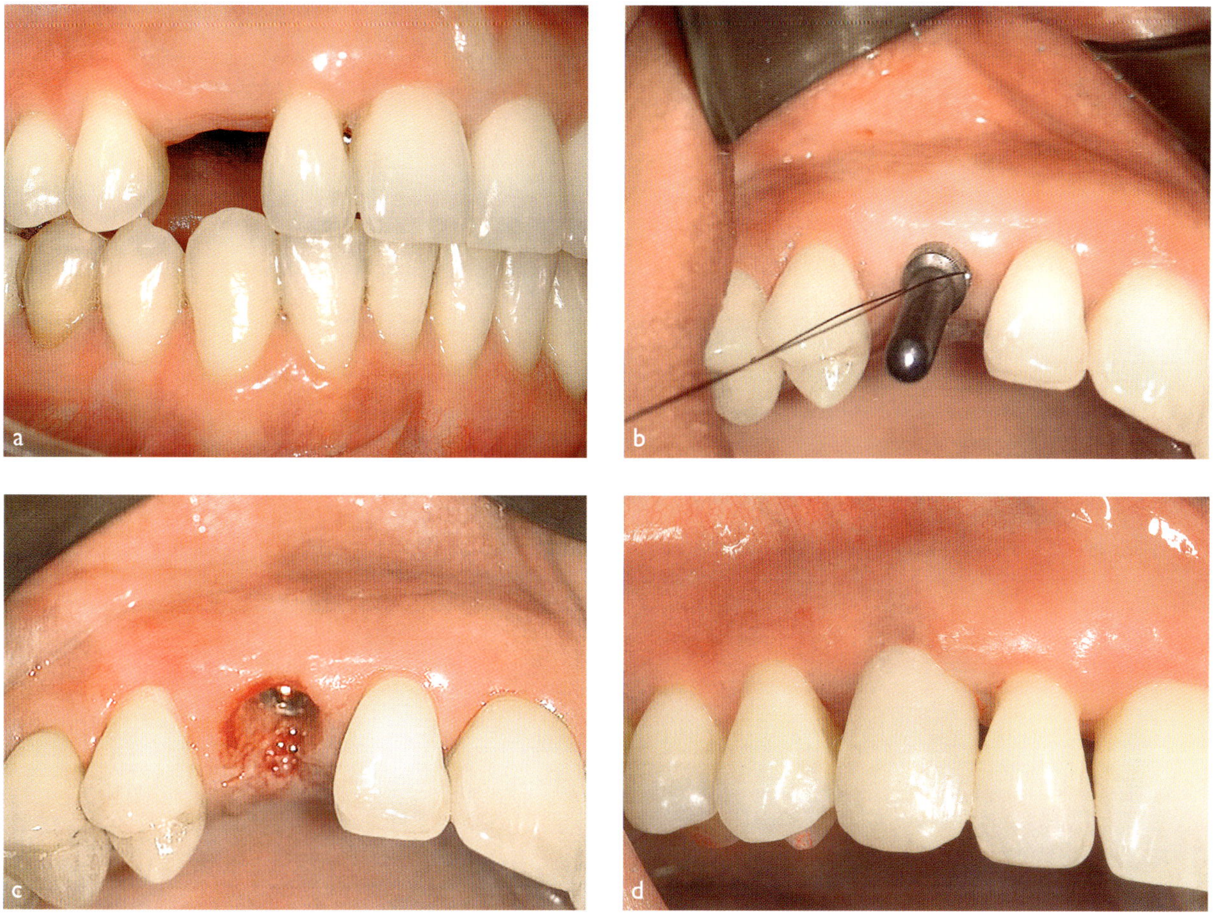

Fig 5-9a to d A 25-year-old woman with an intact alveolar ridge, but revealing a narrow crest with a marked concavity on examination with CBCT. The patient underwent transmucosal surgery, using the 2-mm twist drill with a navigation system to center the perforation on the remaining ridge. The soft tissues were then modified as necessary and a 3.3-mm diameter implant was placed, with the platform placed 4 mm from the future gingival margin of the restoration. Finally, the missing tooth was replaced with an immediate provisional prosthesis.

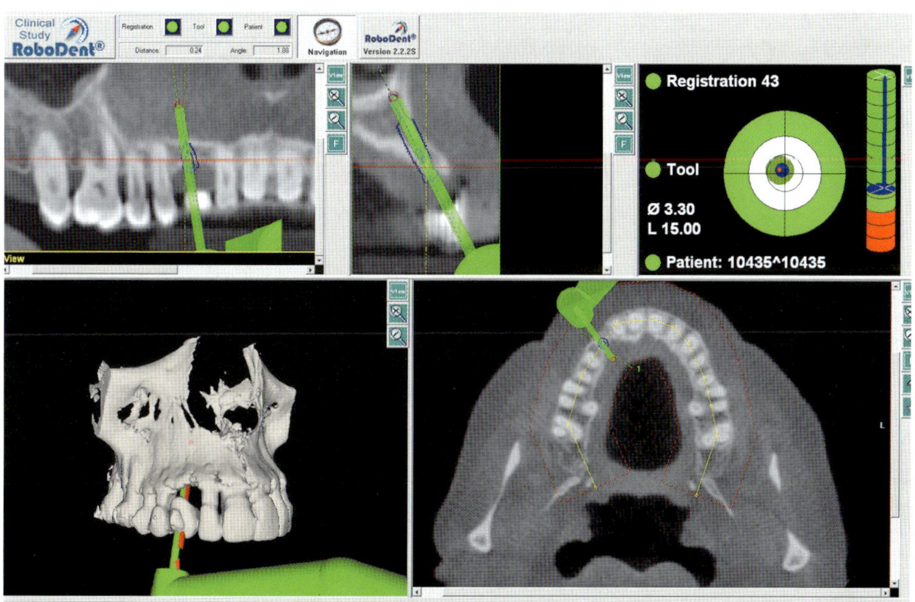

Fig 5-10 View of the CAIS from the case in Fig 5-9, using a navigation protocol (RoboDent®). The position of the drill (green-colored cylinder) can be seen in the three axes of the cavity and in the 3D model. In the upper right side of the screen, an illuminated green target shows that the position and axis of the drill are correct, and a depth gauge with audible alarm indicates the depth of the perforation.

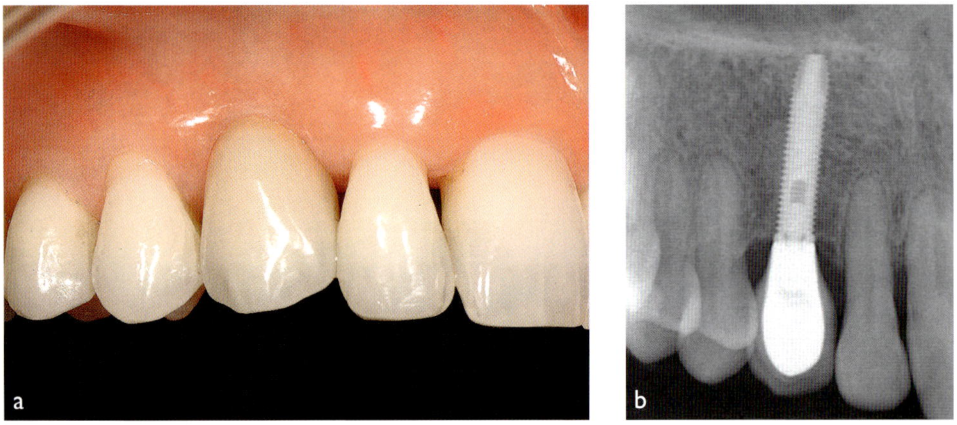

Fig 5-11a and b Final restoration with single screw-retained non-segmented implant-supported prosthesis.

Table 5-1 *Scientific interpretation of the terms precision and accuracy (from Hulley et al.[9])*

	Precision	Accuracy
Definition	The degree to which a treatment has nearly the same result when applied repeated times	The degree to which a treatment produces the result that it is supposed to produce
Best way to assess	Comparison among repeated applications	Comparison with a reference standard
Threatened by	Random error	Systematic error (bias)
	Reproducibility	Validity

5.3 How reliable are CAIS systems?

Computer-aided implant surgery has become a highly accessible technology today, documented by multiple studies.[4,6,8] Some of the systems studied are already implemented in clinical practice, while others are on the way to becoming a routine treatment option. The added safety provided in principle by this technology has made it the standard choice for non-invasive treatments, without the need for flap raising and suturing. It is also the first choice for complex cases such as situations with limited bone availability, or where the implants are to be placed very close to critical anatomical structures.[6] All of the above raise the need for an objective evaluation of the precision and accuracy of these procedures.

The terms precision and accuracy are often confused in the reviewed literature; from a colloquial English point of view, they are almost synonymous. However, when we delve into scientific resources, such as the now classic text by Hulley et al., Designing Clinical Research,[9] we find that they are both noticeably different and complementary concepts (Table 5-1). Precision represents the degree to which a treatment, or a procedure, has nearly the same result when applied several times. The best way to assess precision is to compare among repeated applications. It is affected by random error, and it is a synonymous with reproducibility. On the other hand, accuracy is the degree to which a treatment, or a procedure, produces the result that it is supposed to produce, and no other. The best way to assess accuracy is comparison with a reference standard. It is affected by systematic errors, and it is a synonymous with validity.

Focusing on the field of CAIS, we can try to understand the concept by imagining the behavior of a surgical template for placing six implants in a mandible.

Firstly, let us imagine a surgical template that is very stable in the mouth, which holds its position firmly while scanning and during surgery, but in which the adjustment between drills, implant holders, and drill sleeves and cylinders allows for a certain degree of movement. This lack of adaptation during drilling and positioning of the implant allows for a tilting of the drills and of the implant which, depending on multiple factors such as mouth aperture, bone quality, region of the mouth, skill of the surgeon etc, can lead to slight deviations, in opposing directions, with a different angle and of a different magnitude in each location (Fig 5-12). We would therefore encounter a lack of precision, and if the template was to be used repeatedly

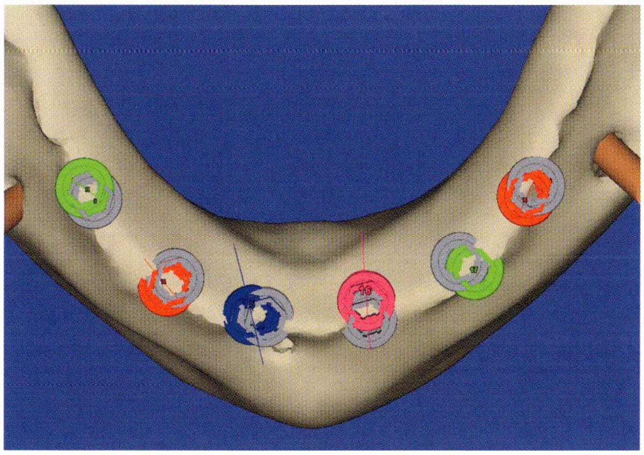

Fig 5-12 Example of lack of precision in the placement of six implants with a drilling template. The implants placed with the template (colored) show random and varied deviations with respect to the planned position (gray color).

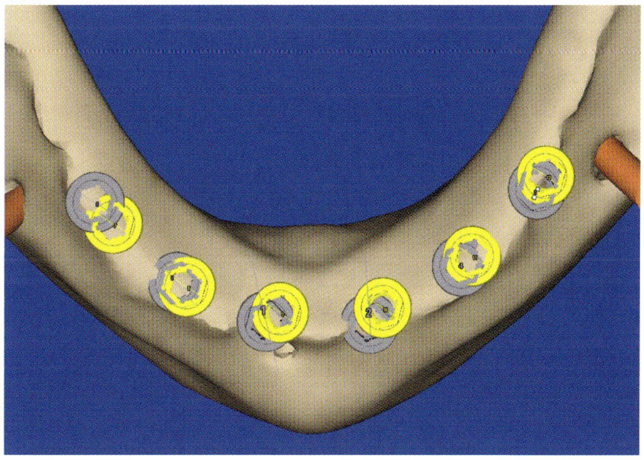

Fig 5-13 Example of lack of accuracy (systematic error) in the placement of six implants with a drilling template. The implants placed with the template (yellow color) show the same type of deviation in all sites with respect to the planned position (gray color).

on different models, the result would change in each case (ie the procedure would not be reproducible).

On the other hand, let's say we have a problem fitting the template into the mouth, which becomes unstable or changes position between scanning and surgery, shifting 1 mm to the left; and, at the same time, the quality of the sleeves of this template results in a perfect seating between the sleeves and drills and consequently the implant can be drilled and positioned without any deviation. In this case, we would be facing a general systematic error, equally affecting all implants which are all shifted 1 mm to the left, maintaining uniformity in all other parameters (Fig 5-13).

In the type of treatment discussed, where both concepts are tightly intertwined, it is difficult to determine when a deviation reported in a study is caused by a problem of precision or accuracy. On the other hand, almost all authors use the term accuracy to encapsulate both concepts, according to the definition of Widmann and Bale:[4] "The accuracy of an image-guided procedure is defined as the deviation in location or angle of the plan compared to the result, and includes all possible individual errors from image acquisition to surgical implant positioning." These types of errors are cumulative and interactive, and range from errors produced by image capturing techniques, possible template instability during x-ray and/or surgery and patient indexing system reliability, to deviations caused by the navigation system or during the surgical template manufacturing process.

Since it is extremely difficult to isolate the effect of each possible source of error, most authors choose to measure the deviations between the position of the planned implant and the position of the implant once placed in the mouth, taking two consecutive CT scans. These scans are then combined and used to evaluate four fundamental variables:

- Deviation at the implant entry point.
- Deviation at the edge of the implant.
- Vertical deviation at the shoulder of the implant.
- Angular deviation of the implant.

A recent meta-analysis from our study group[10] evaluated the precision of these procedures using data from 20 published studies giving information on 12 systems, four of which were based on the use of surgical templates and eight on navigation systems. In total, information was evaluated from 1214 sites (570 implants and 644 drilled alveoli). It is important to bear in mind that the majority of the studies found, particularly those carried out with navigation systems, were performed on cadavers or *in vitro* (14/20), while only six were performed on patients.

Average deviation at the entry point was 0.73 mm (Figs 5-14 and 5-15a), very similar to previous meta-analyses,[6] for which when extrapolated to the general population of patients we could expect a deviation from 0.59 mm to 0.86 mm in 95% of cases. No significant differences were found between the use of template-based systems (average deviation 0.81 mm) and navigation protocols (0.68 mm), although in this second group,

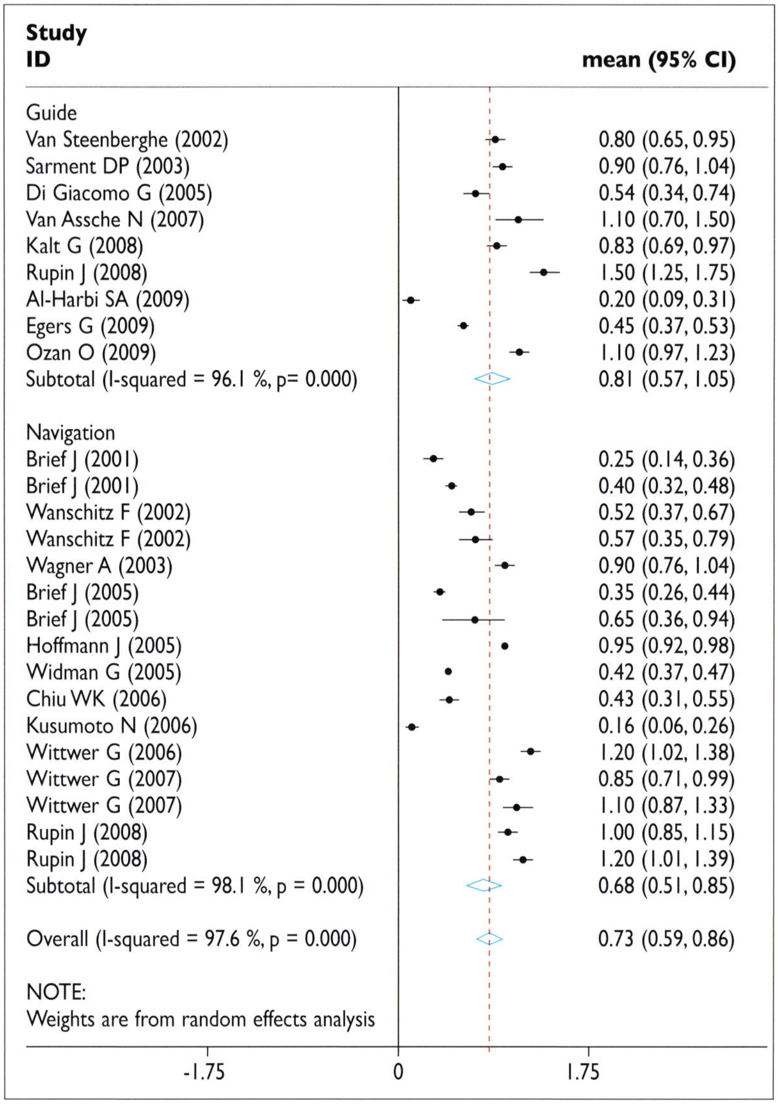

Fig 5-14 Forest plot of deviation analysis at the entry point. The discontinuous vertical red line and the lower diamond indicate the average deviation comprising the studies.[10] Each study is represented by a dot (showing the average) and a horizontal line (showing the standard deviation). The weighted average for each group of studies (template or navigation) is represented by a diamond.

as already mentioned, there are fewer studies on patients. Reliability seems high, although we must consider that in certain cases, the deviations detected could have a significant clinical impact, with the maximum deviation at the point of entry found to be 3.4 mm.[10] Deviation at the apex was 0.85 mm (Fig 5-14), while vertical and angular deviation were 0.3 mm and 5 degrees respectively (Figs 5-15b to 5-15d).[6]

5.3.1 Conclusion

Computer-aided implant surgery is a reliable procedure, with average deviations of less than 1 mm. We must be particularly attentive to factors we can control that can affect the precision of the treatment, such as the correct adaptation of radiographic and surgical templates, adequate patient indexing, and an appropriate image capturing technique. During surgery, the clinician must strive to ensure that the drilling and placement of the implant do not deviate significantly from the plan. Surgery must be guided but must not be blind.

5.4 Is bone density useful as a planning tool?

Primary stability of implants is generally considered an essential factor for osseointegration[11] and capacity to withstand an immediate load, to the extent that if primary stability declines drastically in poor quality bone, osseointegration could be compromised.[12,13] However, primary stability is not only related to bone quantity and quality,

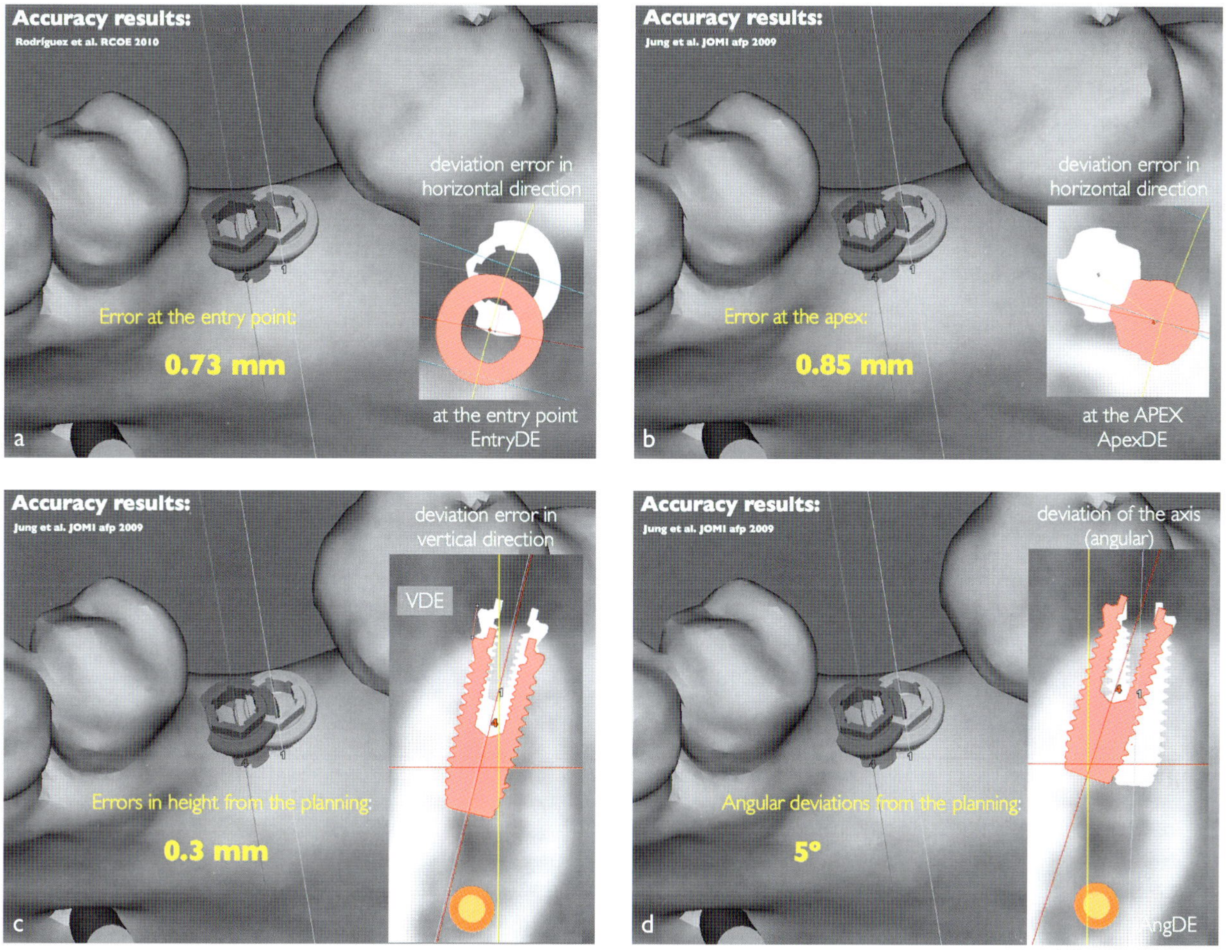

Figs 5-15a to d Measures of precision in CAIS: (a) deviation at entry point, (b) deviation at apex, (c) vertical deviation, and (d) angular deviation.[6]

but also to the morphology of the implant, and the alveoli drilling and the fixture placement techniques.[14,15]

Nowadays, clinicians are forced to make decisions every day during the planning stage, in which they must be able to assess the load capacity of a potential implant that is to be placed at a specific site; patients, meanwhile, expect this decision to be increasingly documented. Consequently, bone density testing of a site where an implant is potentially to be placed could be a parameter of great value.[16]

Bone density is measured in Hounsfield units (HU), which are based on the x-ray attenuation coefficient of the different materials and tissues submitted to x-ray beams. Distilled water at 25°C is defined as zero HU, soft tissues are defined as near-zero HU or negative HU values, while bone, in a CT scan, would fluctuate between 100 and 1900 HU.[16] Trabecular bone would be at the bottom of this scale, and negative values within the space occupied by the bone would represent fatty tissue that has replaced trabecular bone.[17]

Various authors have proposed scales to match HUs and the Lekholm and Zarb bone type classification. One of these is the Fanfani approach.[16]

- 100–350 HU for type IV bone
- 350–700 HU for type III bone
- 700–1200 HU for type II bone
- 1200–1900 HU for type I bone.

Today, the use of CBCT scanners has modified slightly this scale, although there is still a good correlation between bone types and HUs obtained with CBCTs. Like in CT scans, with CBCT studies it is more difficult to distinguish between types II and III bone, though these are clearly differentiated from types I and IV.[18] As a clinical guideline, the authors propose the following scale for CBCT data:

- -50–100 HU for type IV bone
- 100–250 HU for type III bone
- 250–400 HU for type II bone
- > 400 HU for type I bone.

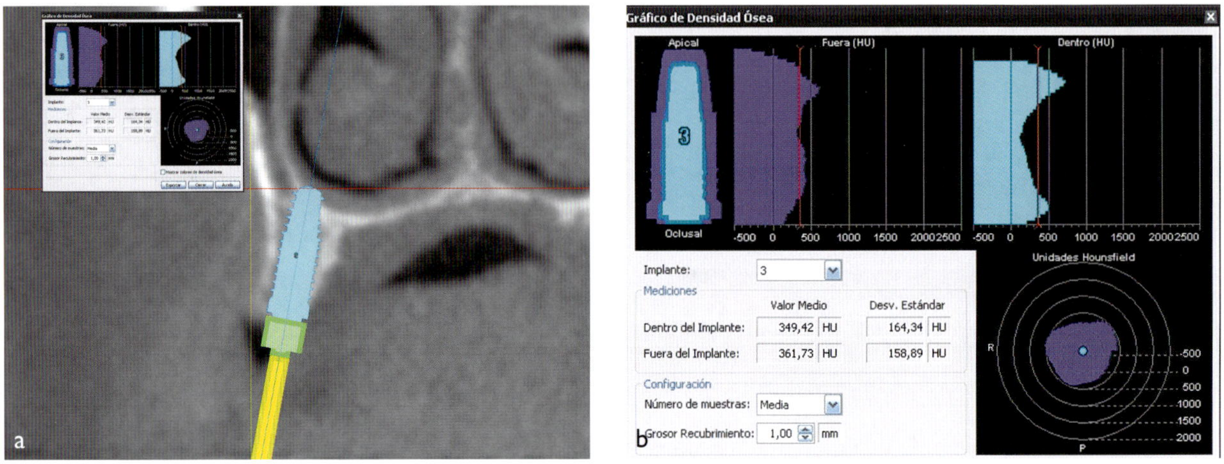

Figs 5-16a and b Bone density analysis obtained using the SimPlant® software in an edentulous area of the alveolar ridge (a). This analysis provides the profile and values of the mean and standard deviation for the osseous portion that will surround the virtually placed implant (blue), and for the bone that is to be removed at the drilling stage (green) (b). The average value in peri-implant bone is 361.73 HU, showing a profile (blue graph) quite balanced with respect to the average (red line) (b).

From a clinical perspective, using CBCT in areas with bone density values over 250 HU gives a good prognosis for primary stability. Greater care must be taken in sites with values of 100 to 250 HU, where good primary stability can be achieved provided that it is performed with carefully customized progressive instrumentation and using an implant with the appropriate morphology (Fig 5-16).

This type of information lets us approach the problem with two different strategies: on the one hand, choosing an implant site that offers optimal immediate load capacity and the best long-term prognosis; on the other hand, establishing the drilling sequence and the type of implant preoperatively, which, given the circumstances, would achieve the best possible primary stability.[15]

One of the drawbacks of measuring bone density in HU is that it is affected by the amount of energy passing through the tissues, which depends on the x-ray technique used with the CT or CBCT. Techniques that use less energy will provide images with higher HU values. As such, studies deriving from different CT or CBCT equipment, set up with different techniques, will give different bone density information in HU. From a research stand point and regarding the publication of results, the solution to this problem may lie in quantitative computerized tomography (QCT).[14] This technique is based on the use of a calibration phantom submitted to CT or CBCT testing at the same time as the patient, which allows calibration of the measuring tool and conversion of HUs into mg of hydroxyapatite per cm^3, or bone mineral density (BMD) units.[14,15] These data can be extrapolated amongst x-ray devices. The clinician can mitigate this problem internally by using the same CT or CBCT device configured using the same technique.

5.4.1 Conclusions

It is advisable to evaluate peri-implant bone density a priori in order to adequately choose the best site for the implant, to optimize the drilling technique, and to select the type of implant in order to obtain the best primary stability, particularly with immediate load methods. All CT or CBCT testing should be performed using the same equipment and configured applying the same technique in order to produce consistent bone density values.

5.5 What are the benefits and drawbacks of each type of system?

Each of the systems evaluated has its own advantages and disadvantages (Tables 5-2 and 5-3), therefore a specialized clinic would benefit from using different systems for different indications, which would broaden its range of use for computer-assisted surgery.

From a practical point of view, clinic and laboratory produced templates offer logistic and economic benefits. Moreover, the Med3D® system, as it is an open technique system, allows the use of cylinders in templates of

Table 5-2 Main differences among the different systems of computer-assisted implant surgery from a clinical point of view

System	Scanning procedure (simple or double)	Fully EP	Perpendicular guide pins to gain stability	Partially EP	Bone-supported templates	Hardware	Facilitates producing immediate provisional prostheses	Open or closed system	Industrial or lab-clinic fabrication of template
NobelGuide®	Double: Pat + Dent and Dent + Fiduc	+++	Yes	+ Scanning of plaster cast	No	+++	+++	Closed	Industrial
SimPlant®	Simple Pat + Dent + RO teeth	+++	Yes	+ Scanning of plaster cast	Yes	++	+++	Open	Industrial
Med3D®	Simple template + teeth + lego brick	+	Difficult	+++ No scanning of plaster cast	No	+++	+++	Open	Lab-clinic
RoboDent®	Simple plastic template + Fiduc	+	No	+++ No scanning of plaster cast	No	No need for special hardware	++	Open	No need

Pat, patient; Dent, denture; EP, edentulous patient; Fiduc, fiducials; RO, radiopaque.

Table 5-3 Main differences among the different systems of computer-assisted implant surgery from a software capabilities point of view

System	Ability to produce a high-quality 3D model	Helpful when exploring the arch anatomy	Helpful when planning implants	Bone density tool	Ability to separate/ highlight anatomic structures	Virtual teeth	Allows precise information of soft tissues	Allows precise information of neighboring crowns/teeth	Planning of bone grafts
NobelGuide®	++ Automatic (editable)	++	++	+	+	No	No	No	No
SimPlant®	+++ (SimPlant Pro or higher version)	+++	+++	+++	+++	Yes	No?	No?	Yes (higher version)
Med3D®	++ Automatic (editable)	++	++	+	+	No	No	No	No
RoboDent®	+ Automatic	+	+	+	+	No	No	No	No

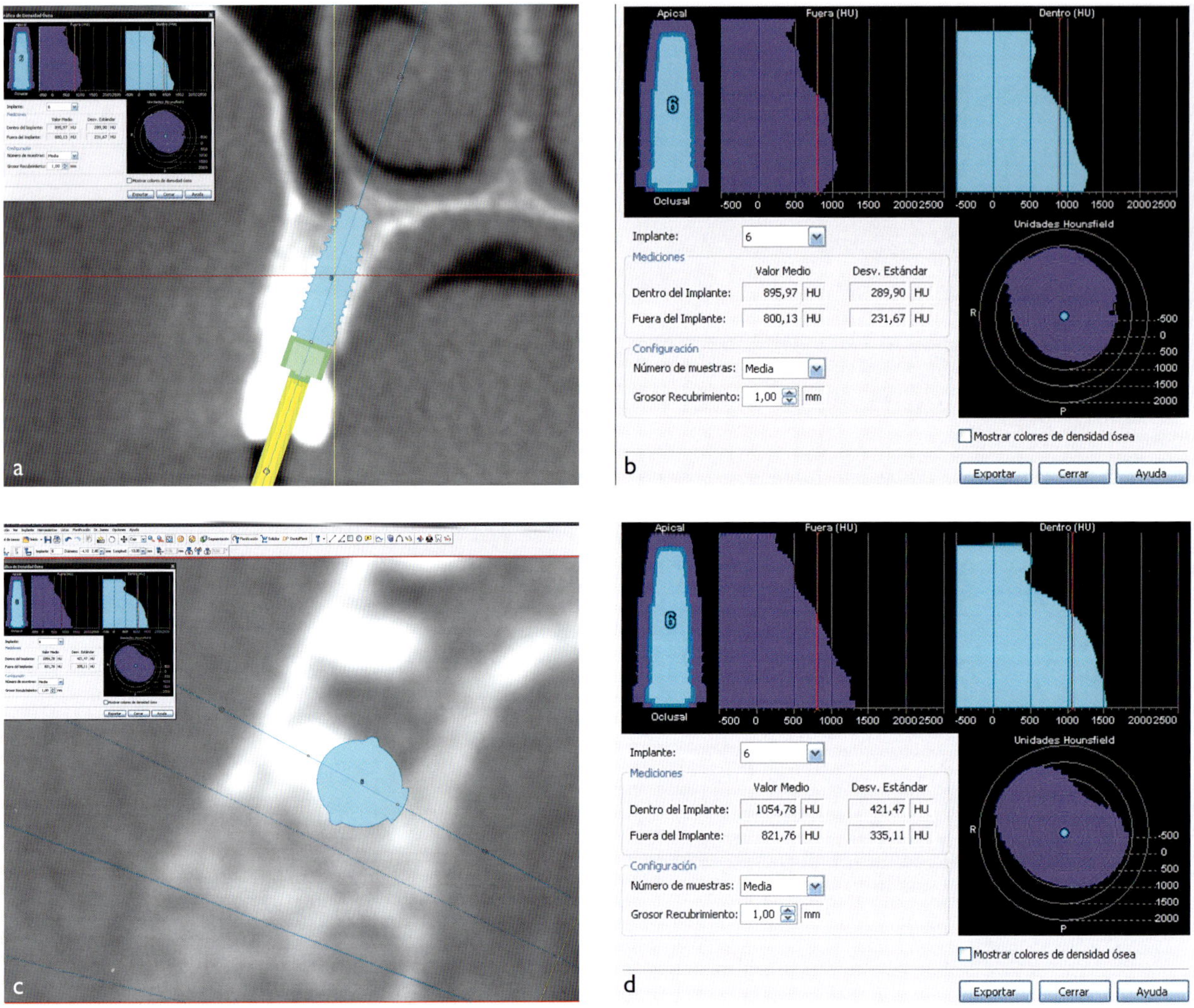

Figs 5-17a to d Bone density analysis in the planning of an immediate post-extraction implant (a). The high density of the tooth (close to 1000 HU; not yet extracted) increases the average density of the future peri-implant bone (800.13 HU) (b), which could lead to clinical confusion. At this point, it is important to observe the profile on the blue graph (b) and assess the bone density apical to the remaining tooth (close to 500 HU) and, from an occlusal perspective (c and d), the density profile of the mesial, distal, and palatine bone.

any implant manufacturer (provided that the company manufactures the corresponding cylinder positioning tool). This, together with its ability to adapt the template to the adjacent teeth (as it is basically created on plaster models, it is not affected by radiographic artifacts), makes this type of mechanical procedure the best choice for building a template for partially edentulous patients (ie to design and fabricate tooth-supported or tooth/mucosa-supported templates [Table 5-2]).

Planning stabilization pins on axes that are nearly perpendicular to those of the implants to be placed is more complex – and sometimes impossible – when using mechanical systems. For this reason, in fully edentulous patients, it seems more appropriate to use procedures based on the use of stereolithographic templates (NobelGuide® and SimPlant®), where stabilization pins can be placed (Table 5-2).

Finally, as it is easy to index patients with a plastic plate securing an arch with markers, and this shows a good stability in partially edentulous patients with teeth at both ends of the edentulous gap, navigation systems such as Robodent® are the most operative procedure. While these procedures reduced costs in each case, because templates are not needed, we do have to consider the cost of purchasing the equipment and tools, which is far greater (Table 5-2).

However, a computer-assisted surgery system needs to provide something more than the mere production of templates or enabling the use of navigators: it needs to facilitate diagnosis and surgery planning. In this sense, it is essential that such a system allows for the creation of high-quality custom 3D models with tools for examining the jaw to be treated (beyond just the placement of implants), providing the clinician with an effective tool for evaluating bone density in each potential implant site (Figs 5-16 and 5-17) and allowing for the separation of the relevant anatomic structures and for virtual dental extractions (Fig 5-2; Table 5-3).

5.5.1 Conclusions

For a specialized center with a significant surgical volume, it may be convenient to use several CAIS systems alongside each other.

- In free-end partially edentulous patients and those requiring multiple implants with just a few remaining teeth, a mechanical system may be the best option.
- In partially edentulous patients with teeth on both sides of the edentulous area, a navigation system would be quicker and more versatile.
- In fully edentulous patients, greater template stability would be observed when using stereolithographic template systems.

5.6 What are the limitations of computer-assisted surgery?

5.6.1 Acceptable reliability, occasional deviations

We have previously reviewed the reliability of CAIS procedures, and reached the conclusion that average reliability is clinically acceptable, with deviations of less than 1 mm. However, we cannot rule out that occasional protocol alterations might cause significant deviations in assisted implant placement. Therefore, the drilling angle and implant placement must be continuously monitored throughout surgery.

5.6.2 A need to combine different systems

Likewise, we have reviewed the CAIS systems and concluded that it would be interesting to use several procedures (mechanical and stereolithographic templates, navigation systems) for different types of clinical scenarios. Unfortunately, this versatility can only be achieved by combining diverse systems, which would multiply the workload and costs for the professional team. Consequently, the ideal situation would be to have a common diagnosis platform that allows for comprehensive diagnosis and planning, and for the creation of any type of template or the use of navigation procedures.

5.6.3 Lack of information on soft tissue

Finally, there is a crucial limitation regarding the information provided by our tomographic research on soft tissue and adjacent teeth morphology, as well as regarding the soft tissue margin position in relation with the position, height, and width of the alveolar crest. It is therefore quite complex to make a precise esthetic evaluation in current 3D models. To overcome this conflict, several experimental procedures have been established where patients' digital imaging and communications in medicine (DICOM) data are assembled with files created from scanning plaster models and pictures of the patient. However, this process shows complications arising from a lack of precision in its analogical factor, as well as from assembling 2D images (eg pictures) on 3D models.

Luckily enough, with the development of intraoral optical scanning technology, such as 3M LAVA (3M, St Paul, MN, USA) systems, information on soft tissue and morphology of adjacent teeth can now be retrieved digitally and in a more precise fashion, and this information can then be brought together in a .stl file that can be "assembled" with DICOM data. This new method of combining information will allow the surgeon to carry out more reliable planning, particularly regarding noninvasive surgical techniques, and a better preoperative assessment of esthetics issues. It could be used to measure esthetic parameters after implant surgery, such as the capacity to preserve the volume of the alveolar ridge after tooth extractions, or the progress of regenerative procedures. Nowadays, this is only possible by analyzing sawn and scanned sections of plaster models, and it will be of great help also in the fabrication of tooth- or mucosa- supported stereolithographic templates (Fig 5-18).

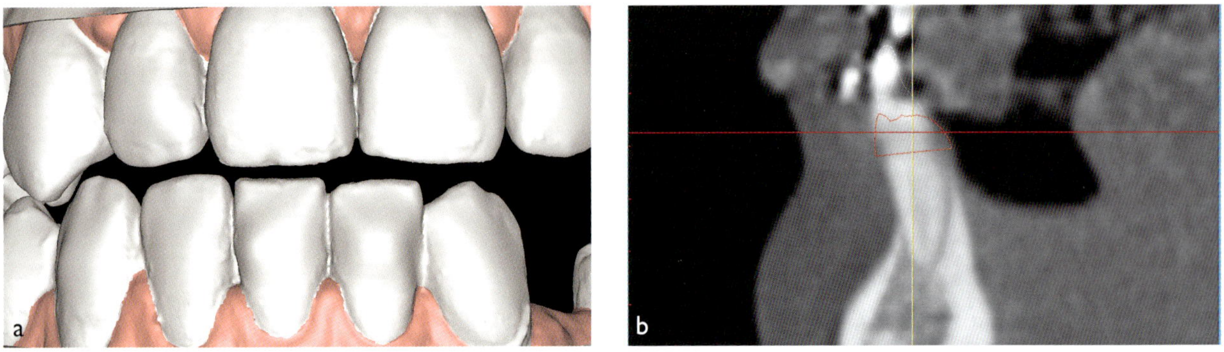

Figs 5-18a and b Resulting images after assembling a DICOM file obtained with a CBCT (iCAT) equipment and a .stl file created from an intraoral optical scanner (3M LAVA). Notice the precise morphology of tooth crowns and soft tissue (a), and its relation with the underlying DICOM data containing information about root morphology and the alveolar bone (b).

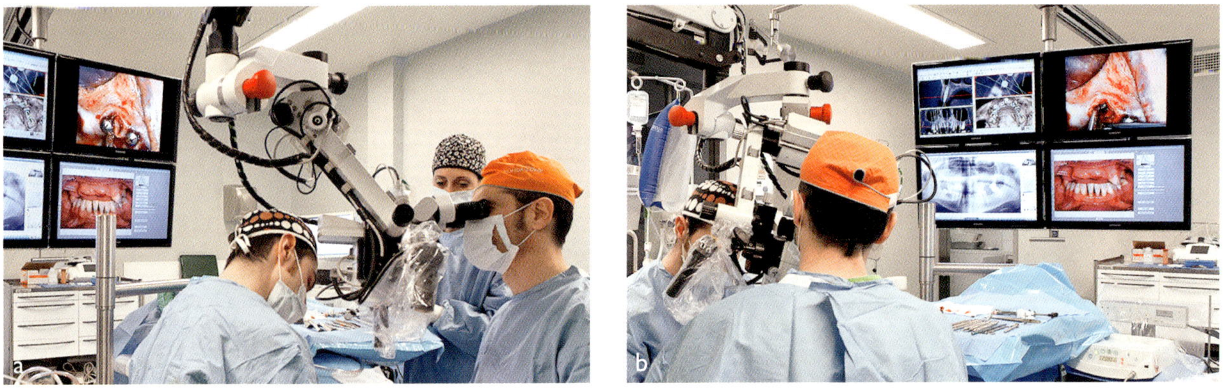

Figs 5-19a and b (a) Surgical environment with multiple screens for COIS. (b) At surgery, the surgeon and his team interactively manage information from the microscope camera, the preoperative intraoral picture, the 2D radiology, the planning information, and the 3D model.

5.7 Computer-oriented surgery: a new dynamic concept

The occasional lack of reliability, the need to use multiple systems in order to approach diverse indications, the scarce information on soft tissue and coronary structure of adjacent teeth, and the need for free, creative, and flexible surgical procedures that can adapt to different intraoral environments and scenarios have encouraged a simultaneous use of information in digital planning, as well as data directly retrieved from clinical reality at surgery, creating the so-called computer-oriented implant surgery (COIS).

In this type of procedure, the surgeon uses digital and analogical information in the planning stage (3D models, planning systems, virtual implant placement, real models, clinical pictures, and standard radiography). Moreover, the surgeon keeps a close rapport with this information during surgery through a computer multi-screen structure, where information from the microscope camera, the preoperative diagnostic picture, standard radiology, and the 3D planning software program are constantly adapted depending on the intraoral site in which the surgeon is working. This technology allows the surgeon to use a template or navigation system at the initial drilling phase using the 2-mm twist drill, in order to establish the position and axis of the future implant, and perform the remaining surgery stages applying a COIS procedure, or the surgery can be entirely carried out using a COIS method. The concept behind this proceeding is the interactive use of information in order to promote at each stage continued "documented real-time decision making" (Fig 5-19).

5.8 Disclosure agreement

The authors of this article declare that at the time of drafting, they had no economic ties whatsoever with any of the companies involved in the design and distribution of the products and equipment of CAIS described herein. Practical statements reflect the authors' experience in the direct use of the various systems analyzed and are merely intended to share their experience with clinicians getting started in this field.

References

1. Sicilia A. Guía rápida para el diagnóstico preoperatorio del paciente de implantes dentales. Barcelona: Ergon, 1993.
2. Sicilia A, Noguerol B, Cobo J, Zabalegui I. Profile surgical template: a systematic approach to precise implant placement. A technical note. Int J Oral Maxillofac Implants 1998;13:109-114.
3. Sicilia A, Enrile FJ, Buitrago P, Zubizarreta J. Evaluation of the precision obtained with a fixed surgical template in the placement of implants for rehabilitation of the completely edentulous maxilla: a clinical report. Int J Oral Maxillofac Implants 2000;15:272-277.
4. Widmann G, Bale RJ. Accuracy in computer-aided implant surgery: a review. Pediatr Nephrol 2006;21:305-307.
5. Tardieu PB, Vrielinck L, Escolano E. Computer-assisted implant placement. A case report: treatment of the mandible. Int J Oral Maxillofac Implants 2003;18:599-604.
6. Jung RE, Schneider D, Ganeles J, Wismeijer D, Zwahlen M, Hämmerle CH, et al. Computer technology applications in surgical implant dentistry: a systematic review. Int J Oral Maxillofac Implants 2009;24(Suppl):92-109.
7. Suarez-Feito JM, Sicilia A, Angulo J, Banerji S, Cuesta I, Millar B. Clinical performance of provisional screw-retained metal-free acrylic restorations in an immediate loading implant protocol: a 242 consecutive patients' report. Clin Oral Implants Res 2010;21:1360-1369.
8. Schneider D, Marquardt P, Zwahlen M, Jung RE. A systematic review on the accuracy and the clinical outcome of computer-guided template-based implant dentistry. Clin Oral Implants Res 2009;20(Suppl 4):73-86.
9. Hulley S, Cummings SR, Browner WS, Grady DG, Hearst N, Newman TB. Planning the measurements: precision and accuracy. In: Designing Clinical Research: An Epidemiologic Approach, 3rd ed. Baltimore: Lippincott, Williams & Wilkins, 2006.
10. Rodríguez-Sánchez A, Cuesta Frechoso S, Tobías A, Sicilia A. Exactitud de los sistemas de cirugía guiada para implantología oral. Revisión sistemática. Revista del Consejo de Odontólogos y Estomatólogos de España 2010;15:301-311.
11. Friberg B, Jemt T, Lekholm U. Early failures in 4,641 consecutively placed Branemark dental implants: a study from stage I surgery to the connection of completed prostheses. Int J Oral Maxillofac Implants 1991;6:142-146.
12. Balshi SF, Allen FD, Wolfinger GJ, Balshi TJ. A resonance frequency analysis assessment of maxillary and mandibular immediately loaded implants. Int J Oral Maxillofac Implants 2005;20:584-594.
13. Balshi SF, Wolfinger GJ, Balshi TJ. A prospective study of immediate functional loading, following the Teeth in a Day protocol: a case series of 55 consecutive edentulous maxillas. Clin Implant Dent Relat Res 2005;7:24-31.
14. Beer A, Gahleitner A, Holm A, Tschabitscher M, Homolka P. Correlation of insertion torques with bone mineral density from dental quantitative CT in the mandible. Clin Oral Implants Res 2003;14:616-620.
15. Homolka P, Beer A, Birkfellner W, Nowotny R, Gahleitner A, Tschabitscher M, et al. Bone mineral density measurement with dental quantitative CT prior to dental implant placement in cadaver mandibles: pilot study. Radiology 2002;224:247-252.
16. Todisco M, Trisi P. Bone mineral density and bone histomorphometry are statistically related. Int J Oral Maxillofac Implants 2005;20:898-904.
17. Shahlaie M, Gantes B, Schulz E, Riggs M, Crigger M. Bone density assessments of dental implant sites: 1. Quantitative computed tomography. Int J Oral Maxillofac Implants 2003;18:224-231.
18. Aranyarachkul P, Caruso J, Gantes B, Schulz E, Riggs M, Dus I. Bone density assessments of dental implant sites: 2. Quantitative cone-beam computerized tomography. Int J Oral Maxillofac Implants 2005;20:416-424.

Chapter 6

Should we really care about peri-implantitis? Can it be successfully treated?

Patricia Anguis Martín, Santiago Mareque Bueno, Hugo Campos Leitão

6.1 Introduction

Replacing a patient's lost teeth is nowadays considered to be as important as obtaining a good esthetic outcome and maintaining implants in adequate health and function.

The literature shows that as the number of dental practices where implants are placed increases, the cases of infection and loss of implants associated with infection increase.

The oral cavity harbors a diverse microbial community, which colonizes different locations and is present in both hard and soft tissues. Therefore, there is a potential for infection due to this bacterial biofilm.

A positive relationship has been established between adequate oral hygiene and prevention of peri-implant diseases. It has been speculated that peri-implant tissues may have a lower capacity of response against external aggressions due to a number of anatomic differences when compared with teeth. It is therefore extremely important to control risk factors and establish an adequate plaque control in order to prevent peri-implant diseases from occurring around dental implants.

There are situations where disease may already be established and clinicians need to be able to correctly diagnose and treat this peri-implant disease. It is important to know the best diagnostic methods, and treatment should be performed according to the diagnosis.

In the first part of this chapter the reader will be guided through the main steps of a proper and accurate diagnosis. Different methods, techniques, and aspects of diagnosis are clarified. Peri-implantitis is multifactorial in nature, and assessment of risk factors is explained.

The last part of this chapter discusses chemical, nonsurgical and surgical treatment of peri-implantitis lesions. Studies both in humans and animals lead the authors to suggest treatment protocols for different situations.

6.2 Background

Peri-implant diseases (peri-implant mucositis and peri-implantitis) are infectious diseases that occur because of an imbalance between bacterial load and host defenses.[1] Peri-implant mucositis describes an inflammatory lesion that resides in the mucosa, while peri-implantitis also affects the supporting bone.[2]

The term "peri-implantitis" was introduced in the late 1980s and was subsequently defined as an inflammatory process affecting the soft and hard tissues around a functioning osseointegrated implant, resulting in loss of supporting bone.[3]

Examples of non-integration or the loss of osseointegration that cannot be considered peri-implantitis include processes that appear during the early stages of *osseointegration*. They are usually the consequence of poor surgical technique (overheating of the bone) or insufficient trabecular bone density in the receptor. In this case, the bone is biologically incapable of bonding to the implant surface, or good primary mechanical stability is impossible at the time of placement as a result of its low density.

Following implant placement, a transmucosal seal is formed around the abutment of the device. The mucosa surrounding the implants and the gingiva surrounding teeth have many features in common. Both tissues are lined with a keratinized oral epithelium; at clinically healthy sites this is continuous with a thin nonkeratinized junctional epithelium that faces the implant or the tooth surface. In the connective tissue immediately lateral to these thin epithelial linings small infiltrates of inflammatory cells (neutrophils, macrophages, T cells, B cells) are frequently seen.[4] The inflammatory cells represent the host's defense against bacterial products and hence they may be considered as one important component of the biological seal that separates the peri-implant and periodontal attachment tissues from the oral cavity.[4]

In order to aid the professional dealing with cases of peri-implantitis, the following topics will be reviewed in this chapter:

- 6.3 What is the cause of peri-implantitis?
- 6.4 Is there a relationship between previous periodontal disease and peri-implantitis?
- 6.5 How can peri-implantitis be diagnosed?
  - 6.5.1 Peri-implant mucositis
  - 6.5.2 Peri-implantitis
- 6.6 Evaluating oral hygiene
  - 6.6.1 Plaque assessment
  - 6.6.2 Mucosal condition
  - 6.6.3 Presence or absence of bleeding
  - 6.6.4 Peri-implant probing depth
  - 6.6.5 Width of peri-implant keratinized mucosa
  - 6.6.6 Suppuration
- 6.7 How can the bone-to-implant interface be evaluated?
  - 6.7.1 Implant mobility and discomfort
  - 6.7.2 Resonance frequency analysis (RFA)
- 6.8 What to look for in x-ray examinations
- 6.9 What are the main risk factors for peri-implantitis?
- 6.10 How should peri-implantitis be treated?
  - 6.10.1 Does antimicrobial treatment work?
  - 6.10.2 How to decontaminate an implant surface
  - 6.10.3 Surgical or nonsurgical treatment?
- 6.11 International University of Catalonia protocol
- 6.12 Clinical cases

6.3 What is the cause of peri-implantitis?

Oral colonization by bacterial species involves a complex relationship of many factors. Several investigations have shown that in a biofilm, microcolonies of mixed species are formed, and through an inter-species mechanism of protection, anaerobes are able to colonize aerobic environments.[5-7] There are higher mean counts of anaerobic species such as *Tannerella forsythia*, *Porphyromonas gingivalis*, *Treponema denticola* and *Prevotella nigrescens* in a supragingival environment of diseased implants when compared with healthy implants (Fig 6-1).

The main difference between healthy and diseased implants is the higher level of some periodontal pathogens and the lower mean proportions of host-compatible microbial complexes in the peri-implantitis affected sites.[8]

Although the microbiology of dental implants in clinically healthy and diseased situations has been studied less intensively than the microbiology of the natural dentition, available data suggest the following:

1. The new "hard tissue" surface presented to the oral environment by the implant provides a surface for the attachment of salivary proteins, peptides, and other substances. These substances rapidly form a pellicle that is probably quite similar to the pellicle formed on natural teeth.
2. The pellicle provides receptors for the adhesions on specific species of oral bacteria that form the early colonizers of the implant. These species appear to be similar to those that colonize the teeth and include members of the genera *Streptococcus*, *Actinomyces*, and *Veillonella*.
3. The insertion of the implant appears to "set the clock back" for the development of the mature biofilm; ie for a number of years the microbiological composition of biofilms on healthy implants may be similar to that observed on the surfaces of periodontally healthy teeth in the adolescent.
4. With time, varying from months to years, the implant microbiota becomes more complex. Pockets may develop around the implant, which harbor increased numbers and proportions of orange and red complex species in a similar way to the increase in these species in deep periodontal pockets adjacent to natural teeth.

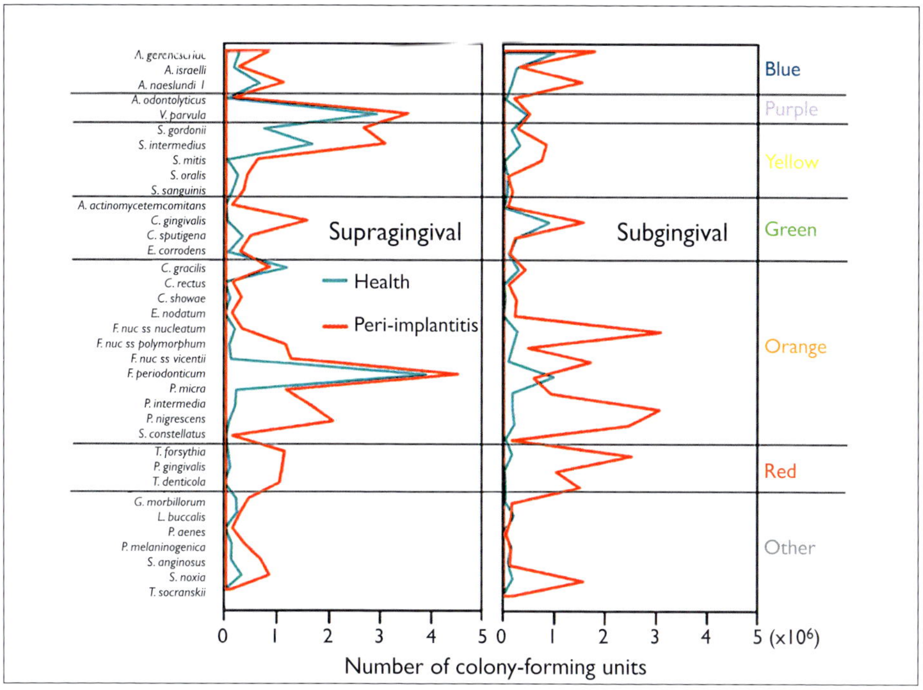

Fig 6-1 Microbial composition of the supragingival biofilmin in periodontally healthy and diseased implant areas.

5. The development of peri-implantitis appears to be related to an increase in bacterial species that have been found to increase in periodontitis.These include periodontal pathogens, such as *P gingivalis*, *T forsythia*, and *Aggregatibacter actinomycetemcomitans*, as well as additional taxa including staphylococci and enteric rods.

6.4 Is there a relationship between previous periodontal disease and peri-implantitis?

Since the remaining dentition has been identified as a source of microorganisms that colonize implants, it might be assumed that higher levels of periodontal pathogens would colonize implants in subjects with periodontal disease.The early colonization of dental implants in subjects treated for aggressive periodontitis was examined in 22 subjects who were on a maintenance program for periods ranging from 12 to 240 months.[9] DNA probes were used to determine the levels of subgingival species such as *A actinomycetemcomitans*, *P gingivalis*, *Prevotella intermedia*, *T forsythia*, and *T denticola*.The implants were colonized by all five periodontal pathogens as early as 10 days after implant insertion and an increase in the frequency of detection of most pathogens was observed over time.

The presence of these species appears to increase the long-term risk for peri-implantitis in subjects with a history of periodontitis.

6.5 How can peri-implantitis be diagnosed?

Correct diagnosis of peri-implant diseases is critical for appropriate management.[10] Periodontal probing should be performed to identify bleeding and/or suppuration. For the assessment of marginal bone loss, radiographs are also needed. It is important, however, to distinguish between bone remodeling that occurs early after implant installation and the loss of supporting bone that may occur due to peri-implantitis.

The so-called apical peri-implantitis or periapical lesion, in which the peri-implant infection is initially located in the apical region of the implant, would also be excluded from the disease category of peri-implantitis. Apical peri-implantitis is due to bacterial contamination of this area by coming in contact with the apex of a tooth that has undergone root canal and without histological signs of healing, even though no clinical or radiological

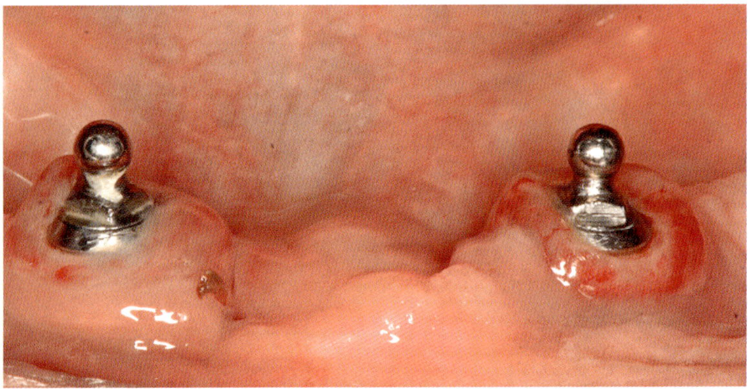

Fig 6-2 Plaque and calculus in implants.

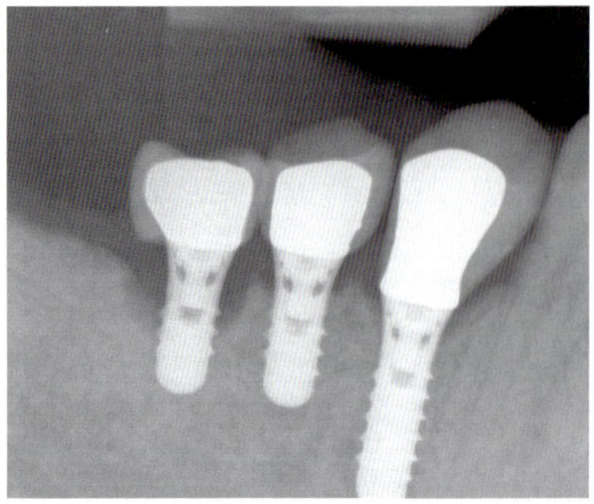

Fig 6-3 Peri-implant defect affecting implants in positions 12 and 13 detected on a periapical radiograph.

symptoms are evident when placing the implant. It may also be the result of implant contamination by epithelial rests of Malassez that remain within the bone despite proper alveolar scaling following extraction of the tooth to be replaced by the implant.

6.5.1 Peri-implant mucositis

The clinical features of peri-implant mucositis are in many aspects similar to those of gingivitis at teeth and include classical symptoms of inflammation, such as swelling and redness. Differences in the morphology of the peri-implant mucosa and the lack of light transmission through the metal of the device, however, may mask visible signs of inflammation. Assessment of peri-implant mucositis must therefore always include assessment of bleeding following probing.

6.5.2 Peri-implantitis

Peri-implantitis is a clinical condition that includes the presence of 1) an inflammatory lesion in the peri-implant mucosa and 2) loss of peri-implant bone. The assessment of the diagnosis of peri-implantitis must consequently require detection of both bleeding on probing (BOP) and bone loss on radiographs. Peri-implantitis initially affects the marginal part of the peri-implant tissues and the implant may remain stable and in function for varying periods of time. Implant mobility is therefore not an essential symptom for peri-implantitis but may occur in a final stage of disease progression and indicates complete loss of integration. As for the clinical characteristics of peri-implant mucositis, various factors such as the morphology of the peri-implant mucosa and position of the implant may also influence the clinical appearance of inflammation in peri-implantitis. Probing is therefore a prerequisite in the examination of peri-implant tissues and should include assessment of both BOP and probing depth (PD).

The clinical appearance of peri-implantitis may therefore vary, and may not always be associated with signs of pathology. Plaque and calculus together with clinical signs of inflammation are present in Figure 6-2, but this does not reveal symptoms of peri-implantitis.

The results of Serino and Stróm[11] show that peri-implant lesions were associated with inadequate plaque control at implant sites, while peri-implantitis was a rare finding around implants when proper plaque control was ensured. These findings are important in the evaluation of risk factors for the development of peri-implantitis. This study shows the importance of giving proper oral hygiene instructions to patients who are rehabilitated with a dental implant as well as performing proper prosthetic constructions that allow accessibility for oral hygiene around implants.

Crater-formed defects around implants are frequently found in radiographs obtained from sites with peri-implantitis (Fig 6-3).

Bone loss in such sites appears also to be symmetric, ie similar amounts of bone loss occur at mesial, distal, buccal, and lingual aspects of the implants. On the other hand, the morphology of the osseous defect may vary depending on the horizontal dimension of the alveolar ridge. Thus, in sites where the buccal–lingual width of the ridge exceeds that of the peri-implantitis lesion, a buccal and lingual bone wall may remain. Conversely, in sites with a narrow ridge the buccal and lingual bone will be resorbed and lost during progression of peri-implantitis (Fig 6-4).

Symptoms of peri-implantitis relate to the infectious/inflammatory nature of the lesion. Thus, there is radiographic evidence of bone loss, and the bone loss often has the shape of a crater. Swelling and redness of the mucosa as well as bleeding on gentle probing occur. Suppuration is also a frequent finding. The implant may remain stable over long periods.[12]

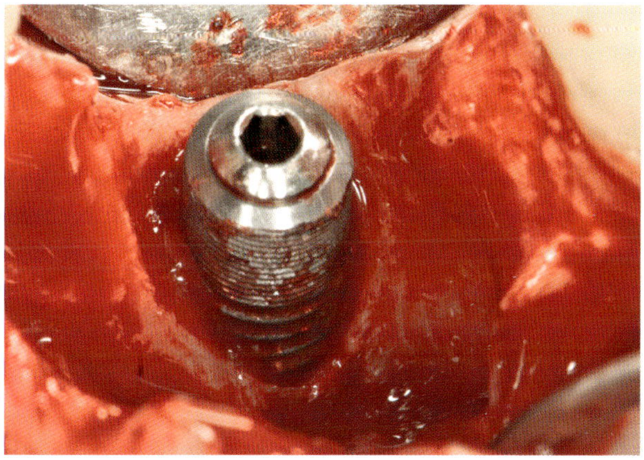

Fig 6-4 Bone loss around implants placed on a narrow ridge due to peri-implantitis.

6.6 Evaluating oral hygiene

6.6.1 Plaque assessment

Microbial biofilms have been shown to form on inert biomaterial surfaces in an aqueous environment. Implants placed in the oral cavity represent artificial surfaces colonized by bacteria from saliva and ecologic niches such as periodontal pockets, tonsils, and crypts of the tongue. Experimental and human studies have provided evidence that formation and development of a microbial biofilm represents an important etiologic factor in the pathogenesis of peri-implant disease.

6.6.2 Mucosal conditions

In addition to redness and swelling of the marginal tissues, BOP, pocket formation, and suppuration have been reported to result from peri-implant infections.[13,14] Assessment of these clinical signs has been considered important in the diagnosis of periodontal diseases. Therefore, the definition of peri-implant parameters based on periodontal indices such as the gingival index (GI) system seems indicated.

Around implants, however, soft tissue texture and color depend on the normal appearance of the recipient tissues before implant placement, and may be influenced by the material characteristics of the implant surface. Furthermore, difficulties in recording mucosal inflammation have been reported, such as nonkeratinized peri-implant mucosa normally appearing redder than keratinized tissue.

6.6.3 Presence or absence of bleeding

Presence of BOP (notated in clinical records as BOP+) elicited after the insertion of a probe into the sulcus with light pressure (ie 0.25 N) has been shown to detect the presence of an inflammatory lesion in the gingiva around teeth with a normal and a healthy but reduced periodontium.[15,16] Absence of BOP (notated BOP–) has been reported to represent peri-implant health with a negative predictive value of 98.5%.[15,16]

The authors reported that BOP alone yielded higher diagnostic accuracy at implant sites compared with tooth sites.[15,16] Furthermore, when combining positive microbiologic test and BOP of 75% or more, the positive predictive values were greater for implants than for teeth. With predictive values of 100% at BOP frequencies of 50% or more at implant sites, this parameter appears to play a central role in monitoring changes in peri-implant tissue conditions.

6.6.4 Peri-implant probing depth

In contrast to natural teeth, for which average PD has been reported, the physiologic depth of the peri-implant sulcus of successfully osseointegrated implants has been a matter of debate. Increasing periodontal PD and loss of clinical attachment are pathognomonic for periodontal diseases. Pocket probing is therefore an important diagnostic process for the assessment of periodontal status and for the evaluation of periodontal therapy. The extent of probe penetration is influenced by factors such as probing force and angulation, probe tip diameter, roughness of the implant or root surface, inflammatory state of the periodontium, and firmness of the marginal tissues. Furthermore, it has to be realized that PD measurements may be affected by compromised access. Data demonstrate that the periodontal probe often fails to locate the histologic level of the connective tissue attachment around teeth.[17,18] The differences with respect to soft tissue composition, organization, and attachment between the gingiva and the root surface on the one hand and between the peri-implant mucosa and the implant surface on the other make the conditions for PD measurements around teeth and implants not fully comparable.[19] One potential explanation influencing the differences in probe penetration is that most collagen fibers in the supracrestal connective tissue compartment have been demonstrated to run mostly in a parallel direction to the implant axis.[20]

However, if healthy peri-implant conditions or mucositis are present, the probe tips may identify the histologic level of the supracrestal connective tissue attachment. One potential explanation for the different outcomes between the two abovementioned studies may be attributed to the different probing forces employed (0.5 N versus 0.2 N). An experimental study in monkeys[19] has documented that PD measurements around teeth and implants are different. While no difference was observed with respect to probe penetration under healthy peri-implant/periodontal conditions, mild and severe marginal inflammation around implants was associated with a significantly deeper probe penetration into the supracrestal connective tissue when compared with that around teeth. The magnitude of probe penetration into a periodontal pocket depends on the force application.[21,22] Furthermore, simultaneous recordings of PD and probing force before and after periodontal therapy have revealed that the force range chosen for repeated probing influences the amount of attachment level change determined.[22,23]

It was concluded that peri-implant PD measurements are more sensitive to force variation than the corresponding measurements around teeth.[24] Correlations between bone levels recorded on radiographs and the extent of peri-implant probe penetration have been observed. In general, studies have indicated that successful implants allow probe penetration of approximately 3 mm.[13,25,26] Implant shape and surface texture influence penetration of the probe tip. Peri-implant probing is impossible around some implant systems because of characteristics of the design (eg concavities, shoulders, suprastructure, or steps). Lack of surface smoothness, as with plasma-coated, sandblasted, acid-etched, or threaded implants, might interfere with probe penetration when bone resorption has reached this level and may lead to underestimation of pocket depth.[27] Although convincing evidence is lacking, some authors have expressed concerns about the possibility of introducing bacteria into the peri-implant tissues and about damaging the implant surface with a metallic periodontal probe.[19,27,28] Other authors concluded that increased pocket depth could be correlated with a higher degree of inflammation of the peri-implant mucosa,[29] but not necessarily with peri-implant bone loss.[30,31]

However, absolute values of PD have to be interpreted in the context of surgical implant positioning, ie submucosal implant placement in esthetic anterior sites versus conventional implant placement in posterior nonesthetic sites. Progressive increases in PD may be an alarming sign. Therefore, the establishment of baseline PD values at the time of delivery of the prosthetic superstructure is of critical importance in allowing comparison with future PD measurements. Peri-implant probing should also include the location of the soft tissue margin relative to a fixed landmark point on the implant (ie implant shoulder for one-stage nonsubmerged implant systems) or its superstructure. Repeated peri-implant PD measurements may be performed with higher reproducibility by means of an automated controlled-force periodontal probe.[32] Furthermore, animal experiments have shown that, as is the case around teeth,[33] peri-implant probing disrupts the epithelial attachment but does not cause permanent damage to the transmucosal soft tissue seal. In one study, complete attachment of the junctional epithelium was re-established after 5 days following probing using a conventional periodontal probe.[34]

6.6.5 Width of peri-implant keratinized mucosa

One animal study showed that the absence of keratinized mucosa around implants seems to increase the susceptibility of plaque-induced peri-implant tissue destruction.[35] These findings have been confirmed in another study,[36] suggesting that the presence of keratinized mucosa around implants is strongly correlated with optimal soft and hard tissue health.

However, longitudinal clinical studies have failed to reveal major differences in the progression of lesions around implants placed in sites with or without keratinized mucosa, or that the lack of an attached portion of masticatory mucosa may jeopardize the maintenance of soft tissue health.[37-39] Furthermore, in the presence of good oral hygiene, the nature of the mucosa may have little influence on the long-term survival of implants. However, suboptimal oral hygiene may lead to greater tissue damage around implants within alveolar mucosa than around implants within keratinized tissue. Proper oral hygiene procedures may also be facilitated in the presence of an adequate band of keratinized mucosa.

6.6.6 Suppuration

High numbers of polymorphonuclear neutrophil (PMN) cells have been detected around implants that are associated with severe signs of mucosal inflammation.[14] Several histopathologic and immunohistochemical analyses of tissues surrounding implants with signs of peri-implantitis, ie clinical signs of inflammation and advanced bone loss, have revealed the presence of large inflammatory cell infiltrates.[40-42] Berglundh et al.[43] analyzed soft tissue biopsies from patients with peri-implantitis and reported that a considerable portion of the connective tissue was occupied by an inflammatory infiltrate. Esposito et al.[40] analyzed the characteristics of soft tissues surrounding failing implants immunohistochemically. They reported that the marginal portion of the specimens was characterized by an "intense inflammatory and immunologic response".

Gualini and Berglundh[41] reported that peri-implantitis lesions contained significantly greater proportions of B-lymphocytes and PMN cells than mucositis lesions.

6.7 How can the bone-to-implant interface be evaluated?

6.7.1 Implant mobility and discomfort

Primary stability at the time of implant placement has been recognized as an important prerequisite for the achievement of osseointegration.[44-46] The establishment and maintenance of direct contact at the bone–implant interface are requirements for long-term implant success. Implant mobility occurs as a result of loss of osseointegration. Even if peri-implant disease has progressed relatively far, implants may still appear immobile because of some residual direct bone-to-implant contact. The recording of implant mobility may be a very specific but not at all sensitive clinical parameter in detecting loss of osseointegration.

Furthermore, pain or discomfort may be associated with implant mobility and could be a symptom indicating failure of an implant.[47,48] Persistent discomfort may be evident long before any radiographic change is detectable.[49]

An electronic device (Periotest; Medizintechnik Gulden, Modautal, Germany), originally designed to measure the damping characteristics of the periodontium around natural teeth,[50,51] has been recommended to monitor initial degrees of implant mobility or horizontal displacement. Despite some positive claims for this method,[31,51,52] the prognostic accuracy of Periotest for the diagnosis of peri-implantitis and early signs of implant failure has been criticized because of the lack of resolution, poor sensitivity, and susceptibility to operator variables.

6.7.2 RFA

A noninvasive device based on the principles of RFA has been developed to measure primary implant stability and to monitor implant stability over time.[53] This method evaluates the stiffness of the bone–implant interface by means of a signal transducer connected to a frequency response analyzer (Ostell ISQ; Ostell, Gothenburg, Sweden).

This may allow detection of an increase in implant mobility before clinical signs are recorded.[54] However, conclusive data on the bone–implant interface and RFA values are still lacking.

6.8 What to look for in x-ray examinations

Long-term preservation of crestal bone height around osseointegrated implants is often used as a primary success criterion for different implant systems. Originally, a mean crestal bone loss ≥1.5 mm during the first year after loading and ≥0.2 mm/year after had been proposed as one of the major success criteria.[45] This success criterion, however, has recently been questioned, because longitudinal studies have provided evidence that crestal bone loss around osseointegrated implants in well maintained patients may be minimal.[55]

Conventional radiography represents a widely accepted technique for the long-term evaluation of marginal bone changes at interproximal sites of osseointegrated implants. In general, the long-cone paralleling technique, supported by positioning devices, is used. It should be noted that conventional radiography yields a high proportion of false negative findings, ie it has low sensitivity in the detection of early pathologic and/or bone remodeling changes.[56] Therefore, radiographic assessment should be performed in conjunction with assessment of clinical parameters.[57]

- Probing is essential for diagnosis of peri-implant diseases.
- Conventional probing using a light force (0.25 N) does not damage the peri-implant tissues.
- BOP indicates the presence of inflammation in the peri-implant mucosa.
- BOP may be used as a predictor for loss of tissue support.
- An increase in PD over time is associated with the loss of attachment and supporting bone.
- The PD, the presence of BOP and suppuration should be assessed regularly for the diagnosis of peri-implant diseases.
- Radiographs are required to evaluate supporting bone levels around implants.

6.9 What are the main risk factors for peri-implantitis?

The oral status, the implant configuration, and the surface in particular have an impact on the pathogenicity of the peri-implant flora. Whether osseointegration is at risk depends on the defense mechanism, the duration of the infection, the implant design, and its surface characteristics. Indeed, some implants seem to be more at risk for occlusal overload, while other systems are more prone to plaque build-up.

Implants in partially edentulous patients, in contrast to fully edentulous subjects, will easily be colonized by putative periodontal pathogens. It seems therefore reasonable that every partially edentulous patient receives appropriate periodontal screening and treatment prior to placement of dental implants and is maintained on an individualized recall schedule for supportive periodontal therapy afterwards. Patients with a history of periodontitis may exhibit significantly greater long-term PD, peri-implant marginal bone loss and incidence of peri-implantitis compared with periodontally healthy subjects. Even though the short-term implant prognosis for patients treated for aggressive periodontitis is acceptable, on a long-term basis the matter is open to question. Alterations in clinical parameters around implants and teeth in aggressive periodontitis patients may not follow the same pattern, in contrast to what has been reported for chronic periodontitis patients.[58]

Karbach et al.[59] demonstrate in their study that smoking was the most important risk factor for the formation of peri-implant mucositis. Second, radiation therapy was an explanatory variable for the occurrence of inflammation. Implant surface roughness, augmentation at the implant site, and type of dentition had little influence on clinical signs of inflammation of peri-implant tissue. Linear logistic regression analysis showed that the type of dentition influences the periodontal microbiota at the impant site.[59]

In conclusion, a number of risk indicators should be taken into account for a correct diagnosis of peri-implant diseases.[2] There is evidence that the following indicators are associated with peri-implant diseases:

- Poor oral hygiene.
- History of periodontitis.
- Cigarette smoking; a significant increase in marginal bone loss exists in smokers compared with non-smokers.

There is limited evidence that the following indicators are associated with peri-implant diseases:

- Diabetes with poor metabolic control.
- Alcohol consumption.

There is conflicting and limited evidence for an association with peri-implant diseases for the following:

- Genetic traits: there is evidence for a synergism between genetic traits and smoking.
- Implant surface: rough surface was worse than smooth, moderately rough was similar to smooth.

Where clinical assessment indicates the presence of peri-implant disease, a radiograph should be taken in order to determine the extent of bone loss.[10]

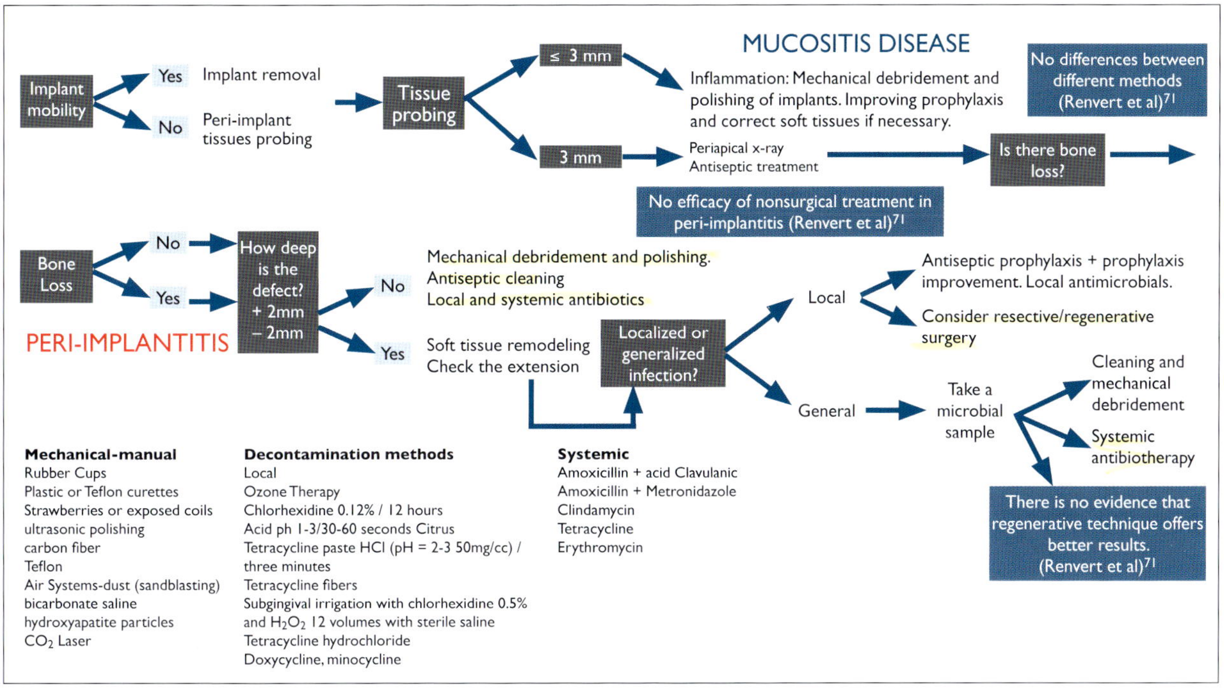

Fig 6-5 Performance chart peri-implant lesion.

6.10 How should peri-implantitis be treated?

As long as the implant surface is contaminated with soft tissue cells, bacteria, or bacterial byproducts, wound healing is compromised. The nonsurgical treatment for peri-implant infection involves removing plaque deposits with plastic instruments to avoid damaging the implant surface and polishing all accessible surfaces with pumice. The patient may also be treated with subgingival irrigation with 0.12% chlorhexidine and must be encouraged to improve home oral hygiene practice when needed. The initial phase of therapy may be sufficient to reestablish gingival health. If not, a surgical procedure may be required. The surgical techniques currently advocated for controlling peri-implant lesions are modifications of techniques used to treat bone defects around teeth. The type and size of bone defects must be identified before deciding on the appropriate treatment modality. This determines whether the implant should be removed or a regenerative procedure undertaken. Regenerative therapy is used to reduce pockets, but with the ultimate goal of regenerating lost bone tissue. Also, systemic antibiotics have been advocated as a supportive regimen during the treatment phase of peri-implant disease.

For implant surface preparation, mechanical devices and chemotherapeutics have been evaluated *in vitro* and *in vivo*. Conventional and ultrasonic instruments are not suitable for preparing and detoxifying the implant surface. Mechanical instrumentation may damage the implant surface if performed with metal instruments harder than titanium. The method of choice involves a high-pressure, air-powered abrasive comprising a mixture of sodium bicarbonate and water. This method completely removes microbial deposits from titanium surfaces, does not significantly change the surface topography, and does not adversely affect cell adhesion.[60]

The flowchart (Fig 6-5) aids the choice of consequent treatment depending on the case.

6.10.1 Does antimicrobial treatment work?

The antibiotic regimens used vary between studies with respect to type of antibiotic, dosage, delivery system, duration, and start of antibiotic therapy. Adverse effects related to the antimicrobial agents and patient compliance were not considered. Antimicrobial susceptibility testing should be performed prior to selection of the antibiotic. There is insufficient evidence to recommend a particular anti-infective protocol for the treatment of peri-implantitis. All experimental studies resulted in resolution of the inflammatory lesion and new bone formation, while some protocols demonstrated varying degrees of re-osseointegration. The most common choice of systemic antibiotic was metronidazole and amoxicillin combined, or metronidazole alone. However, there are no animal studies comparing local therapy with or without systemic antibiotics, and hence the value of adjunctive antimicrobial therapy cannot be evaluated.

6.10.2 How to decontaminate an implant surface

It has been suggested that the establishment of an implant surface favorable to bone formation is a prerequisite for successful regenerative treatment of peri-implantitis. Contaminants such as bacteria and their products, calculus, and soft tissue cells should be removed without modifying the implant surface. However, it is still unknown to what extent these contaminants have to be removed to achieve a successful treatment outcome.[22]

It has been concluded that several methods are inappropriate for implant surface cleaning, especially metal curettes for hand scaling, conventional sonic/ultrasonic scalers, and some types of lasers, which may severely damage the implant surface.

Animal models of experimental peri-implantitis have been useful for the evaluation of various implant surface decontamination methods in the surgical treatment of peri-implantitis.[61-65] No difference could be demonstrated regarding the degree of osseointegration with implants that were cleaned either with cotton pellets soaked in saline or with a rotating brush with pumice during regenerative surgery. Furthermore, no difference could be detected when decontamination by a carbon dioxide laser and/or an air-powder abrasive unit was done during flap surgery with or without coverage of the defect by an expanded polytetrafluoroethylene (e-PTFE) membrane.[61] Air-powder abrasive units are often recommended for the surgical treatment of peri-implantitis. The influence of various air-powder abrasive systems on the titanium surface has been evaluated in vitro and was previously reviewed.[62-65]

Decontamination of peri-implantitis affected implants may be achieved most easily and effectively by applying gauze soaked alternately in chlorhexidine and saline during surgical treatment.[66]

6.10.3 Surgical or nonsurgical treatment?

Nonsurgical treatment of peri-implant diseases

Treatment of peri-implant mucositis

Benefits of antimicrobial rinsing with essential oil-containing mouthwashes were demonstrated by Ciancio et al.[67] Local delivery antimicrobials have not been shown to be beneficial in the treatment of peri-implant mucositis, neither has a single professional irrigation of the sulcius with chlorhexidine.[68,69] On the other hand, self-administered irrigation with chlorhexidine has been found to be useful.[70]

Treatment of peri-implantitis

Mechanical nonsurgical therapy alone does not seem to be effective to treat peri-implantitis lesions.[2] Only minor changes in bleeding tendency are generally reported and PDs either do not seem to improve in the long term or worsen.[71] Mechanical therapy with an adjunct of systemic antimicrobials includes both local antimicrobial irrigation and administration of antimicrobials systemically. While short-term improvements have been noted for measurements such as PDs, GI, and microbiological parameters, these case reports do not allow definite conclusions on the effects of systemic antimicrobials alone.[2]

Mechanical therapy with an adjunct of local antimicrobials: with the use of tetracycline containing fibers, Mombelli et al.[72] demonstrated some clinical improvement of clinical parameters such as PDs and bleeding index. In a controlled study, Bücher et al.[73] demonstrated clinical benefits of the adjunctive use of a slow release doxycycline-containing preparation. In two of these case series it was suggested that the adjunctive use of either chlorhexidine gel or minocycline microspheres improved both clinical and microbiological parameters following treatment.[74] In a series of randomized controlled studies, Renvert et al.[71] found benefits of the adjunctive use of minocycline-containing microspheres. Although all studies included in the review employing local antimicrobials as an adjunct to mechanical treatment demonstrated mean improvements of BOP and PDs, this therapy did not resolve the lesion in all cases.

Laser therapy: the outcome data on laser therapy are incomplete and do not show benefits as compared with conventional mechanical therapy.

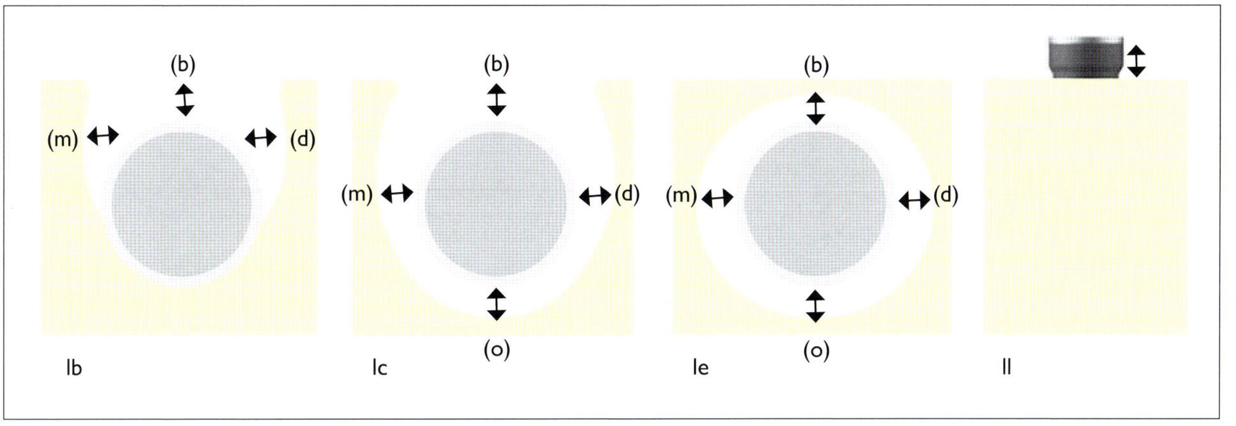

Fig 6-6 Intra-operative assessment of the defect components. Class Ib (buccal dehiscence + semicircular bone resorption to the middle of the implant body). Class Ic (buccal dehiscence + circular bone resorption under maintenance of the lingual compacta). Class Ie (circular bone resorption under maintenance of the buccal and oral compacta); intrabony component (i), blue circles; circumferential (width) component s(c), arrows, Class II: supraalveolar component s(a), arrow. b, buccal aspect; d, distal aspect; m, mesial aspect; o, oral aspect.

Conclusions

- Mechanical nonsurgical therapy is effective in the treatment of peri-implant mucositis lesions. Furthermore, the adjunctive use of antimicrobial mouth rinses enhanced the outcome of mechanical therapy of such mucositis lesions.
- In peri-implantitis lesions, treatment with nonsurgical therapy was not found to be effective. Adjunctive chlorhexidine application had only limited effects on clinical and microbiological parameters. However, adjunctive local or systemic antibiotics were shown to reduce BOP and PDs.
- Minor beneficial effects of laser therapy on peri-implantitis have been shown; this approach needs to be further evaluated. Reports do not allow definite conclusions on the effects of systemic antimicrobials.[71]

Surgical treatment of peri-implant diseases

Surgical treatment of peri-implantitis lesions can be performed in cases with considerable pocket formation (larger than 5 mm) and bone loss after the acute infection has been resolved and proper oral hygiene has been instituted.

Therefore, further long-term studies in humans involving sufficient numbers of subjects are needed to provide a solid basis for recommendations regarding the surgical treatment of peri-implantitis. Moreover, the encouraging treatment outcomes of regenerative procedures recently revealed in animal experiments and applied in the treatment of peri-implantitis around implants with sandblasted/acid-etched surfaces have not yet been documented for implants with other surfaces, especially turned surfaces. Numerous implant surface decontamination methods have been suggested as part of the surgical treatment of peri-implantitis. Decontamination of affected implants with titanium plasma-sprayed (TPS) or sandblasted/acid-etched surfaces may most easily and effectively be achieved by applying gauze soaked alternately in chlorhexidine and saline.[66]

Recently studies demonstrate that defect configuration of peri-implant defects may have an impact on the clinical outcome following surgical regenerative therapy of these peri-implant lesions. Schwarz et al.[75] investigated the clinical outcome of surgical regenerative therapy using natural bone mineral in combination with a collagen membrane. The classification of lesions described in Figure 6-6 was used.

The authors observed that while Class Ie defects seem to be promising in conjunction with natural bone mineral and a native collagen membrane, Class Ib and Class Ic must be considered as unfavorable. From both a clinical and a scientific point of view, future studies aimed at investigating any type of surgical treatment of peri-implantitis are encouraged to properly report on the specific configuration of the included defects.

The use of autogenous bone grafts with or without membrane coverage in humans was also evaluated. A clinically healthy peri-implant mucosa was a consistent finding after treatment, but the amount of bone regeneration varied widely among studies. As an example, 25 implants with a TPS surface were analyzed in one study.[76] The surgical treatment involved placement of blocks or particles of autogenous bone without membrane coverage after cleaning of the implant surface with an air-powder abrasive unit. A mean radiographic bone gain of 4.2 mm, corresponding to 100% regeneration, was observed after 3 years.[76]

Membranes are applied to stabilize the blood clot and to prevent growth of connective tissue and epithelium into the peri-implant bone defect during surgical therapy.[77,78] Various grafting materials have been combined with membranes to maintain the space created under the membrane and to serve as an osteoconductive scaffold to promote bone regeneration.

Findings from animal studies have indicated that the combination of grafting materials and a membrane is preferable in the surgical treatment of the osseous defects in peri-implantitis.[62-65] However, membrane exposure is a frequent complication after such procedures.

6.11 International University of Catalonia protocol

The following protocol has been created by the International University of Catalonia (Universitat Internacional de Catalunya [UIC]) to treat mucositis and peri-implantitis. It has been developed in order to control, check, and improve the state of implants over time. Protocol phases are based on various investigations that help to conclude and standardize the methodology.

Mucositis

Mucositis is diagnosed when there is:

- BOP.
- Absence of progressive bone loss.

Treatment: mechanical debridement with plastic, Teflon®, or metal curettes, plastic tips for ultrasound,[79] combined with good oral hygiene.[80] However, if conditions are more severe the treatment below should be considered:

- BOP.
- Peri-implant sulcus over 4 to 5 mm.
- Absence of progressive bone loss.

Treatment: mechanical debridement with plastic or Teflon® curettes, ultrasonic plastic tips for ultrasound,[79] antiseptic prophylaxis (chlorhexidine rinses for 7 days), combined with oral hygiene instruction.[80] Re-evaluation at 6 weeks.

Peri-implantitis

To understand how to treat peri-implantitis it is important to understand the types of defect that could occur as a result of disease. In 1997, Mombelli[81] categorized the peri-implant defects into four groups:

- Minimum horizontal bone loss with early signs of peri-implant vertical resorption.
- Moderate horizontal bone loss with peri-implant vertical resorption located.
- Horizontal bone loss with moderate to advanced vertical resorption.
- Horizontal bone loss with moderate to advanced vertical circumferential.

Peri-implantitis surgical treatment

According to the Sixth European Workshop on Periodontology,[2] nonsurgical treatment is not effective in peri-implantitis. Surgical treatment will depend on the type of defect and the walls that are affected: this could be 1, 2, or 3 walls, circumferential defects, or a combination of these.

1. Mobility: implant removal.[22]
2. No mobility.

- Loss of bone support >50%: implant removal.
- Horizontal bone loss (supra-alveolar defect):
  - Removal of plaque and supra- and subgingival calculus.
  - Debridement and degranulation, plus detoxification of the implant surface: decontamination is via gauze soaked with saline for 5 minutes and a further 5 minutes with chlorhexidine 0.1%, followed by irrigation 10 times alternating between each solution. Schou et al.[63] demonstrated that this treatment is as effective as any other decontamination method tested.
  - Modification of bone architecture with a round bur and saline irrigation.
  - Modification of the implant surface with a diamond bur of 30 µm in a handpiece (15000 rev/min), followed by use of a diamond bur of 15 µm, an Arkansas bur, and silicone polishers, leaving a polished surface.[82]
  - Apically repositioned flap.
  - Regular plaque control.[82]

- Infrabony defects (1, 2, or 3 walls):
  - Removal of plaque and supra- and subgingival calculus.
  - Debridement and degranulation plus detoxification of the implant surface: decontamination is via pellets soaked with saline for 5 minutes and a further 5 minutes with chlorhexidine 0.1%, followed by irrigation 10 times alternating between each solution.
  - Buccal or lingual dehiscences may be additionally treated by means of implantoplasty, since they seem to respond worse to regenerative therapy.[75]
  - Guided bone regeneration (GBR) with a biomaterial plus resorbable collagen membrane. Results of GBR show no differences between using resorbable or non-resorbable membranes; the main complication with the reinforced membranes is membrane exposition.
  - Repositioned flaps.
- Combination defects (supra-alveolar and infrabony defects): The supra-alveolar portion of the implant may be treated by means of implantoplasty, whereas the portion of the implant exhibiting an infrabony defect may be treated by means of GBR.[75]

Supportive therapy

- Control at 3, 6, and 12 months post-loading, with annual controls.
- Oral hygiene reinforcement if plaque is present.
- Periapical radiographs.
- Clinical evaluation:
  - Visual exploration (peri-implant mucosal inflammation, presence of plaque).
  - Palpation (suppuration, abscess, implant mobility).
  - PD (BOP + 3 mm).
- If progressive bone loss in the presence of inflammation is present (ie BOP, suppuration), retreatment might be necessary.

6.12 Clinical cases

Case 1

An 80-year-old patient presented with two implants affected by peri-implantitis (Fig 6-7). Periodontal probing revealed deep probing depths and bleeding on probing (Fig 6-8). Bone loss was evident on the preoperative radiograph (Fig 6-9), and around both implants after flap

Figs 6-7 to 6-12 Case 1

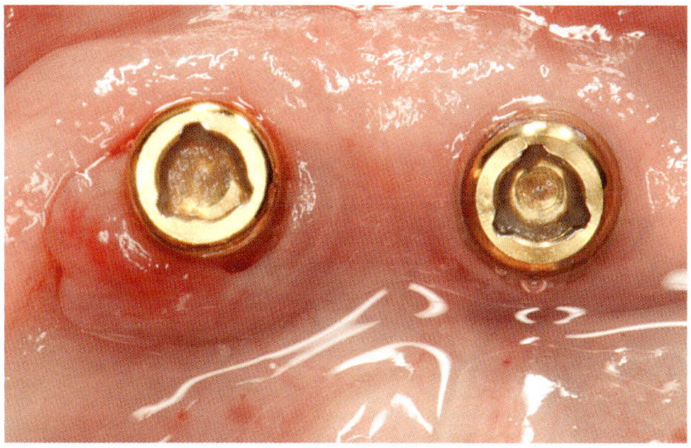

Fig 6-7 Occlusal view of the affected implants.

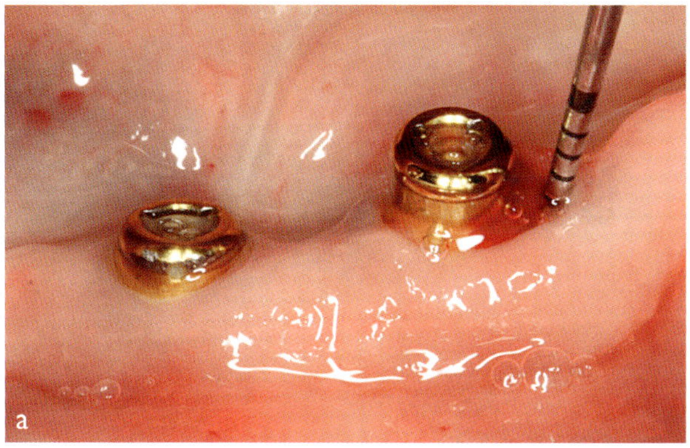

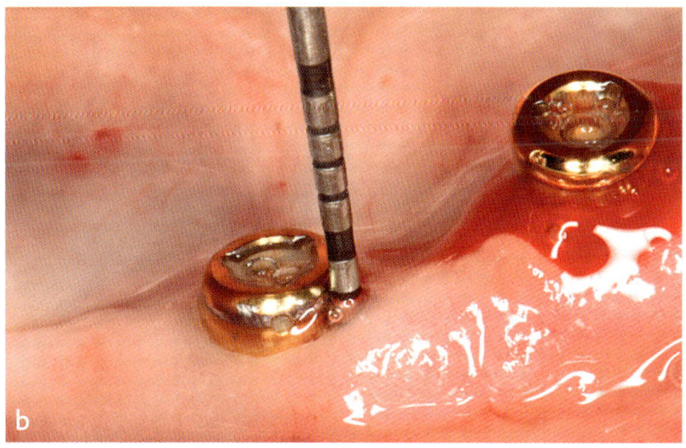

Figs 6-8a and b Deep probing depth and bleeding on probing present on both implants.

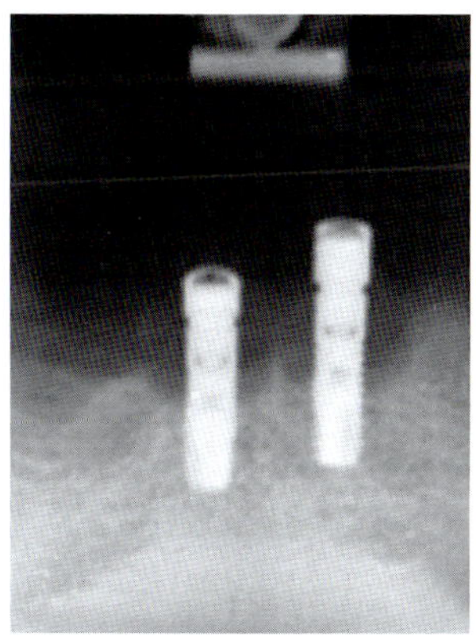

Fig 6-9 Preoperative radiograph.

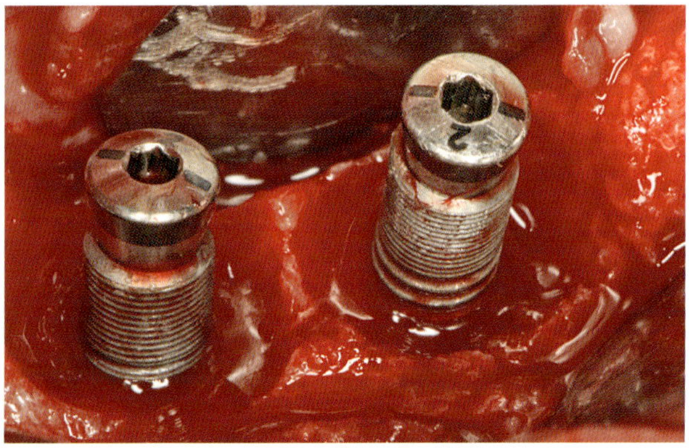

Fig 6-10 Notice the peri-implant bone loss and defect configuration around both implants after flap elevation and defect debridement.

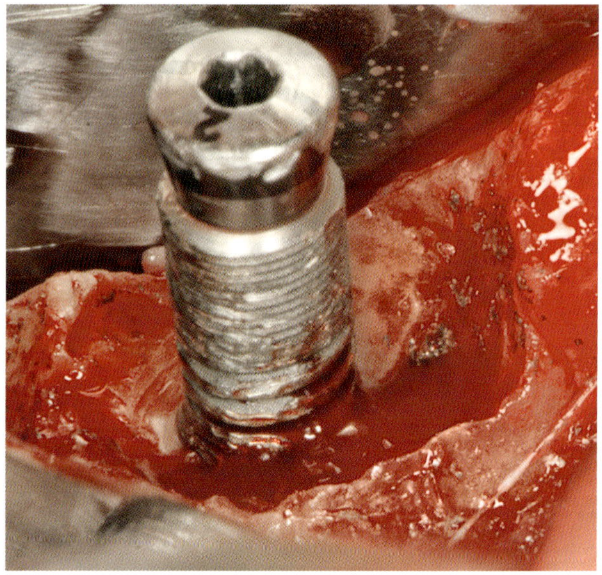

Fig 6-11 Anterior view of the implant during implantoplasty.

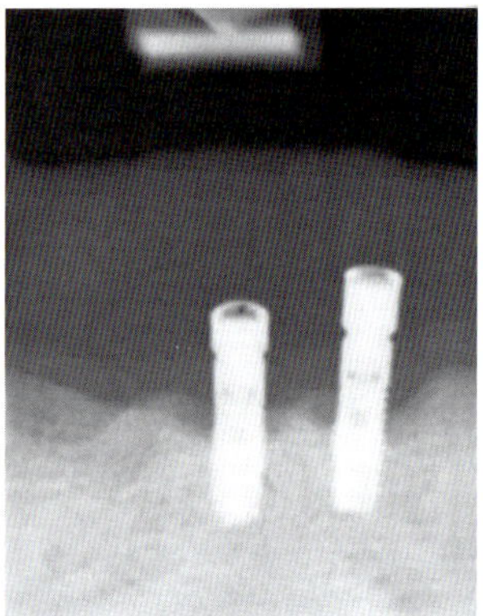

Fig 6-12 A slight gain can be observed only 3 months postoperatively.

elevation and defect debridement (Fig 6-10). Implantoplasty was performed (Fig 6-11) and a slight gain was observed 3 months later (Fig 6-12).

Case 2

A 41-year-old patient presented with peri-implantitis. Probing revealed a 7-mm probing depth with suppuration (Fig 6-13), and bone loss was confirmed by a radiograph (Fig 6-14). Flap elevation and debridement were performed (Fig 6-15), revealing calculus on the implant. Implantoplasty was performed (Fig 6-16) and the defect was grafted with demineralized bovine bone (Fig 6-17). The graft was covered with a resorbable membrane (Fig 6-18) and the flap closed (Fig 6-19). The postoperative radiograph revealed that the defect was successfully filled with bone 6 months later (Fig 6-20).

Figs 6-13 to 6-20 Case 2

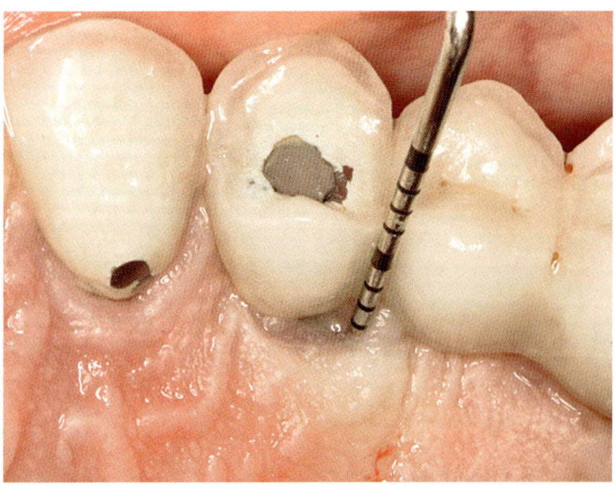

Fig 6-13 Suppuration and a 7-mm probing depth can be observed on the palatal aspect of the affected implant.

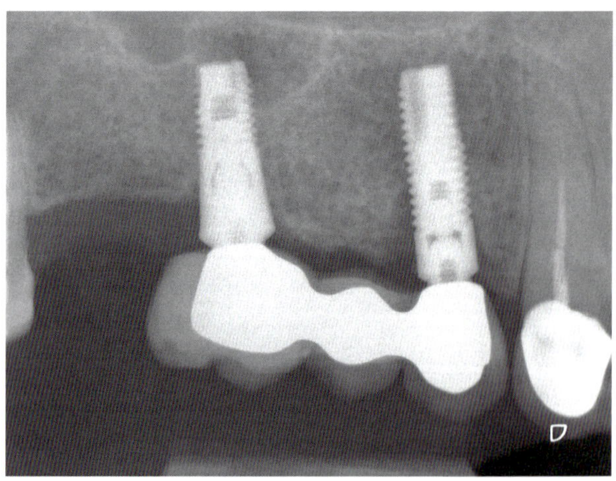

Fig 6-14 Radiographic view prior to treatment.

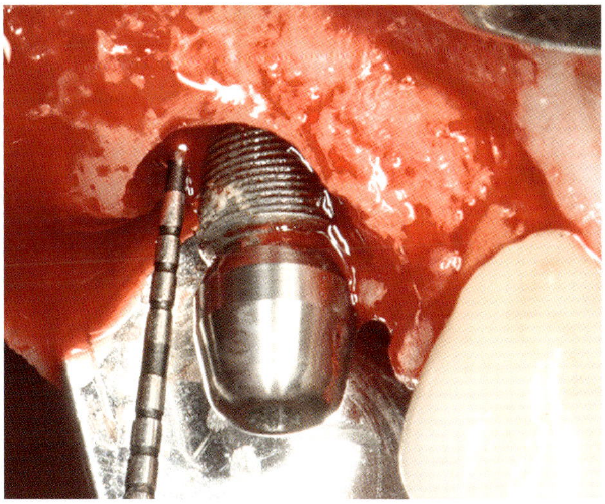

Fig 6-15 Peri-implant defect after flap elevation and debridement of the defect. Notice calculus present on the distal aspect of the implant.

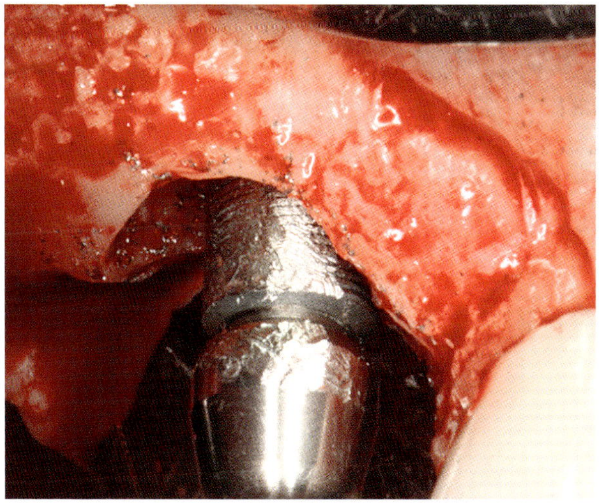

Fig 6-16 Implantoplasty.

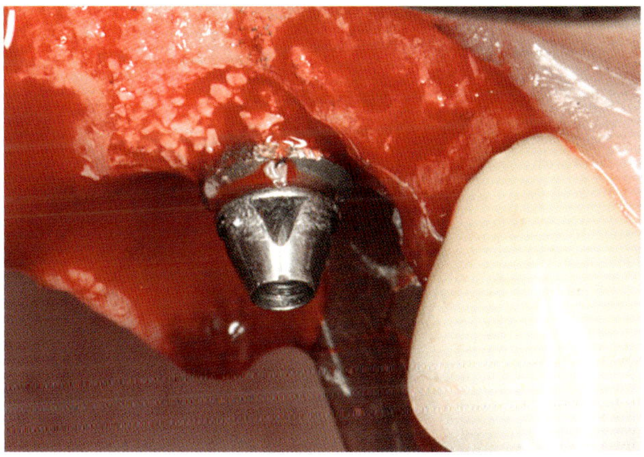

Fig 6-17 The defect was grafted with demineralized bovine bone.

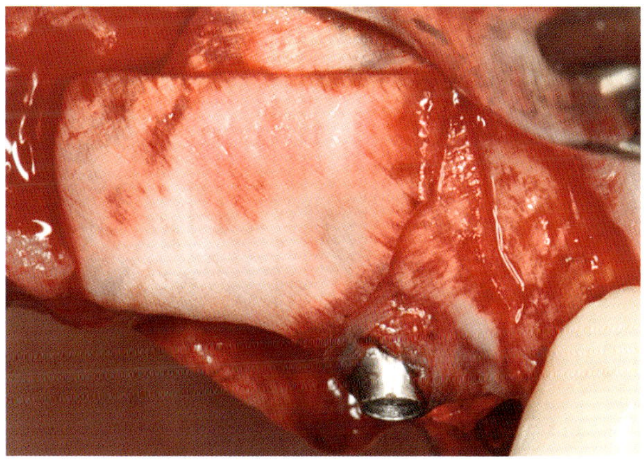

Fig 6-18 Graft covered with a resorbable collagen membrane.

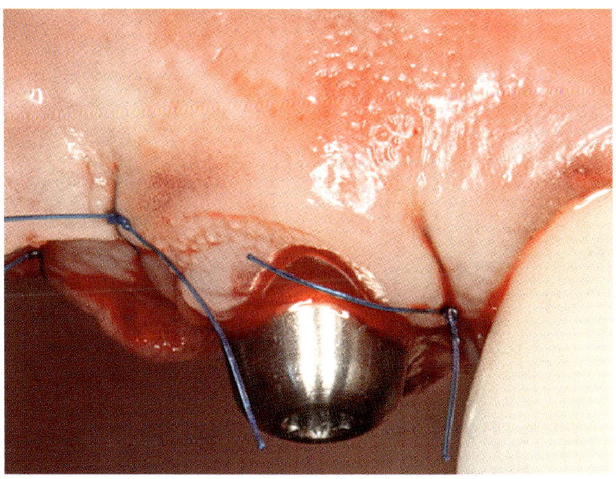

Fig 6-19 Flap closure.

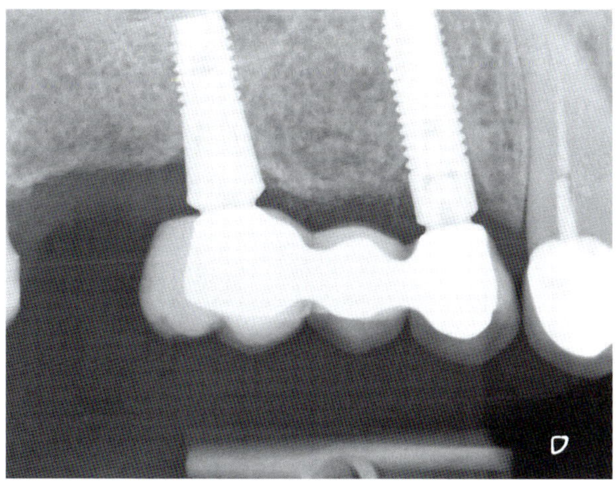

Fig 6-20 Six-months postoperative radiograph illustrating successful bone fill of the peri-implant defect.

References

1. Zitzmann NU, Berglundh T. Definition and prevalence of periimplant diseases. J Clin Periodontol 2008;35(Suppl 8):286-291.
2. Lindhe J, Meyle J, Group D of European Workshop on Periodontology, 2008. Peri-implant diseases: Consensus Report of the Sixth European Workshop on Periodontology. J Clin Periodontol 2008;35(Suppl 8):282-285.
3. Albrektsson T, Isidor F. Consensus Report of Session IV. In: Lang NP, Karring T (eds). Proceedings of the 1st European Workshop on Periodontology. London: Quintessence Publishing, 1994:365-369.
4. Berglundh T, Lindhe J, Ericsson I, Marinello CP, Liljenberg B. Soft tissue reactions to de novo plaque formation on implants and teeth. An experimental study in the dog. Clin Oral Implants Res 1992;3:1-8.
5. Costerton JW, Lewandowski Z, DeBeer D, Caldwell D, Korber D, James G. Biofilms, the customized microniche. J Bacteriol 1994;8:2137-2142.
6. Socransky SS, Haffajee AD. Dental biofilms: difficult therapeutic targets. Periodontol 2000 2002;28:12-55.
7. Socransky SS, Haffajee AD. Periodontal microbial ecology. Periodontol 2000 2005;38:135-187.
8. Shibli JA, Melo L, Ferrari DS, Figueiredo LC, Faveri M, Feres M. Composition of supra- and subgingival biofilm of subjects with healthy and diseased implants. Clin Oral Implants Res 2008;19: 975-982.
9. De Boever AL, De Boever JA. Early colonization of non-submerged dental implants in patients with a history of advanced aggressive periodontitis. Clin Oral Implants Res 2006;17:8-17.
10. Heitz-Mayfield LJA. Periimplant diseases: diagnosis and risk indicators. J Clin Periodontol 2008;35(Suppl 8):292-304.
11. Serino G, Strŏm C. Peri-implantitis in partially edentulous patients: association with inadequate plaque control. Clin Oral Implants Res 2009;20:169-174.
12. Lindhe J (ed). Proceedings of the 3rd European Workshop on Periodontology. Berlin: Quintessence Books, 1999;281-303.
13. Mombelli A, Van Oosten MAC, Schürch E, Lang NP. The microbiota associated with successful or failing osseointegrated titanium implants. Oral Microbiol Immunol 1987;2:145-151.
14. Rams TE, Roberts TW, Tatum H Jr, Keyes PH. The subgingival microbial flora associated with human dental implants. J Prosthet Dent 1984;51:529-534.
15. Luterbacher S, Mayfield L, Brägger U, Lang NP. Diagnostic characteristics of clinical and microbiological tests for monitoring periodontal and peri-implant mucosal tissue conditions during supportive periodontal therapy (SPT). Clin Oral Implants Res 2000;11:521-529.
16. Lang NP, Wetzel AC, Stich H, Caffesse RG. Histologic probe penetration in healthy and inflamed peri-implant tissues. Clin Oral Implants Res 1994;5:191-201.
17. Armitage GC, Svanberg GK, Löe H. Microscopic evaluation of clinical measurements of connective tissue attachment levels. J Clin Periodontol 1977;4:173-190.
18. Magnusson I, Listgarten MA. Histological evaluation of probing depth following periodontal treatment. J Clin Periodontol 1980;7:26-31.
19. Schou S, Holmstrup P, Stoltze K, Hjørting-Hansen E, Fiehn NE, Skovgaard LT. Probing around implants and teeth with healthy or inflamed periimplant mucosa/gingiva. A histologic comparison in cynomolgus monkeys (*Macaca fascicularis*). Clin Oral Implants Res 2002;13:113-126.
20. Listgarten MA, Lang NP, Schroeder HE, Schroeder A. Periodontal tissues and their counterparts around endosseous implants. Clin Oral Implants Res 1991;2:1-19.
21. van der Velden U. Probing force and the relationship of the probe tip to the periodontal tissues. J Clin Periodontol 1979;6:106-114.
22. Mombelli A, Mühle T, Frigg R. Depth-force patterns of periodontal probing. Attachment gain in relation to probing force. J Clin Periodontol 1992;19:295-300.
23. Mombelli A, Mühle T, Brägger U. Probing force dependence of attachment level measurement in the assessment of effects of surgical periodontal treatment with or without NSAID. Acta Med Dent Helv 1996;1:34-39.
24. Gerber JA, Tan WC, Balmer TE, Salvi GE, Lang NP. Bleeding on probing and pocket probing depth in relation to probing pressure and mucosal health around oral implants. Clin Oral Implants Res 2009;20:75-78.
25. Apse P, Zarb GA, Schmitt A, Lewis DW. The longitudinal effectiveness of osseointegrated dental implants. The Toronto study: periimplant mucosal response. Int J Periodontics Restorative Dent 1991;11:95-111.
26. Buser D, Weber HP, Lang NP. Tissue integration of nonsubmerged implants. 1-year results of a prospective study with 100 ITI hollow-cylinder and hollow-screw implants. Clin Oral Implants Res 1990;6:55-61.
27. Bauman GR, Mills M, Rapley JW, Hallmon WH. Clinical parameters of evaluation during implant maintenance. Int J Oral Maxillofac Implants 1992;7:220-227.
28. Lekholm U, Adell R, Lindhe J, Brånemark PI, Eriksson B, Rockler B, et al. Marginal tissue reactions at osseointegrated titanium fixtures. (II) A cross-sectional retrospective study. Int J Oral Maxillofac Surg 1986;15:53-61.
29. Quirynen M, van Steenberghe D, Jacobs R, Schotte A, Darius P. The reliability of pocket probing around screw-type implants. Clin Oral Implants Res 1991;2:186-192.
30. Spiekermann H, Jansen VK, Richter EJ. A 10-year followup study of IMZ and TPS implants in edentulous mandibles using bar-retained overdentures. Int J Oral Maxillofac Implants 1995;10:373-378.
31. Behneke A, Behneke N, d'Hoedt B, Wagner W. Hard and soft tissue reactions to ITI screw implants: 3-year longitudinal results of a prospective study. Int J Oral Maxillofac Implants 1997;12:749-757.
32. Christensen MM, Joss A, Lang NP. Reproducibility of automated periodontal probing around teeth and osseointegrated oral implants. Clin Oral Implants Res 1997;8:455-464.
33. Taylor AC, Campbell MM. Reattachment of gingival epithelium to the tooth. J Periodontol 1972;43:281-293.
34. Etter TH, Håkanson IH, Lang NP, Trejo PM, Caffesse RG. Healing after standardized clinical probing of the periimplant soft tissue seal. Clin Oral Implants Res 2002;13:571-580.
35. Warrer K, Buser D, Lang NP, Karring T. Plaque-induced peri-implantitis in the presence or absence of keratinized mucosa. An experimental study in monkeys. Clin Oral Implants Res 1995;6:131-138.
36. Block MS, Gardiner D, Kent JN, Misiek DJ, Finger IM, Guerra L. Hydroxyapatite-coated cylinder implants in the posterior mandible: 10-year observations. Int J Oral Maxillofac Implants 1996;11:626-633.
37. Zitzmann NU, Schärer P, Marinello CP. Long-term results of implants treated with guided bone regeneration: a 5-year prospective study. Int J Oral Maxillofac Implants 2001;16:355-366.
38. Bengazi F, Wennström JL, Lekholm U. Recession of the soft tissue margin at oral implants. Clin Oral Implants Res 1996;7:303-310.
39. Wennström JL, Bengazi F, Lekholm U. The influence of the masticatory mucosa on the periimplant soft tissue condition. Clin Oral Implants Res 1994;5:1-8.
40. Esposito M, Thomsen P, Mölne J, Gretzer C, Ericson LE, Lekholm U. Immunohistochemistry of soft tissues surrounding late failures of Brånemark implants. Clin Oral Implants Res 1997;8:352-366.
41. Gualini F, Berglundh T. Immunohistochemical characteristics of inflammatory lesions at implants. J Clin Periodontol 2003;30:14-18.
42. Piattelli A, Scarano A, Piattelli M. Histologic observations on 230 retrieved dental implants: 8 years' experience (1989–1996). J Periodontol 1998;69:178-184.

43. Berglundh T, Gislason O, Lekholm U, Sennerby L, Lindhe J. Histopathological observations of human periimplantitis lesions. J Clin Periodontol 2004;31:341-347.
44. Adell R, Lekholm U, Rockler B, Brånemark P-I. A 15-year study of osseointegrated implants in the treatment of the edentulous jaw. Int J Oral Surg 1981;10:387-416.
45. Albrektsson T, Zarb GA, Worthington DP, Eriksson R. The long-term efficacy of currently used dental implants. A review and proposed criteria of success. Int J Oral Maxillofac Implants 1986;1:11-25.
46. Brånemark P-I, Hansson BO, Adell R, Breine U, Lindström J, Hallén O, Ohman A. Osseointegrated implants in the treatment of the edentulous jaw. Experience from a 10-year period. Scand J Plast Reconstr Surg 1977;16(Suppl):1-132.
47. Lekholm U, van Steenberghe D, Herrmann I, et al. Osseointegrated implants in the treatment of partially edentulous jaws: a prospective 5-year multicenter study. Int J Oral Maxillofac Implants 1994;9:627-635.
48. Gröndahl K, Lekholm U. The predictive value of radiographic diagnosis of implant instability. Int J Oral Maxillofac Implants 1997;12:59-64.
49. Worthington P, Bolender CL, Taylor TD. The Swedish system of osseointegrated implants: problems and complications encountered during a 4-year trial period. Int J Oral Maxillofac Implants 1987;2:77-84.
50. Olivé J, Aparicio C. The Periotest method as a measure of osseointegrated oral implant stability. Int J Oral Maxillofac Implants 1990;5:390-400.
51. Van Steenberghe D, Tricio J, Naert I, Nys M. Damping characteristics of bone-to-implant interfaces. A clinical study with the Periotest device. Clin Oral Implants Res 1995;6:31-39.
52. Aparicio C. The use of the Periotest value as the initial success criteria of an implant: 8-year report. Int J Periodontics Restorative Dent 1997;6:151-161.
53. Meredith N, Alleyne D, Cawley P. Quantitative determination of the stability of the implant-tissue interface using resonance frequency analysis. Clin Oral Implants Res 1996;7:261-266.
54. Friberg B, Sennerby L, Meredith N, Lekholm U. A comparison between cutting torque and resonance frequency measurements of maxillary implants. A 20-month clinical study. Int J Oral Maxillofac Surg 1999;28:297-303.
55. Feloutzis A, Lang NP, Tonetti MS, Bürgin W, Brägger U, Buser D, et al. IL-1 gene polymorphism and smoking as risk factors for periimplant bone loss in a well-maintained population. Clin Oral Implants Res 2003;14:10-17.
56. Brägger U, Pasquali L, Rylander H, Carnes D, Kornman KS. Computer-assisted densitometric image analysis in periodontal radiography. J Clin Periodontol 1988;15: 27-37.
57. Lang NP, Hill RW. Radiographs in periodontics. J Clin Periodontol 1977;4:16-28.
58. Karoussis IK, Kotsovilis S, Fourmousis I. A comprehesnsive and critical review of dental implant prognosis in periodontally compromised partially edentulous patients. Clin Oral Implants Res 2007;18:669-679.
59. Karbach J, Callaway A, Kwon Y, d'Hoedt B. Int J Oral Maxillofac Implants 2009;24:491-496
60. Rose LF, Mealey BL. Periodontics: Medicine, Surgery, and Implants. St Louis: Mosby, 2004:664.
61. Deppe H, Horch H-H, Henke J, Donath K. Peri-implant care of ailing implants with the carbon dioxide laser. Int J Oral Maxillofac Implants 2001;16:659-667.
62. Schou S, Holmstrup P, Jørgensen T, et al. Anorganic porous bovine-derived bone mineral (Bio-Oss) and ePTFE membrane in the treatment of peri-implantitis in cynomolgus monkeys. Clin Oral Implants Res 2003;14:535-547.
63. Schou S, Holmstrup P, Jørgensen T, Skovgaard LT, Stoltze K, Hjørting-Hansen E, Wenzel A. Implant surface preparation in the surgical treatment of experimental periimplantitis with autogenous bone graft and ePTFE membrane in cynomolgus monkeys. Clin Oral Implants Res 2003;14:412-422.
64. Schou S, Holmstrup P, Jørgensen T, Stoltze K, Hjørting Hansen E, Wenzel A. Autogenous bone graft and ePTFE membrane in the treatment of peri-implantitis. I. Clinical and radiographic observations in cynomolgus monkeys. Clin Oral Implants Res 2003;14:391-403.
65. Schou S, Holmstrup P, Skovgaard LT, Stoltze K, Hjørting- Hansen E, Gundersen HJG. Autogenous bone graft and ePTFE membrane in the treatment of peri-implantitis. II. Stereologic and histologic observations in cynomolgus monkeys. Clin Oral Implants Res 2003;14:404-411.
66. Schou S, Berglundh B, Lang NP. Surgical treatment of peri-implantitis. Int J Oral Maxillofac Implants 2004;19(Suppl):140-149.
67. Ciancio SG, Lauciello F, Shibly O, Vitello M, Mather M. The effect of an antiseptic mouthrinse on implant maintenance: plaque and peri-implant gingival tissues. J Periodontol 1995;66:962-965.
68. Schenk G, Flemmig TF, Betz T, Reuther J, Klaiber B. Controlled local delivery of tetracycline HCl in the treatment of periimplant mucosal hyperplasia and mucositis. A controlled case series. Clin Oral Implants Res 1997;8:427-433.
69. Porras R, Anderson GB, Caffesse R, Narendran S, Trejo PM. Clinical response to 2 different therapeutic regimens to treat peri-implant mucositis. J Periodontol 2002;73:1118-1125.
70. Felo A, Shibly O, Ciancio SG, Lauciello FR, Ho A. Effects of subgingival chlorhexidine irrigation on peri-implant maintenance. Am J Dent 1997;10:107-110.
71. Renvert S, Roos-Jansaker A-M, Claffey N. Non-surgical treatment of peri-implant mucositis and peri-implantitis: a literature review. J Clin Periodontol 2008;35(Suppl 8):305-315.
72. Mombelli A, Feloutzis A, Brägger U, Lang NP. Treatment of peri-implantitis by local delivery of tetracycline. Clinical, microbiological and radiological results. Clin Oral Implants Res 2001;12:287-294.
73. Buchter A, Meyer U, Kruse-Losler B, Joos U, Kleinheinz J. Sustained release of doxycycline for the treatment of peri-implantitis: randomized controlled trial. Br J Oral Maxillofac Surg 2004;42:439-444.
74. Gerber J, Wenaweser D, Heitz-Mayfield L, Lang NP, Persson RG. Comparison of bacterial plaque samples from titanium implant and tooth surfaces by different methods. Clin Oral Implants Res 2006;17:1-7.
75. Schwarz F, Sahm N, Schwarz K, Becker J. Impact of defect configuration on the clinical outcome following surgical regenerative therapy of peri-implantitis. J Clin Periodontol 2010;37:449-455.
76. Behneke A, Behneke N, d'Hoedt B. Treatment of periimplantitis defects with autogenous bone grafts: six-month to 3-year results of a prospective study in 17 patients. Int J Oral Maxillofac Implants 2000;15:125-138.
77. Hämmerle CHF, Karring T. Guided bone regeneration at oral implant sites. Periodontol 2000 1998;17:151-175.
78. Hämmerle CHF. Membranes and bone substitutes in guided bone regeneration. In: Lang NP, Karring T, Lindhe J (eds). Proceedings of the 3rd European Workshop on Periodontology. Implant Dentistry. Berlin: Quintessence, 1999:468-499.
79. Matarasso S, Quaremba G, Coraggio F, Vaia E, Cafiero C, Lang NP. Maintenance of implants: an in vitro study of titanium implant surface modifications subsequent to the application of different prophylaxis procedures. Clin Oral Implants Res 1996;7:64-72.
80. Lang NP, Berglundh T, on behalf of Working Group 4 of the Seventh European Workshop on Periodontology. Periimplant disease: where are we now? Consensus of Seventh European Workshop on Periodontology. J Clin Periodontol 2011;38(Suppl 11):178.
81. Mombelli A, Mühle T, Brägger U, Lang NP, Bürgin WB. Comparison of periodontal and periimplant probing by depth-force pattern analysis. Clin Oral Implants Res 1997;8:448-455.
82. Romeo E, Ghisolfi M, Murgolo N, Chiapasco M, Lops D, Vogel G. Therapy of periimplantitis with resective surgery. A 3-year clinical trial on rough screw-shaped oral implants. Part I: clinical outcome. Clin Oral Implants Res 2005;16:9-18.

Chapter 7

Limitations of guided bone regeneration

Jose Nart, Andres Pascual La Rocca, Hugo Campos Leitão

7.1 Introduction

Guided bone regeneration (GBR) refers to the techniques and procedures indicated in the guided growth of new bone at sites with insufficient dimensions or volumes of bone. Nowadays, GBR techniques are mainly indicated in the oral cavity to support new bone growth on an alveolar ridge to enhance the site for a future stable placement of dental implants. There is evidence that when soft tissue is mechanically excluded from the healing of osseous defects, bone regeneration is significantly enhanced.

On the cellular level, bone regeneration is a complex coordinated proliferation process where different types of cells including osteoblasts, bone-lining cells, osteoclasts, and osteocytes regulate bone formation. At the same time, angiogenesis is vital to provide blood support for development, maintenance, and repair of the bone.

In this chapter, the following topics will be assessed in order to understand GBR:

- 7.2 Is the exclusion of epithelial and connective tissue cells necessary?
- 7.3 How to begin GBR therapy
- 7.4 Which membrane is recommended?
  - 7.4.1 Resorbable or non resorbable membrane?
- 7.5 What are the options for grafting materials?
  - 7.5.1 Are there any differences between block and particulate grafts?
  - 7.5.2 Will using a mineralized or demineralized graft improve results?
- 7.6 Clinical cases
- 7.7 Conclusions

7.2 Is the exclusion of epithelial and connective tissue cells necessary?

In periodontal regeneration, the exclusion of the epithelial and connective tissue cells from the root surface, using a membrane during the healing of the wound, favors the migration of cells from the periodontal ligament and the bone to the defect, resulting in a gain in attachment and periodontal regeneration of the lost tissues.[1,2]

The GBR concept is born from the guided tissue regeneration (GTR) principle regarding the exclusion of the undesirably soft tissues from growing into the osseous wound space,[3,4] by the application of occlusive membranes that mechanically exclude the non-osteogenic cells from the surrounding soft tissues, thereby allowing osteogenic cell populations originating from the parent bone to inhabit the osseous wound.[5]

7.3 How to begin GBR therapy

When choosing a GBR procedure, prior analysis of the bone defect (Figs 7-1 to 7-4) is essential for selection of the technique and the materials required. Present protocols are based on two main objectives: GBR for preservation of the alveolar ridge, and GBR for the augmentation or reconstruction of the ridge.

Procedures can be carried out in two steps (first the regeneration, and the implant in a second stage) or in one step (combining the GBR with the implant placement). The one-stage procedure is preferred when the bone morphology offers primary stability and ideal prosthetic positioning of the implant. In cases where the defect morphology impedes stability of the implant or a non-prosthetically driven position, a two-staged procedure is recommended.

As previously mentioned, GBR therapy includes the use of occlusive membranes above the bone defect to physically create and maintain the necessary space for regeneration, achieve wound stability, and exclude undesirable cells.

7.4 Which membrane is recommended?

A wide variety of membranes is available and new materials are continually introduced. It is necessary to understand the basic requirements of a membrane to select those that adjust better to the necessities of each procedure and case.

The standard characteristics of a membrane include biocompatibility, cell occlusion, tissue integration, space making and maintenance, and clinical handling.

Different materials are suggested in the elaboration of membranes, and accordingly they can be divided into two major groups, resorbable and non-resorbable.

7.4.1 Resorbable or non-resorbable membranes?

During the 1980s, expanded polytetrafluoroethylene (ePTFE) became the standard non-resorbable membrane for GBR procedures. This is a polymer with a high biologic stability, and numerous investigations demonstrate the effects of ePTFE membranes.[3,6-8]

Two versions are available according the type of defect: a regular e-PTFE membrane that needs support from bony walls or grafting materials, which can be used in 4-, 3-, or 2-wall narrow defects. Today this membrane is widely replaced by resorbable membranes. A second version of the membrane is reinforced with titanium, which provides space maintenance regardless of the bony walls of the defect. It can be used in large 1- or 2-wall defects and supracrestal areas.

The practice of GBR with e-PTFE membranes is technique-sensitive and it is based on complete stabilization and coverage during the healing process.

This technique may present some postoperative complications. The most common complication is the exposure of the membrane, with up to 45.5% of incidence,[9] reducing the amount of total regenerated bone. A recent modification of the material is the non-expanded PTFE, also called dense PTFE (d-PTFE). The benefit of using this type of membrane is the possibility of leaving it intentionally exposed.

Because of the low porosity (0.2 nm) of the material, the membrane resists the incorporation of bacteria, with a low risk of infection. This was shown in a report of 420 cases where the membrane was left intentionally exposed in combination with freeze-dried bone allograft (FDBA) for the treatment of fresh extraction sockets.[8] Results showed formation of a ridge contour with appropriate conditions for implant placement, and also soft tissue formation with similar characteristics to healthy keratinized gingiva. On the other hand, the use of these types of membranes requires a second surgery for removal of the membrane.[8]

To avoid the possible complications originating from non-resorbable membranes, the use of bioresorbable membranes is increasing in GBR procedures.

The materials used for the elaboration of these membranes are numerous, but the most commonly used and investigated are made of collagen lyglycolic acids (PGAs) and/or polylactic acids (PLAs).[10]

The use of PGA and PLA membranes has shown good durability of the membrane[11] and bone formation, but also the presence of giant cells and encapsulation in some parts of the membrane was observed. In cases where the membrane was exposed, a rapid resorption process began immediately, with total degradation after 3 to 4 weeks.[12]

Collagen membranes are made from bovine and porcine type III and type I collagen. They present the following advantages: hemostasis, weak immunogenicity, easy manipulation, and bone formation. Unfavorable mechanical properties and limited barrier function have also been reported.[10]

To improve the barrier function time, cross-linked collagen is used to delay the resorption process and increase the stability of the membrane.[11] However, cross-linked membranes show only limited tissue integration, vasculari-

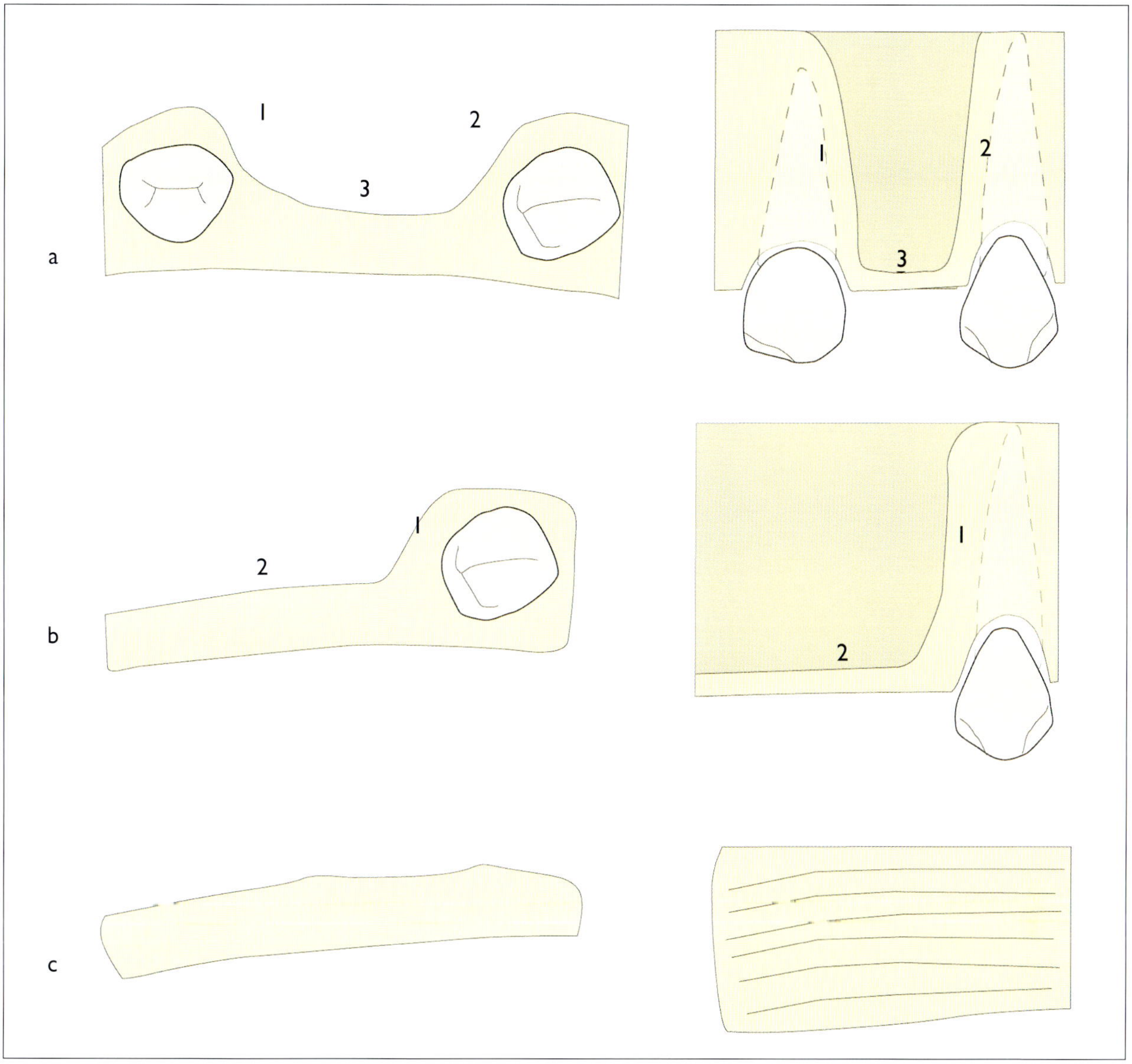

Fig 7-1 Horizontal ridge defects: (a) 3-wall, (b) 2-wall, and (c) 1-wall defects.

zation, and enhanced foreign body reaction. This could be of importance to the primary wound closure during the healing period.[13] Other animal investigations have shown that when healing occurs with exposure, bone regeneration is higher when using a cross-linked membrane.[14]

In general, the use of bioresorbable membranes results in the integration of the tissues with a good healing response.[15] A few complications are associated with this type of membrane, and if they become exposed or infected, rapid resorption will occur with minor consequences. For these reasons, resorbable membranes have become the standard in most clinical situations.

The principal inconvenience of the bioresorbable membranes is the difficulty in maintaining adequate space for bone regeneration, which limits the use for bone defects with adequate walls (4- and 3-wall defects) for the maintenance of the space.[15] Although some studies found no differences when comparing bioresorbable and non-resorbable membranes,[16,17] most clinical studies show higher bone gain with non-resorbable membranes. Following the recommendations of Buser et al.,[18] bioresorbable membranes are recommended to treat 3- and 2-wall horizontal defects, contained 4- and 3-wall vertical defects, dehiscenses, fenestrations, and sinus floor elevation surgeries. The non-resorbable PTFE membranes are recommended for 1-wall horizontal defects and vertical augmentation procedures (Figs 7-1 and 7-5).

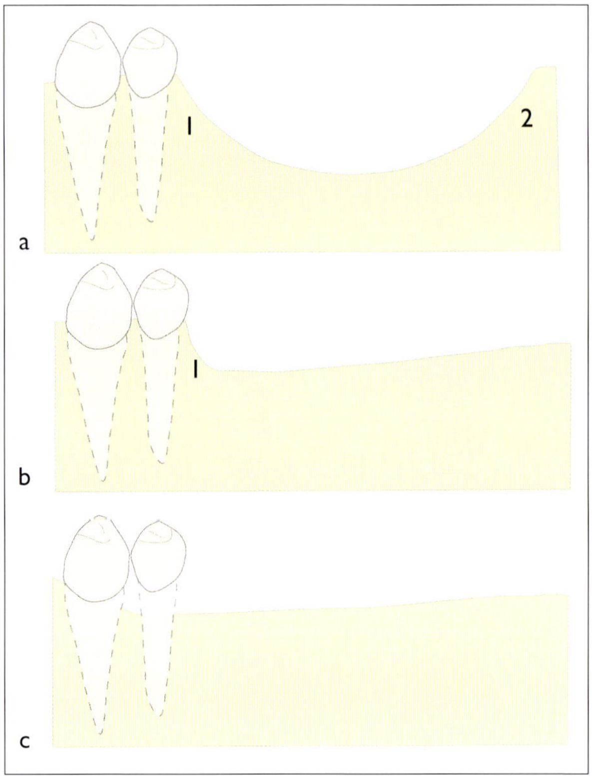

Fig 7-2 Vertical ridge defects: (a) 2-wall, (b) 1-wall, and (c) supracrestal defects.

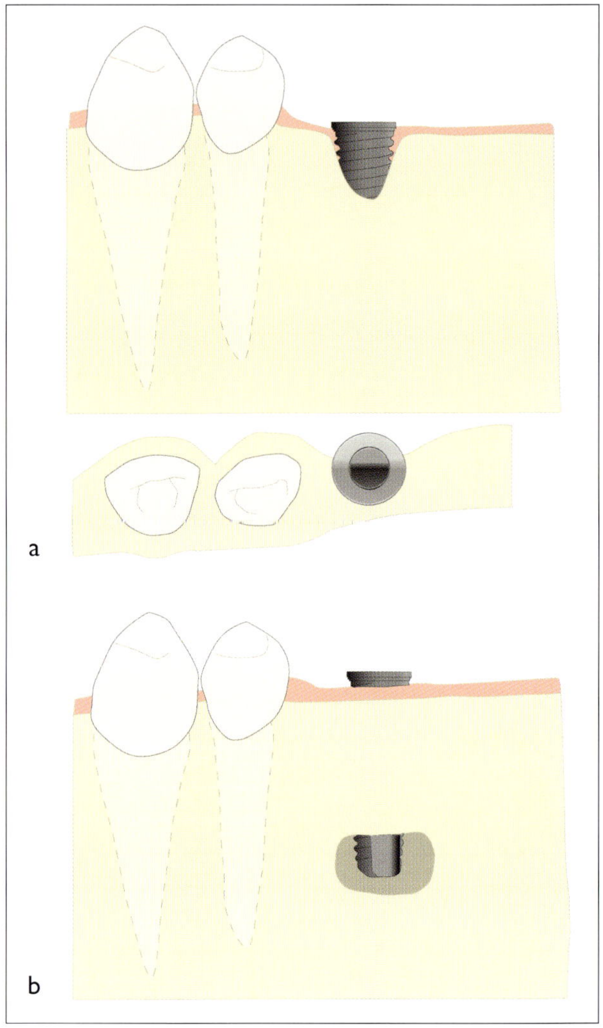

Fig 7-3 Implant dehiscence (a) and fenestration (b).

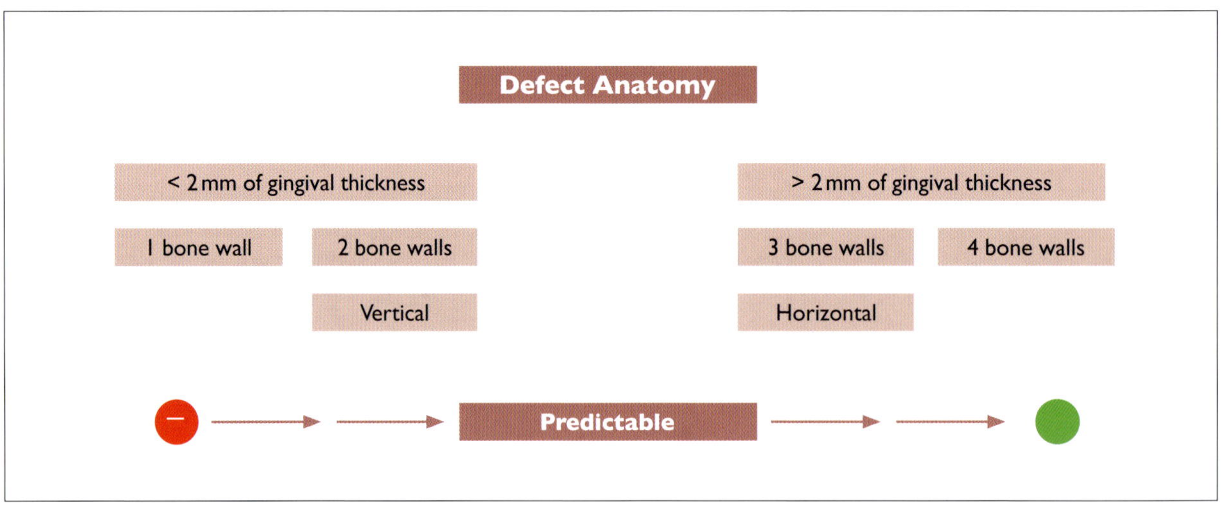

Fig 7-4 Bone defect anatomy and predictability.

7.5 What are the options for grafting materials?

A wide variety of materials is available and can be classified in two major groups.

Autogenic grafts are when the bone is obtained and transplanted from the same individual, and xenogenic grafts are when the origin is a different individual or species. This latter group can also be divided into allografts when the graft is obtained from another individual within the same species, and xenografts when obtained from a different species. Alloplastic materials are synthetically derived.

A second classification divides grafts in three groups based on the bone formation properties. These are termed osteogenic when they induce the formation of new bone, osteoinductive when they induce osteogenesis, and osteoconductive when they induce the growth of bone on a surface.[19] The graft provides support to the membrane to preserve the volume and also serves as a scaffold for the vascular ingrowth between the particles to permit the new bone formation.

The type of surface of the particles is likewise important since this will determine the attachment of bone cells and subsequent apposition of newly formed bone.[20]

Autogenous bone grafts can be harvested intraorally from donor areas including the chin, the ramus, or the retromolar area, and also can be obtained extraorally from the iliac crest, the calvaria, or the tibia among other areas.

When autogenous bone is transplanted, the stimulating growth factors and osteogenic cells are carried to the receiver site. The growth factors include bone morphogenetic proteins (BMPs), insulin-like growth factors, platelet derived growth factors, transforming growth factor β and fibroblast growth factors A and B. The cells included are osteocytes, osteoblasts, osteoclasts, and bone-lining cells. For this reason the autogenous bone is considered osteogenic.

7.5.1 Are there any differences between block or particulate grafts?

Autogenous bone can be used in block or particulate form. Blocks confer mechanical stability when immobilized with fixation screws, and if the technique is combined with the use of a membrane, a deceleration in the vascularization may occur,[21] but less resorption is observed.[22] Depending on the origin of the graft, a varying number of osteogenic cells are present, for example there is an increased number in the bone from the iliac crest.

The autogenous particulate grafts offer better osteoinductive and osteoconductive properties than blocks. This characteristic is related to the larger surface of the graft exposed to growth factors.[23] The osteogenic capacity is well demonstrated in the literature.[24]

Harvesting bone with bone scrapers is also recommended, but the obtained graft has a low number of osteocytes and osteoblast-like cells, limiting the growth potential.[25] Autogenous particulate grafts are rarely used alone because of their limited dimensional stability combined with their resorption properties, and they are most often mixed with other bone grafting materials such as xenografts.

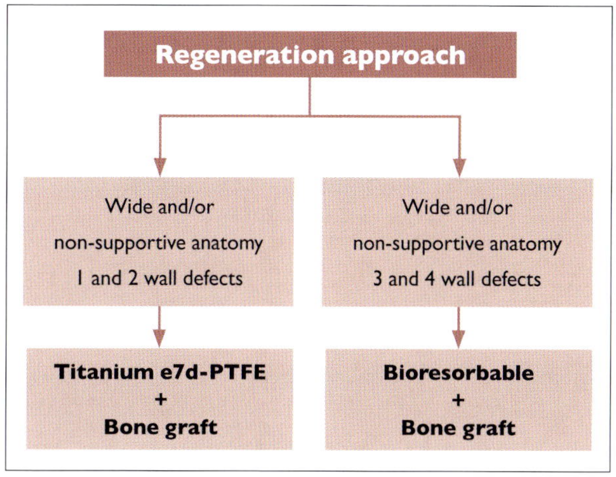

Fig 7-5 Regenerative approach: decision making tree.

7.5.2 Will the use of a mineralized or demineralized graft improve the results?

The use of allografts is also very common in GBR and other oral surgery techniques. Allografts come from a bone bank and are normally used as a FDBA or demineralized freeze-dried bone allograft (DFDBA), to eliminate the risk of disease transmission and immunogenic responses. Allografts are available from cortical or cancellous bone and presented in blocks or particulate forms.

The demineralized form exposes the BMPs on the surface, increasing the osteoinductive potential.[26,27] However, it should be noted that some studies only report the osteoconductive potential.[28] While DFDBA has been mostly used in GTR, it has also been suggested for use in GBR combined with a xenograft due to the rapid resorption rate of the DFDBA enhancing vascularity in the whole particulate graft.[29] Depending on its origin (cancellous, cortical, or mixed), FDBA has been widely used alone for GBR and may have a faster resorption rate than a xenograft.

Natural bone-derived xenografts are extensively used in GBR techniques. Bovine bone minerals are biocompatible and osteoconductive, but there is controversy as to whether they are truly resorbable. One study found bovine-derived bone substitutes remained up to 10 years post-operatively.[30] These have the highest level of evidence in sinus lift procedures and are also frequently used in vertical augmentation as well as in demanding horizontal regenerations due to the maintenance of the volume the material.[31]

The xenogenic/allopastic grafts are derived from other species like coral or algae, or originated from natural bone mineral. These materials have shown biocompatibility and osteoinductive potential. The resorption of some of these materials is limited and it is too rapid in others. Encapsulation of some of these materials in connective tissue has also been described.[32,33]

7.6 Clinical cases

Case 1: May a collagen membrane be left exposed in ridge preservation on a 3-wall socket?

A healthy patient had tooth 21 with history of periapical pathology and apicoectomy along with repeated abscesses (Figs 7-6 and 7-7). After atraumatic extraction, the presence of the buccal plate was checked with a periodontal probe and was clearly absent. A full-thickness buccal flap was raised from the mesial line angle of tooth 11 to the distal line angle of tooth 22, where a vertical releasing incision was made to gain access. A complete dehiscence of the buccal plate can be observed (Fig 7-8). This was a contained 3-wall defect as the buccal plate was absent. In order to gain bone horizontally, GBR was performed with FDBA and a cross-linked collagen membrane (Figs 7-9 and 7-10). We recommend loosely packing the bone grafting particles in order to allow vascularization. It is also advised to slightly overbuild the defect with the bone particles as a certain amount of contraction is expected. The membrane has to extend about 3 mm from the margins of the defect and undermine the palatal flap. The buccal flap was replaced to its original position and the cross-linked collagen membrane was left exposed over the crestal area (Figs 7-11 and 7-12). It is unclear whether for ridge preservation the membrane needs to be completely covered on the crestal area by advancing the flap. This was a contained defect on an extraction socket. It is not recommended to leave the membrane exposed on a more demanding defect. After 3.5 months, healing was uneventful and the crestal area had epithelialized with keratinized mucosa (Figs 7-13 and 7-14). When raising an envelope flap for implant placement, complete regeneration of the defect can be seen horizontally and vertically. Clinically the bone appears to bleed normally and residual grafting particles can rarely be seen just 3.5 months after the regeneration (Figs 7-15 and 7-16).

As illustrated, regeneration of 3-wall contained horizontal defect is very predictable.

Figs 7-6 to 7-16 Case 1

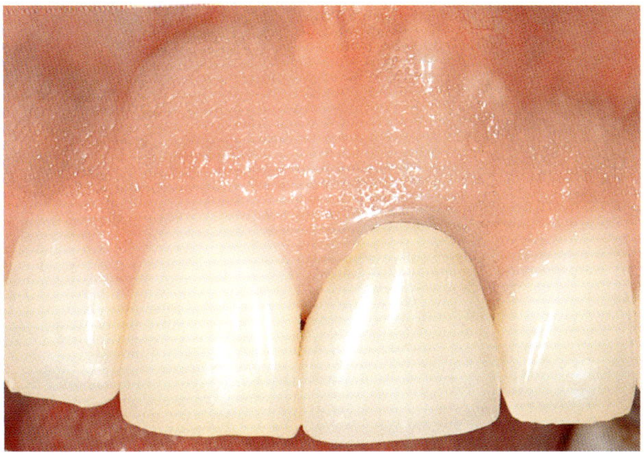

Fig 7-6 Anterior view of tooth 21.

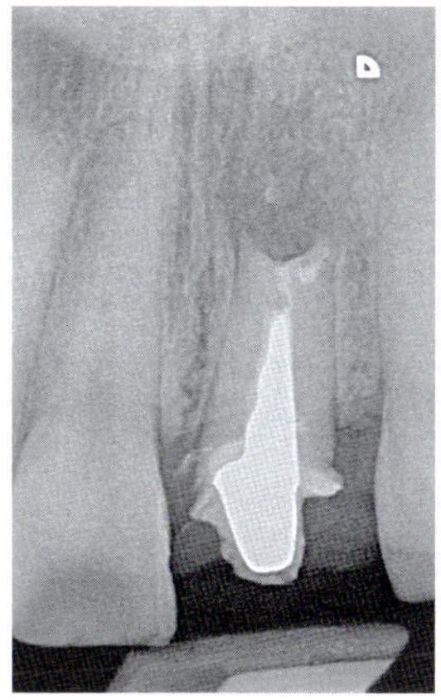

Fig 7-7 Tooth 21 with periapical pathology and apicoectomy.

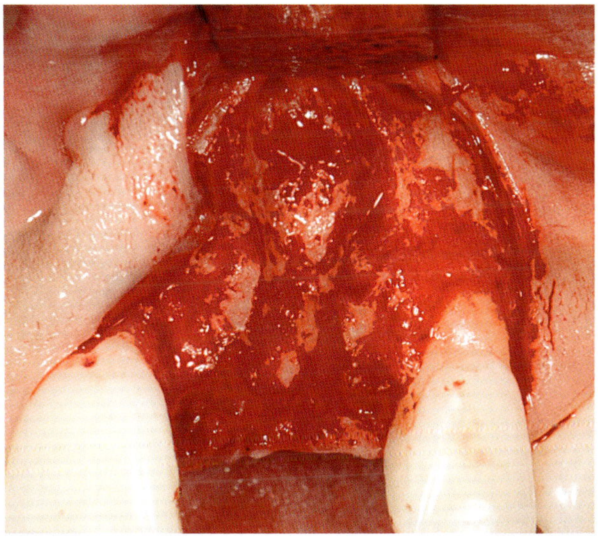

Fig 7-8 Complete dehiscence of the buccal plate.

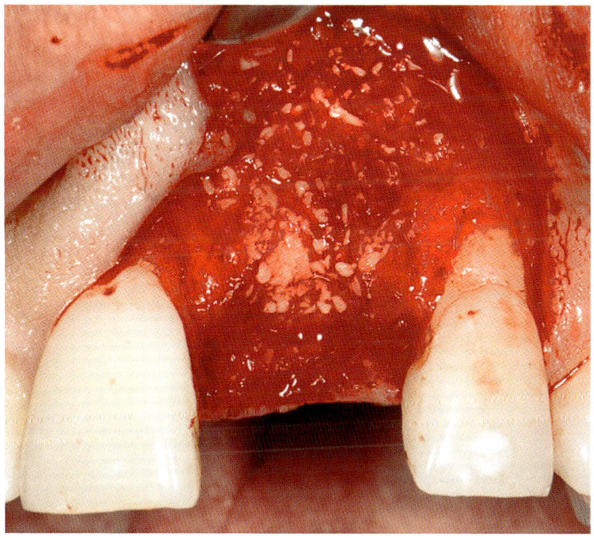

Fig 7-9 FDBA loosely packed in the socket.

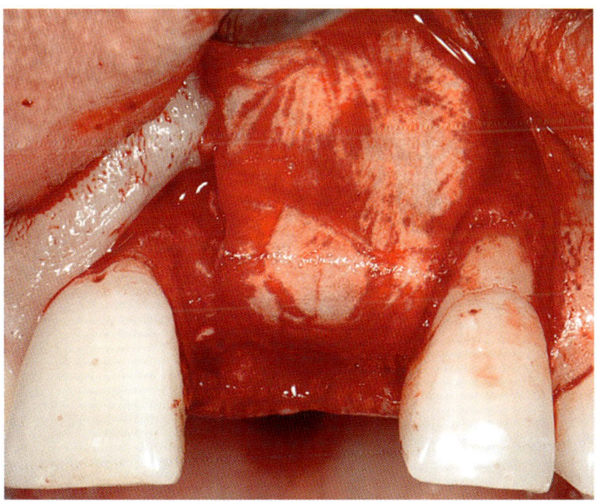

Fig 7-10 A cross-linked membrane is extended 2–3 mm over the defect.

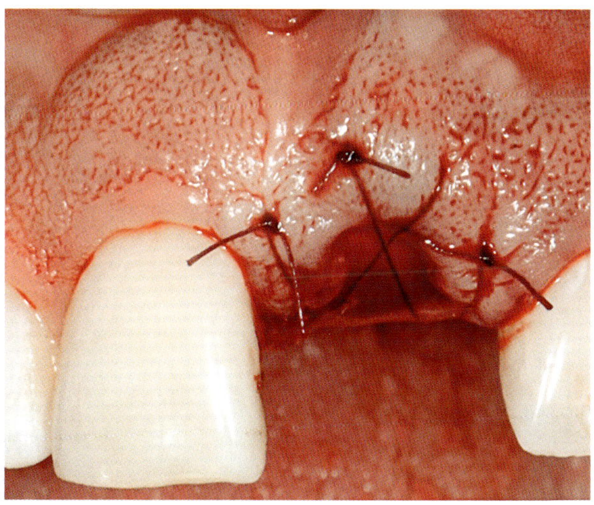

Fig 7-11 The flap is replaced to its original position.

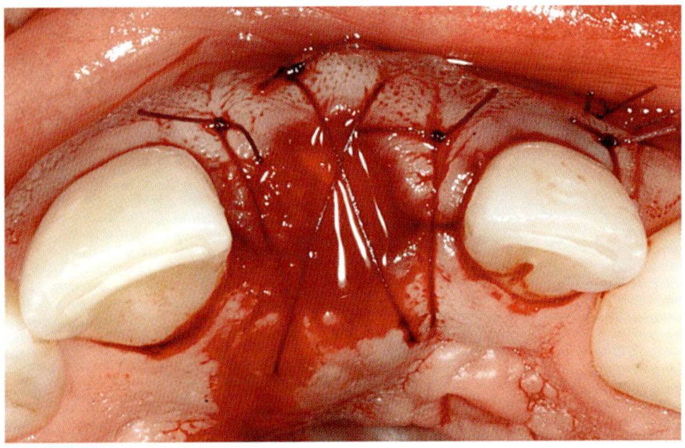

Fig 7-12 Occlusal view with the exposed membrane.

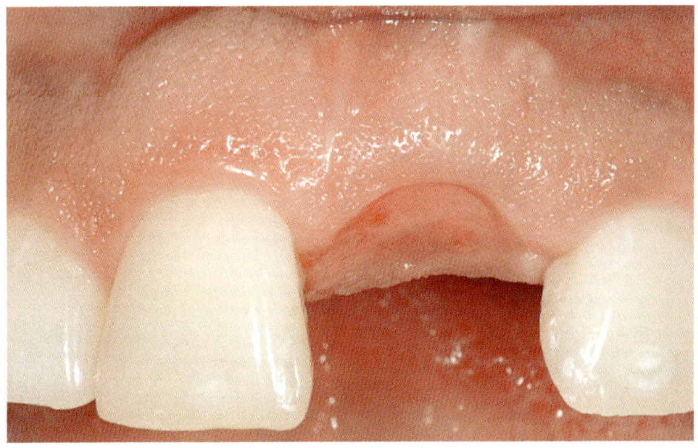

Fig 7-13 Anterior view of healing at 4 months.

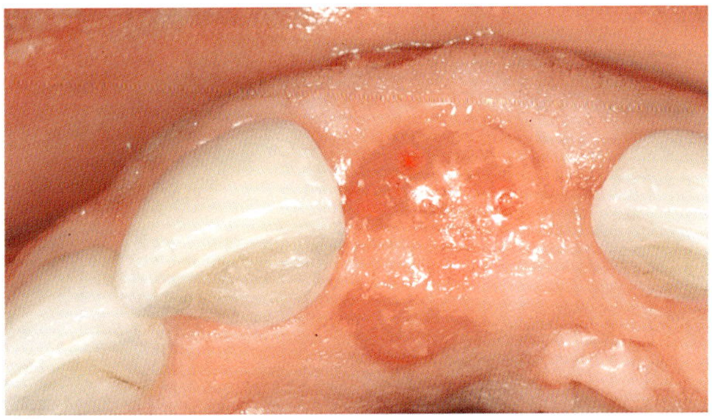

Fig 7-14 Occlusal view of healing at 4 months.

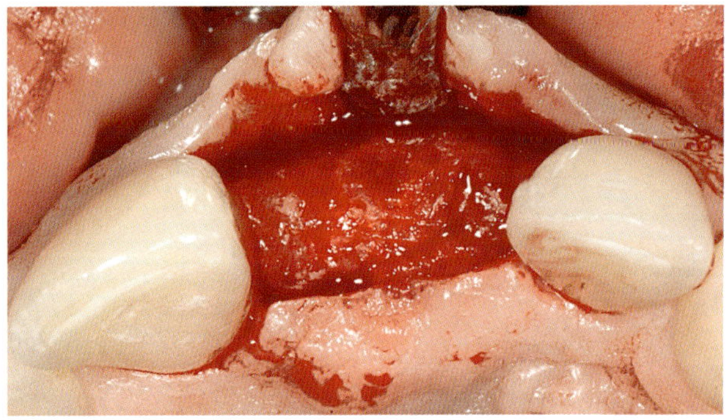

Fig 7-15 Re-entry anterior view at 4 months.

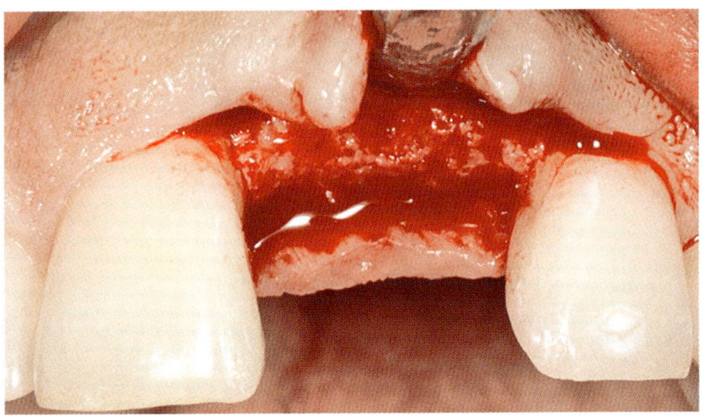

Fig 7-16 Re-entry occlusal view at 4 months.

Case 2: How much bone width can be achieved with resorbable membranes?

(Courtesy of Fabio Mazzocco DDS, MS, Private Practice, Padova, Italy)

An implant was planned for the edentulous space of 24 to 25, which had a Seibert class III defect, mainly horizontal (Fig 7-17). A crestal incision in the edentulous area was followed by an intrasulcular incision distal of 26 and mesial of 23, where a vertical releasing incision was raised to gain access to the osseous defect. A full-thickness flap was raised and a wide poorly contained 3-wall defect was observed. The mesial, palatal, and distal bone walls were present (Figs 7-18 and 7-19). A cortico-cancellous mineralized allograft was placed in the defect overbuilding the site in thickness to compensate for shrinkage during healing (Fig 7-20). A cross-linked collagen membrane covered the particulate bone graft and extended 2 to 3 mm over the defect, ending below the palatal flap (Fig 7-21). Buccal and occlusal views show how the flap was advanced coronally to cover the membrane completely and was sutured without tension (Figs 7-22 and 7-23). The incision line remained closed during the 5 months of healing, and at re-entry bone width gain was observed (Figs 7-24 and 7-25). Some bone grafting particles were observed although bone texture was not soft. Waiting longer periods of healing may reduce the number of residual grafting particles that can be seen. Bone width gain would have been higher with a non-resorbable membrane but chances of complication are also increased.

Case 3: Is there a predictable treatment for implant dehiscence?

An implant was placed in the area of tooth 23 following a prosthetic stent. Although the implant was

Figs 7-17 to 7-31 Cases 2 and 3

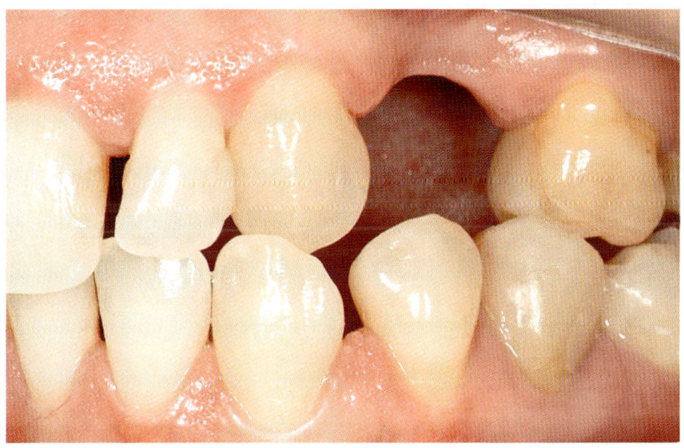

Fig 7-17 Horizontal and vertical ridge defect of tooth 24.

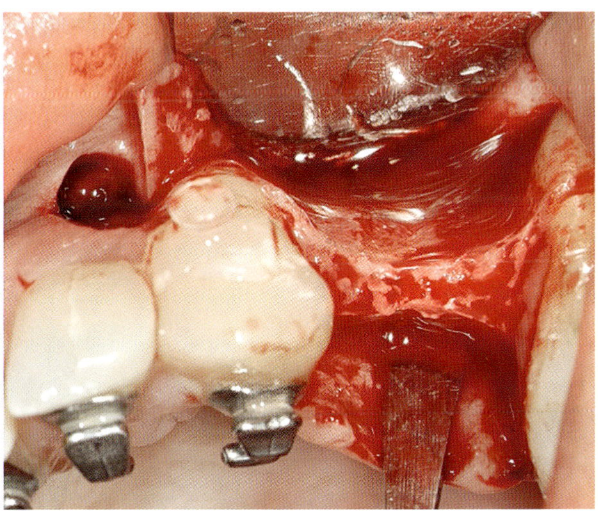

Fig 7-18 Buccal view of the horizontal bone defect.

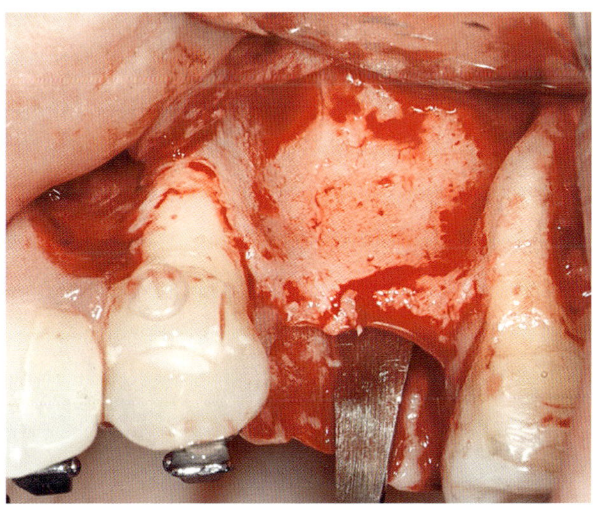

Fig 7-19 Occlusal view of the horizontal bone defect.

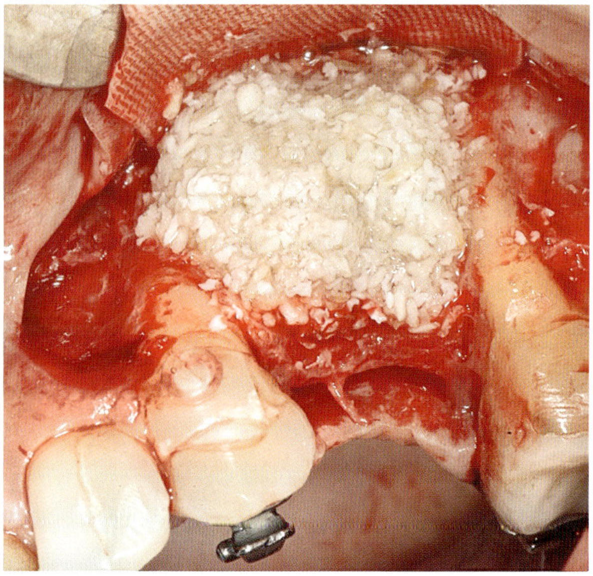

Fig 7-20 Bone allograft placed in the area to be regenerated.

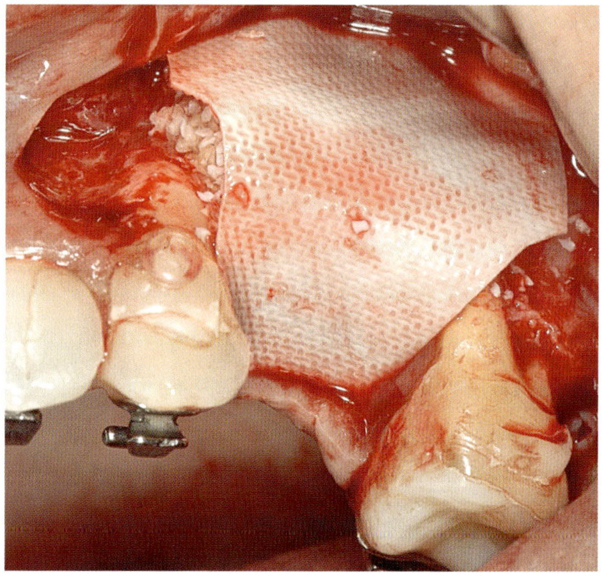

Fig 7-21 Collagen cross-linked membrane extended apically underneath the periosteum.

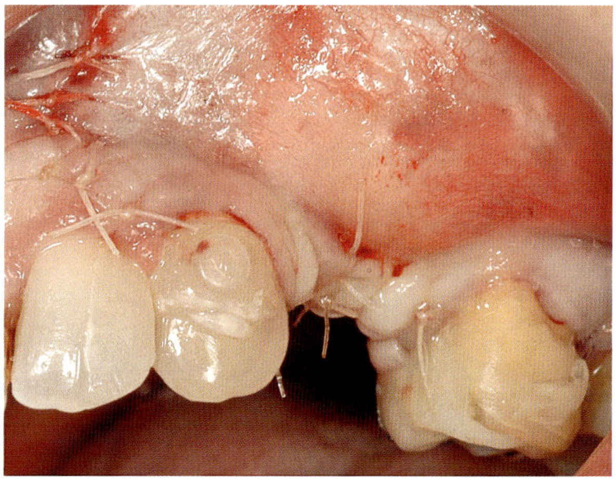

Fig 7-22 Buccal view of the sutured tension free flap.

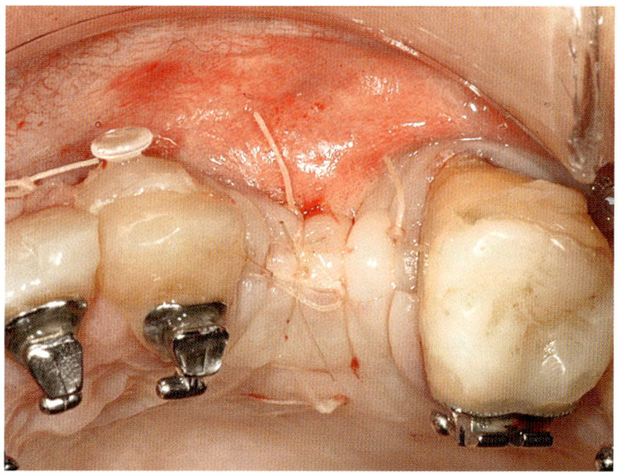

Fig 7-23 Occlusal view of the sutured tension free flap.

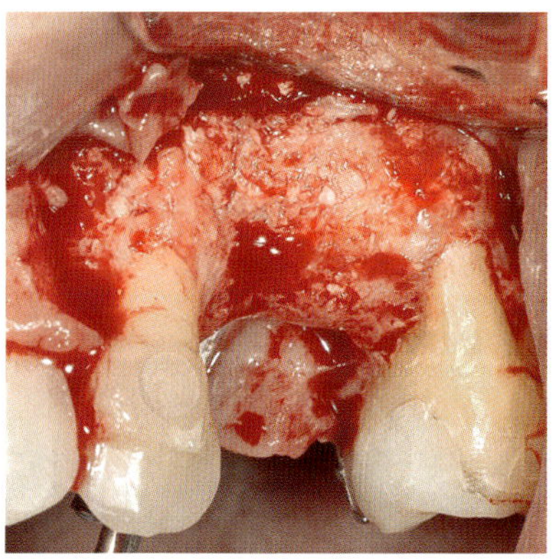

Fig 7-24 Re-entry anterior view.

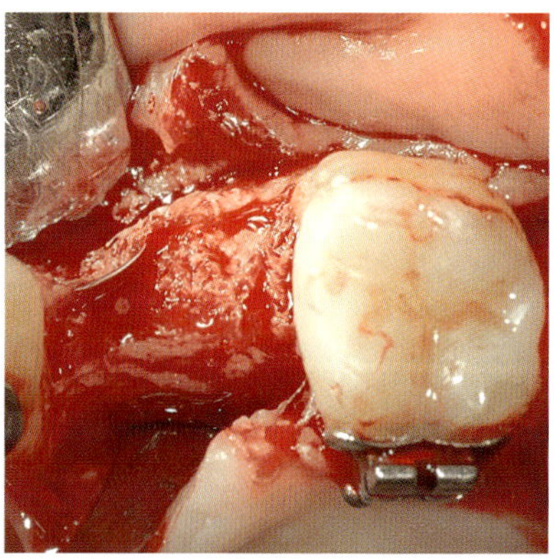

Fig 7-25 Re-entry occlusal view.

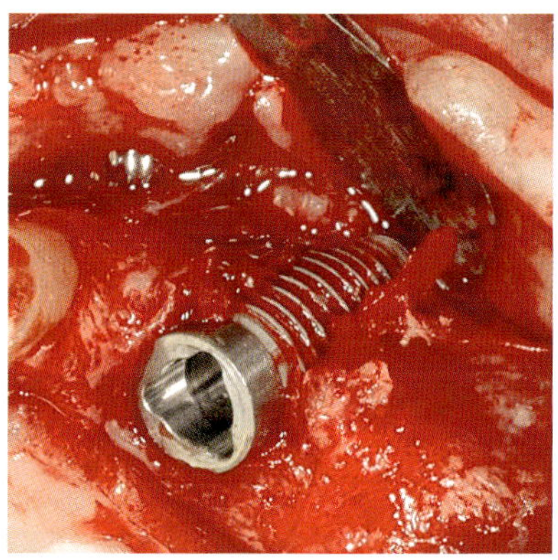

Fig 7-26 Complete buccal dehiscence of the implant.

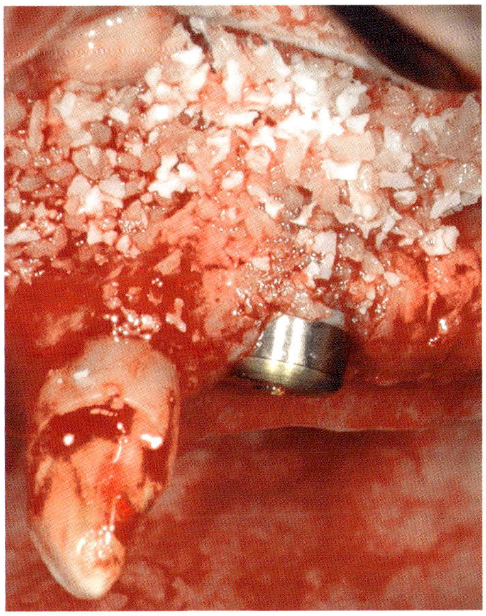

Fig 7-27 Xenograft and DFDBA under a collagen membrane are used to regenerate bone over the implant.

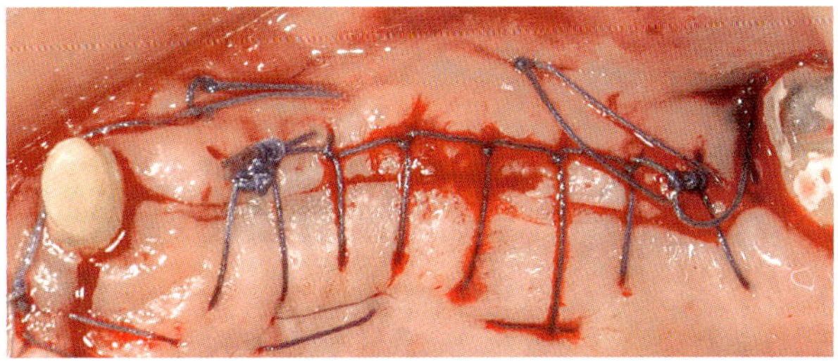

Fig 7-28 Suture technique.

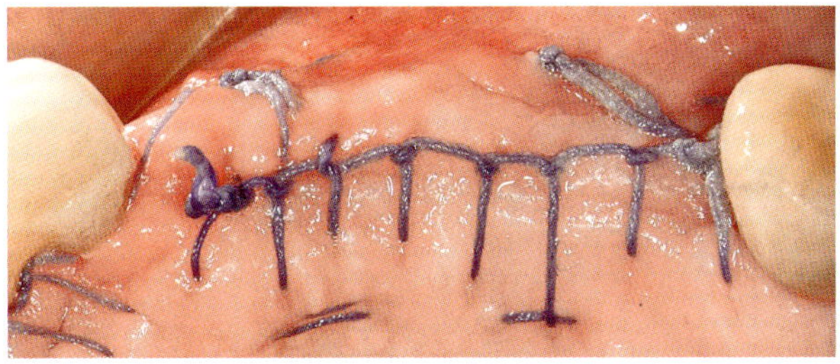

Fig 7-29 At 2 weeks after surgery the healing is uneventful.

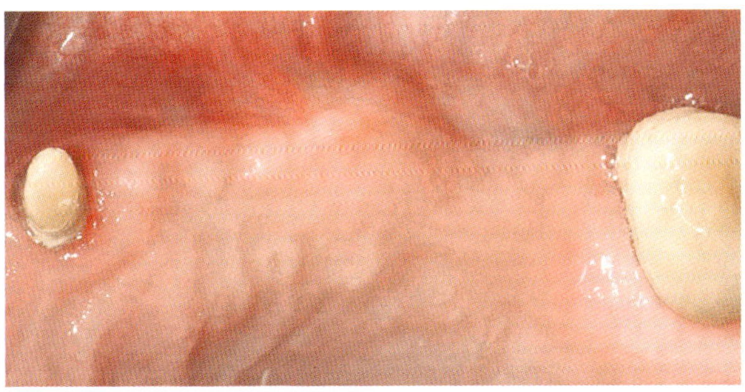

Fig 7-30 The flap remains closed during the healing.

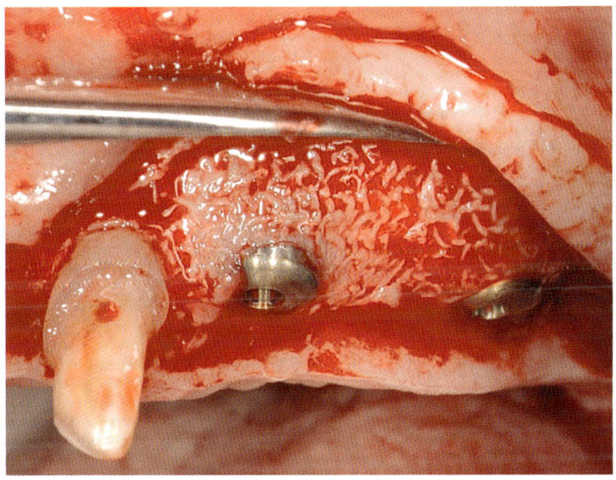

Fig 7-31 Re-entry at 6 months.

stable, a complete dehiscence of the implant threads had occurred on the buccal wall (Fig 7-26). A mixture of particulate xenograft and DFDBA was used to cover the implant threads and a collagen membrane was placed over it to secure the bone graft in position and exclude cells from the soft tissue. The membrane should always extend 2 to 3 mm from the bone graft or defect (Fig 7-27). Releasing incisions in the periosteum are critical to achieve primary closure without tension. A horizontal mattress suture was placed at the area of the implant dehiscence to assure tension free closure. A continuous interlocking suture was then performed (Fig 7-28). At 2 weeks of healing the complete closure of the flap was observed, which leads to proper bone regeneration if pressure on the area is prevented and flap closure is maintained during healing (Figs 7-29 and 7-30). Four months later, at implant stage two, complete regeneration of the dehiscence had occurred (Fig 7-31). The regenerated bone presented the indentations of the cross-linked collagen membrane used, which may show its long-lasting capability.

The regeneration of dehiscences, fenestrations and 4-wall defects is very predictable because of the large amount of vascularity present.

Case 4: Are decortications necessary?

The edentulous area of teeth 35 to 38 presented a combined horizontal and vertical ridge deformity (Figs 7-32 and 7-33). The radiographs show sufficient bone height to the mental foramen and mandibular canal for implant placement was present (Figs 7-34 and 7-35). Clinically there was a severe horizontal bone defect. The treatment plan was to perform GBR with non-resorbable e-PTFE titanium-reinforced membrane in combination with particulate FDBA and xenograft (2:1), with the surgical technique described by Buser et al.[34] A perpendicular incision to the bone was made at the mucogingival junction (MGJ) of the edentulous area and a full thickness flap was raised on the lingual side. A partial thickness flap was created at the buccal part, achieving a periosteal flap and a mucosal tension-free flap. No vertical releasing incisions were made and an envelope flap was extended to the distal of tooth 33 (Fig 7-36). It was a one-wall defect (lingual wall) in most areas and a two-wall defect at the mesial part (mesial and lingual bony walls present). Decortications were made with a #6 carbide bur in order to obtain blood supply from the marrow for the bone graft particles. Scientific evidence shows that decortication may not be necessary[35] although some animal studies demonstrate earlier bone healing and graft maturation (Fig 7-37).[36] The empiric mixture of FDBA and xenograft (2:1) was used in this defect (Fig 7-38). The xenograft will not be resorbed and might be the best bone graft for maintaining volume. When using a stiff membrane, which maintains the space per se, there is no need for overbuilding with the bone graft. The titanium-reinforced membrane was fixed to the periosteum with two horizontal mattress sutures, with the knot on the lingual flap (Fig 7-39). Then the buccal flap was easily advanced over and sutured with a continuous interlocking suture; a simple suture was made in the papilla between teeth 33 and 34. Some vertical volume gain was also observed (Figs 7-40 and 7-41). After 6 months of healing, bone width and height gain were clinically and radiographically observed (Figs 7-42 and 7-43). At re-entry the non-resorbable membrane was well

Figs 7-32 to 7-45 Case 4

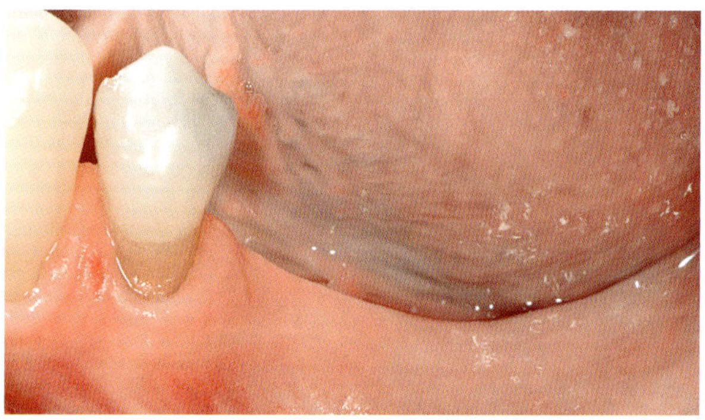

Fig 7-32 Buccal view of the horizontal and vertical ridge deformity.

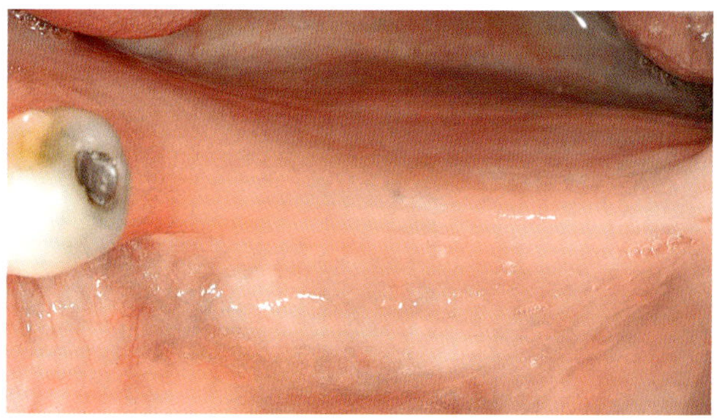

Fig 7-33 Occlusal view of the horizontal ridge deformity.

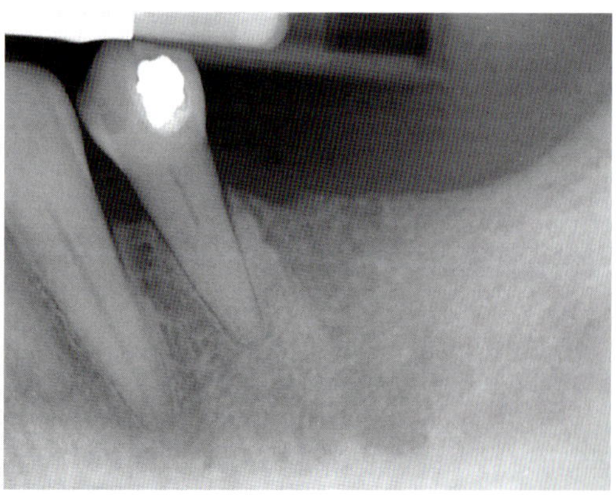

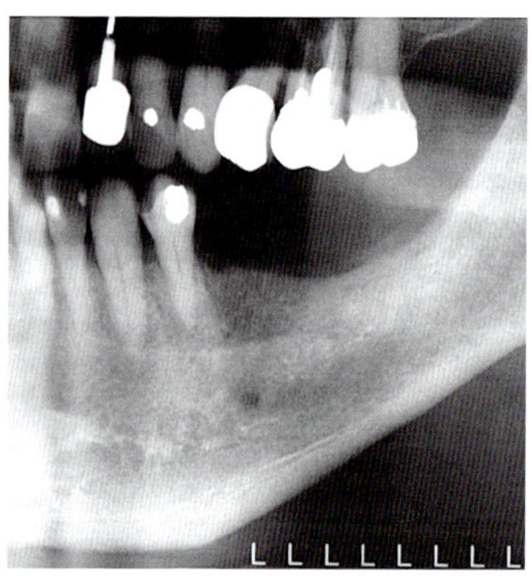

Fig 7-34 (left) Periapical radiography.

Fig 7-35 (right) Panoramic radiograph view.

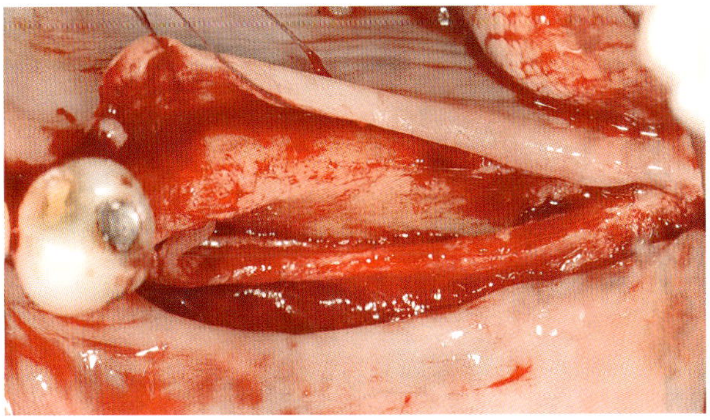

Fig 7-36 Occlusal view of the horizontal bone resorption. The technique was described previously by Buser et al.[34]

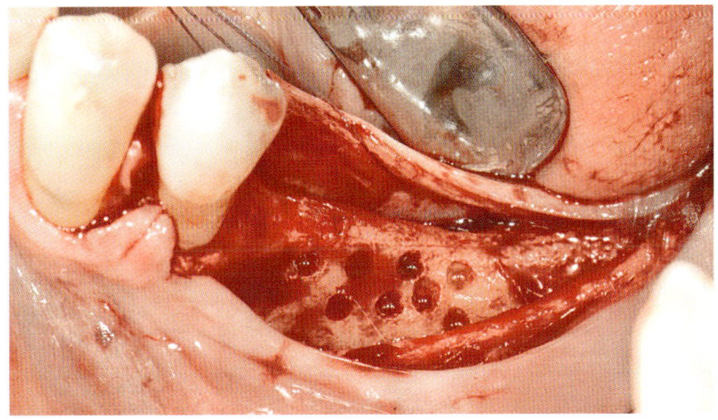

Fig 7-37 Bone decortications.

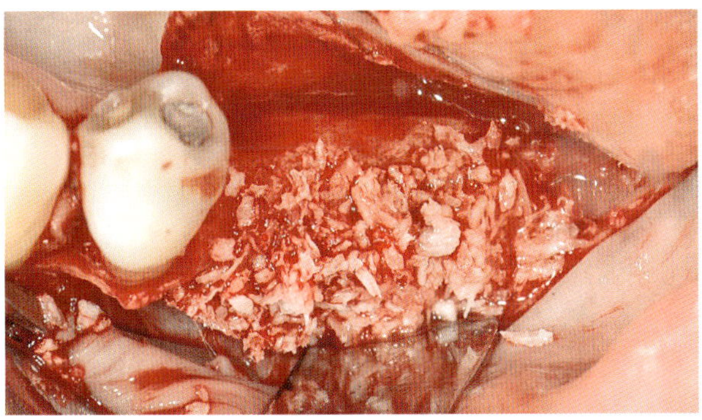

Fig 7-38 FDBA is placed in the defect.

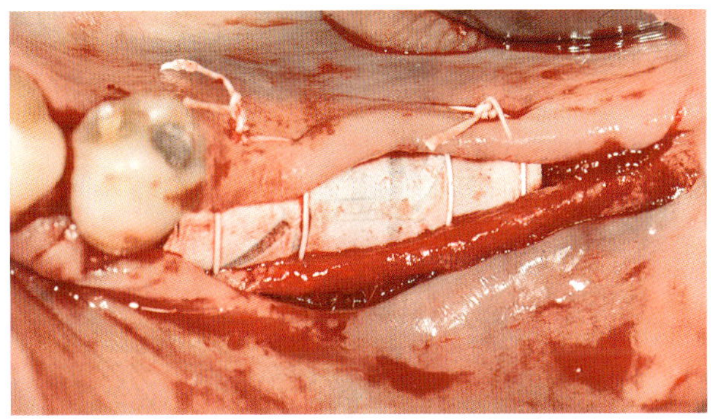

Fig 7-39 A titanium-reinforced membrane is secured with the periosteum.

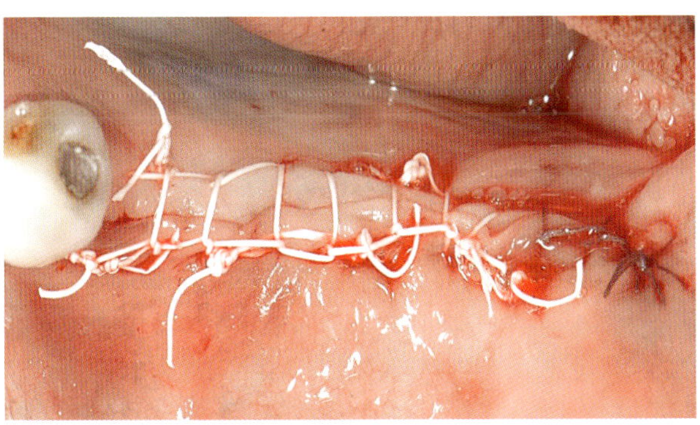

Fig 7-40 The buccal flap is advanced and sutured (occlusal view).

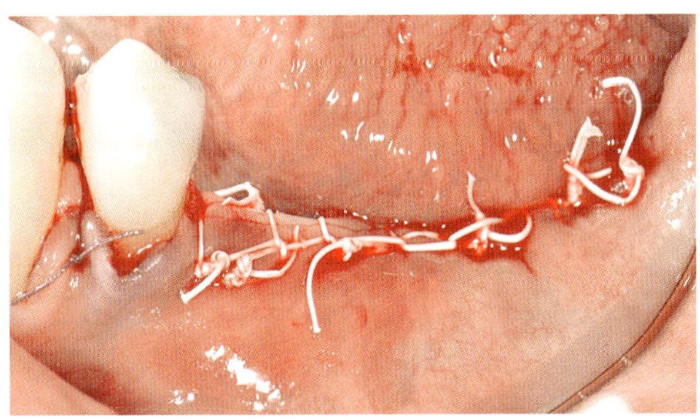

Fig 7-41 The buccal flap is advanced and sutured (buccal view).

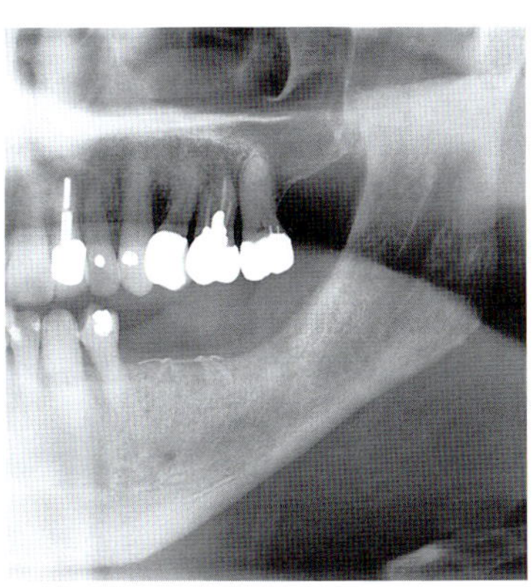

Fig 7-42 Panoramic radiograph view after 6 months of healing.

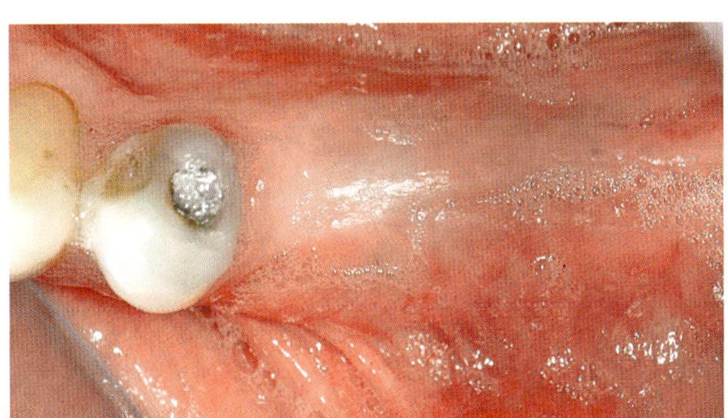

Fig 7-43 Occlusal view after 6 months of healing..

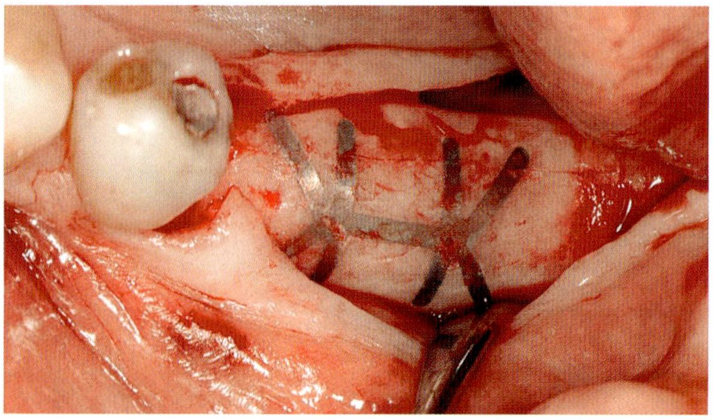

Fig 7-44 Re-entry before removing the membrane.

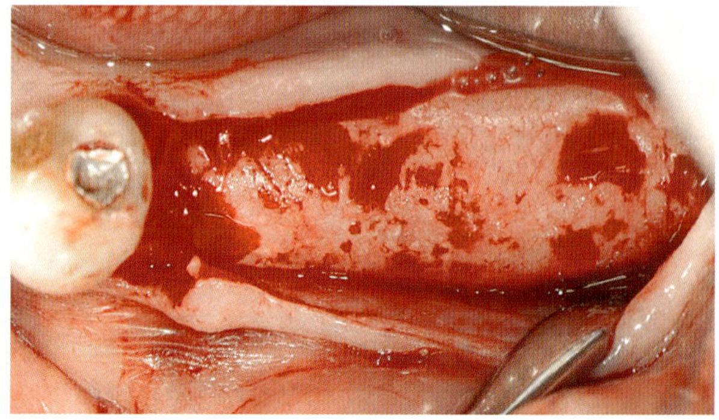

Fig 7-45 Occlusal bone view after 6 months of healing.

adapted to the bone crest and had to be raised with an elevator (Fig 7-44). An important amount of bone width was achieved. Clinically the bone bled naturally and a small amount of residual bone grafting particles was seen (Fig 7-45). The double buccal flap technique allows the buccal flap to be advanced easily as well as allowing primary closure, yet causes a lot of swelling to the patient. Releasing incisions in the periosteum may achieve the same primary closure with less swelling.

Case 5: Reacting to non-resorbable membrane exposure

This patient presented a horizontal and vertical ridge deformity in the edentulous area of teeth 44 to 48. The horizontal defect seemed to be more obvious than the vertical one (Figs 7-46 and 7-47). The computed tomographic (CT) scan showed a ridge width of 2 to 3 mm in the mesial part and 4 to 5 mm in the distal area with an included root tip. There was about 10 mm of bone height to the mental foramen and mandibular canal in the whole edentulous area (Fig 7-48). A crestal incision was performed to raise a full thickness envelope flap, extended intrasulcularly bucally and lingually to the distal side of tooth 42. Extraction of the root tip was performed (Fig 7-49). After decortications on the mesial part of the defect to achieve blood supply were performed, FDBA and a non-resorbable titanium-reinforced membrane were used (Fig 7-50). Periosteal releasing incisions were performed to mobilize the buccal flap and the lingual full thickness flap was raised at least past the MG; we advise not to perform periosteal releasing incisions in the lingual flap because of the anatomical risks. Two horizontal mattress sutures were made along with single interrupted sutures. The suture bites had to be at least 5 mm away from the incision line. Note some suture tension on the mesial part of the defect, corresponding to a titanium-free membrane area (Figs 7-51 and 7-52). The healing was uneventful until 7 weeks after the GBR when the patient presented swelling on the distal part of the regenerated area. On exploration, exposure of the membrane could not be seen but inflammatory tissue, which bled easily on palpation, was present on the distal part (Fig 7-53). Differentiation of mesenchymal cells occurs approximately 6 weeks after GBR,[37] so this is the minimum time for the non-resorbable membrane to remain under the gingiva. Thus the membrane was removed and a soft osteoid tissue was seen underneath the mesial regenerated area. Inflammatory bleeding tissue was observed on the distal part (Fig 7-54). Then a resorbable collagen membrane was placed over to prevent soft tissue cells from migrating into the regenerating tissue (there is no scientific evidence to know if this is better than not placing the collagen membrane). Four more months of healing were permitted (Fig 7-55) and at re-entry, bone width gain was observed on the whole ridge. There was less bone width gain at the mesial part, where tension with suturing was present and it partially collapsed the membrane (Fig 7-56). We understand that bone width gain would have been higher without the infection that occurred at the beginning of the healing, nevertheless the early response to the complication allowed partial regeneration.

Fig 7-46 to 7-56 Case 6

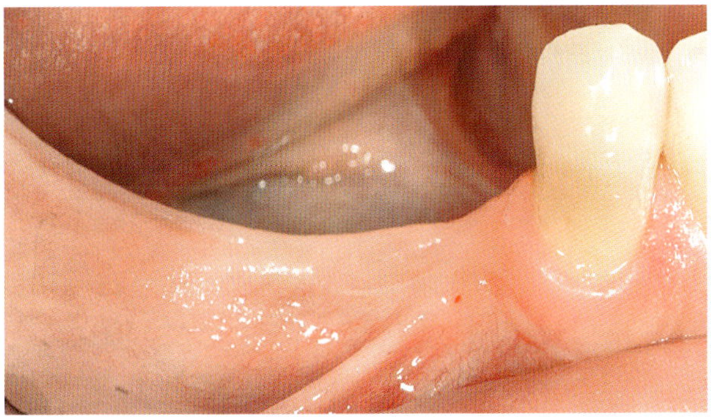

Fig 7-46 Buccal view of the horizontal and vertical ridge deformity.

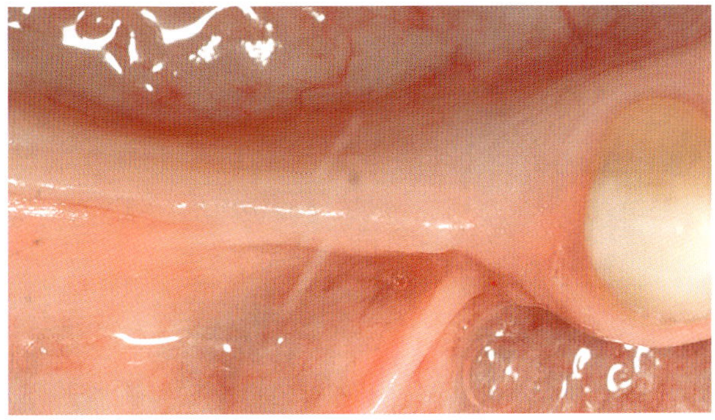

Fig 7-47 Occlusal view of the horizontal ridge deformity.

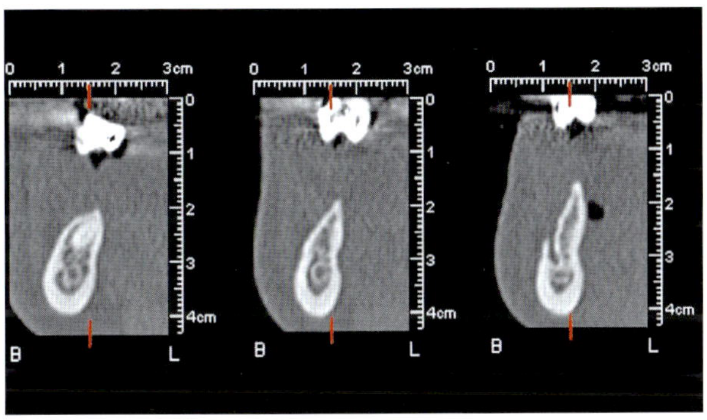

Fig 7-48 Computerized tomography scan.

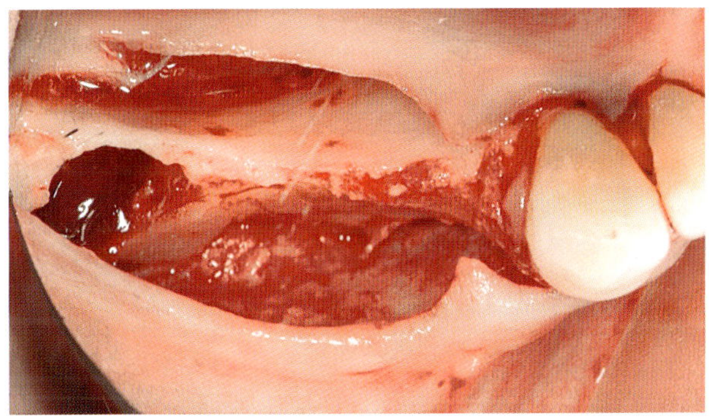

Fig 7-49 Occlusal view of the horizontal bone resorption.

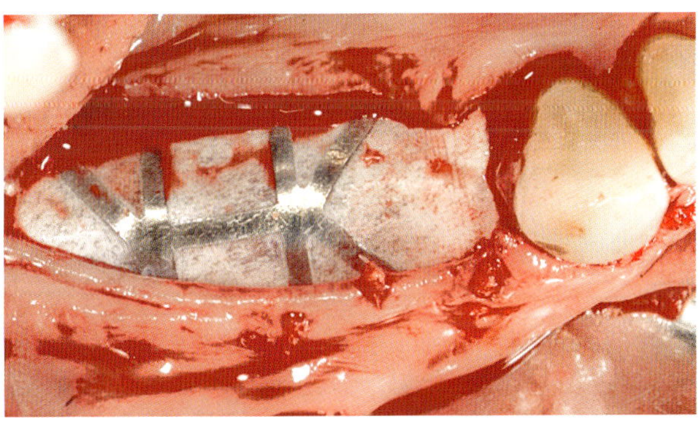

Fig 7-50 Occlusal view of the titanium-reinforced membrane in place.

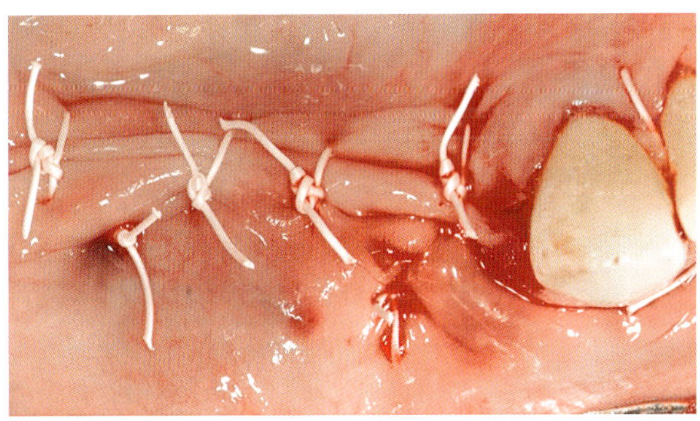

Fig 7-51 The buccal flap is advanced and sutured (occlusal view).

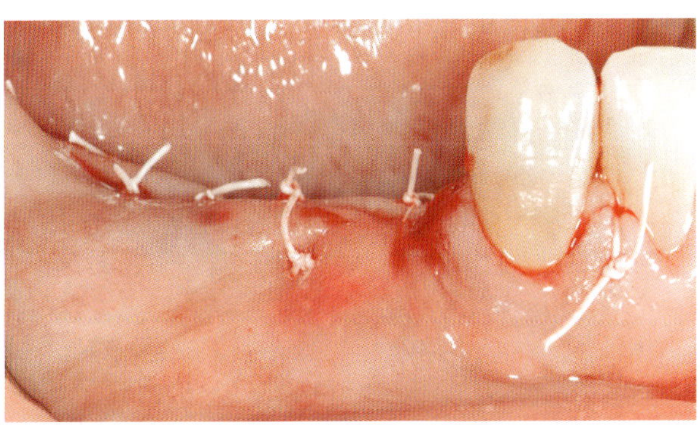

Fig 7-52 The buccal flap is advanced and sutured (buccal view).

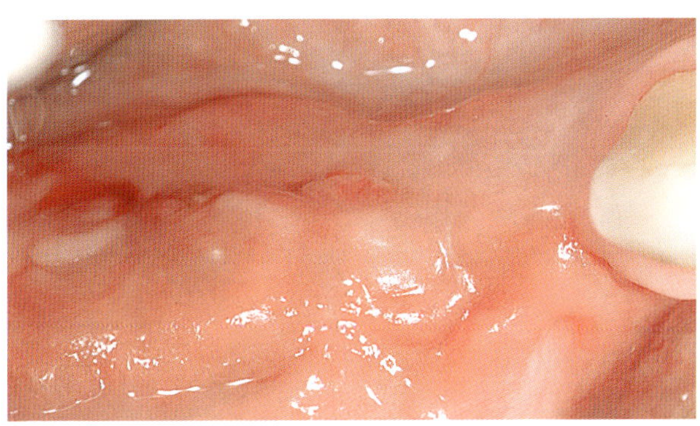

Fig 7-53 Occlusal clinical view of the edema during healing.

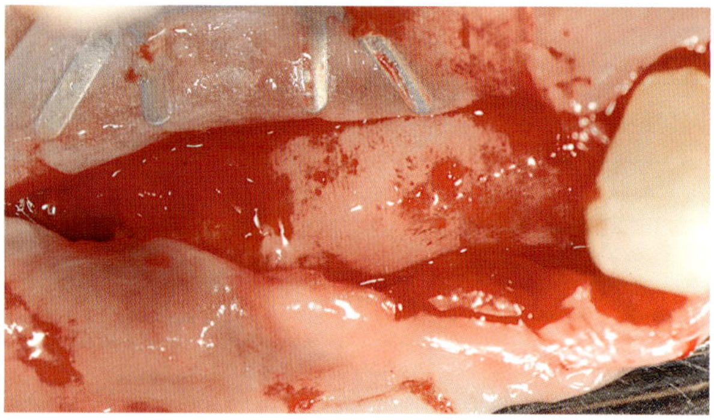

Fig 7-54 Occlusal view of the infected site after 2 months of healing.

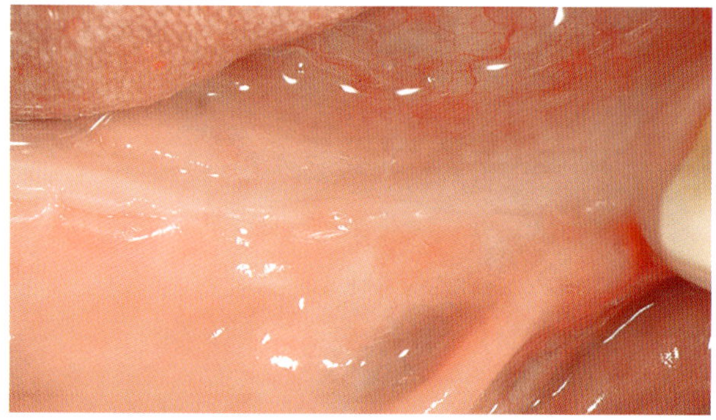

Fig 7-55 Occlusal soft tissue view after 4 months more of healing.

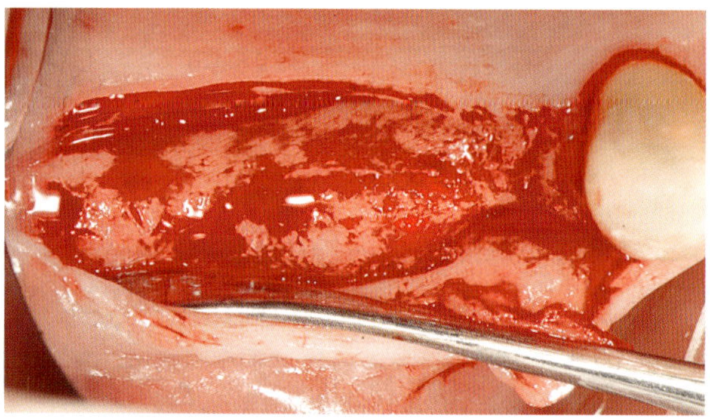

Fig 7-56 Occlusal bone view after 6 months of healing.

Case 6: What is the limit of vertical GBR?

(Courtesy of Fabio Mazzocco DDS, MS, Private Practice, Padova, Italy.)

The edentulous area of teeth 35 to 38 clinically and radiographically presented a horizontal and a vertical ridge deformity. Severe vertical bone loss was seen distal of tooth 34 with about 7 mm of bone above the mandibular canal and mental foramen (Figs 7-57 to 7-60). Vertical defects are the most challenging to regenerate. This was a 2-wall wide supracrestal defect, where the height of the distal bone picks of tooth 34 and at the third molar region determines the limit of the amount of vertical regeneration that can be achieved. "V"-shaped defects would regenerate better than wide "U"-shaped defects or flat defects because of the amount and proximity of blood supply to the grafting material. There is no question that short implants can be predictably used these days and that a poor crown-to-implant ratio may not affect the success rate of implants. This was concluded in a systematic review based on just two clinical studies and it has to be taken into consideration.[38]

A crestal incision was performed and extended intrasulcularly two teeth mesially, and a full thickness flap was raised bucally and lingually (Figs 7-61 and 7-62). As the defect was not self-contained, either a block graft and a resorbable membrane or a titanium-reinforced membrane with particulate graft could be used. The bone graft or the membrane would need to hold the space for regeneration. In this case a mixture of xenograft and autogenous particulate bone was used, combining the low/non-substitution of the former with the cellular activity and rapid resorption of the latter (Fig 7-63). The non-resorbable membrane was fixed with four tacks at the corners of the membrane. The membrane has to be stable during healing for cells to differentiate to osteoblasts and not fibroblasts. A distance of about 1.5 mm has to be left from the distal of the adjacent tooth to the non-resorbable membrane to avoid contamination (Fig 7-64). Flaps were advanced coronally by periosteal releasing incisions on the buccal side and superficial incisions on the most coronal part of the lingual side. Horizontal mattresses sutures were performed to compensate for the tension, as well as a single interrupted suture (Fig 7-65). If the edges of the flaps approximate gently when sutured without any tension, most probably the membrane will remain covered for the healing (Fig 7-66). When advancing flaps,

Figs 7-57 to 7-69 Case 6

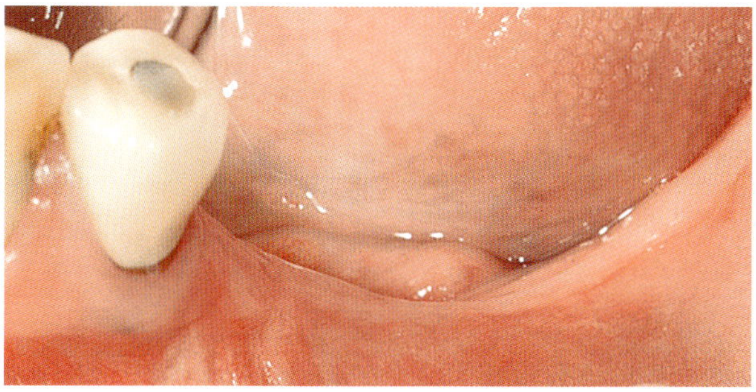

Fig 7-57 Buccal view of the horizontal and vertical ridge deformity.

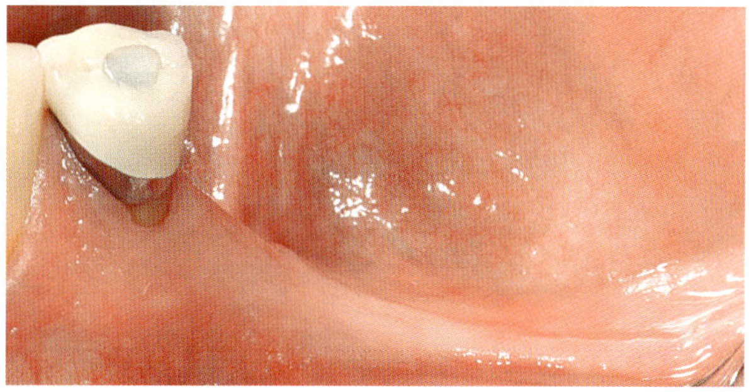

Fig 7-58 Lingual view of the horizontal and vertical ridge deformity.

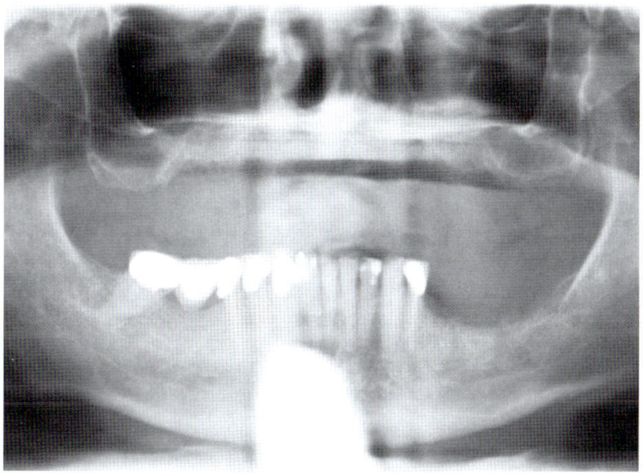

Fig 7-59 Panoramic radiograph view.

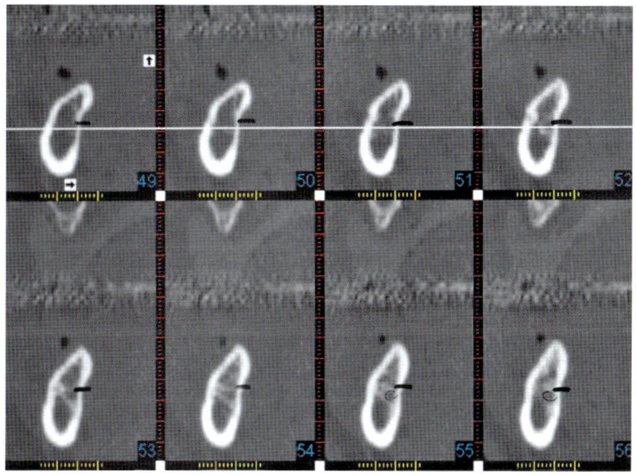

Fig 7-60 Computerized tomography scan.

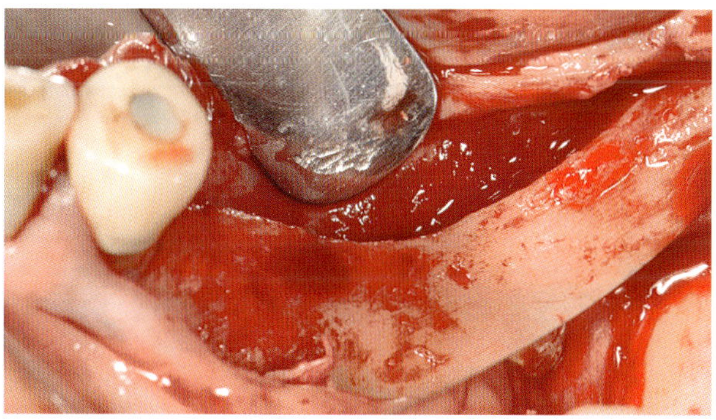

Fig 7-61 Buccal view of the horizontal and vertical bone resorption.

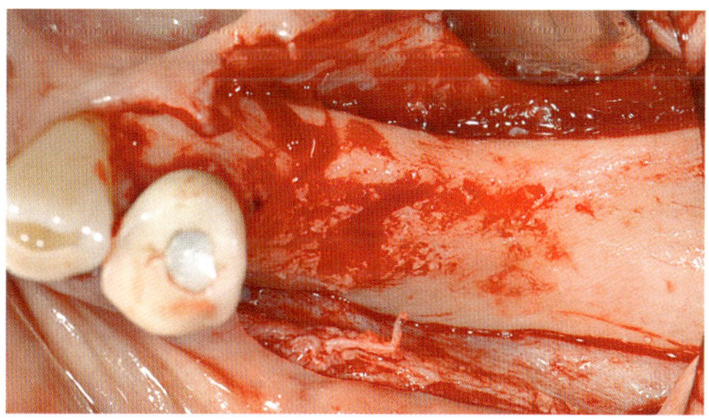

Fig 7-62 Occlusal view of the horizontal bone resorption.

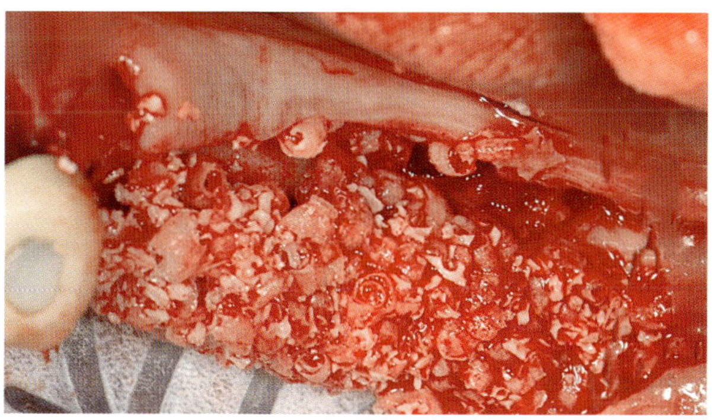

Fig 7-63 A xenograft and autogenous graft are mixed.

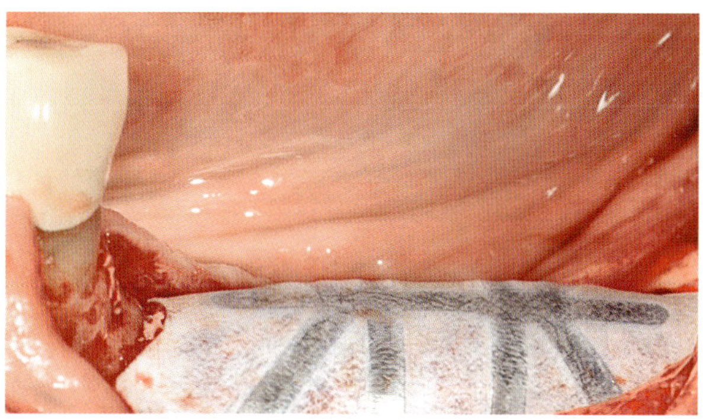

Fig 7-64 A titanium-reinforced membrane is fixed with screws.

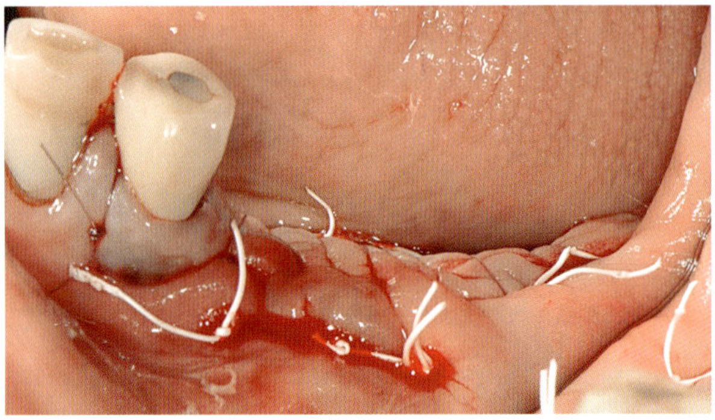

Fig 7-65 Suturing technique.

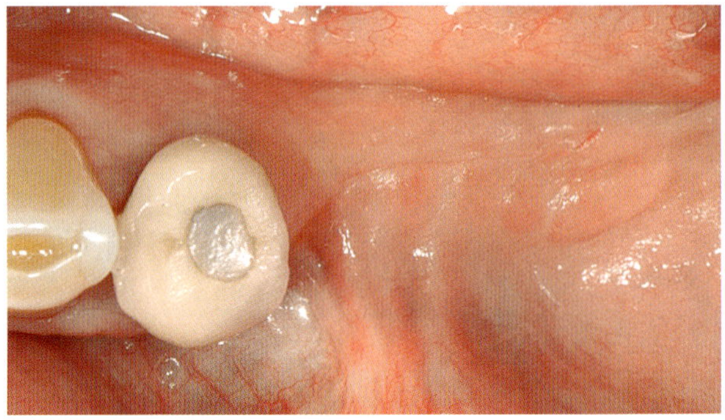

Fig 7-66 Occlusal soft tissue healing after 6 months.

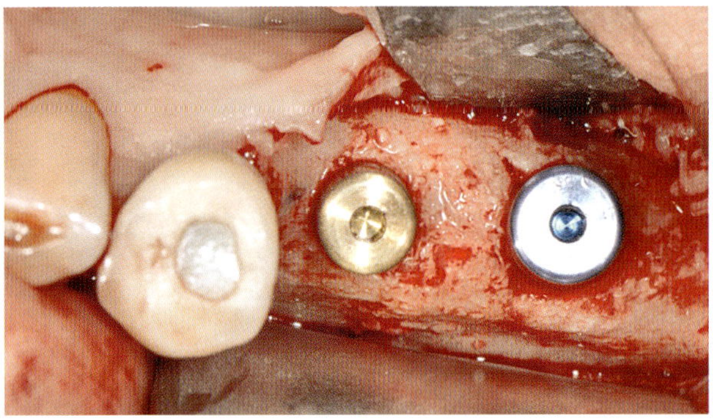

Fig 7-67 Occlusal view of the implants placed.

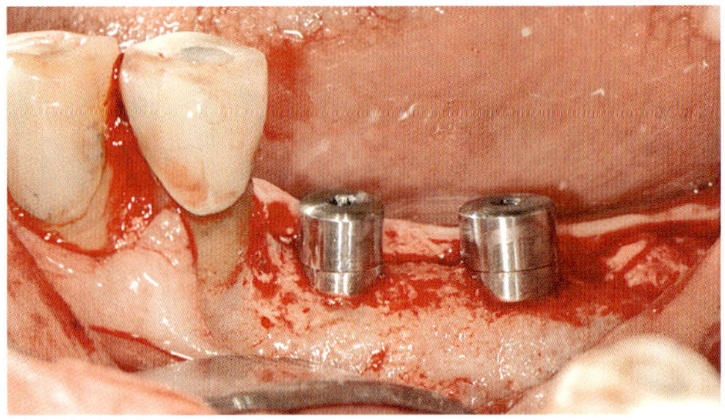

Fig 7-68 Buccal view of the inserted implants.

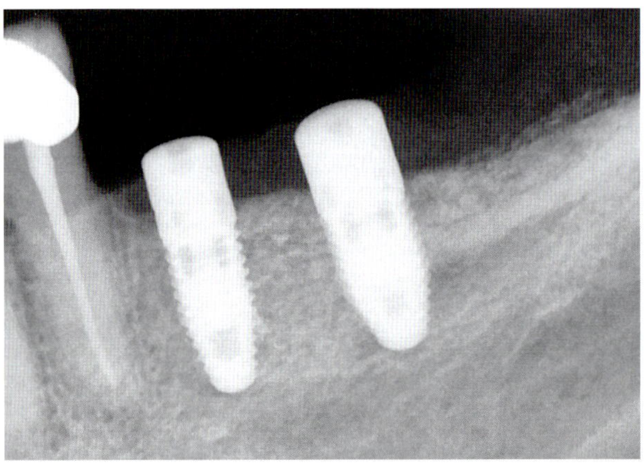

Fig 7-69 Final periapical radiograph.

keratinized tissue is normally lost. However, it can be compensated for at a later stage. The necessary healing period may vary from 6 to 9 months depending on the bone grafting materials used. In this case a xenograft and an autogenous graft were mixed in order to achieve earlier healing. Re-entry took place at seven months and both vertical and horizontal bone regeneration were achieved (Figs 7-67 and 7-68). The regenerated bone was sufficiently hard to achieve primary stability of the implants (Fig 7-69).

7.7 Conclusions

- Regeneration of 3-wall contained horizontal defects is very predictable.
- Bone width gain might be higher with a non-resorbable membrane but chances of complications are also higher.
- The regeneration of dehiscences, fenestrations, and 4-wall defects is very predictable because of the huge amount of vascularity present.

- Double buccal flap technique allows advancing the buccal flap easily and achieving primary closure yet causes a lot of swelling to the patient.
- Releasing incisions in the periosteum may achieve the same primary closure with less swelling.
- Differentiation of mesenchymal cells occurs approximately 6 weeks after GBR,[37] so this is the minimum time suggested for the non-resorbable membrane to remain under the gingiva.
- Vertical defects are the most challenging to regenerate.
- "V"-shaped defects would regenerate better than wide "U"-shaped defects or flat defects because of the amount and proximity of blood supply to the grafting material.

References

1. Gottlow J, Nyman S, Lindhe J, Karring T, Wennström J. New attachment formation in the human periodontium by guided tissue regeneration. Case reports. J Clin Periodontol 1986;13:604-616.
2. Stahl SS, Froum S. Histologic healing responses in human vertical lesions following the use of osseous allografts and barrier membranes. J Clin Periodontol 1991;18:149-152.
3. Dahlin C, Linde A, Gottlow J, Nyman S. Healing of bone defects by guided tissue regeneration. Plast Reconstr Surg 1988;81:672-676.
4. Hammerle CH, Schmid J, Lang NP, Olah AJ. Temporal dynamics of healing in rabbit cranial defects using guided bone regeneration. J Oral Maxillofac Surg 1995;53:167-174.
5. Retzepi M, Donos N. Guided Bone Regeneration: biological principle and therapeutic applications. Clin Oral Implants Res 2010;21:567-576.
6. Urban IA, Jovanovic SA, Lozada JL. Vertical ridge augmentation using guided bone regeneration (GBR) in three clinical scenarios prior to implant placement: a retrospective study of 35 patients 12 to 72 months after loading Int J Oral Maxillofac Implants 2009;24:502-510.
7. Buser D, Dula K, Belser U, Hirt HP, Berthold H. Localized ridge augmentation using guided bone regeneration. 1. Surgical procedures in the maxilla. Int J Periodontics Restorative Dent 1993;13:29-45.
8. Barboza EP, Stutz B, Ferreira VF, Carvalho W. Guided bone regeneration using nonexpanded polytetrafluoroethylene membranes in preparation for dental implant placements: a report of 420 cases. Implant Dent 2010;19:2-7.
9. Rocchietta I, Fontana F, Simion M. Clinical outcomes of vertical bone augmentation to enable dental implant placement: a systematic review. J Clin Periodontol 2008;35(Suppl 8):203-215.
10. Hutmacher D, Hürzeler MB. Biologisch abbaubare Polymere und Membranen für die gesteurte Gewebe- und Knochenregeneration. Implantologie 1995;1:21-37.
11. von Arx T, Broggini N, Jensen SS, Bornstein MM, Schenk RK, Buser D. Membrane durability and tissue response of different bioresorbable barrier membranes: a histologic study in the rabbit calvarium. Int J Oral Maxillofac Implants 2005;20:843-853.
12. Simion M, Maglione M, Iamoni F, Scarano A, Piattelli A, Salvato A. Bacterial penetration through Resolut resorbable membrane in vitro. An histological and scanning electron microscopic study. Clin Oral Implants Res 1997;8:23-31.
13. Hürzeler M, Thalmair T, von Mohrenschildt S, Fickl S. Double-layer technique for alveolar ridge augmentation: a case presentation. Pract Proced Aesthet Dent 2009;21:185-191.
14. Tal H, Kozlovsky A, Artzi Z, Nemcovsky CE, Moses O. Cross-linked and non-cross-linked collagen barrier membranes disintegrate following surgical exposure to the oral environment: a histological study in the cat. Clin Oral Implants Res 2008;19:760-766.
15. Oh TJ, Meraw SJ, Lee EJ, Giannobile WV, Wang HL. Comparative analysis of collagen membranes for the treatment of implant dehiscence defects. Clin Oral Implants Res 2003;14:80-90.
16. Zitzmann NU, Schärer P, Marinello CP. Long-term results of implants treated with guided bone regeneration: a 5-year prospective study. Int J Oral Maxillofac Surg 2001;16:355-366.
17. Christensen DK, Karoussis IK, Joss A, Hammerle CH, Lang NP. Simultaneous or staged installation with guided bone augmentation of transmucosal titanium implants. A 3-year prospective cohort study. Clin Oral Implants Res 2003;14:680-686.
18. Buser D, Dahlin C, Schenk RK. Bone grafts and bone substitute materials. In: Guided Bone Regeneration in Implant Dentistry, 2nd edn. Chicago: Quintessence Publishing, 2009:71-96.
19. Albreksson T, Johansson C. Osteoinduction, osteoconduction and osseointegration. Eur Spine J 2001;10:S96-101.
20. Berube P, Yang Y, Carnes DL, Stover RE, Boland EJ, Ong JL. The effect of sputtered calcium phosphate coatings of different crystallinity on osteoblast differentiation. J Periodontol 2005;76:1697-1709.
21. De Marco AC, Jardini MA, Lima LP. Revascularization of autogenous block grafts with or without an e-PTFE membrane. Int J Oral Maxillofac Implants 2005;20:867-874.
22. Antoun H, Sitbon JM, Martinez H, Missika P. A prospective randomized study comparing two techniques of bone augmentation: onlay graft alone or associated with a membrane. Clin Oral Implants Research 2001;12:632-639.
23. Jensen SS, Bornstein MM, Dard M, Bosshardt D, Buser D. Comparative study of biphasic calcium phosphates with different HA/TCP ratios in mandibular bone defects. A long-term histomorphometric study in minipigs. J Biomed Mater Res B Appl Biomater 2009;90B:171-181.
24. Jensen SS, Broggini N, Hjortinq-Hansen E, Schenk R, Buser D. Bone healing and graft resorption of autograft, anorganic bovine bone and ß-tricalcium phosphate. A histologic and histomorphometric study in the mandibles of minipigs. Clin Oral Implants Res 2006;17:237-243.
25. Johansson B, Grepe A, Wannfors K, Hirsch JM. A clinical study of changes in the volume of bone grafts in the atrophic maxilla. Dentomaxillofac Radiol 2001;30:157-161.
26. Urist MR. Bone: Formation by autoinduction. Science 1965;150:893-899.
27. Pacaccio DJ, Stern SF. Demineralized bone matrix: basic science and clinical applications. Clin Podiatr Med Surg 2005;22:599-606.
28. Boyan BD, Ranly DM, Schwartz Z. Use of growth factors to modify osteoinductivity of demineralized bone allografts: lessons for tissue engineering of bone. Dent Clin North Am 2006;50:217-228, viii.
29. Noumbissi SS, Lozada JL, Boyne PJ, Rohrer MD, Clem D, Kim JS, Prasad H. Clinical, histologic, and histomorphometric evaluation of mineralized solvent-dehydrated bone allograf (Puros) in human maxillary sinus grafts. J Oral Implantol 2005;31:171-179.
30. Mordenfeld A, Hallman M, Johansson CB, Albrektsson T. Histological and histomorphometrical analyses of biopsies harvested 11 years after maxillary sinus floor augmentation with deproteinized bovine and autogenous bone. Clin Oral Implants Res 2010;21:961-970.
31. Tonetti MS, Hammerle CHF. Advances in bone augmentation to enable dental implant placement: Consensus Report of the Sixth European Workshop on Periodontology. J Clin Periodontol 2008;35(Suppl 8):168-172.

32. Stahl SS, Froum S. Histological evaluation of human intraosseous healing responses to the placement of tricalcium phosphate ceramic implants. I. Three to eight months. J Periodontoln 1986;57:211-217.
33. Shepard WK, Bohat O, Joseph CE, LoPiccolo P, Bernick S. Human clinical and histological responses to a Calcitite implant in intraosseous lesions. Int J Periodontics Restorative Dent 1986;6:46-63.
34. Buser D, Dula K, Belser UC, Hirt HP, Berthold H. Localized ridge augmentation using guided bone regeneration. II. Surgical procedure in the mandible. Int J Periodontics Restorative Dent 1995;15:10-29.
35. Greenstein G, Greenstein B, Cavallaro J, Tarnow D. The role of bone decortication in enhancing the results of guided bone regeneration: a literature review. J Periodontol 2009;80:175-189.
36. Verdugo F, D'Addona A, Pontón J. Clinical, tomographic, and histological assessment of periosteal guided bone regeneration with cortical perforations in advanced human critical size defects. Clin Implant Dent Relat Res 2012;14:112-120.
37. El-Fayomi S, El-Shahat A, Omara M, Safe Ikram. Healing of bone defects by guided bone regeneration (GBR): an experimental study. Egypt J Plast Reconstr Surg 2003;27:159-166.
38. Blanes RJ. To what extent does the crown-implant ratio affect the survival and complications of implant-supported reconstructions? A systematic review. Clin Oral Implants Res 2009;20(Suppl 4): 67-72.

Chapter 8

Biomaterials: which to use and when?

Anna Mañes Medina, Elvira Ferres Amat, Eduard Ferres Padró

8.1 Introduction

In a significant proportion of cases, bone availability is insufficient to allow implant placement. One solution is to collect the patient's bone from a different location (autogenous) and graft the area to augment. Even today this is one of the most commonly used procedures. However, it is time consuming, technique sensitive, and requires extra training. It may also cause morbidity, which can lead to poor patient acceptance when this technique is used.

Interestingly, the availability of different biomaterials from different sources has increased the acceptance of advanced surgical treatments previously refused. The limitation of the quantity of bone available from the donor site has also been overcome, since biomaterials can be almost limitless.

These materials have been subjected to countless animal and human studies that have proved the efficacy, biocompatibility, and other properties suitable for the regeneration of lost hard and soft tissue. An enormous choice of biomaterials has burst onto the market making it difficult for the practitioner to decide on the best and most appropriate for the procedure being performed.

This chapter explains the available biomaterials and their properties, to aid selection of the most appropriate. This includes clinical examples, where the use of one type of biomaterial may have advantages over others.

8.2 Background

In the body two types of processes may be carried out in those cases with loss of tissue substance: regeneration and reparation. It is known as regeneration when the new tissue has the same properties and characteristics as the previous tissue. By contrast, in reparation the newly formed tissue can have altered functions or morphology when compared with the primary tissue, a situation that is more commonly known as healing. It often involves a reduction in the volume of damaged tissue secondary to its contraction, and an increased collagen deposition. Some tissues have the ability to regenerate spontaneously, especially in the embryonic stage. Achieving a controlled regeneration in adults is the main goal of biomaterials. To achieve this, the mechanisms responsible for the repairing and regeneration processes should be understood.[1,2]

Biomaterials have been developed due to the need to regenerate bone defects in different anatomical regions. In the oral cavity, these defects may have been caused by various reasons, including trauma, atrophy by tooth loss, or resection of tumors or cysts. Traditionally the type of graft used was autologous bone. The main objective of biomaterials is to allow regeneration of these defects, reducing morbidity in the patient.

Ridge augmentation procedures using autogenous bone from both intraoral and extraoral regions have provided favorable results. However, the availability (in intraoral grafts), the need for hospitalization, and the high morbidity (for extraoral grafts) are factors that are disadvantageous to the use of this kind of graft.[3-5] Autologous bone has several properties that are imitated by the biomaterials: osteoconduction, osteogenesis, and osteoinduction, with varying success depending on the biomaterial. The main objective in the use of biomaterials in the orofacial area will be to restore the normal contour and function of bone tissue.

In the bone tissue a permanent cycle of remodeling, consisting of apposition and resorption phenomena, is produced. There are certain factors that can affect the turnover between formation and resorption, inducing alterations that can lead both to the emergence of bony exostoses and to decreased bone volume and density. Under normal conditions both processes are in balance. For this reason, the bone mass of a healthy adult should not be altered. The remodeling process has several stages, the first of which is a migration of osteoblasts and a replacement by osteoclasts. These cells will join the bone, starting the reabsorption process, after which the cells will be released. In the resorption zones, osteoclasts will form Howship's lacunae. In these areas, bone apposition by osteoblasts takes place.[2]

Among the techniques that can be performed with biomaterials, we find ridge augmentation techniques for allowing implant placement, regeneration of periodontal defects, peri-implant defect treatment, and treatment of pathological processes associated with implants (peri-implantitis) (Fig 8-1).

In order to establish the best choice of biomaterial depending on the treatment, the following topics will be discussed in this chapter.

- 8.3 Which biomaterials are available according to their proprieties?
- 8.4 Which biomaterial should be used?
  - 8.4.1 Sinus lift
  - 8.4.2 Horizontal regenerations and crestal split
- 8.5 In which situations may biomaterials be used for vertical regeneration in the mandible?
  - 8.5.1 Onlay
  - 8.5.2 Inlay
  - 8.5.3 Guided bone regeneration (GBR)
  - 8.5.4 Socket preservation
  - 8.5.5 Peri-implantitis
- 8.6 Conclusions

Table 8-1 Classification of bone substitutes

Bone substitute	Types available
Xenografts	Hydroxyapatite
	Bovine hydroxyapatite
	Equine hydroxyapatite
	Porcine hydroxyapatite
	Coralline hydroxyapatite
Alloplastic materials	Beta tricalcium phosphate
	Hydroxyapatite with collagen
	Calcium sulfate
	Bioglass
Allografts	
Other materials	Collagen
	Synthetic polymers of polylactic acid and polyglycolic acid
Non-resorbable membranes	
Resorbable membranes	
Materials for soft tissue augmentation	

8.3 Which biomaterials are available according to their properties?

Research has led to the development of a variety of materials (Table 8-1). However, none of them has achieved the three conditions that enable bone regeneration under physiological conditions: osteogenesis, osteoinduction, and osteoconduction. Apart from these features, another important factor that a biomaterial must have is the ability to chemically bond to the surface of bone without an intervening layer of fibrous tissue, known as osseointegration.

According to the reaction that they induce in the native bone, biomaterials can be classified into three groups. The first corresponds to the osteoconductive materials, among which are included the main biomaterials used today, such as hydroxyapatite or tricalcium phosphate (Table 8-2). The second group consists of those materials that have the ability to induce bone formation through activation of different pathways involved in the processes of apposition and bone regeneration. Plasma rich in growth factors and bone morphogenetic proteins (BMPs) have been proposed among the materials that are able to activate osteoinduction, with varying degrees

Figs 8-1a to g Types of bone defect.

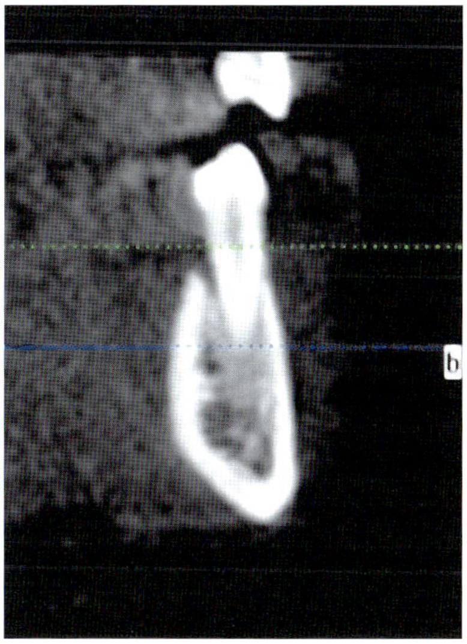

Fig 8-1a Periodontal defects: supra- or infraosseous; from one to three walls.

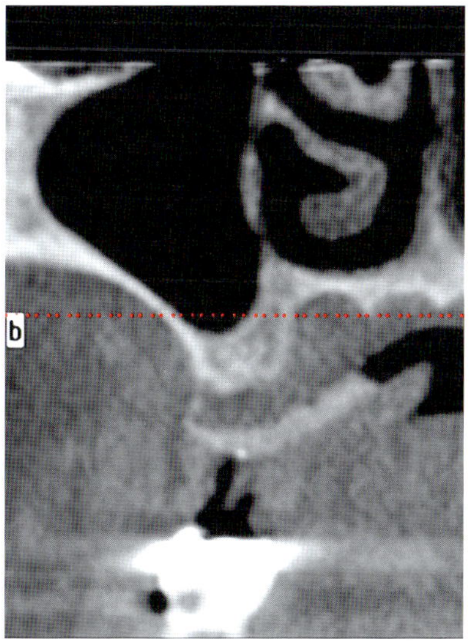

Fig 8-1b Maxillary sinus pneumatization.

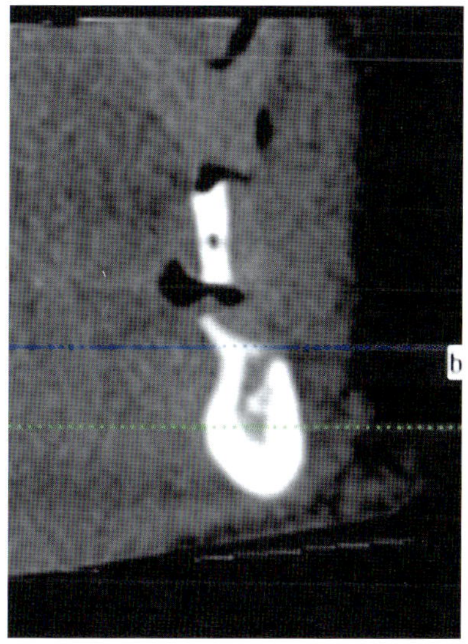

Fig 8-1c Insufficient bone height of the residual crest.

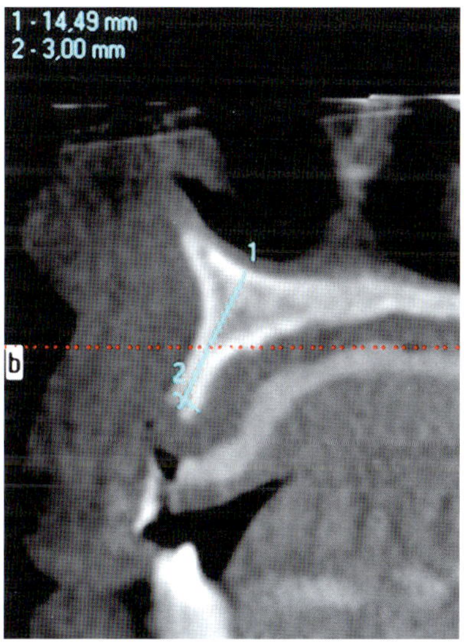

Fig 8-1d Insufficient bone width of the residual crest.

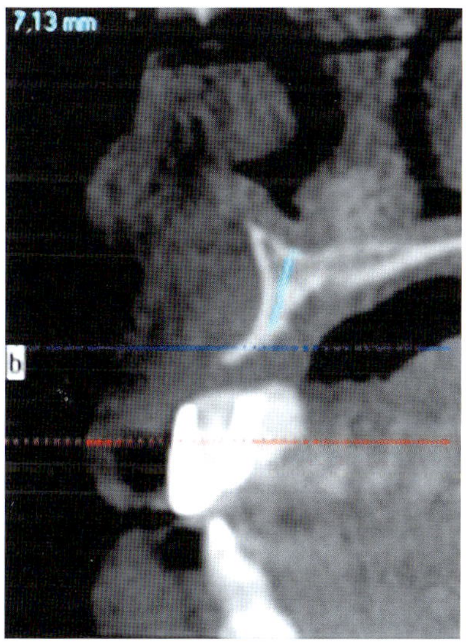

Fig 8-1e Insufficient bone height and width of the residual crest.

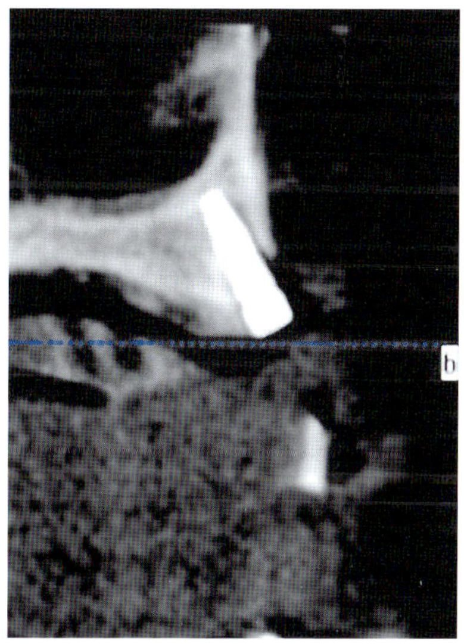

Fig 8-1f Peri-implant defects: dehiscences and fenestrations.

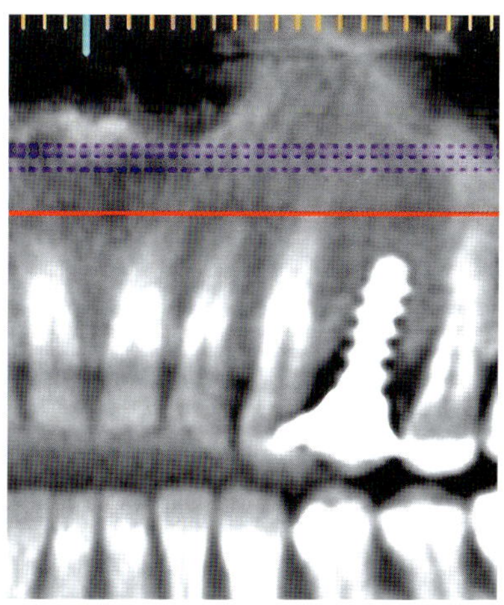

Fig 8-1g Pathological processes associated with implants (peri-implantitis).

Table 8-2 Types of bone substitutes according to their properties

	Types	Subtypes	Properties
Xenografts	Hydroxyapatite	Bovine hydroxyapatite	Osteoconduction
		Equine hydroxyapatite	Osteoconduction
		Porcine hydroxyapatite	Osteoconduction
		Coralline hydroxyapatite	Osteoconduction
Alloplastic materials		Beta tricalcium phosphate	Osteoconduction
		Hydroxyapatite with collagen	Osteoconduction
		Calcium sulfate	Osteoconduction
		Bioglass	Osteoconduction
Allografts			Osteoconduction
Other materials	Collagen		Osteoconduction
	Synthetic polymers	Polyglycolic acid	Osteoconduction
		Polylactic acid	Osteoconduction

of agreement in the scientific literature. The third group, and perhaps the most interesting at the present time, is composed of those materials capable of producing the process of osteogenesis directly. In this regard, research is paying special attention to stem cells for tissue repair, with the long-term goal of achieving complete organ reproduction in a controlled laboratory environment. This field requires more research and development, since current technology is inadequate.[3]

8.4 Which biomaterial should be used?

8.4.1 Sinus lift

One of the great controversies in the world of biomaterials is the sinus lift procedure, one of the most widely used bone grafting treatments. The type of graft needed to carry out this treatment has been discussed many times: biomaterial, autologous graft, or a combination of both?

Among the most studied biomaterials in sinus lift is hydroxyapatite, alone or in combination with autologous bone. Several authors have demonstrated similar implant survival rates, regardless of the filler material grafted and proportions when combined with autogenous bone. Likewise, the survival rate is similar to implants placed in non-grafted areas.[6]

The use of biomaterials when remaining autologous bone is present is recommendable. Otherwise combinations can be performed with particulate autologous bone, which will reduce the total healing time of the graft. A healing time of around 4 months for sinus elevations made with 100% autologous bone is also advised, while for xenografts it is preferable to wait between 6 and 9 months.

The use of resorbable membranes in the lateral sinus wall is recommended to prevent ingrowth of connective tissue inside the regenerated sinus. In the systematic review by Wallace and Froum[7] a higher survival rate of implants placed in sinus where the lateral window had been covered by membranes was found. However, in Nkenke and Stelzle[8] no differences in the use or non-use of membranes were reported.

In implants placed in regenerated sinus, more time is needed before prosthetic loading of the implant to allow graft consolidation. Depending on the previous residual bone, the sinus pneumatization and the grafting material, a time ranging between 4 and 9 months is needed (see Case 1).

8.4.2 Horizontal regeneration and crestal split

There are several options for horizontal bony defect correction (Table 8-3). These include GBR, autologous bone blocks, or crestal split.[9] GBR for the treatment of localized jaw bone defects is well documented. GBR procedures can be used with simultaneous or staged approaches. The implant survival rate of implants placed in these regenerated areas is similar to those placed in pristine bone.[10] Several graft types are used in GBR:

Table 8-3 Horizontal reconstructions

	Resorbable membrane	Non resorbable membrane	Bone gain	Advantages	Disadvantages
Block allografts	Recommended	Not recommended	4-5 mm	Lack of morbidity Good stability Similar gain that with autologous bone.	Cost Steep learning curve to allow primary closure Lack of studies
Autologous bone blocks combined with biomaterials	Recommended	Not recommended	4-5 mm	Predictable results Less costly than block allografts High gain values	Steep learning curve to extract, adapt the grafts, and allow primary closure.
GBR	Necessary	Not recommended, similar results and less complications with resorbable membranes	3 mm	Well documented techniques	Technically sensitive Less bone gain Not for extensive reconstructions
Crestal split	Recommended	Not necessary	3–5 mm	Predictable results in maxilla Creation of contained defect (well regeneration of the gap)	Steep learning curve, especially in mandible (less recommended) Need to stage implant placement if primary stability is not allowed or the position is not correct

autogenous bone, xenografts, allografts, or alloplastic materials. The need for a good graft resorption rate, the availability of the intraoral grafts, and the future rehabilitation will determine the choice.

Bone blocks

One technique used for horizontal reconstruction is regeneration with bone allografts. Wallace and Gellin[11] reported a gain of 4.6 mm when cancellous block allografts were used. They were covered with a cross-linked collagen resorbable membrane and adapted with particulate bone. The healing time was 5 months before implant placement and 4 months before prosthetic loading. An implant success rate of a 100% was obtained.

Particulate bone with membrane

The classic technique of GBR is with particulate bone and a resorbable or non-resorbable membrane (Fig 8-2). The main problem is membrane exposure (in non-resorbable membranes), the lack of mechanical properties of the resorbable membranes, and less bone gain than with autologous bone blocks.

In moderate defects, particulate xenografts with a resorbable membrane can be used. Three millimeters of bone gain is expected with this treatment, not differing from the use of non-resorbable membranes (see Case 2).[12]

Crestal split

The goal of the lateral ridge expansion technique is to increase the total amount of available bone, creating a new bed by longitudinal osteotomy of alveolar bone thanks to a green stick fracture which displaces the buccal cortical bone. The created gap can be filled with autologous bone or biomaterials (Figs 8-3 and 8-4).[9] This technique is especially recommended in the maxilla, when insufficient bone width is found but the cortical plates are not yet fused. In the mandible this technique should be performed carefully due to the high risk of cortical bone fracture and the high possibility of bad fractures. The implants may be placed if primary stability can be achieved. Several factors should also be considered, like the learning curve of the surgeon, the esthetic component of the implant, and the proper amount of soft tissue.

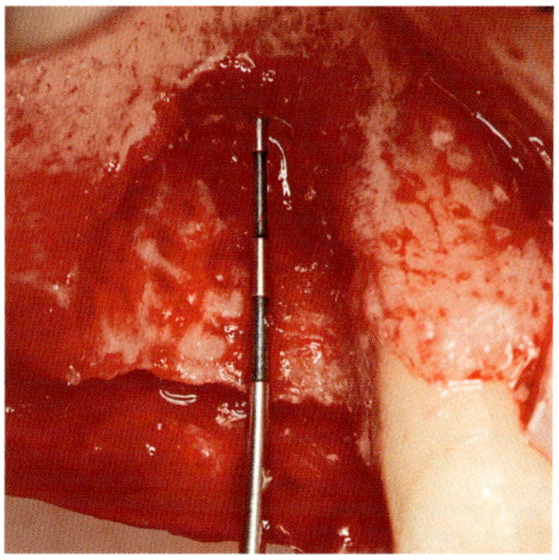

Figs 8-2a Horizontal defect after tooth extraction.

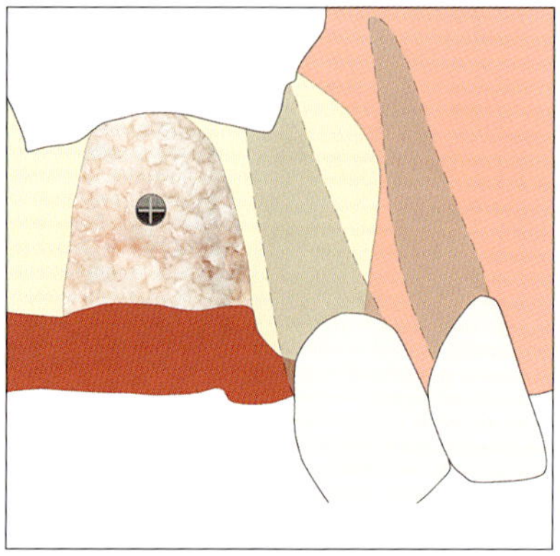

Fig 8-2b Regeneration with Bio-Oss® (Geistlich, Wolhusen, Switzerland).

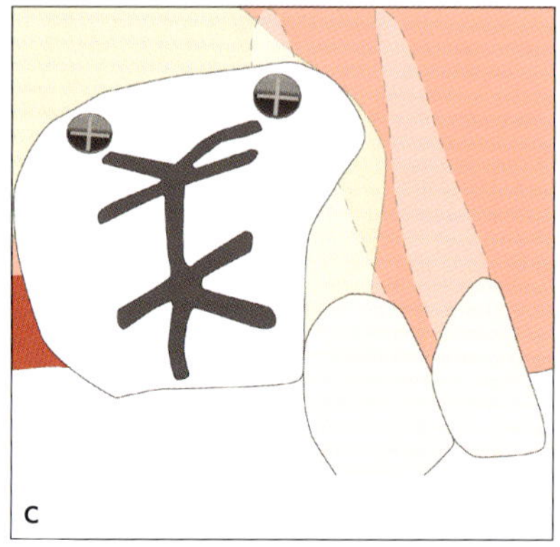

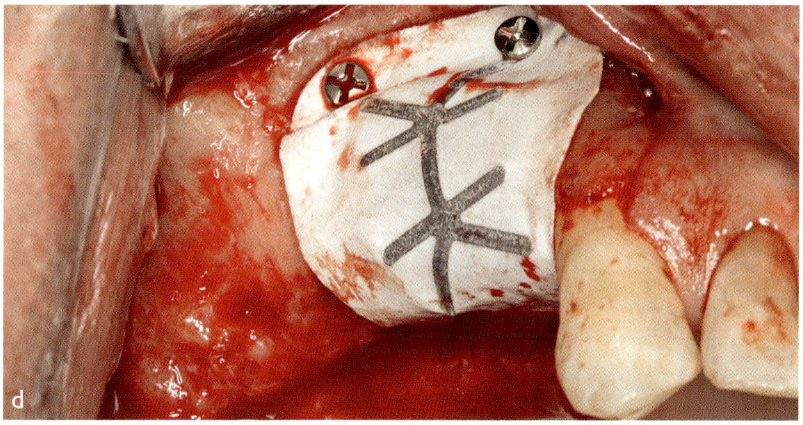

Figs 8-2c and d Non-resorbable membrane of Gore-Tex® reinforced with titanium.

Figs 8-3a to d Sequence of crestal split.

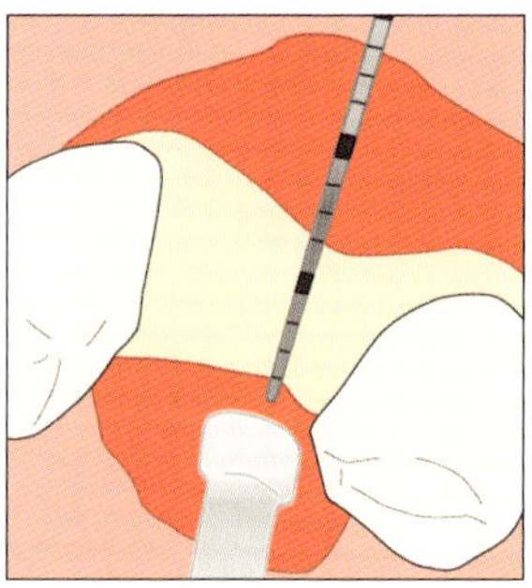

Fig 8-3a Pristine bone.

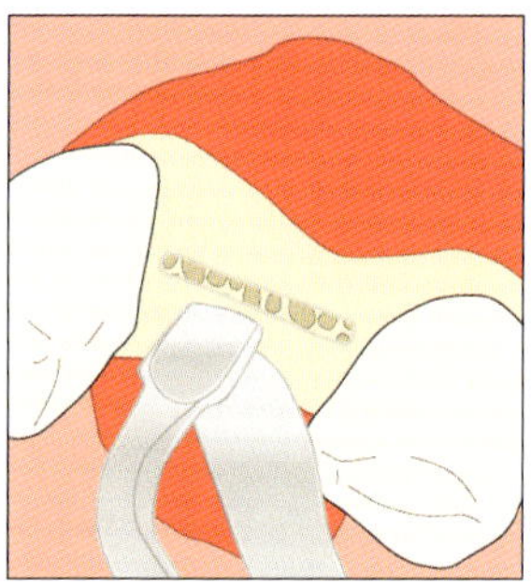

Fig 8-3b Ostectomy done with a piezoelectric device or fissure burn.

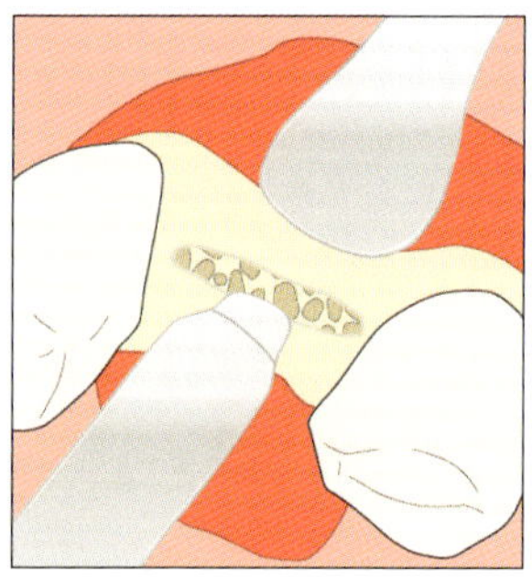

Fig 8-3c Bone fracture and separation with a chisel.

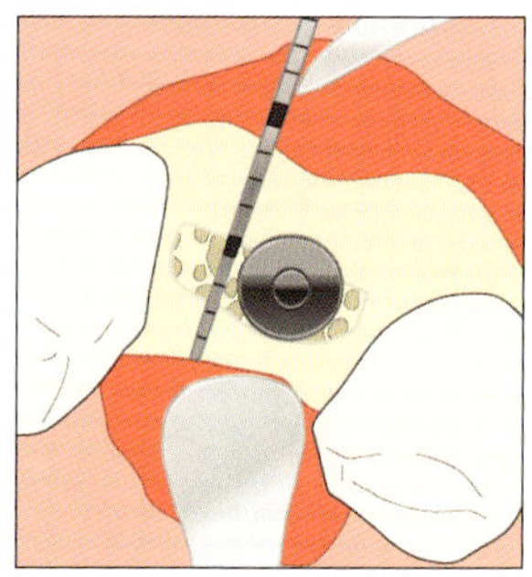

Fig 8-3d Total horizontal gain after implant placement.

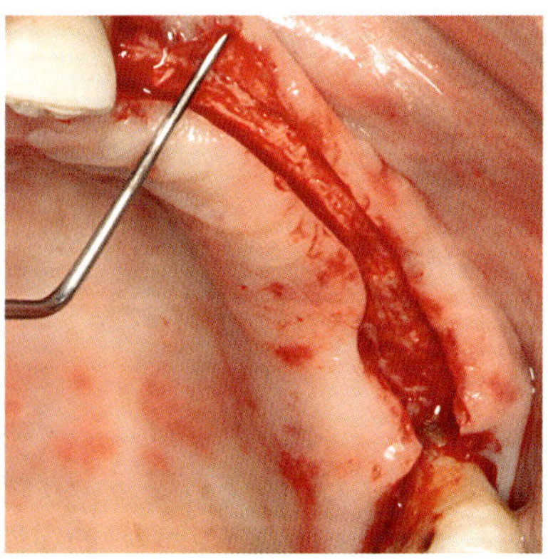

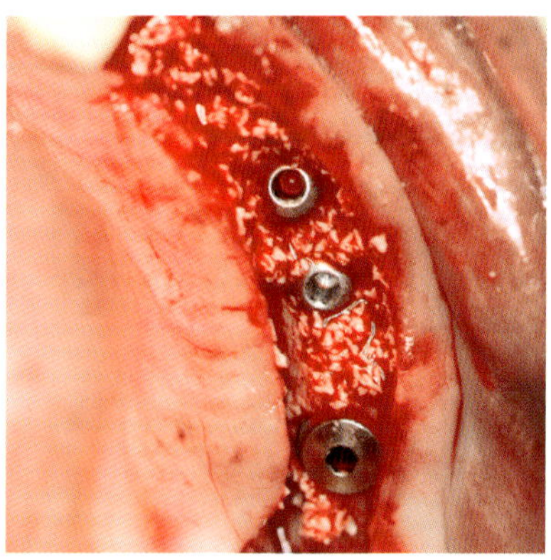

Fig 8-4a (left) Crestal split with immediate implant placement.

Fig 8-4b (right) The gap was filled with bovine hydroxyapatite.

8.5 In which situations may biomaterials be used for vertical regeneration in the mandible?

There are several situations where standard implant placement is not possible. In many of these cases short implants can be placed with high success rates, but when the distance to the inferior alveolar nerve is less than 7 mm a vertical bone augmentation should be considered (Table 8-4).

8.5.1 Onlay

Onlay bone graft was the first procedure to be used in the correction of vertical atrophies. It is a well documented procedure according to the follow-up of implants placed in the reconstructed areas, but due to the lack of homogeneity the comparison of results is difficult.

The use of biomaterials with onlay bone graft is recommended to reduce the gap between the recipient bed and the graft, permitting a better adaptation between them.

A resorbable membrane should be placed over the reconstruction to reduce the infiltration of connective tissue (see Case 3).

Some studies in animals have evaluated vertical augmentation with equine blocks and recombinant human platelet-derived growth factor-BB (rhPDGF-BB). The results show a vertical gain with dense, well-vascularized bone, and that was greater when non-resorbable membrane was placed over the grafts. More studies are needed to follow this line of investigation.[13]

8.5.2 Inlay

When the bone fragment is displaced coronally, the created gap needs to be filled with something that impedes the proliferation of soft tissue between the two parts of the bone and maintains the volume. Several materials such as particulate hydroxyapatite or blocks of the same material have been used. Again it s preferable to place a resorbable membrane on the vestibular wall, and in the lingual one if needed, to contain the particulate bone. Six months, approximately, of healing time are required before implant placement (see Case 3).

8.5.3 GBR

Several techniques have been proposed to allow vertical reconstruction of the atrophic ridges. The main problem that needs to be solved is the need for mechanical support to impede the collapse, by gravity or by chewing

Table 8-4 Vertical augmentation treatments

Treatment	Situation A	Situation B	Use of barriers
Sinus lift	Very pneumatized sinus: hydroxyapatite in combination with autologous bone	Sinus with residual autologous bone: hydroxyapatite	Recommended in both cases
3 wall defects	To maintain volume: hydroxyapatite + membrane	To regenerate the defect to allow implant placement: autologous bone in combination with biomaterials	Recommended in both cases
Horizontal regeneration	For esthetic reasons: hydroxyapatite	To allow implant placement: autologous bone or mixture to reduce the treatment time	Recommended in both cases
Crestal split	Use of hydroxyapatite to maintain the space. Delayed implants.	Immediate implants with or without additional bone graft.	Recommended, especially if delayed implant placement
Vertical regeneration	GBR: biomaterials + reinforced membrane		Recommended
Bone blocks	Use of biomaterials to adapt the graft and to protect it from resorption		Recommended

Table 8-5 The choice of the biomaterial for socket preservation

Situation	Biomaterial characteristics	Type of biomaterial recommended
The restoration will have a fixed partial prosthesis (pontic) over the preserved area	Low resorption rate	Bovine hydroxyapatite
An implant will be placed on the regenerated area	Medium/fast resorption rate	DFDBA β–tricalcium sulfate
An extensive rehabilitation will be effectuated with a fixed prosthesis over implants, without implant placement over the regenerated area	Low resorption rate	Bovine hydroxyapatite
No treatment will be performed in the near future	Low resorption rate	Bovine hydroxyapatite

DFDBA, demineralized freeze-dried bone allograft

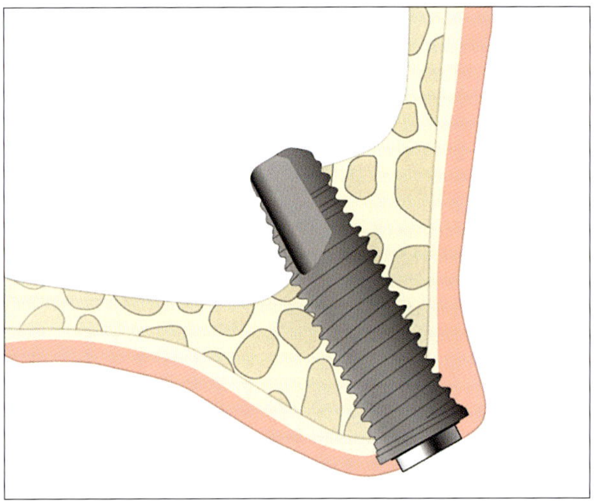

Fig 8-5 Peri-implant defect, dehiscenses, and fenestrations.

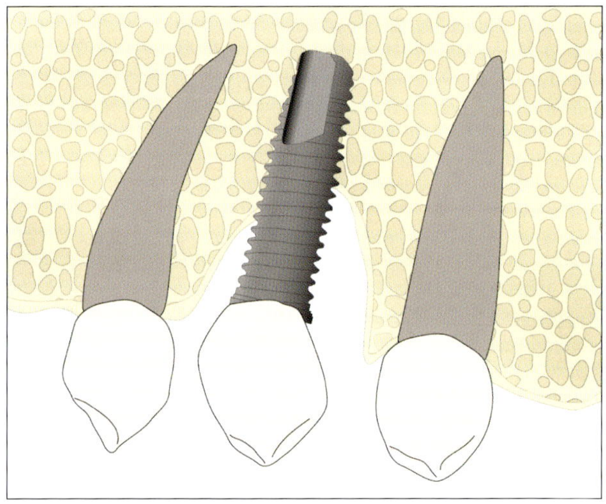

Fig 8-6 Pathological resorption of the bone (peri-implantitis).

forces, of the regenerated areas. This problem is partially solved with reinforced membranes. The problem that this type of barrier presents is the high incidence of exposure, which can compromise the results of the regeneration. The closure of the flap without tension is the other point that has to be considered, especially in areas that are difficult to reach (posterior mandibular areas).

8.5.4 Socket preservation

The choice of the biomaterial for socket preservation should be made according to the treatment option that will be applied in the area (Table 8-5). Different characteristics are desirable depending on the future rehabilitation option. Four situations can be found, as described in Table 8-5.

According to the situation, different treatment options with a faster or lower resorption rate will be needed. If no treatment is to be applied over the regenerated area, a biomaterial with a low resorption rate should be used to maintain the volume of the alveolar ridge. If an implant placement is going to be performed, a material with a faster resorption time is preferable, with the aim to reduce the total treatment time (see Case 2).

8.5.5 Peri-implantitis

Defect regeneration of peri-implant bone loss caused by peri-implantitis is commonly performed (Figs 8-5 to

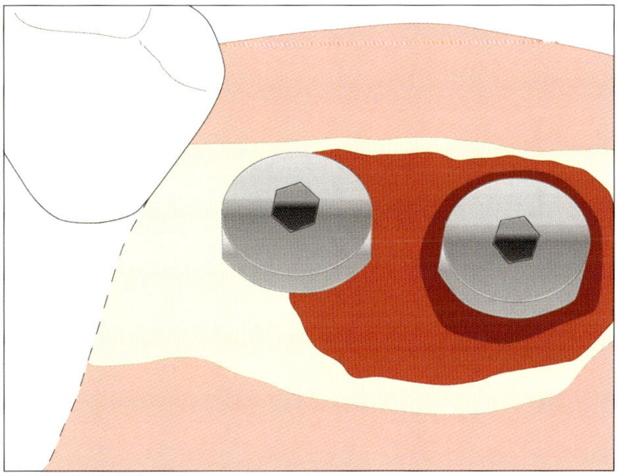

Fig 8-7a Bone defect that affects the distal implant and the distal aspect of the mesial implant.

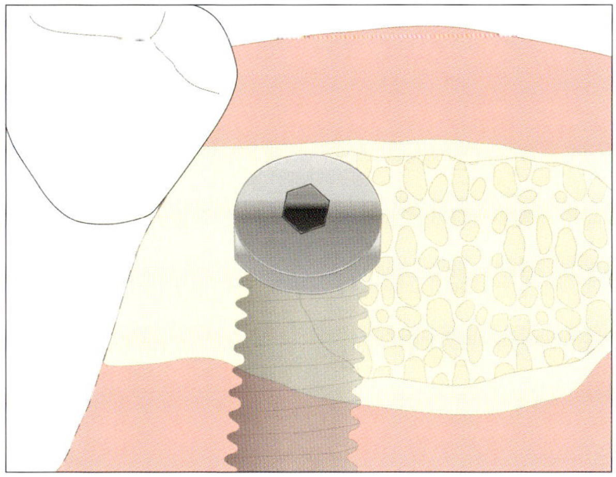

Fig 8-7b After curettage.

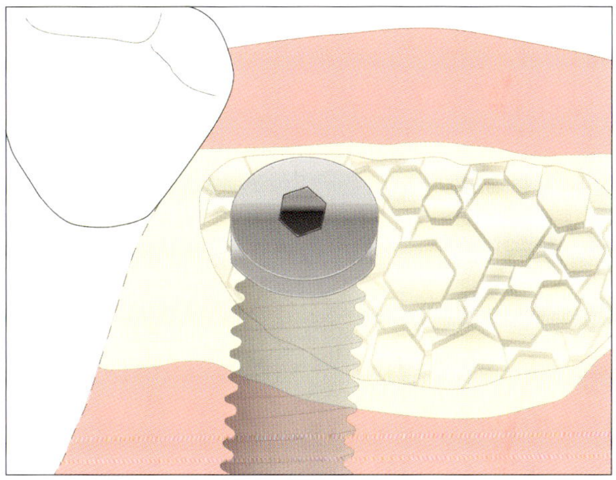

Fig 8-7c Regenerated defect.

8-7). It has been demonstrated that new ossification can be produced inside the defects. After establishment of good hygiene technique, a surgical phase can be planned. Several biomaterials are used to fill the pathological gap after implant surface decontamination, especially if the gap is greater than 5 mm. Of the desirable characteristics, a low resorption rate of the material is required. Several techniques have been used in peri-implant lesion treatment: resorbable/non-resorbable membranes with or without bone grafts. The rough or machined surface of the implants can influence the success of the regeneration. Although there is difficulty in decontaminating rough surfaces, good results in terms of bone regeneration are found in the literature.

The characteristics of the peri-implant defects (circumferential) are favorable in the regeneration of these lesions. When horizontal bone loss or craters with a narrow crestal opening are present, decontamination and regenerative therapy are more difficult.

Better results have been found in bone filling and re-osseointegration with GBR procedures when compared with surgical debridement and decontamination, especially when bone graft is combined with a membrane. When it is compared with guided tissue regeneration alone and bone graft material alone, the results from the studies are not homogenous in terms of the amount of bone filling.[14] No method resolves the peri-implant defect predictably.

8.6 Conclusions and prospects

- Current literature does not provide sufficient data to determine the best material for bone regeneration.
- There is no scientific evidence to support or refute the superiority of autologous bone graft over other materials in relation to the implant survival rate or complications associated with the grafted area.
- There are more reports of sinus lifts than other treatments, and it is considered a very predictable treatment. However, it is difficult to determine, with current data, which graft material is the most predictable.
- There is a large disparity in GBR. The studies are not homogenous and, again, it is difficult to establish what type of material is the most suitable, and to evaluate what kind of membrane achieves more regeneration of the defect. Likewise, there are few studies that report long-term stability of the bone level reached.[6,15] Also, the influence of regeneration in peri-implant tissues has not been fully studied.
- One of the main goals in the research on the use of biomaterials should be to improve knowledge about the behavior and cellular interactions with signals and markers, both external and internal, and how they can alter the biologic response in the host.[15] Also required are a greater number of multicenter, randomized, well-designed clinical studies, to determine the pros and cons of each material in each one of the possible clinical situations.

Membranes:
- Similar bone gain in horizontal reconstructions.
- If mechanical support is not needed, no advantages of non-resorbable membranes.

Horizontal augmentations:
- Predictable.
- Use of biomaterials in moderate defects.
- For larger defects: autologous bone blocks in combination with bio-materials and membranes.

Vertical defects:
- The most predictable treatment is sinus lift.
- Less predictability in posterior areas.
- Need for mechanical support, use of autologous bone blocks or inlays.

Peri-implantitis:
- The use of bone grafts with or without membranes improves bone filling and reduces probing depth.

Sinus lift:
- Similar survival rates of implants compared with non-grafted sites.
- No superiority of one biomaterial over another one or autologous bone grafting.
- Hydroxyapatite is the most studied biomaterial.

8.7 Clinical cases

Case 1 (Figs 8-8 to 8-17)

A sinus lift was performed to allow implant placement in position 26, as shown on the initial panoramic radiograph (Fig 8-8). As there was sufficient bone remaining to allow primary stability, a simultaneous implant placement was performed in this patient.

The sinus lift (Figs 8-9 to 8-11) was grafted with bovine hydroxyapatite (Figs 8-12 and 8-13) and a resorbable membrane was placed inside the sinus (to cover a

Figs 8-8 to 8-17 Case 1

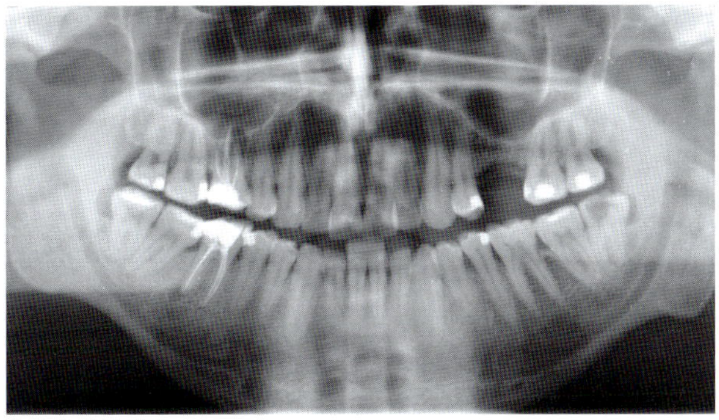

Fig 8-8 Initial panoramic radiograph.

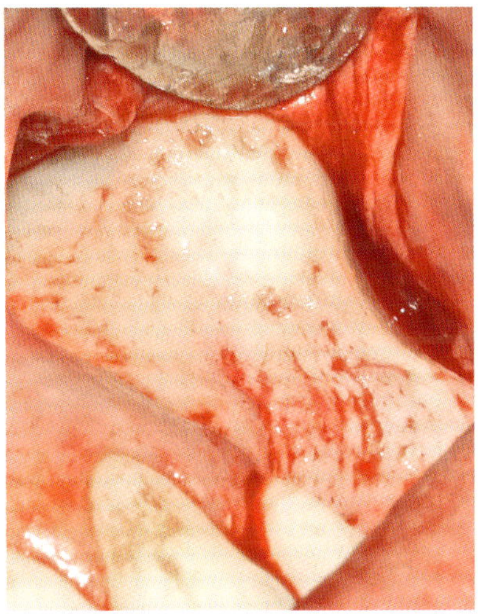

Fig 8-9 Window design.

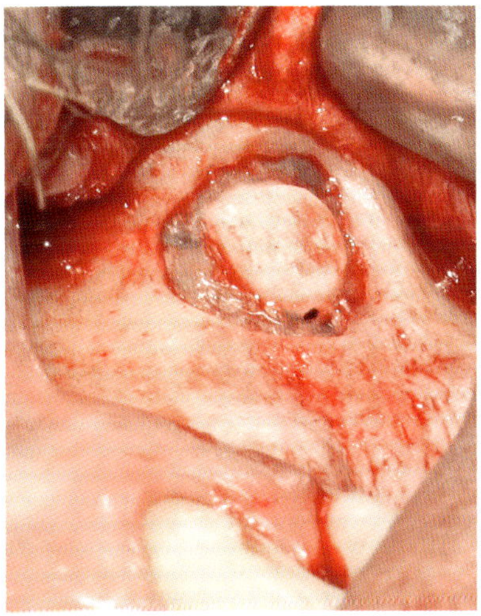

Fig 8-10 Ostectomy: a membrane perforation can be observed.

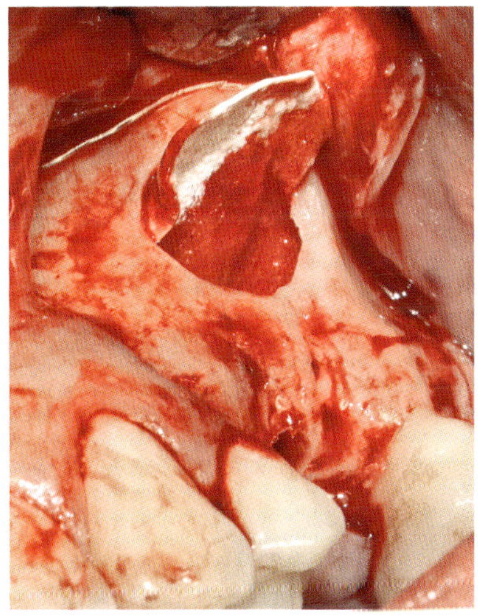

Fig 8-11 Elevation of the Schneiderian membrane. A collagen membrane was placed inside the sinus to cover the membrane perforation.

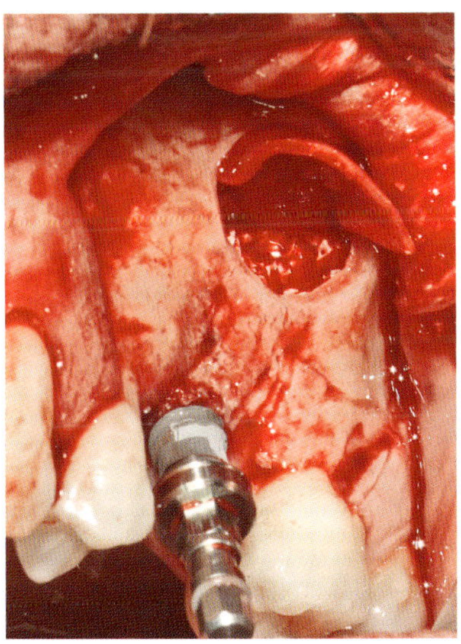

Fig 8-12 Implant placement.

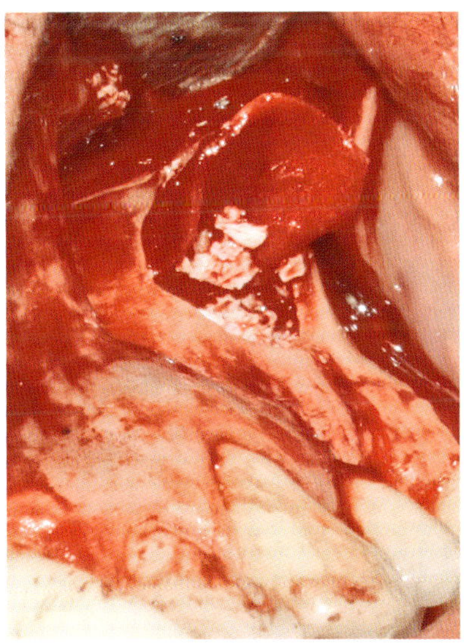

Fig 8-13 The sinus was filled with bovine hydroxyapatite.

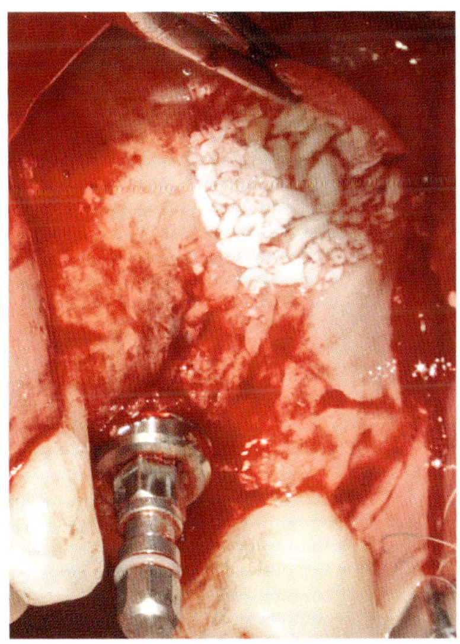

Fig 8-14 Coverage with the same collagen membrane.

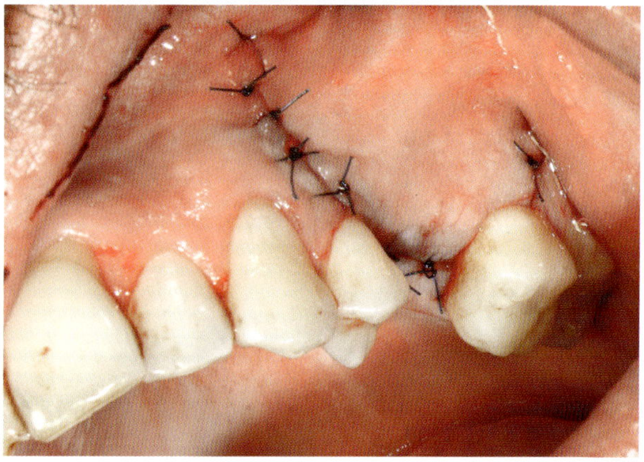

Fig 8-15 Suturing was performed.

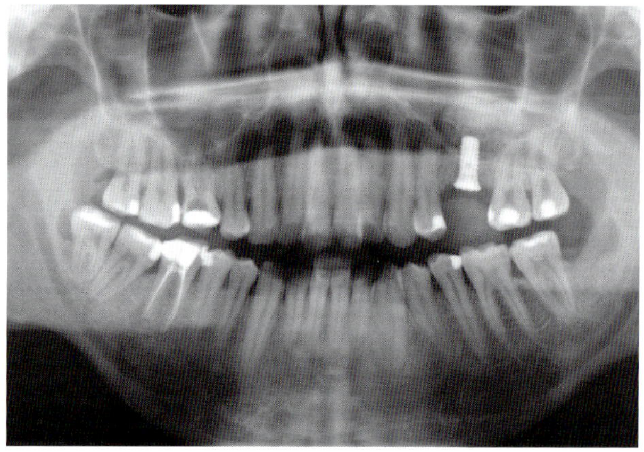

Fig 8-16 Final panoramic radiograph.

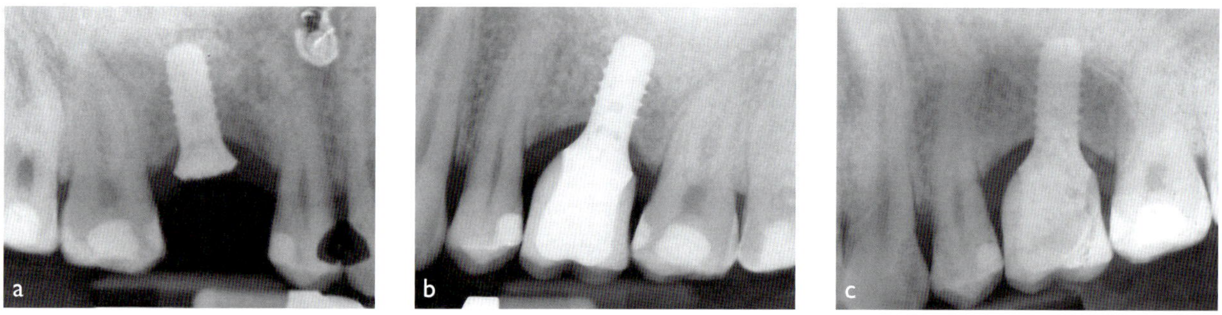

Figs 8-17a to c Periapical radiographs showing (a) the initial situation, (b) the final situation, and (c) 6 months after the restoration.

membrane perforation) as well as in the lateral wall (Figs 8-14 and 8-15).

Six months of healing was allowed before the start of the prosthetic rehabilitation.

The postoperative status is shown in the panoramic and periapical radiographs (Figs 8-16 and 8-17).

Case 2 (Figs 8-18 to 8-29)

The patient's preoperative status is shown in Figs 8-18 and 8-19. Socket preservation was performed on teeth 11 and 22. Simultaneous to implant placement a horizontal regeneration of the vestibular wall was performed to cover the fenestration and correct the bone concavity of the area. No membrane was placed over the alveolar preservation (with β-tricalcium phosphate; Fig 8-20), and a collagen resorbable membrane was placed to cover the horizontal regeneration done with hydroxyapatite (Fig 8-23).

Six months of healing was allowed after each surgery (Fig 8-24). The final situation is shown in Figs 8-26 to 8-29.

Figs 8-18 to 8-29 Case 2

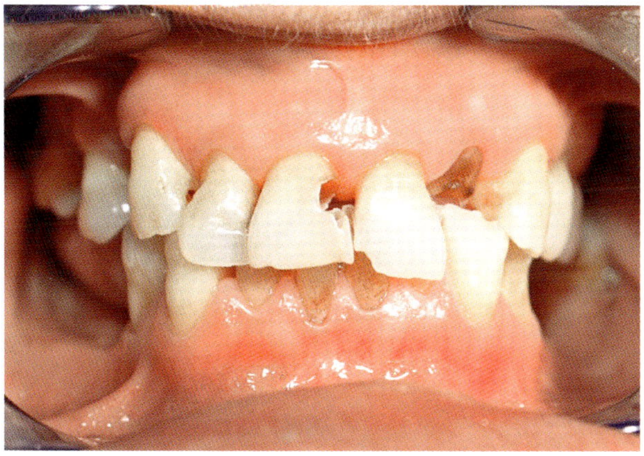

Fig 8-18 Preoperative situation.

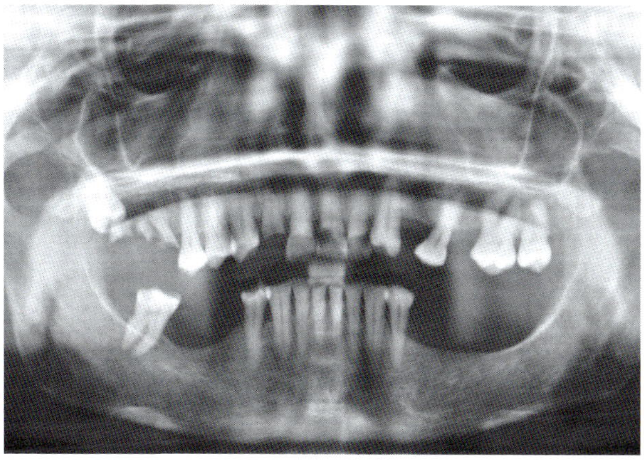

Fig 8-19 Initial panoramic radiograph.

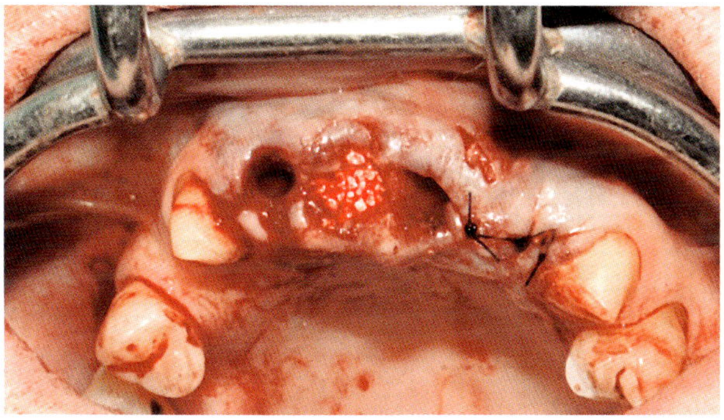

Fig 8-20 Tooth extraction and alveolar preservation with tricalcium phosphate.

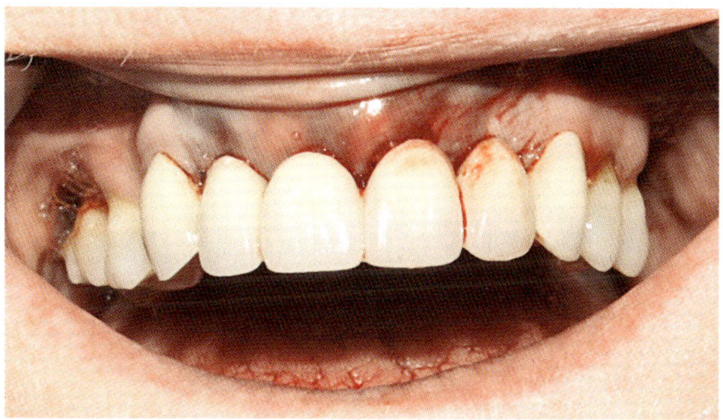

Fig 8-21 Placement of the provisional restoration.

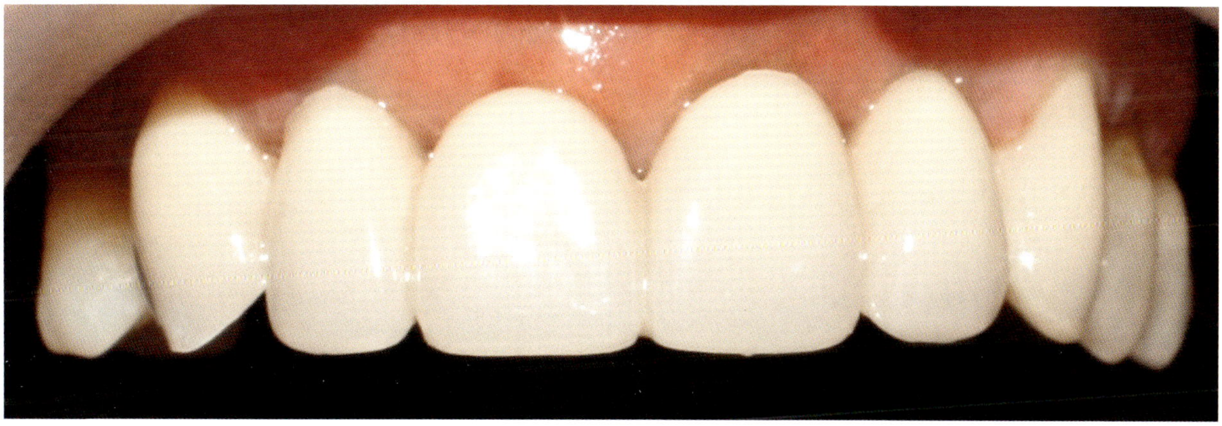

Fig 8-22 Provisional restoration after one week.

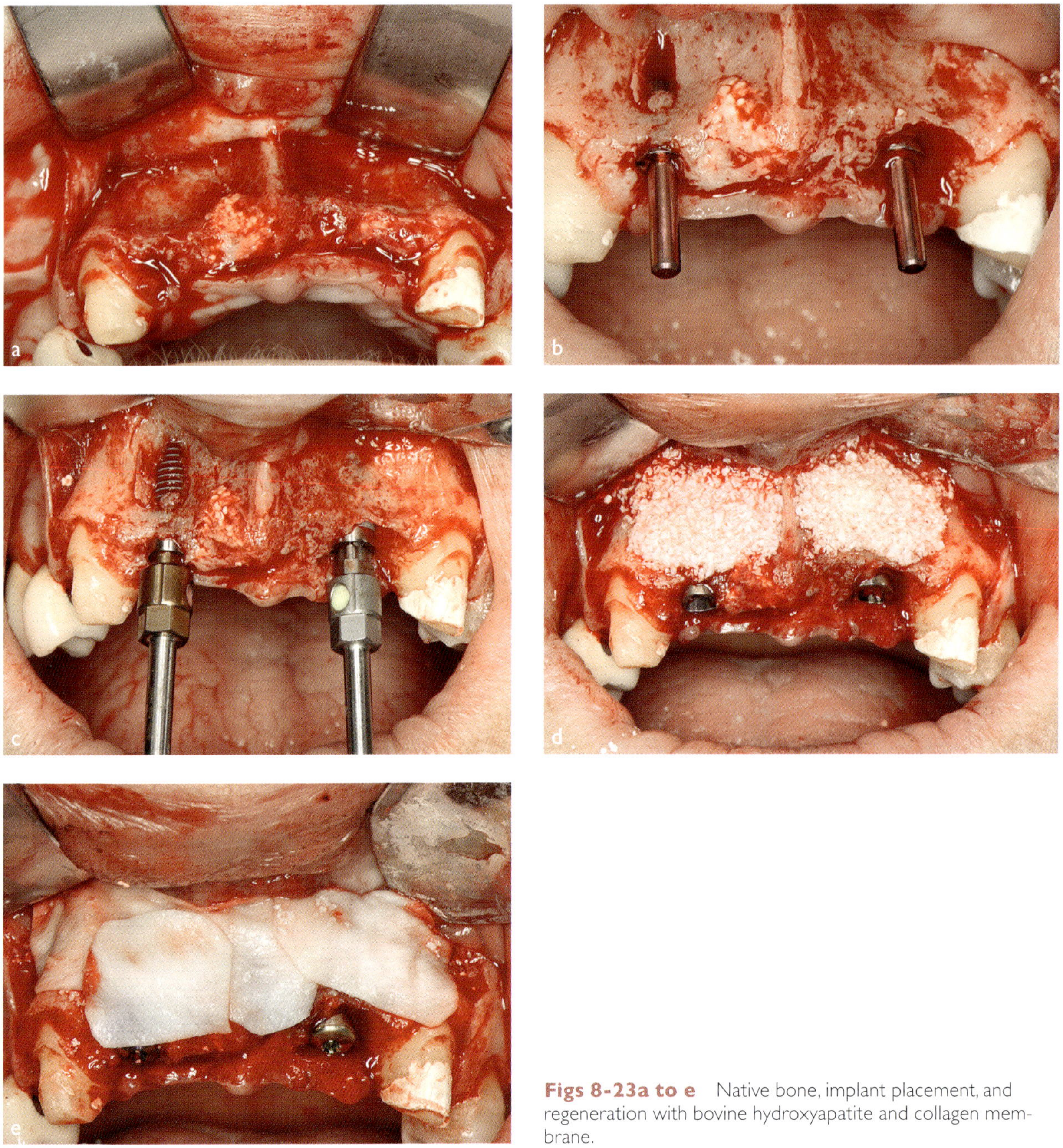

Figs 8-23a to e Native bone, implant placement, and regeneration with bovine hydroxyapatite and collagen membrane.

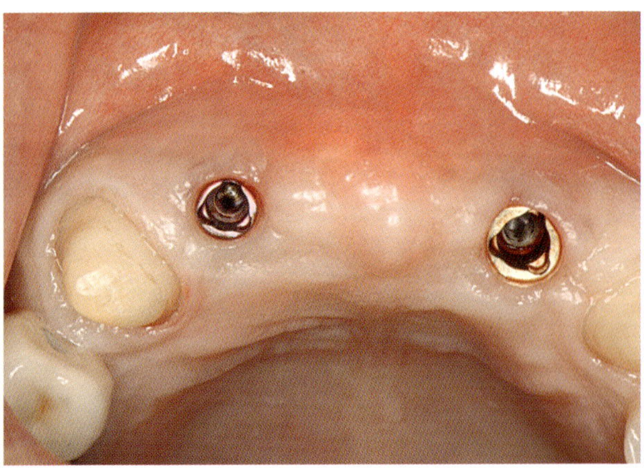

Fig 8-24 Bone volume after 6 months.

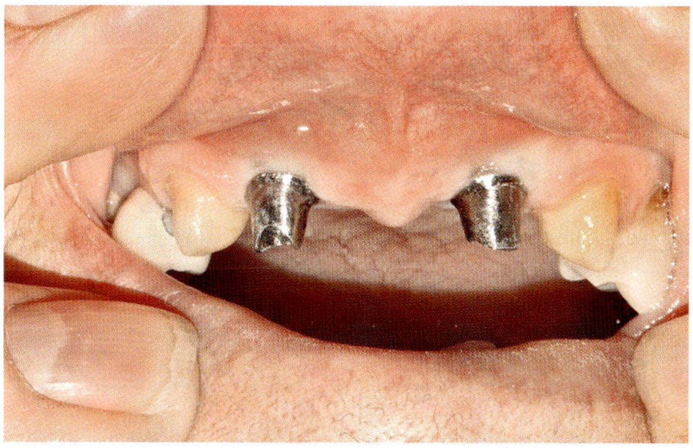

Fig 8-25 Soft tissue with the abutments.

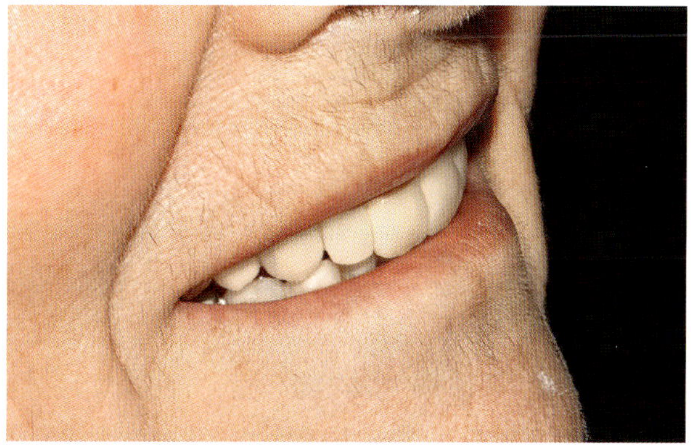

Fig 8-26 Lateral view of try-in.

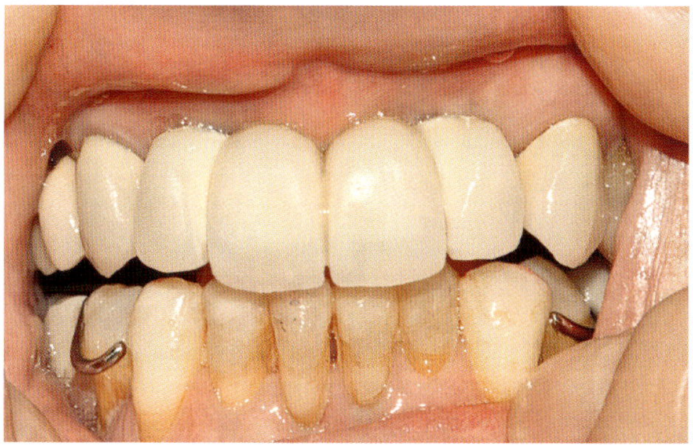

Fig 8-27 Anterior view of try-in.

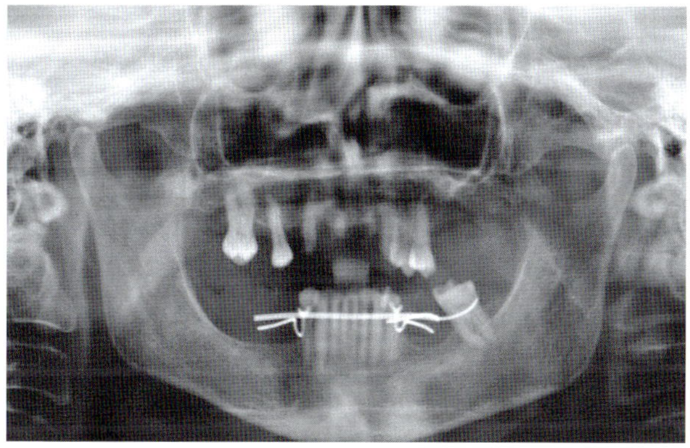

Fig 8-28 Panoramic radiograph after tooth extraction.

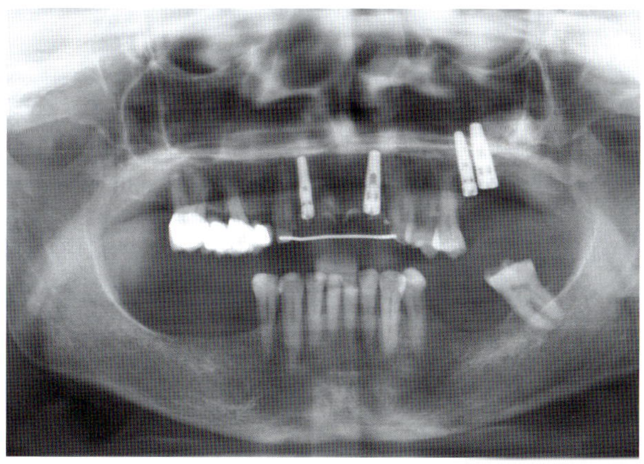

Fig 8-29 Final panoramic radiograph.

Case 3 (Figs 8-30 to 8-39)

In this patient two sinus lift procedures, each with different implants, were performed on the maxilla (Figs 8-32 and 8-33). In the posterior regions of the mandible an onlay graft on the fourth quadrant (Fig 8-34) and an inlay graft on the third quadrant (Fig 8-35) were performed.

The gaps between the native bone and the graft were filled with bovine hydroxyapatite and covered with a resorbable membrane. The created space after the coronal bone displacement in the inlay technique was also regenerated with the same materials.

The implants were placed at 5 months (Figs 8-36 to 8-38) and loaded after 6 months. The final situation can be seen in Fig 8-39.

Figs 8-30 to 8-39 Case 3

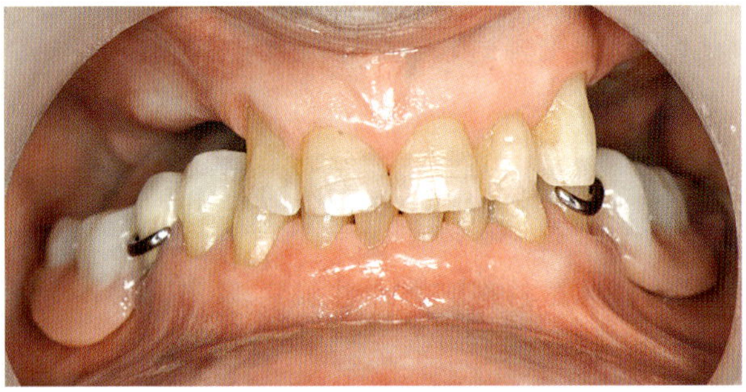

Fig 8-30 Initial situation.

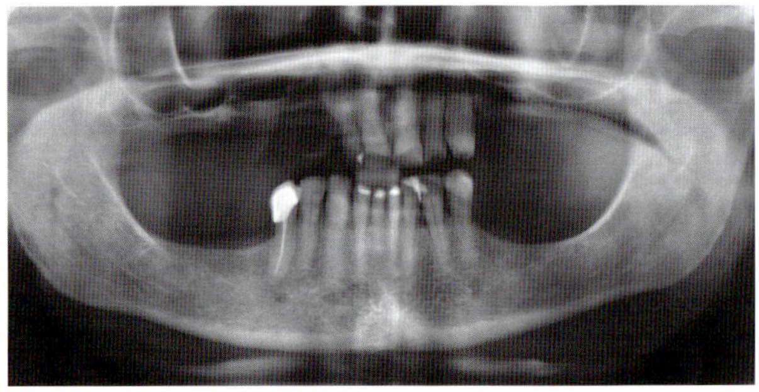

Fig 8-31 Preoperative panoramic radiograph.

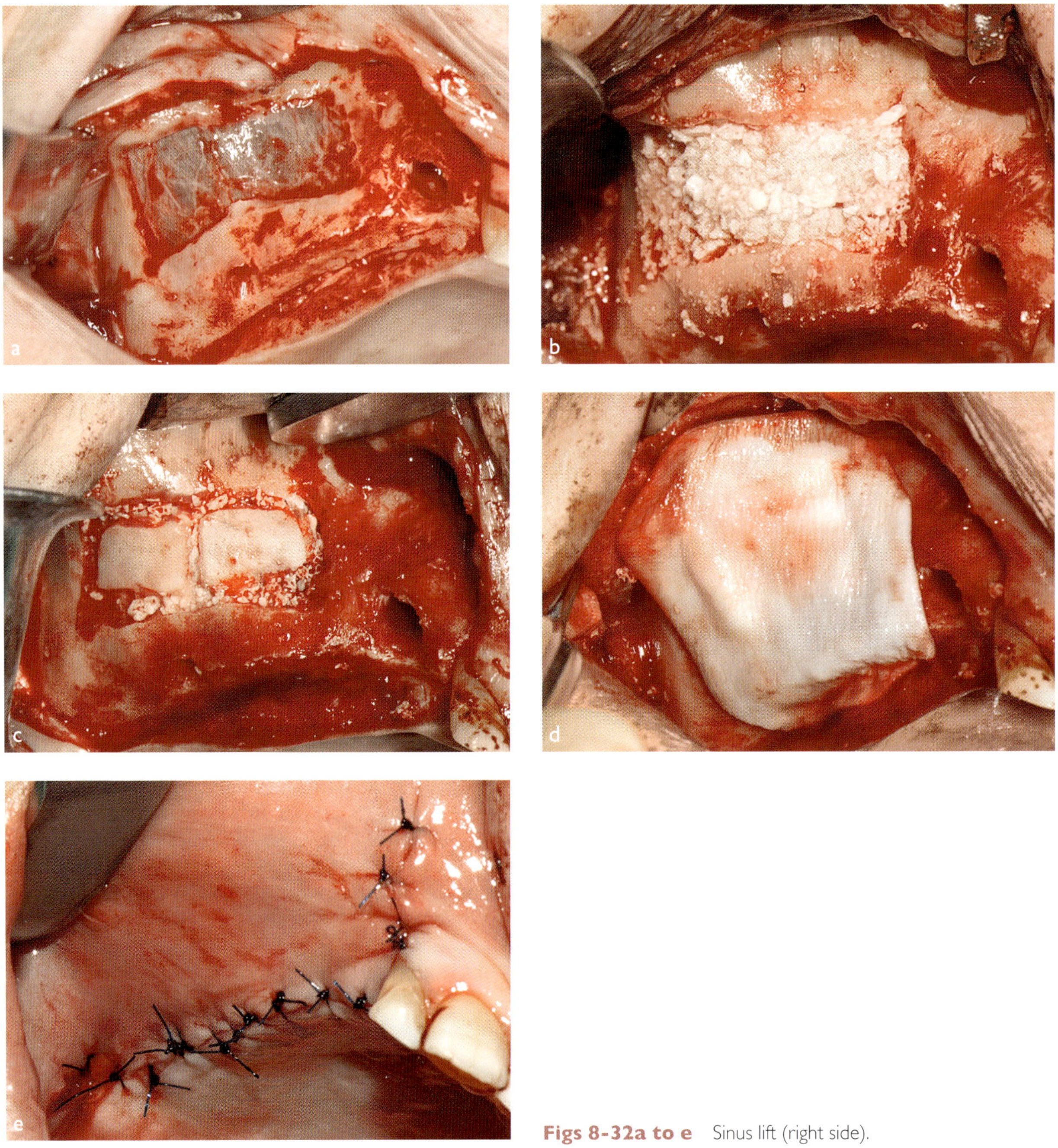

Figs 8-32a to e Sinus lift (right side).

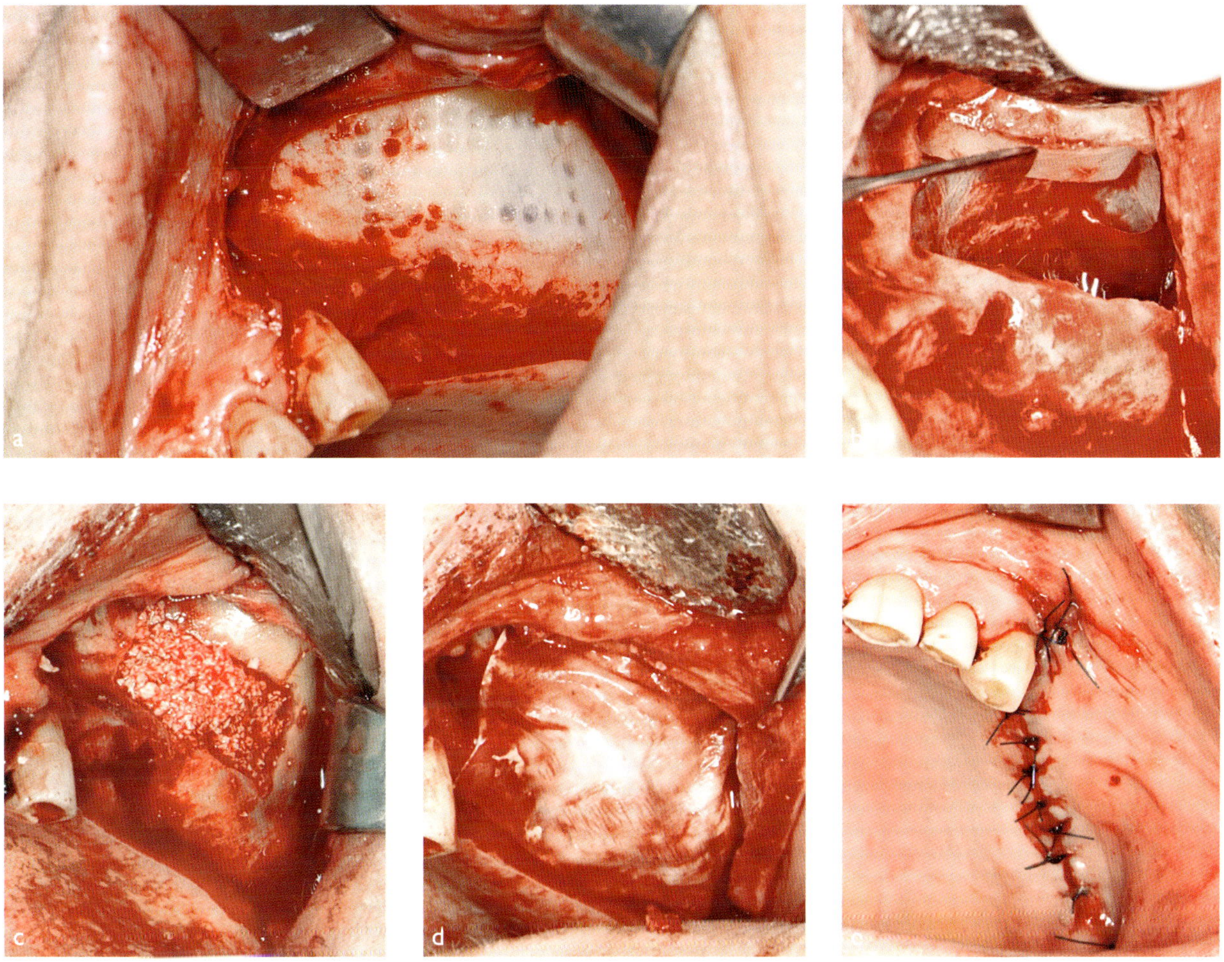

Figs 8-33a to e Sinus lift (left side).

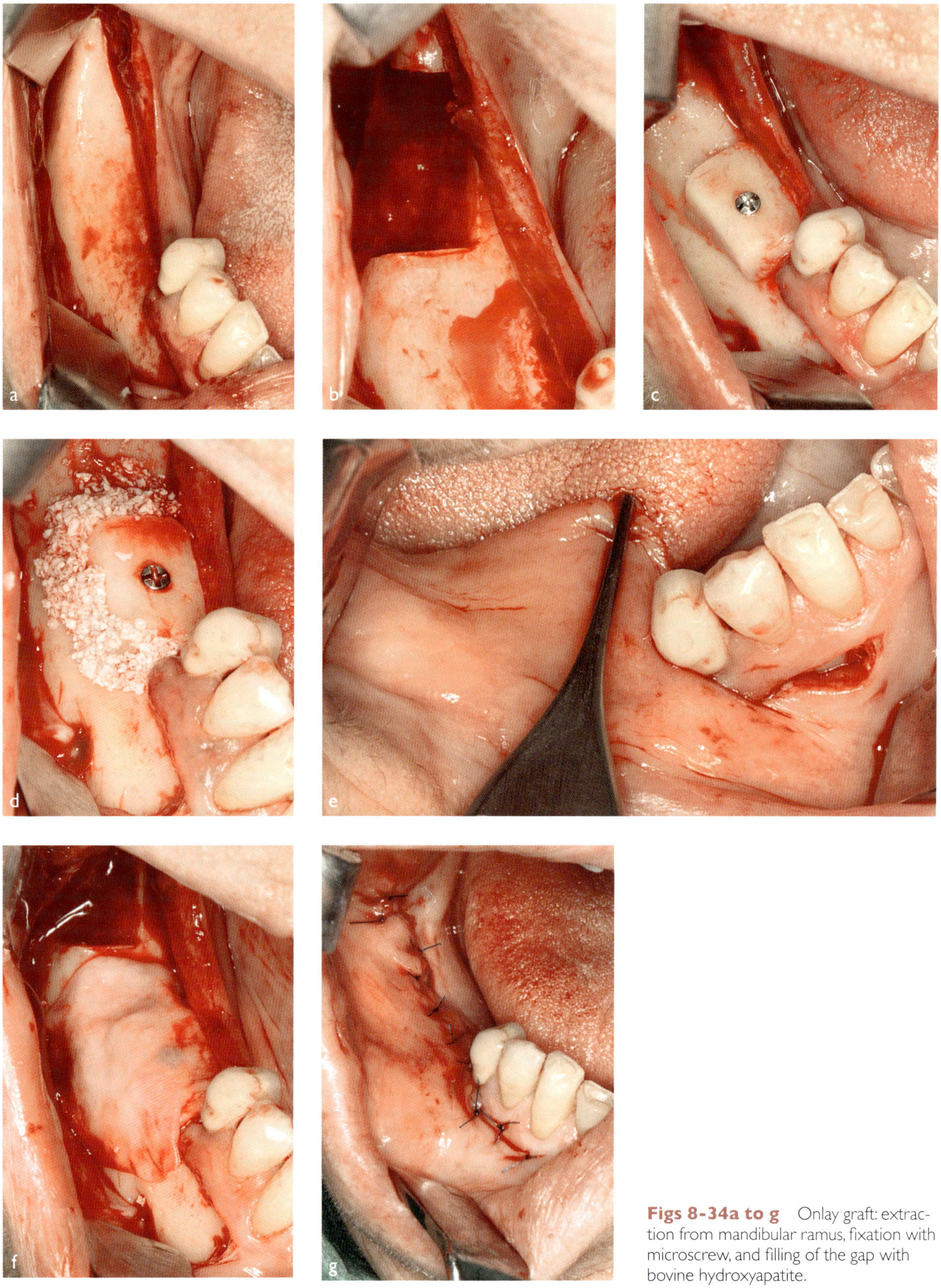

Figs 8-34a to g Onlay graft: extraction from mandibular ramus, fixation with microscrew, and filling of the gap with bovine hydroxyapatite.

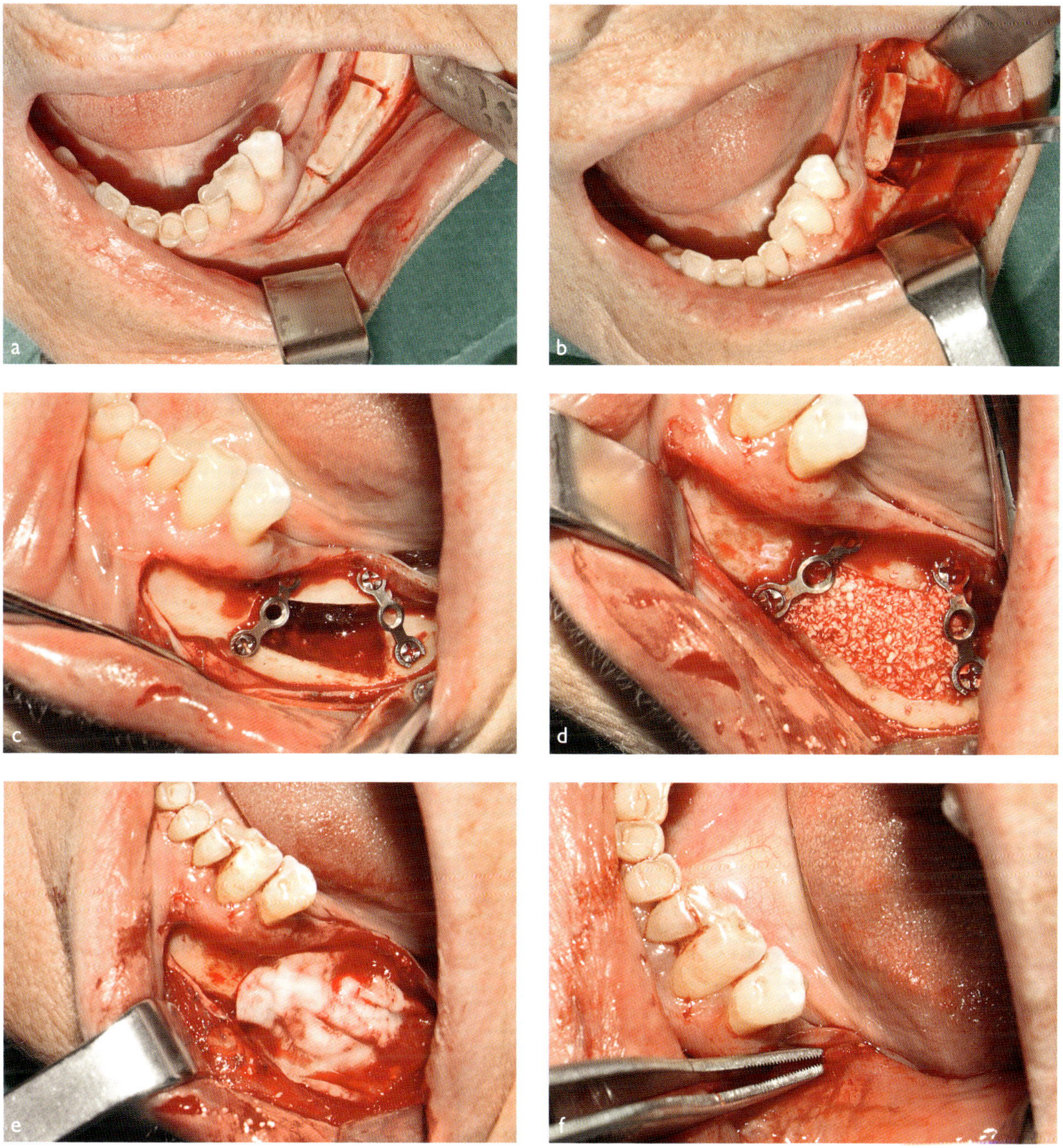

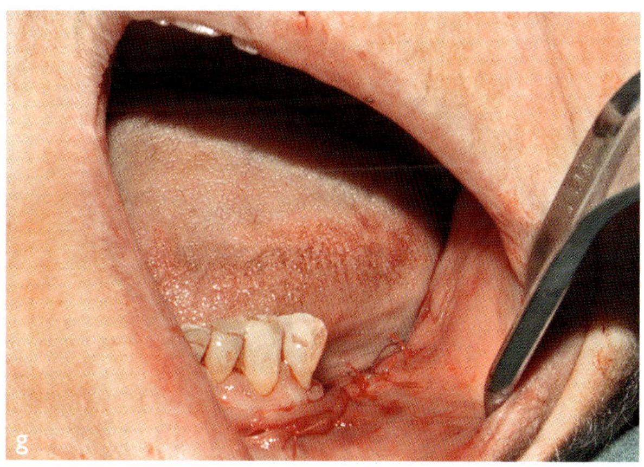

Figs 8-35a to g Inlay graft, and filling of the gap with bovine hydroxyapatite.

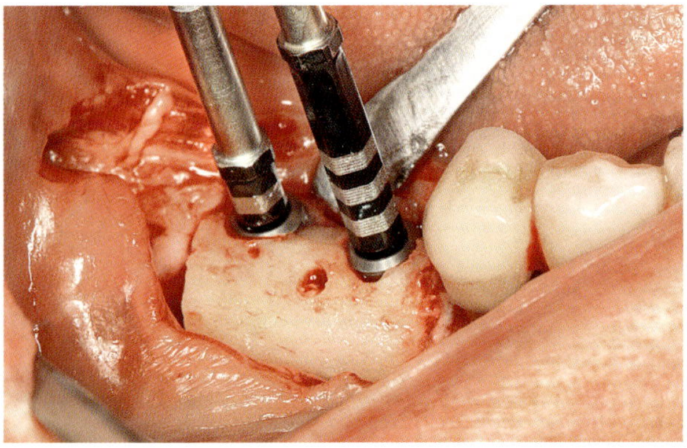

Fig 8-36 Implant placement after onlay healing.

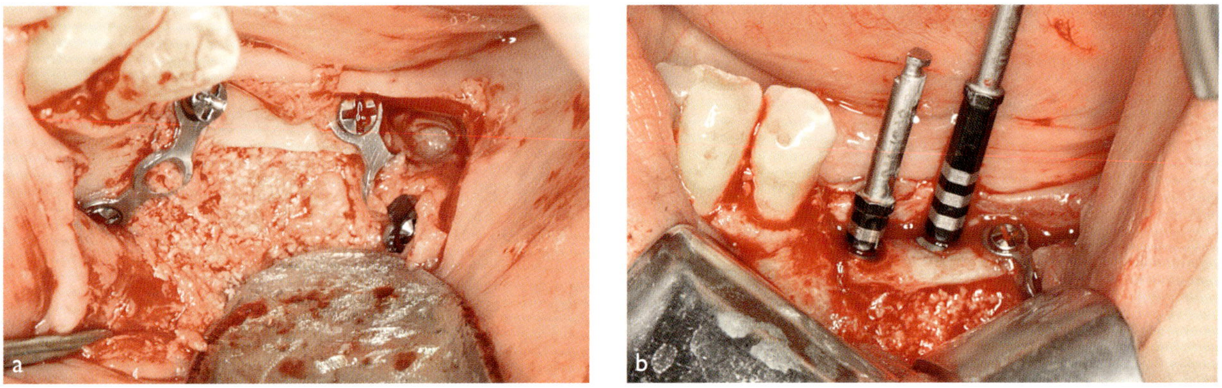

Figs 8-37a and b Implant placement after inlay healing.

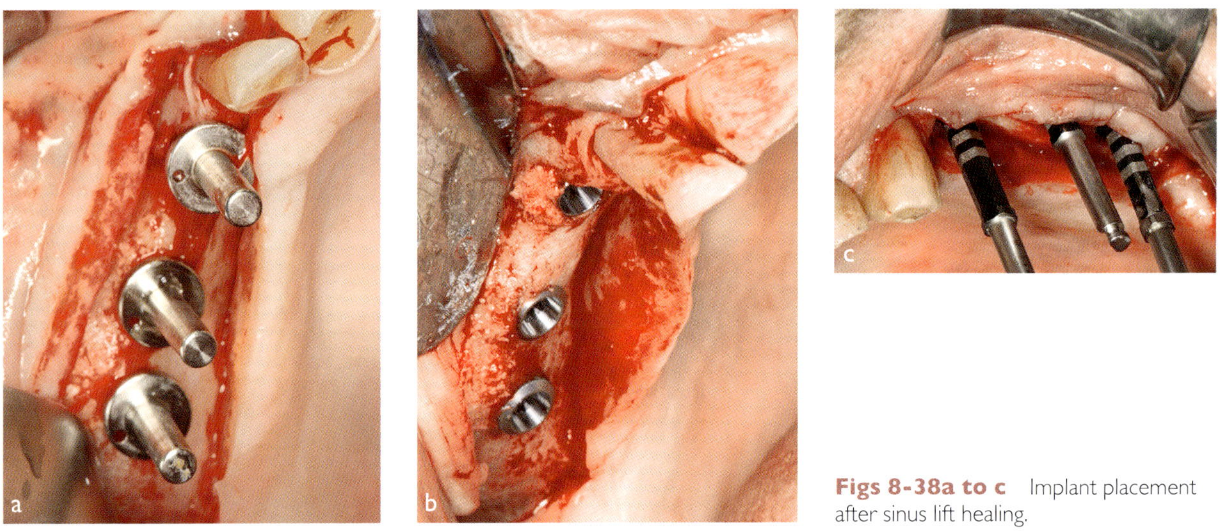

Figs 8-38a to c Implant placement after sinus lift healing.

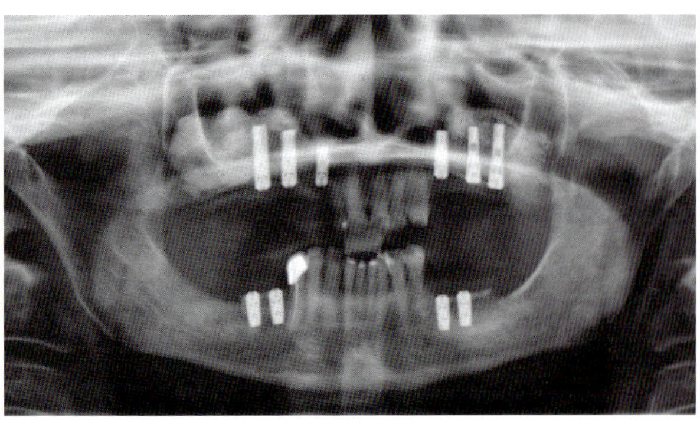

Fig 8-39 Final panoramic radiograph.

References

1. Beare AH, Metcalfe AD, Ferguson MW. Location of injury influences the mechanisms of both regeneration and repair within the MRL/MpJ mouse. J Anat 2006;209:547-559.
2. Anitua E, Sanchez M, Orive G, Andia I. The potential impact of the preparation rich in growth factors (PRGF) in different medical fields. Biomaterials 2007;28:4551-4560.
3. Ward BB, Brown SE, Krebsbach PH. Bioengineering strategies for regeneration of craniofacial bone: a review of emerging technologies. Oral Dis 2010;21:71-80.
4. Scarano A, Degidi M, Iezzi G, Pecora G, Piattelli M, Orsini G, et al. Maxillary sinus augmentation with different biomaterials: a comparative histologic and histomorphometric study in man. Implant Dent 2006;15:197-207.
5. Fontana F, Santoro F, Maiorana C, Iezzi G, Piattelli A, Simion M. Clinical and histologic evaluation of allogeneic bone matrix versus autogenous bone chips associated with titanium-reinforced e-PTFE membrane for vertical ridge augmentation: a prospective pilot study. Int J Oral Maxillofac Implants 2008;23:1003-1012.
6. Aghaloo TL, Moy PK. Which hard tissue augmentation techniques are the most successful in furnishing bony support for implant placement? Int J Oral Maxillofac Implants 2007;22(Suppl):49-70.
7. Wallace SS, Froum SJ. Effect of maxillary sinus augmentation on the survival of endosseous dental implants. A systematic review. Ann Periodontol 2003;8:328-343.
8. Nkenke E, Stelzle F. Clinical outcomes of sinus floor augmentation for implant placement using autogenous bone or bone substitutes: a systematic review. Clin Oral Implants Res 2009;20:124-133.
9. Sohn DS, Moon JW, Moon KN, Cho SC, Kang PS. New bone formation in the maxillary sinus using only absorbable gelatin sponge. J Oral Maxillofac Surg 2010;68:1327-1333.
10. Christensen DK, Karoussis IK, Joss A, Hammerle CH, Lang NP. Simultaneous or staged installation with guided bone augmentation of transmucosal titanium implants. A 3-year prospective cohort study. Clin Oral Implants Res 2003;14:680-686.
11. Wallace S, Gellin R. Clinical evaluation of freeze-dried cancellous block allografts for ridge augmentation and implant placement in the maxilla. Implant Dent 2010;19:272-279.
12. Thoma DS, Benic GI, Zwahlen M, Hammerle CH, Jung RE. A systematic review assessing soft tissue augmentation techniques. Clin Oral Implants Res 2009;20(Suppl 4):146-165.
13. Simion M, Nevins M, Rocchietta I, Fontana F, Maschera E, Schupbach P, et al. Vertical ridge augmentation using an equine block infused with recombinant human platelet-derived growth factor-BB: a histologic study in a canine model. Int J Periodontics Restorative Dent 2009;29:245-255.
14. Schwarz F, Ferrari D, Balic E, Buser D, Becker J, Sager M. Lateral ridge augmentation using equine- and bovine-derived cancellous bone blocks: a feasibility study in dogs. Clin Oral Implants Res 2010;21:904-912.
15. Del Fabbro M, Testori T, Francetti L, Weinstein R. Systematic review of survival rates for implants placed in the grafted maxillary sinus. Int J Periodontics Restorative Dent 2004;24:565-577.

Chapter 9

Atrophic maxilla: to use what is available or reconstruct?

Jorge Bertos, Pau Altuna, Jose M Lluch, Federico Hernández Alfaro

9.1 Introduction

Oral rehabilitation with osseointegrated dental implants is nowadays a highly predictable procedure. Treatment quality has been improved, offering different treatment options that were previously not only unfeasible but also impossible. Implant placement is now possible as long as there is sufficient three-dimensional bone quantity. Bone quality is also crucial for treatment predictability.

When dealing with maxillary bone atrophy, it should be remembered that there are not only bone resorption patterns, as described Cawood and Howell,[1] but also variable relationships between different anatomic structures in the maxilla, and continuous alveolar bone changes due to bone atrophy that come with tooth loss and aging. Thus, maxillary sinus pneumatization combined with the presence of nostrils, the nasopalatine nerve channel, and the centripetal maxillary bone resorption pattern, results in a drastic reduction in alveolar bone volume that compromises dental implant placement.

To aid management of maxillary atrophy, different surgical approaches are described in this chapter, divided into the following topics:

- 9.2 Maxillary sinus lift
  - 9.2.1 How can the sinus be accessed?
  - 9.2.2 How can the sinus be filled?
- 9.3 Le Fort I osteotomy plus inlay bone grafting
  - 9.3.1 Indications
  - 9.3.2 Contraindications
  - 9.3.3 Technique
  - 9.3.4 Conclusions
- 9.4 Zygomatic implants
  - 9.4.1 Indications
  - 9.4.2 Contraindications
  - 9.4.3 Technique
  - 9.4.4 Advantages
  - 9.4.5 Disadvantages
  - 9.4.6 Conclusions
- 9.5 Pterygoid implants
  - 9.5.1 Anatomical considerations
  - 9.5.2 Indications
  - 9.5.3 Technique
  - 9.5.4 Advantages
  - 9.5.5 Disadvantages
  - 9.5.6 Conclusions
- 9.6 Autogenous bone block grafts
  - 9.6.1 Indications
  - 9.6.2 Advantages of GBR with autogenous block grafts
  - 9.6.3 Advantages of GBR with autogenous block grafts
  - 9.6.4 Extraoral donor sites
  - 9.6.5 Intraoral donor sites
  - 9.6.6 Recipient sites
  - 9.6.7 When should implants be placed?
- 9.7. Clinical cases

9.2 Maxillary sinus lift

There are many well-described techniques for the maxillary sinus lifting procedure.[2-4] There is a common

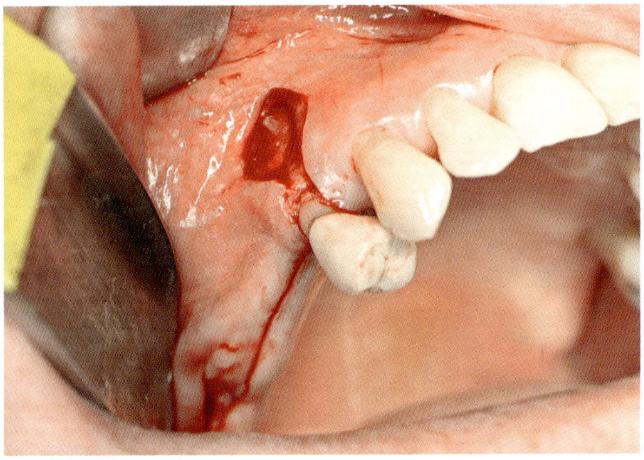

Fig 9-1 Triangular flap to access the lateral wall of the maxillary sinus.

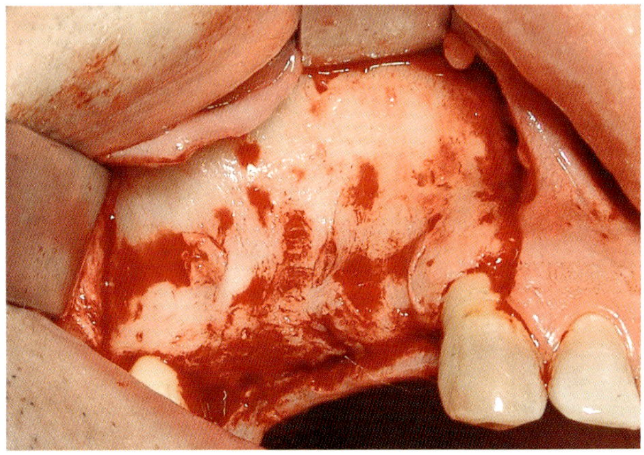

Fig 9-2 Trapezoidal flap to access the lateral wall of the maxillary sinus.

denominator among all its modalities: the elevation of the sinus membrane and filling with grafting material. The main difference among the techniques is in the sinus approach, where a crestal or a lateral approach is made.

This technique of maxillary sinus lifting for the purpose of implant placement was first described in 1977 by Tatum,[5] and first published in 1980 by Boyne and James.[6] This lateral approach technique is considered a Caldwell-Luc's technique modification. It is used in pathologic sinus treatment where an anterior approach of the sinus is made followed by a thorough curettage of its contents, and creation of a drainage opening in the middle meatus of the nasal cavity.[7]

9.2.1 How can the sinus be accessed?

Maxillary sinus access

Flap design

A mucoperiosteal flap must be reflected and its size should depend on the sinus volume desired to graft. The flap design must allow correct blood supply from its base, so oral and maxillofacial flap design principles must be followed. The most common flap designs are a trapezoidal flap or a triangular flap (Figs 9-1 and 9-2).

The trapezoidal flap is composed of three incisions; one crestal incision on the top of the crest limited by two vertical mesial and distal oblique releasing incisions. When performing a triangular flap, note that one releasing incision is omitted. This reduces the flap reflection capacity and therefore the visibility of the area. To minimize this added handicap the incisions should be made longer.

This flap design is made when only sinus lifting and no implant placement is planned due to the insufficient residual bone height in posterior areas. In cases where sinus lifting and implant placement is possible, as for a fully edentulous maxilla, a wider flap design including the whole maxilla is needed. In cases where as well as sinus lifting, implant placement in posterior and anterior areas is planned, an incision from tuberosity to tuberosity with a vertical releasing incision in the midline of the maxilla is the best option to provide good access and visibility (Fig 9-3).

Access bony window

Osteotomy

Once the flap is raised, the maxillary lateral wall is found, and through its width the maxillary sinus is located. An opening that allows the most comfortable and least aggressive approach to the sinus possible should be done.

The access window's design can be square, rectangular, ovoid, circular, or semicircular (Figs 9-4 to 9-7). It must be remembered that sinus membrane is lining the inside of the sinus so at the time of performing the access window it is crucial not to lacerate it to avoid sinus membrane perforations.

The access window can be created with various instruments, such as:

- Handpiece and tungsten carbide or diamond round bur, number 8 usually. With diamond burs, sinus membrane laceration is minimized but the cutting speed is diminished compared with tungsten carbide burs. This is due to the morphology of tungsten carbide burs; because it is comprised of multiple

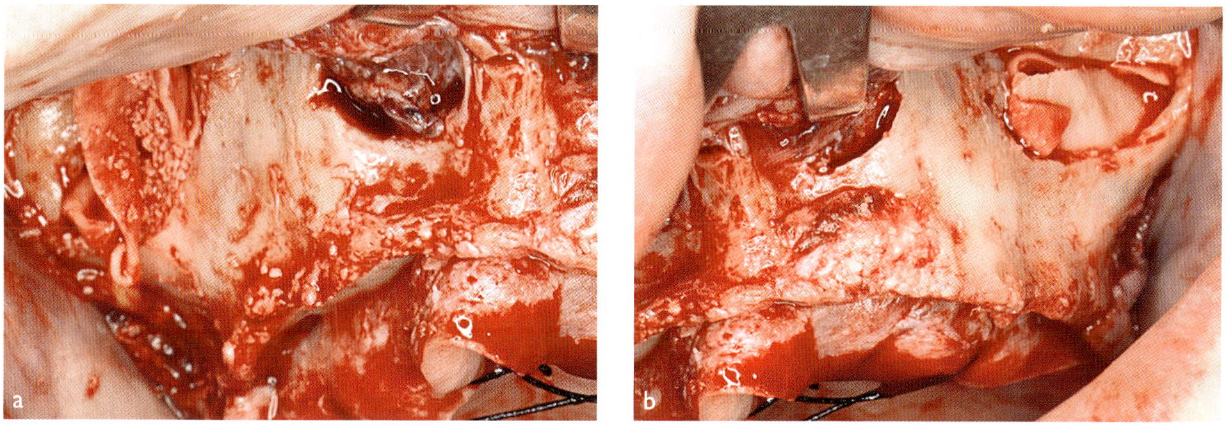

Figs 9-3a and b Bilateral sinus lift with particulate xenograft and autogenous chips. The incision from tuberosity to tuberosity can be seen.

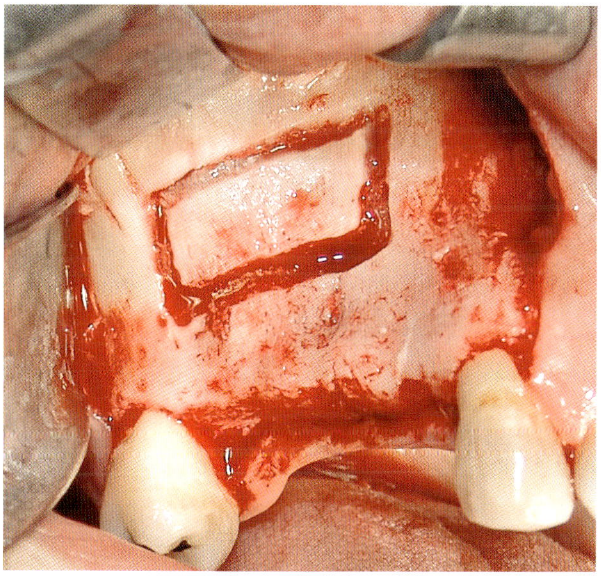

Figs 9-4 Rectangular design of the maxillary sinus access window.

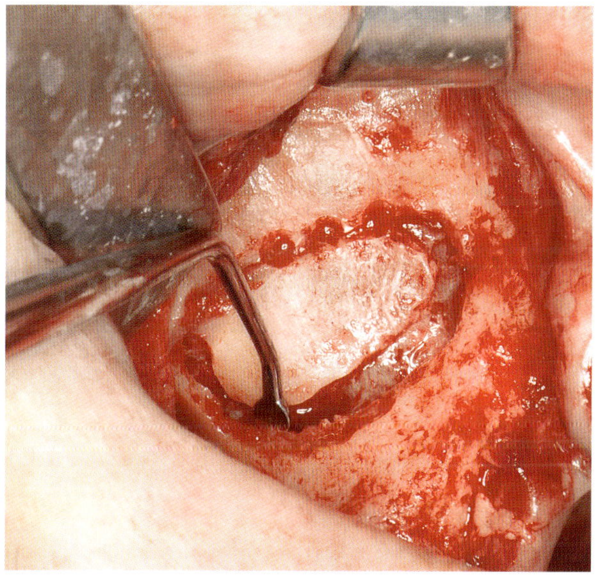

Figs 9-5 Ovoid design of the maxillary sinus access window.

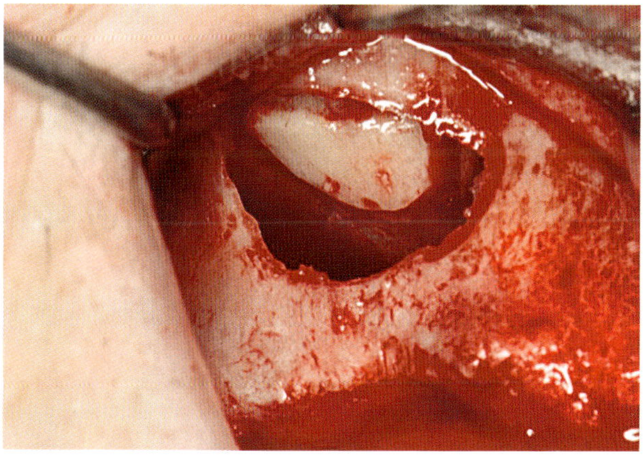

Fig 9-6 Semicircular design of the maxillary sinus access window.

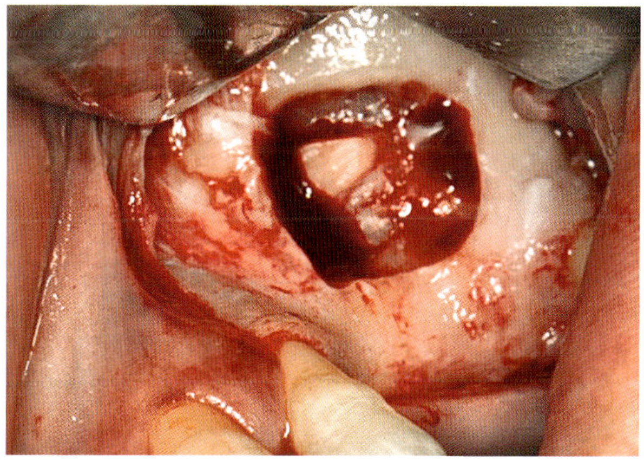

Fig 9-7 Square design of the maxillary sinus access window.

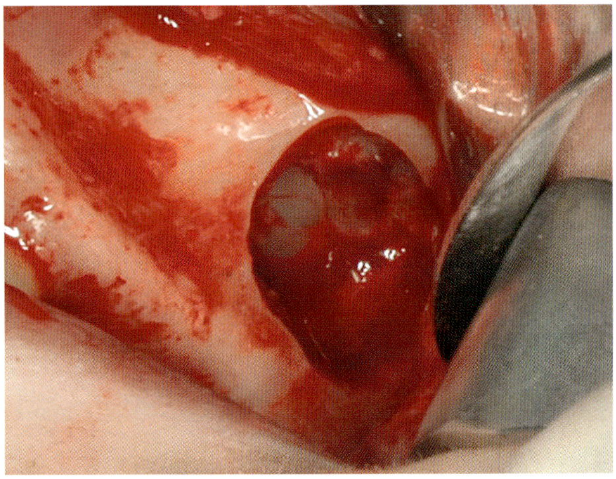

Fig 9-8 Extraction of the window and sinus membrane exposure.

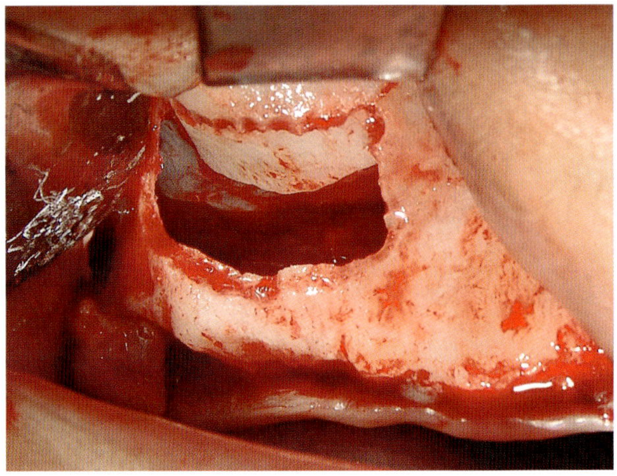

Fig 9-9 Mediocranial rotation of the window and the membrane.

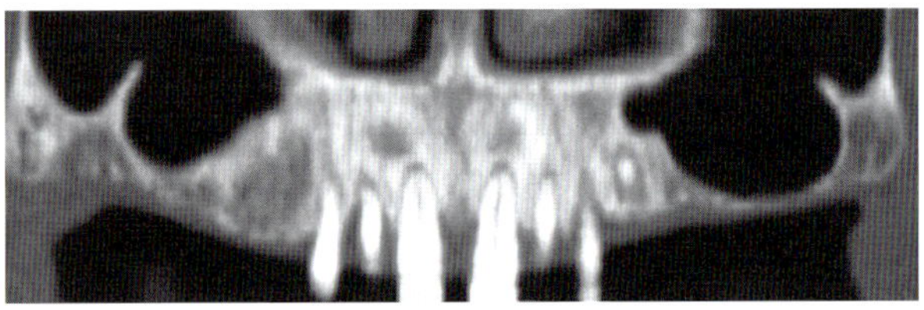

Fig 9-10 Underwood septa are well defined in the first quadrant.

sheets it has a greater cut efficacy compared with diamond burs.

- Piezoelectric device. The advantage of this device is the proved effectiveness in bone cutting while the soft tissue is not affected. This minimizes the risk of sinus membrane tearing.

Once the osteotomies are finished, it must be checked that the window is completely free from the remaining maxillary lateral wall and that the sinus membrane is intact.

Membrane lifting

At this point it is possible to access the sinus interior. However, first a decision must be made regarding the bony lateral window. Two options are available:

- Remove the lateral window with careful dissection from the sinus membrane and elevate the membrane with specific curettes. While lifting the sinus membrane, the active portion of the curette should always be in direct contact with the bone surface. This will guarantee lifting success (Fig 9-8).
- Maintain the bony lateral window and perform a mediocranial rotation of the window and the membrane, as explained above. The grouping formed by the bony lateral wall and the sinus membrane become the new sinus floor (Fig 9-9).

Another modality in maxillary sinus access is performing a selective and progressive scraping of the lateral wall of the maxillary bone until the Schneiderian membrane is localized. Afterwards, the sinus membrane can be lifted as explained above. This technique can be performed with different instruments, such as:

- Handpiece and round bur.
- Scraping with piezoelectric device.
- Scraping with a conventional scraper.

The scraped bone can be kept and later mixed with the desired biomaterial for use in grafting.

While lifting the sinus membrane, some obstacles inside the sinus may be found. For example, it is frequent to find partitions called "Underwood's septa"[8] (Fig 9-10) that can divide the sinus into two or more compartments. Usually these septa appear to be in a buccopalatal direction, being wider in the base than in the distal portion, and rarely fully divide the sinus.[9]

The presence of Underwood's septa will force the clinician to make different maneuvers to overcome these anatomical structures, such as creating two different windows to exclude the sinus septum from the bony window.[10] It must be considered that insertion of the sinus membrane in the septum cranial portion

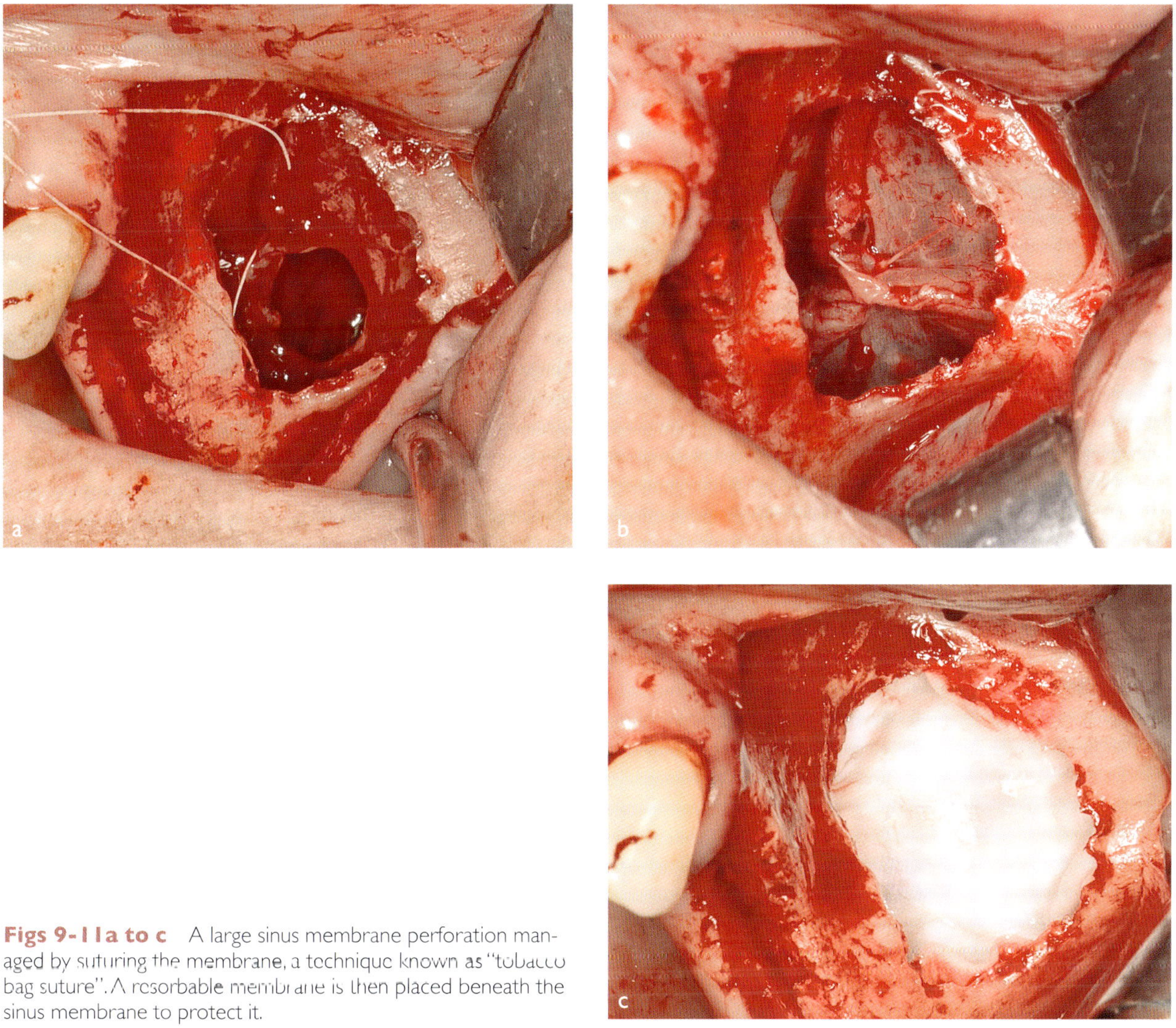

Figs 9-11a to c A large sinus membrane perforation managed by suturing the membrane, a technique known as "tobacco bag suture". A resorbable membrane is then placed beneath the sinus membrane to protect it.

(opposite side from its base) increases the risk of membrane tearing.

Another possible obstacle is the presence of sinus floor irregularities where the membrane has a greater insertion. These will make sinus membrane lifting more challenging and a source of possible membrane tearing. They are usually found when recent dental extractions with periapical infection or root tips with sinus floor intimate contact have been performed.

Once the membrane is lifted and there is no membrane perforation the clinician may proceed with sinus grafting.

In case of a membrane perforation, it is vital to know how to manage it properly. Several publications report how to manage these perforations according to their location[11] and size[12] (Figs 9-11 and 9-12).

9.2.2 How can the sinus be filled?

There are several types of grafting materials, among which are:

- Autograft – own patient bone.
- Xenograft – animal bone origin.
- Allograft – human bone origin from tissue bank.
- Alloplastic materials – inert metals, ceramics or plastics.

Once the grafting material has been chosen, the sinus lift may be performed. The most difficult access areas should be filled with the grafting material first, finishing with the most accessible areas (Fig 9-13). This allows visual checking that there are no gaps during sinus grafting.

Controversy about ideal grafting material particle size exists. Ideally, the grafting material particle size should be

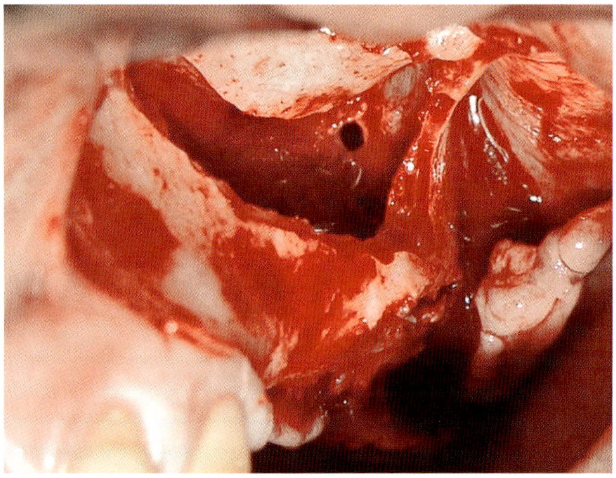

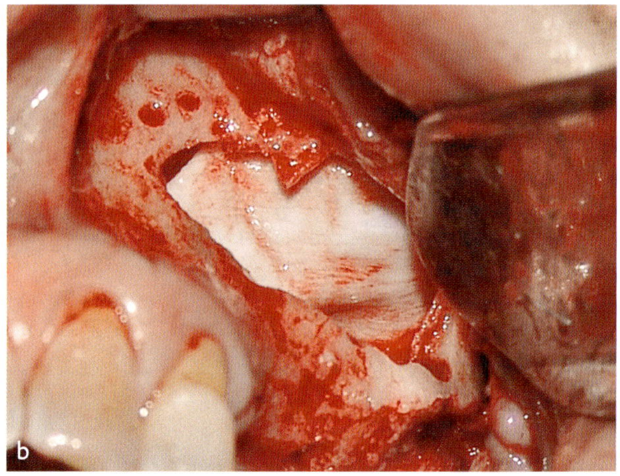

Figs 9-12a and 9-12b Small sinus membrane perforation managed by applying directly a resorbable collagen membrane.

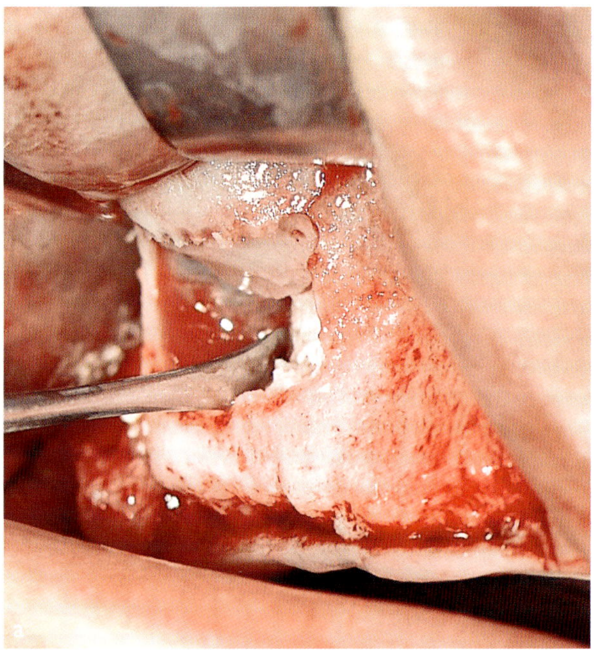

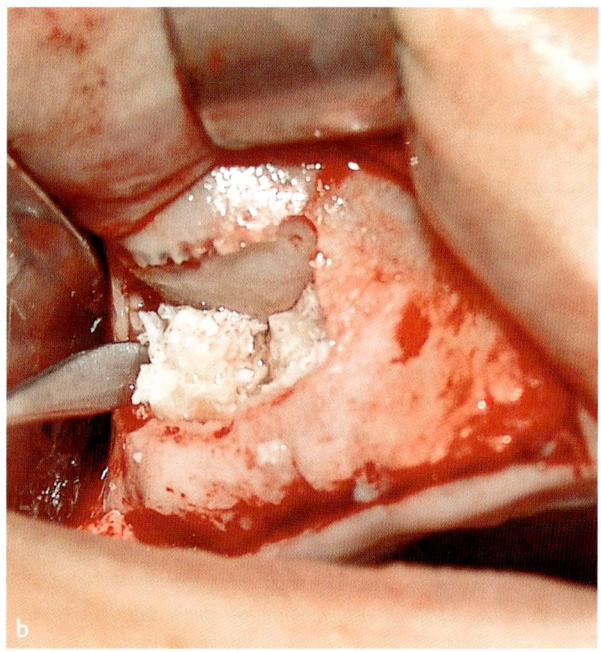

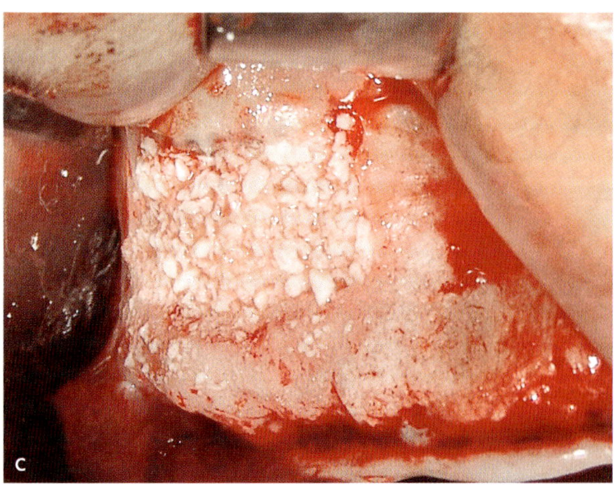

Figs 9-13a to c The sinus is filled in order, first by filling the sinus medial wall, then the anterior (a) and distal walls (b), ending with the lateral wall (c).

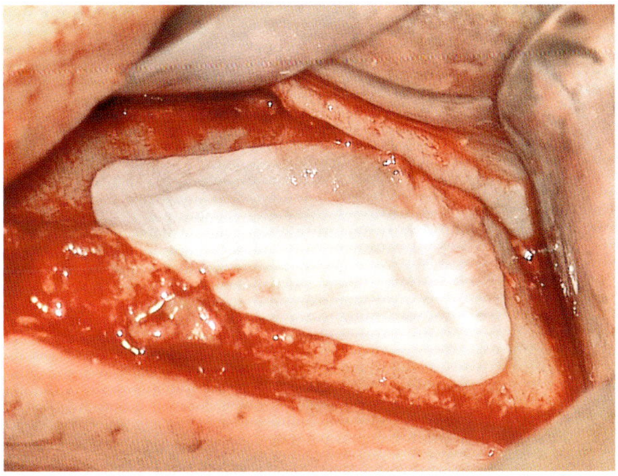

Fig 9-14 Resorbable membrane placed in the lateral wall of the maxilla and covering the grafting material.

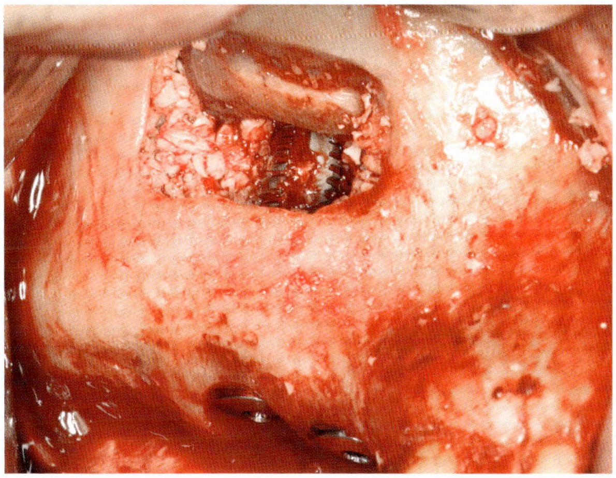

Fig 9-15 Medial, anterior, posterior, and cranial sinus walls are filled. Following this, implants are placed and the most lateral aspect of the sinus is filled, covering the implants.

thick, approximately 1 to 2 mm in diameter. Thus, sinus bone grafting is faster and cheaper, because a smaller quantity of grafting material is needed.[4]

Ideally, once the sinus is completely grafted a membrane is placed in the lateral wall of the maxilla, covering the grafting material (Fig 9-14). This promotes blood supply from inside the sinus, avoiding soft tissue invagination that could compromise overall grafted bone volume.[3]

If sinus volume is considerable, some authors advocate the use of biomaterial and autologous bone mixture. In large sinuses, grafting with only biomaterial has been observed to leave some areas where bone formation has not occurred at the end of the grafting consolidation time, located mainly in the center of the overall bone grafting volume. This could compromise implant placement. By incorporating small chips of autogenous bone, the osteogenic and osteoinductive cells will promote a better and more homogenous ossification.

Between 7 and 9 months should be allowed to obtain optimal bone graft consolidation.[4]

When can simultaneous implants be placed?

There is controversy in the literature regarding the placement of simultaneous implants. Some authors report a minimum bone height of about 5 mm, and others advocate 4 mm. Another important factor is bone quality, which is important to provide good implant anchorage.[13-15]

Once it is confirmed that simultaneous implant placement is possible, the situation can be managed in two ways:

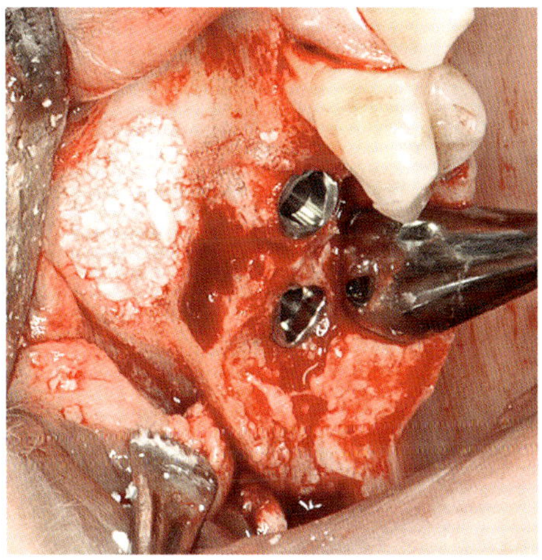

Fig 9-16 The sinus is completely filled and the implants are placed normally.

- Filling medial, anterior, posterior, and cranial sinus walls. The implants may then be placed, ending with filling of the most lateral aspect of the sinus, and covering the implants (Fig 9-15).
- Fully filling the sinus and then placing the implants normally (Fig 9-16).

To complete this surgical procedure, the wound should be sutured. If the bone volume has not been bucally overcorrected and the flap has been correctly hydrated, a tension-free closure of the wound should be performed, which will guarantee a correct cicatrization. However, if a tension-free closure cannot be achieved, a technique called "Rehrmannplasty" or "Rehrmann maneuver" should be performed. It consists in making several releasing incisions in the periosteum to elongate the soft tissue flap in order to achieve tension-free wound closure.

9.3 Le Fort I osteotomy plus inlay bone grafting

This technique allows implant placement in atrophic maxillary bone, although nowadays there are different treatment options for rehabilitation of this type of atrophy, such zygomatic implants and pterygoid implants, or bone block grafting. One of the advantages of this technique is that the maxilla can be moved three-dimensionally to correct maxillary retrusion due to centripetal resorption in maxillary atrophy (see Case 1, Figs 9-17 to 9-26, and Case 2, Figs 9-27 to 9-35).

9.3.1 Indications

Le Fort I osteotomy plus inlay bone grafting is used mainly in the surgical treatment of maxillary class V and VI Cawood and Howell atrophy classification,[1] where there is a moderate to severe increase in interarch distance. Not only the vertical defect can be corrected, but also the horizontal defect and maxillary retrusion due to atrophy.[16,17]

9.3.2 Contraindications

There are no absolute contraindications, other than those that medically could compromise general anesthesia.

9.3.3 Technique

Maxillary bone access: incision

A high sublabial incision from molar to molar should be performed in cases where no vestibular onlay block bone grafting is required, and a crestal incision if bone blocks are needed.

A periosteal reflection up to the infraorbital foramen, the pterygo-maxillary suture, and the piriform aperture should be made, leaving nasal mucosa exposed to be carefully reflected from the nasal floor later. Once the nasal mucosa is reflected it is recommended to apply an hemostatic gauze in both nasal fossae to control bleeding and to protect nasal mucosa from the osteotomy.

Osteotomy

The osteotomy should be from the tuberosity to the nasal cavity. At this point, it is not necessary to preserve the sinus mucosa from the osteotomy, but any mucosa remaining should be removed from the sinus floor because it will be the recipient area of the bone graft.

The nasal septum and both nasal walls should be cut with a chisel, taking care not to damage the nasal mucosa. A curved chisel can be used to cut the pterygo-maxillary suture. Then the maxillary bone can be mobilized, a technique known as "maxillary down-fracture". The first force vector in the maxillary down-fracturing has to be in a superior-inferior direction following a saggital movement frequently more limited by soft tissue. At this point it is important to identify and protect the palatine arteries that will nourish the maxillary bone.

Final maxillary positioning

The final maxillary position will be given by the positioning splint. All the time needed should be spent to adapt the bone grafts to give the complex the maximum stability, reshaping if necessary the nasal and sinus floor. The maxilla–block grafts complex should be stabilized to the remaining craniofacial structures by miniplates and screws, without gaps if possible. If gaps are present they should be corrected by applying particulate bone graft (autologous bone chips or particulate biomaterial). Good stability can usually be achieved by placing a minimum of two miniplates in the maxillary posterior thirds and also two miniplates in the maxillary medium-anterior thirds.

In those cases for which a large maxillary advancement and down-fracturing is required, a modified vestibuloplasty is needed, leaving the bloody surface to heal by secondary intention and letting the soft tissue develop an epithelial metaplasia.

In some cases it will be necessary to level the occlusal plane, so that a maxillary segmented osteotomy can be performed, stabilizing the fragments with miniplates.

In cases with horizontal atrophy, a crestal incision should be made in order to manage the vertical atrophy and the horizontal atrophy by placing onlay block bone grafting.

Suturing

Once the stability of the whole craniofacial complex, the bone grafts, and the hemostasis are checked, the wound may be sutured. It should be tension-free and tight. Nylon sutures or resorbable sutures should preferably be used.

Implant placement can be done simultaneously in cases where good stability has been achieved, or deferred for 3 to 5 months.

9.3.4 Conclusions

- This technique is indicated in the correction of the completely atrophic maxilla and allows three-dimensional correction of the maxillary position as well as creating a good intermaxillary relationship.
- It is a very predictable technique once the necessary skills have been acquired.
- Two different surgical fields are needed when using autologous bone grafts, and one when using biomaterials.
- General anesthesia is required.

9.4 Zygomatic implants

Zygomatic implants are another alternative in the treatment of moderate to severe maxillary atrophy. They can achieve excellent anchorage even in severe alveolar atrophy. Implant lengths vary from 30 to 52.5 mm and they anchor in the residual alveolar process, passing through the maxillary sinus and reaching the zygomatic bone[18] (see Case 3, Figs 9-36 to 9-42, and Case 4, Figs 9-43 to 9-45).

9.4.1 Indications

- Partial or complete resections of maxilla, although in these cases it is recommended to perform bone block grafts to regenerate maxillary defects.
- Maxillary posterior atrophy with a minimum residual bone height and width of 5 mm. In these cases zygomatic implants in posterior areas can be combined with standard implants in anterior areas.
- In cases where there is anterior and posterior moderate to severe atrophy, the situation can be dealt with as follows:
- one bilateral posterior zygomatic implant and anterior block bone grafting plus standard implants
- one bilateral posterior zygomatic implant and one bilateral anterior zygomatic implant.
- The patient must be able to open their mouth wide, and two basic anatomic structures must be taken into consideration: the orbital cavity and infratemporal fossae.

9.4.2 Contraindications

Zygomatic implants are contraindicated in Cawood and Howell[1] class V, mainly because of antero-posterior and vertical interarch discrepancy. In these cases it is recommended to perform a Le Fort I osteotomy plus inlay grafts.

9.4.3 Technique

Specific instruments include a specific bur ranging from 30 mm to 52.5 mm in length, a direction- and depth-checking probe, and zygomatic implants.

It is recommended to perform this surgery under general anesthesia and nasotracheal intubation to leave the oral cavity free from any kind of devices that can disturb the surgeon during the procedure.

A crestal incision with a mesial and distal vertical oblique releasing incision should be made to achieve a good surgical field. While raising a mucoperiosteal flap some anatomical structures should be identified, such as: the lateral inferior orbital rim, inferior orbital rim base, infraorbital nerve, temporal apophysis of the zygomatic bone, and its lateral and medial part.[19]

Parameters to follow in the implant insertion axis

Implant emergence at the crestal level should be as central as possible, and also as distal as possible, at the first molar level, although in some cases the emergence is towards the palatine vault because of the implant direction and the atrophy pattern.

The implant has to be in direct contact or as close as possible to the lateral-distal maxillary sinus wall, although in some cases it can be left exterior to the maxillary sinus.[20]

The apex of the implant should be placed in the angle formed by the zygomatic arch with the anterior apophysis of the zygomatic bone, since this is where more bone can be found.

Bone drilling follows the same protocol as for standard implants. First, an initial bur is used to control the correct direction in order to avoid infratemporal fossae and orbital cavity penetration. Should this occur, complex complications can arise.

Once the drilling phase is finished, the implant placement phase begins. This implant has the crestal module angulated to compensate the implant angulation and make the emergence of the platform suitable for prosthetic rehabilitation. The remaining implants are placed, the healing abutments are screwed and the wound is sutured tension-free.

To evaluate the success of these implants, the same evaluation parameters as for conventional implants are followed. Success rates are similar to those of conventional implants.[21]

Infraorbitary paresthesia appears frequently, but will disappear after a few months.

9.4.4 Advantages

- No surgical reconstruction of posterior maxillary atrophic area is needed so the overall treatment time is reduced.
- Excellent anchorage can be achieved due to the large volume of zygomatic bone.
- Biologic cost is reduced because there is no need for bone grafting.

9.4.5 Disadvantages

- The placement of zygomatic implants is more challenging than conventional implants.
- Experience is needed for their placement.
- General anesthesia is recommended.
- Possible infraorbitary nerve paresthesia.
- The palatine emergence can be corrected, placing the implant exteriorly to the sinus or giving the implant less angulation (more vertical) but lateral orbital wall invasion is possible.

9.4.6 Conclusions

Zygomatic implants are a good option in the treatment of atrophic maxillary posterior areas, with advantages in terms of bone reconstruction, but they are not risk free. Risks can be minimized with good technique and experience.

9.5 Pterygoid implants

Pterygoid implants are another treatment option in cases of maxillary atrophy. The technique was first described by Tulasne.[22]

These implants may be used in cases where large sinus pneumatization makes it impossible to place implants without any kind of reconstructive approach. Moreover, with this technique distal cantilevers that could compromise the prosthesis integrity are avoided.[23]

Placement of pterygoid implants is highly predictable, because the implants are placed in the buttress formed by the maxilla, the pyramidal aspect of the palatine bone, and the pterygoid apophysis of the sphenoid bone.

In the region of the maxillary tuberosity there is type III or IV quality bone whereas in the pyramidal and pterygoid apophyses, type I or II quality bone is present (see Case 3, Figs 9-38 to 9-40).

9.5.1 Anatomical considerations

The maxillary artery crosses above the pterygomaxillary suture, which leaves a risk-free area of about 25 mm for implant placement.[24]

Bleeding can occur while drilling due to veins of the internal pterygoid muscle. This bleeding stops at implant placement.

9.5.2 Indications

- Molar absence that prevents standard implant placement.
- Totally edentulous patients that require posterior prosthesis fixation.
- Cases where sinus lifting is contraindicated or refused by the patient.

9.5.3 Technique

This surgical procedure can be performed under local anesthesia.

A crestal incision, from the maxillary tuberosity to the molar or premolar region is made and a mucoperiosteal flap is raised. The implant angulation is given by maxillary sinus and tuberosity morphology, and pterygoid plate location. The drilling should be mesially angulated about 45 degrees with respect to the occlusal plane and about

10 to 15 degrees laterally to find the most dense part of the pterygoid plate.

The surgical procedure should be finished by suturing the wound. Since there is a large amount of soft tissue present in this area, it could be surgically reduced in order to make elaboration of the prosthesis easier.

Cicatrization time is around 4 to 6 months due to the poor bone density.

9.5.4 Advantages

- Bone grafts are avoided.
- Maxillary sinus integrity is maintained.
- Predictable results.
- Prosthetic cantilever is avoided.
- Low morbidity.
- Treatment time is shortened.
- Prosthetic restoration is relatively easy.

9.5.5 Disadvantages

- The technique is challenging.

9.5.6 Conclusions

The pterygoid implant is another option in the treatment of the atrophic maxilla limited to posterior regions. It has high predictability, it reduces treatment time compared with reconstructive procedures, and it permits distal anchorage pillars to avoid cantilevers.

9.6 Autogenous bone block grafts

Autogenous bone block grafts represent the gold standard in the reconstruction of the maxillofacial area. In recent years, many efforts have been made to replace this technique with bone substitutes. However, none has achieved the same advantages and long-term predictability.[25]

Autogenous bone block grafting usually involves a donor site and a receptor site. The size of the defect is the key element to choose one donor site or another. When large reconstructions are needed, the iliac crest is the main donor area for large amounts of cancellous blocks. The major problems of the iliac crest are hospitalization needs, morbidity, and resorption rate of the blocks. Calvarium is an excellent source of large amounts of membranous bone, but patients are difficult to convince of such a procedure. In cases of moderate to severe atrophic maxillas, intraoral donor sites are the main source of autogenous blocks for the great majority of defects. Ramus, retromolar, and symphysis areas of the mandible are good sources of cortical bone to reconstruct a great variety of defects. The oral surgeon is well familiarized with the buccal cavity and has new tools, such as piezosurgery instruments, which allow for predictable, precise, and safe intervention.

9.6.1 Indications

Depending on the size and amount of bone needed in the receptor site, there are several intraoral and extraoral donor areas. Anatomy and access to the donor site are also important. Limitation in mouth opening or the proximity of the inferior alveolar nerve would seriously compromise the surgery. The cost of the intervention and the time taken might also have to be considered in the choice of one donor site over another.

For small and contained defects (class II and III of the Cawood and Howell classification[1]; 3-wall defects, 1 to 2 teeth), biomaterials in combination with collagen or expanded polytetrafluoroethylene (ePTFE) membranes may be used. In some cases it might be convenient to combine autogenous blocks with biomaterials, as described later. Bone blocks for lateral augmentation have their main indication in class IV, V, and VI of the Cawood and Howell[1] classification. When the bone available is less than 4 mm in width and an implant of a diameter larger than 3.5 mm should be placed, it is necessary to augment the alveolar crest.[26]

When a ≤5-mm-wide crest is found in association with a high lip line, this technique is recommended.

When vertical augmentation is desired, bone blocks can be an alternative to guided bone regeneration (GBR) with bone substitutes or distraction osteogenesis. Resorption rates increase in vertical augmentation with the onlay block technique.

9.6.2 Advantages of GBR with autogenous block grafts

Autogenous bone block grafts are the gold standard in the reconstruction of the maxillofacial area. The main reasons for their success are their osteogenic, osteoconductive, and osteoconductive properties. On the other hand, the use of bone from the same patient allows a non-allergenic graft without the risk of contagious diseases.

The autogenous block is space-maintaining so there is no need for a titanium mesh or reinforcement. If proper fixation is provided with screws, it offers excellent mechanical stability.

After a long healing period, creeping substitution will replace the original grafted bone for newly formed bone. This is possible when adequate vascularization is provided by the surrounding tissues.

9.6.3 Disadvantages of GBR with autogenous block grafts

Morbidity at the donor site is still the main disadvantage. Ramus and calvarium are the sites with less morbidity, compared with the chin and the iliac crest. The use of allografts or xenografts combined with a titanium-reinforced membrane is the alternative treatment option.

Resorption of the block grafts is one of the most discussed points. Resorption rates of 20% for lateral augmentation and up to 40% in the vertical dimension have been described in the literature for cortical intraoral grafts. Resorption rates of up to 60% are described in the literature with corticocancellous bone grafts.

Wearing a removable denture with mucosal support will increase the risk of resorption of the graft.

For extraoral donor sites like the iliac crest, hospitalization needs make the procedure time-consuming and expensive.

9.6.4 Extraoral donor sites

Calvarium

Calvarium is an excellent source of membranous bone and it has very low morbidity, but its major drawback is that patients are often difficult to convince to undergo this surgical technique.

Surgical technique

Under general anesthesia, an incision is performed in the parietal area and a full thickness flap is raised. Ostectomy is performed using piezoelectric surgery and several rectangular cortical bone blocks are obtained. To prevent complications, the blocks must be obtained preserving the internal cortical integrity at all times and good hemostasis is needed (Figs 9-46 and 9-47).

Iliac crest

When large amounts of bone are needed for a complex reconstruction, the iliac crest is the best option (see Case 5, Figs 9-48 to 9-59). Severe maxillary, mandibular, or combined atrophies are the main indication for this donor site. Bone obtained from this area has a large amount of cancellous bone and a relatively thin cortical plate. Resorption rate is more pronounced than in blocks from cranial sites. General anesthesia and hospitalization are needed, thus increasing the costs of the procedure. The main complications of this technique are pain and transient alteration of deambulation for a considerable amount of time.

Surgical technique

Two separate surgical fields are needed to perform this procedure: the intraoral and the extraoral. While the recipient site is exposed, access to the donor site in the iliac crest is performed. Detailed aspects of this intervention exceed the aim of this chapter and other sources must be consulted.

As a general description of the procedure, an incision to the anterior aspect of the iliac crest is created to expose the bone. The antero-superior iliac spine, the crest, and the tubercle of the crest should be localized in order to perform the incision, no longer than 5 cm in order not to damage the femorocutaneous nerve. Hemostasis is needed throughout the procedure. Careful dissection of the muscles attached is done to expose the bone. At this point, there are two techniques to obtain bone blocks: the trap door and the split techniques.

Once the desired blocks are obtained, hemostasis and drainage is recommended. Abdominal muscles, fat, and fascia are sutured in layers with resorbable materials, followed by the subcutaneous cellular tissue. Continuous intradermic suture is performed in the skin layer.

9.6.5 Intraoral donor sites

Ramus and body of the mandible (retromolar area donor site)

Since the ramus and body of the mandible is an intraoral area with very low morbidity, this donor site is becoming very popular (see Case 6, Figs 9-60 to 9-75).[27] The piezoelectric device makes it easier to obtain a graft than previously possible with conventional and dangerous rotating instruments.[28,29] Moderate to severe atrophy and a segment of the arch of up to four teeth are the main indications. A cone-beam computed tomographic (CBCT) scan is recommended to evaluate the anatomy (thickness, safety margins to the mandibular canal, etc).

Surgical technique

The limits of the donor site are the coronoid process, the mandibular canal, the molar teeth, and the width of the posterior mandible.[30]

The mandibular body is the most anterior harvest site, located lateral to the first and second mandibular molars. The ramus has maximum thickness in contact with the ramus and the body. Piezosurgery is a key instrument when performing the osteotomies to avoid damaging the soft tissues such as blood vessels and nerves.

Several incisions have been described:

- Intrasulcular incision from the distal line angle of the second premolar and extending posteriorly lateral to the retromolar pad and medial to the external oblique ridge.
- Submarginal incision along the mucogingival line with a posterior extension as in the previous case.
- Crestal incision made in edentulous ridges or when implants are planned in the same edentulous crest.
- Under local anesthesia, intrasulcular and crestal incisions are performed and a full thickness flap is raised. Care should be taken to protect the mental nerve in the anterior area.

Bone grafts can be harvested with drills, trephines, or piezoelectric surgery. Piezoelectric devices are a good option: they minimize the risk of damaging nerves and simplify the lower horizontal bone cut thanks to an angulated insertion. They also provide a clean operating area with profuse irrigation and the cavitation effect and extra illumination if equipped.

The block is removed with a chisel, and the holes for the screws must be made at this point with a handpiece and the suitable bur.

Hemostatic biomaterials are used to control bleeding before closure with monofilament 4/0 non-resorbable sutures.

Complications

Wound dehiscence, prolonged postoperative pain, hematoma infection, ptosis of chin, altered chin sensation, and altered pulpal sensitivity are some of the complications described when autogenous blocks are obtained.

Mandibular symphysis

Once considered one of the best intraoral sites from which to obtain corticocancellous bone blocks, the symphysis has several disadvantages compared with the retromolar area (Figs 9-76 to 9-78).[31] The access to the area is convenient; cortical and cancellous bone, along with cancellous chips, can be obtained. A CBCT scan is recommended to evaluate the anatomy (thickness, safety margins, etc.). Bone deficiencies of up to six teeth can be corrected using this area.

Surgical technique

With local anesthesia, a full mucoperiosteal flap is raised. Two different techniques have been proposed:

- With a no. 15 or 15c surgical blade, an intrasulcular incision is performed from teeth 33 to 43 in cases of dentate patients. Two vertical releasing incisions are then performed in the canine areas. Extending these releasing incisions distally can damage mental foramen nerve fibers and could cause mental nerve paresthesia.
- With a no. 15 or 15c scalpel, a submarginal incision of attached gingiva is performed with two releasing incisions in the canine area.

The first technique could be chosen in patients with a healthy periodontal status, reduced depth of the vestibule, and without fixed partial dentures showing the gingival margin. On the other hand, a submarginal incision should be performed in cases with a periodontally compromised patient with an appropriate depth of the vestibule.

Osteotomy design

Traditionally the "rule of fives" was used to avoid complications: a 5 mm safety margin to the mental foramina, to the apex of the mandibular teeth,[32] and to the inferior border of the mandible.

In recent studies, these safety margins have changed. Eight millimeters are recommended as a safety margin to the apex of mandibular teeth. Osteotomy should never be deeper than 4 mm to avoid damage to the incisal nerve and bleeding complications due to lingual cortex perforation.

Irrigation with cool sterile saline should be used whether piezoelectric or conventional instruments are used.

When the osteotomy has been performed, the block is loosened from the chin with a chisel. Before removing it from the site, the osteosynthesis screw holes should be drilled. At this point, the block is removed along with some cancellous chips if desired. Harvesting of cancellous chips should be performed with caution.

Collagen plugs or biomaterials along with a membrane might be used before suturing the muscular layer with a resorbable material and the mucosal layer.[33] If a one-layer technique is used, mattress sutures are recommended.

Complications

Ptosis of the chin and neurosensory disturbance are among the complications of using the mandibular symphysis as donor site.

9.6.6 Recipient sites

Good exposure of the recipient site can be obtained with a good mucoperiosteal flap. Lateral releasing incisions according to the surgical needs of the reconstruction should be made. The area must be cleared of any granulation or periosteal tissues. The autogenous block is presented and adapted to the recipient site.

Small perforations or decortication of the recipient wall are recommended to improve vascularization of the graft. A new perforation should be made through the block into the recipient site for the placement of a compression osteosynthesis screw. The block should be stable and with close contact to the pristine bone. If there is any movement of the autogenous graft, additional screws must be placed. Self-tapping ostheosynthesis screws usually do not need this kind of drilling when the cortical plate is thin.

The sharp edges of the block should be rounded and modeled with a bur or piezoelectric device. Then the gaps are filled with autogenous bone chips or bone substitutes and covered with a collagen membrane. Periosteal releasing incisions should be performed to facilitate a tension-free closure of the wound. Monofilament 4/0 nonresorbable sutures are recommended. Antibiotic, antiseptic, and anti-inflammatory medications should be prescribed.[34] The patient should be instructed not to use a removable denture during the healing period. Sutures must be removed 7 to 10 days after the surgery.

9.6.7 When should implants be placed?

If corticocancellous blocks from the iliac crest are performed, the reentry surgery to place the implants should take place 3 to 4 months after the grafting procedure. If cortical blocks from the calvarium or the mandible are placed, the consolidation period can be from 4 to 6 months.[35]

Implant insertion must be performed using the protocol for dense or cortical bone (including thread formation and profile drills), to prevent the fracture or detachment of the block graft.

9.7 Clinical cases

Case 1 (Figs 9-17 to 9-26)

The patient was a 60-year-old woman, with a completely edentulous maxilla. Class V Cawood and Howell atrophy with an arch defect in the first quadrant that needs to be level. Split Le-Fort I plus inlay autogenous bone block grafting was performed, with prosthetic metal-ceramic rehabilitation.

Figs 9-17 to 9-26 Case 1

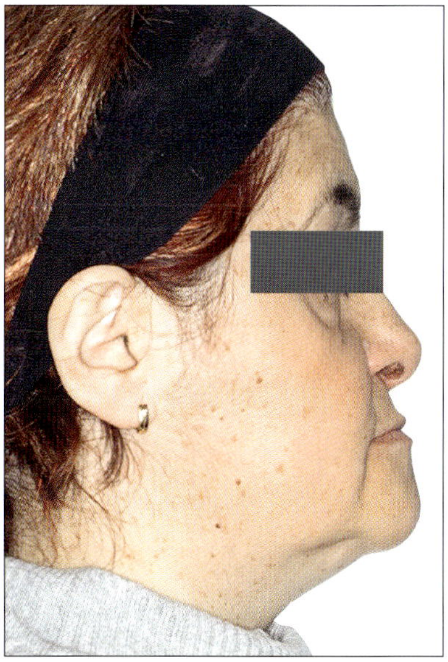

Fig 9-17 Cawood and Howell[1] class VI maxillary atrophy with oral and facial failure.

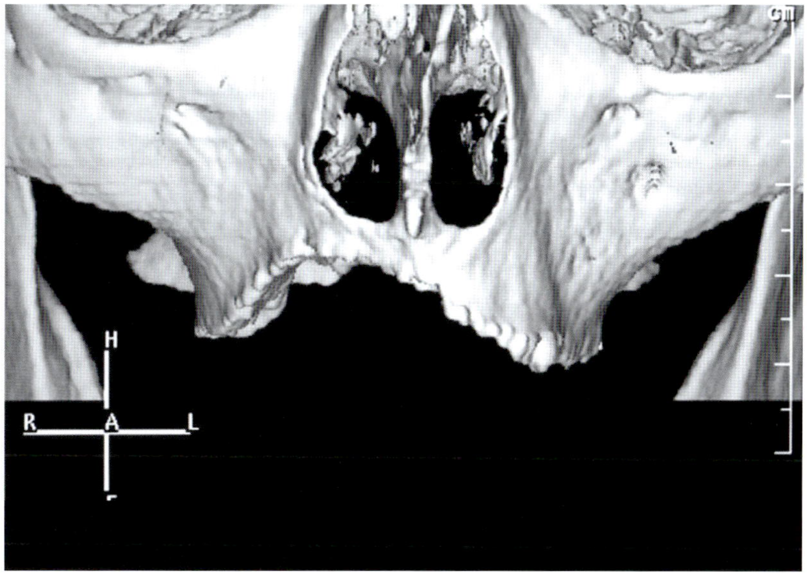

Fig 9-18 Three-dimensional image of maxillary atrophy.

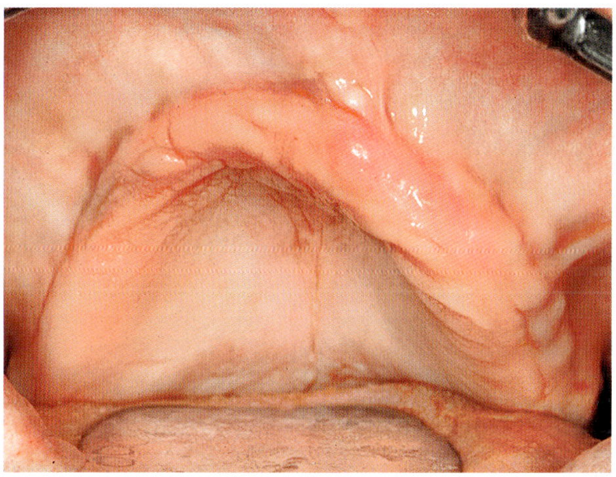

Fig 9-19 Clinical preoperative occlusal view of maxillary atrophy.

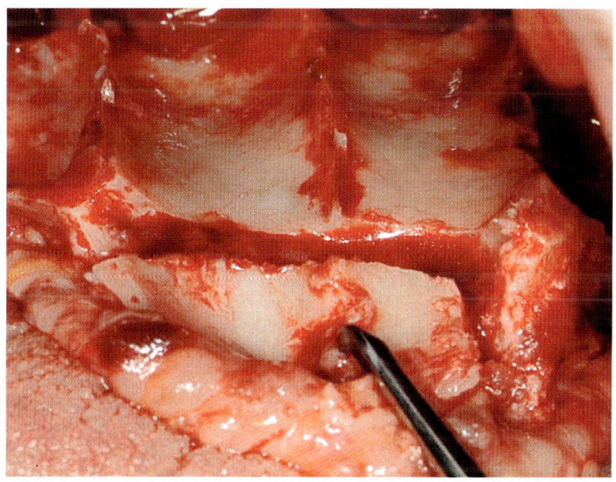

Fig 9-20 Split Le Fort I.

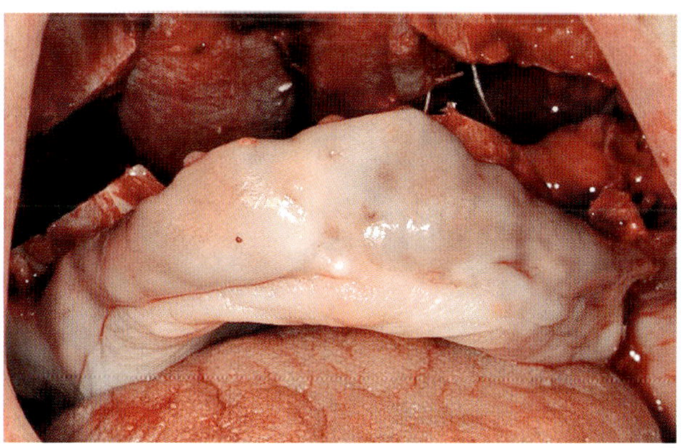

Fig 9-21 Anterior and inferior repositioning of the maxilla to normalize interarch relationships.

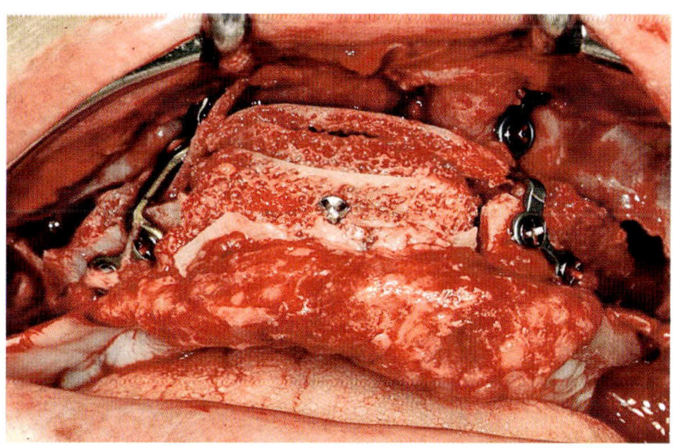

Fig 9-22 Maxillary down-fracture plus interpositional iliac crest bone block grafts.

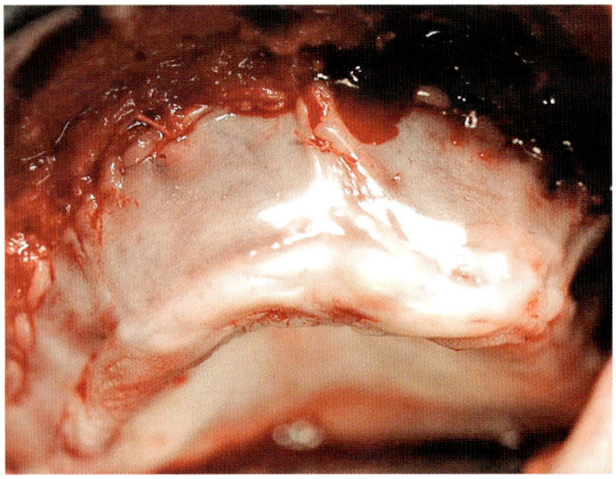

Fig 9-23 Vestibuloplasty.

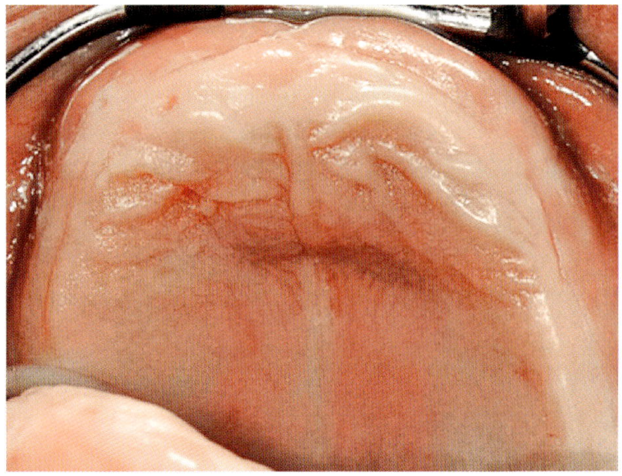

Fig 9-24 Postoperative occlusal view.

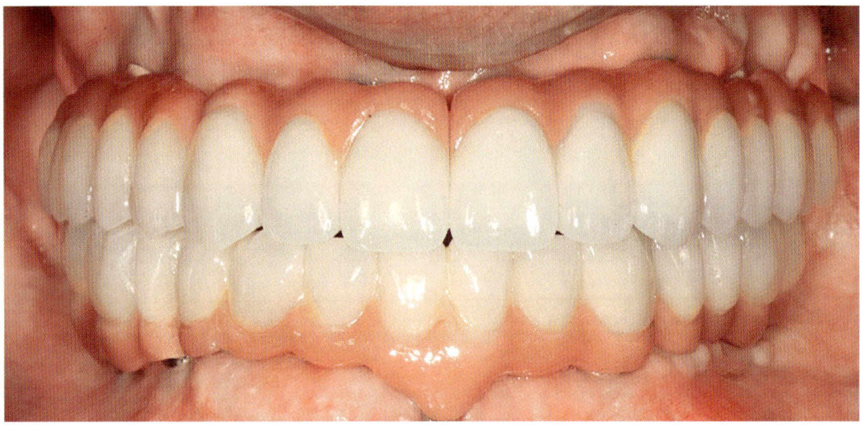

Fig 9-25 Anterior view of prosthetic rehabilitation.

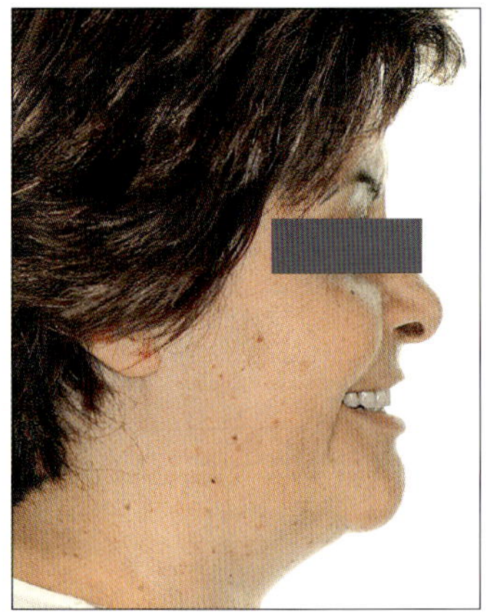

Fig 9-26 Restoration of facial harmony.

Figs 9-27 to 9-35 Case 2

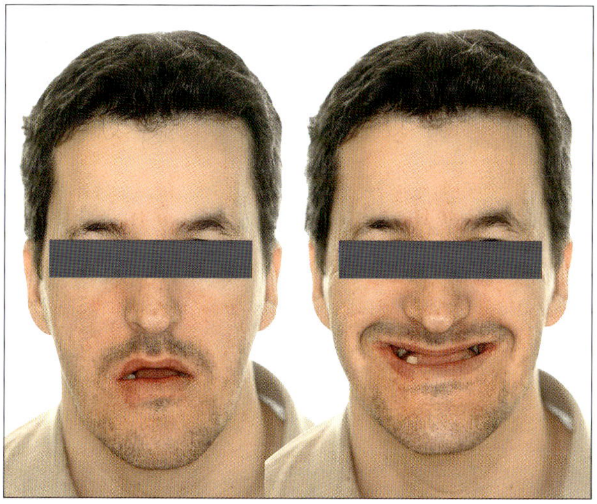

Fig 9-27 Class III skeletal relationship with edentulism and intermaxillary bone atrophy.

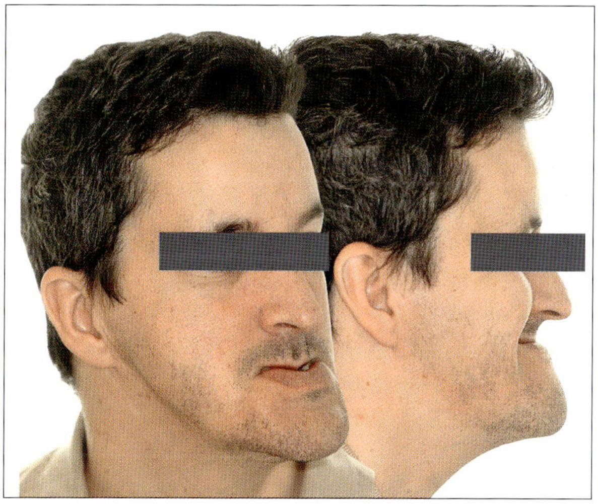

Fig 9-28 Class III skeletal relationship with edentulism and intermaxillary bone atrophy.

Case 2 (Figs 9-27 to 9-35)

The patient was a 43-year-old man, with a Class III skeletal relationship with edentulism and intermaxillary bone atrophy. Bimaxillary orthognathic surgery with maxillary advancement, mandibular set back, and simultaneous bone reconstruction was performed, with implant placement at the second stage.

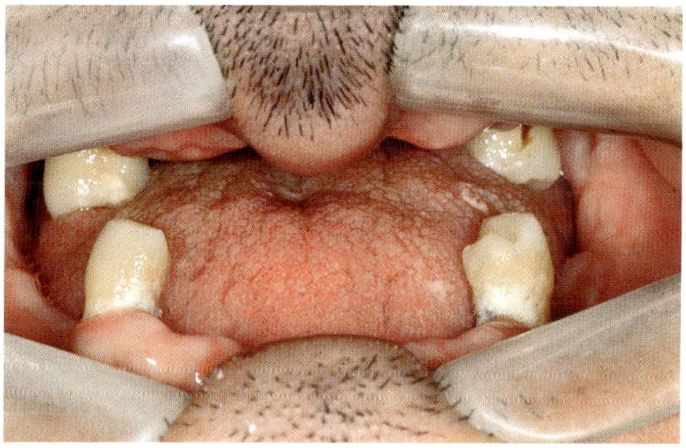

Fig 9-29 Anterior view showing bone atrophy and edentulism.

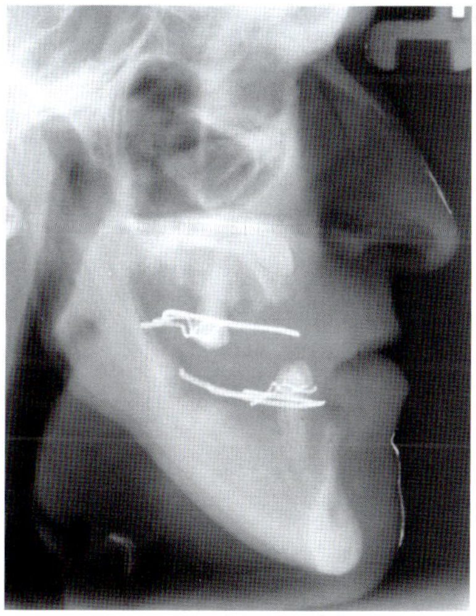

Fig 9-30 Lateral cephalometry showing skeletal class III, bone atrophy, and edentulism.

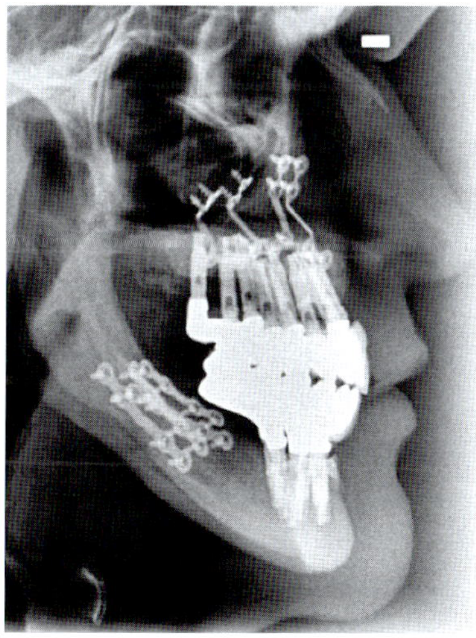

Fig 9-31 Bimaxillary orthognathic surgery with maxillary advancement, mandibular set back, and simultaneous bone reconstruction. Implant placement at second stage.

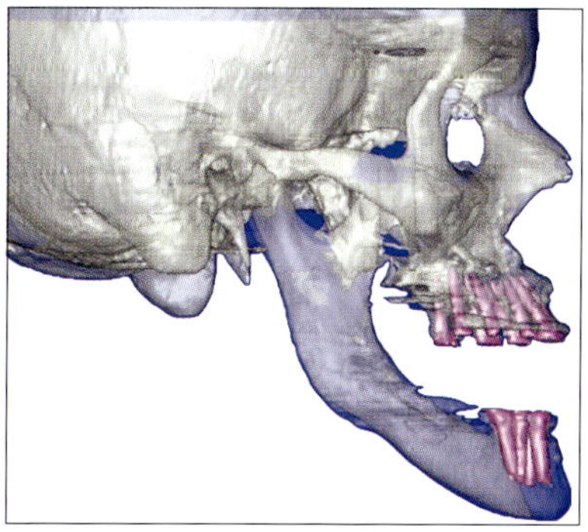

Fig 9-32 Three-dimensional reconstruction of bimaxillary orthognathic surgery and implant placement.

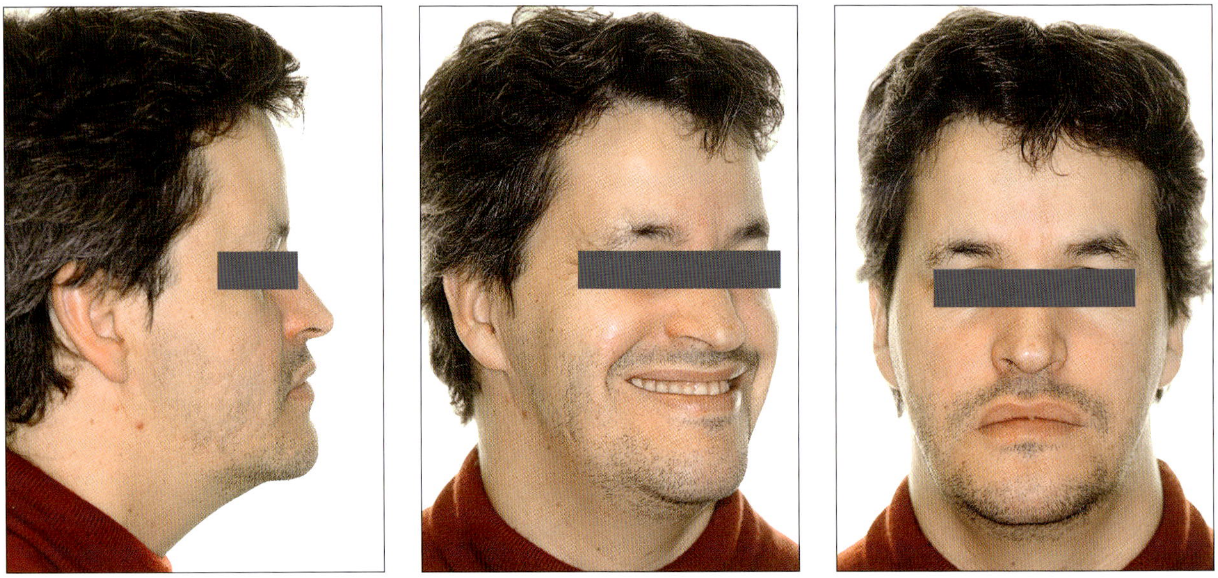

Fig 9-33 to 9-35 Facial and oral rehabilitation.

Case 3 (Figs 9-36 to 9-42)

The patient was a 52-year-old woman, with atrophy of the maxilla after multiple surgeries in childhood. Treatment was placement of two bilateral zygomatic implants plus two pterygoid implants, with an implant-retained removable prosthesis.

Figs 9-36 to 9-42 Case 3

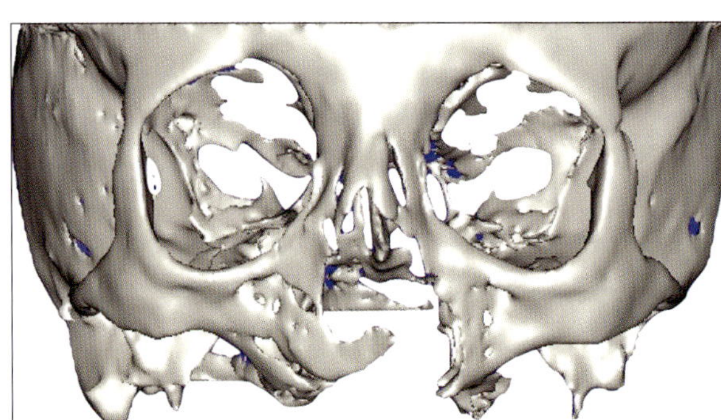

Fig 9-36 Maxilla vanishing after multiple surgeries in childhood.

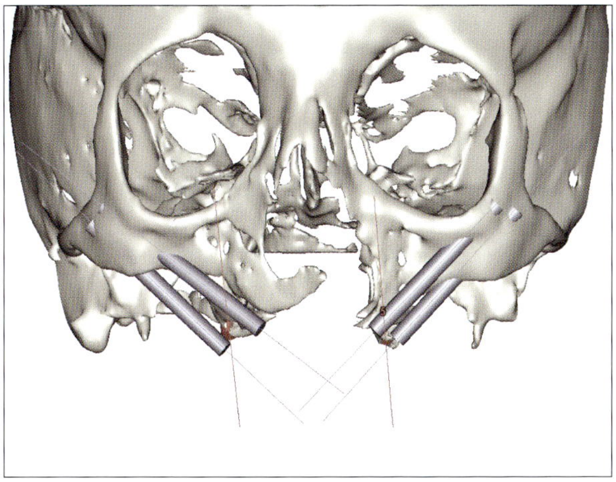

Fig 9-37 Three-dimensional planning of four zygomatic and two pterygoid implants. Anterior view.

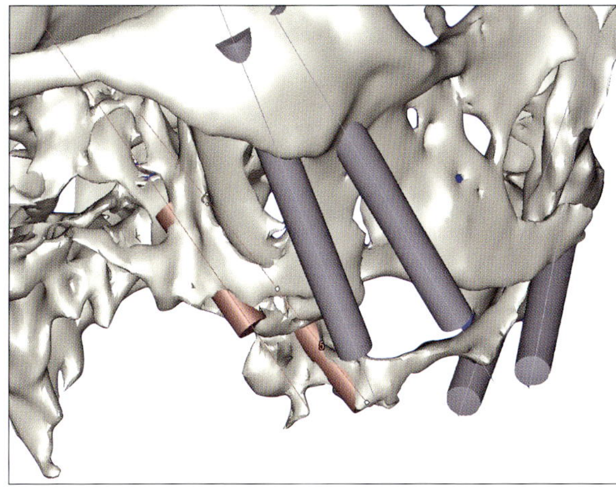

Fig 9-38 Three-dimensional planning of four zygomatic and two pterygoid implants. Lateral view.

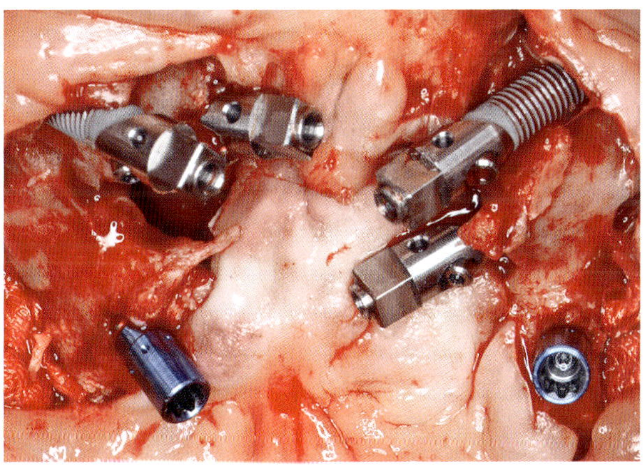

Fig 9-39 Clinical intraoperative occlusal view showing four zygomatic and two pterygoid implants.

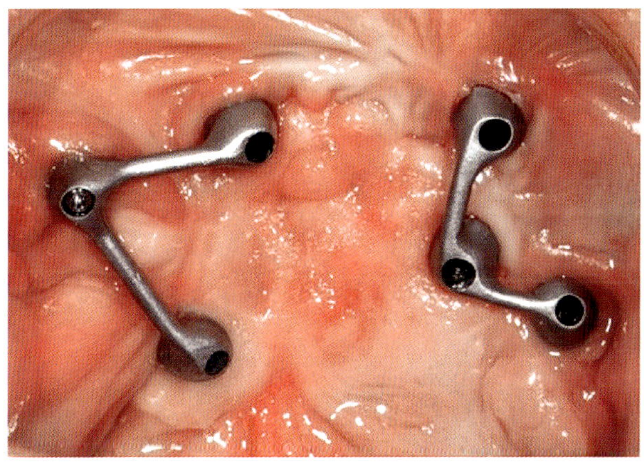

Fig 9-40 Prosthetic rehabilitation with removable overdenture.

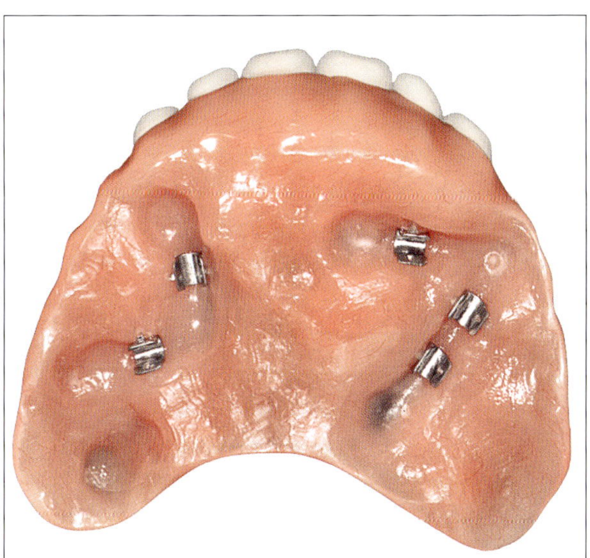

Fig 9-41 Prosthetic rehabilitation with removable overdenture.

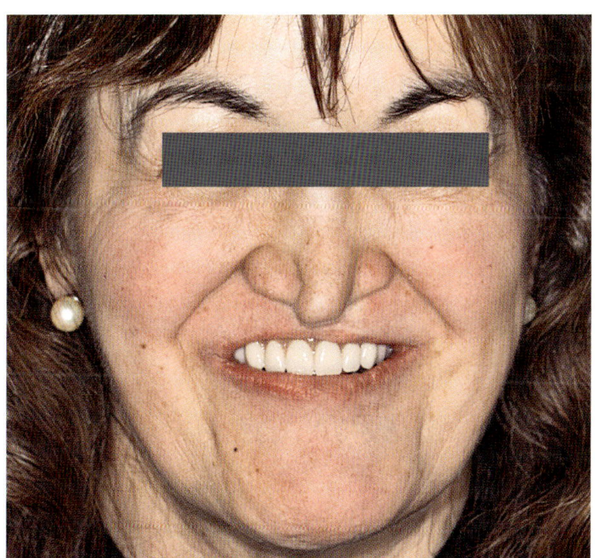

Fig 9-42 Facial and oral rehabilitation.

Case 4 (Fig 9-43 to 9-45)

Pterygoid implant drilling, length measuring, and implant placement.

Fig 9-43 to 9-45 Case 4

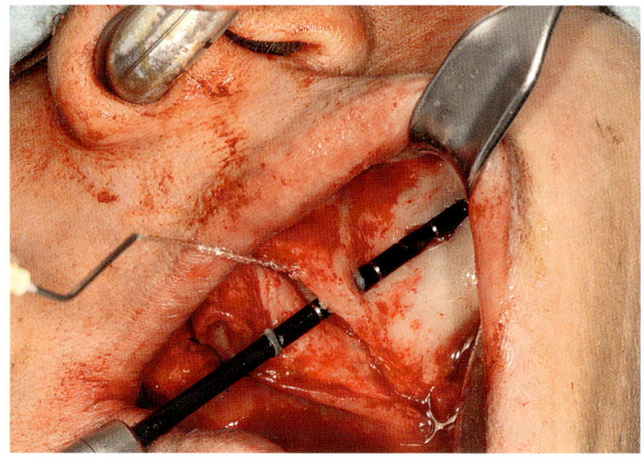

Fig 9-43 Drilling a zygomatic implant.

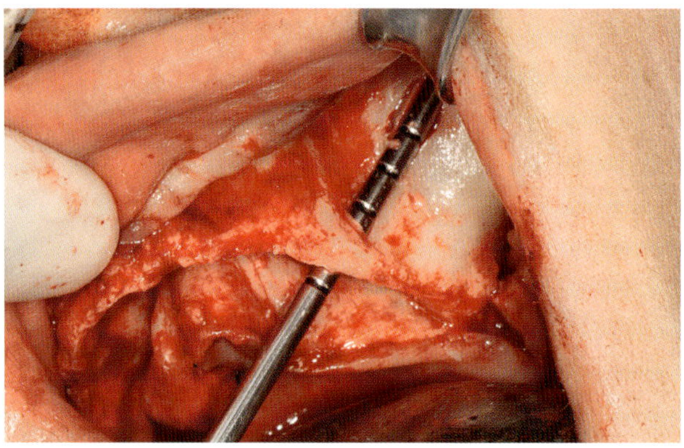

Fig 9-44 Zygomatic implant depth measurement.

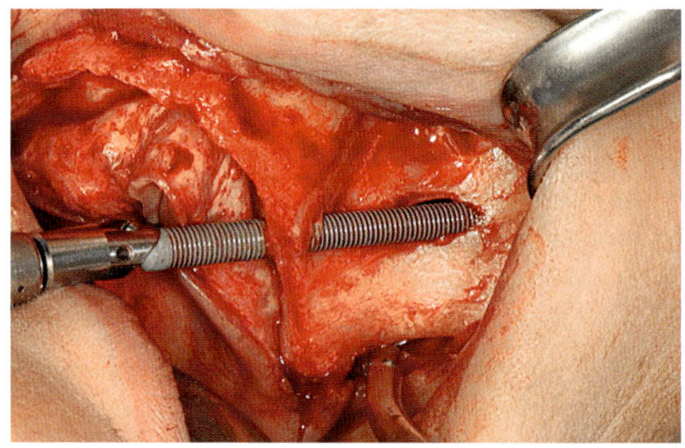

Fig 9-45 Placing a zygomatic implant.

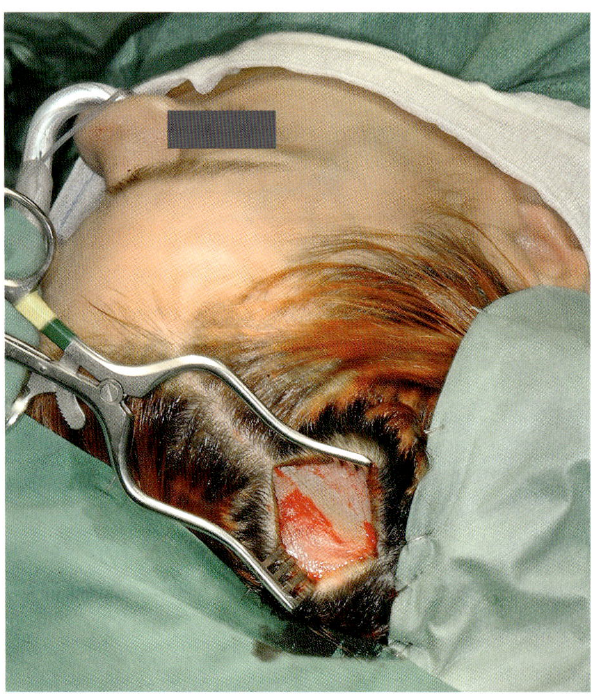

Fig 9-46 Calvaria approach.

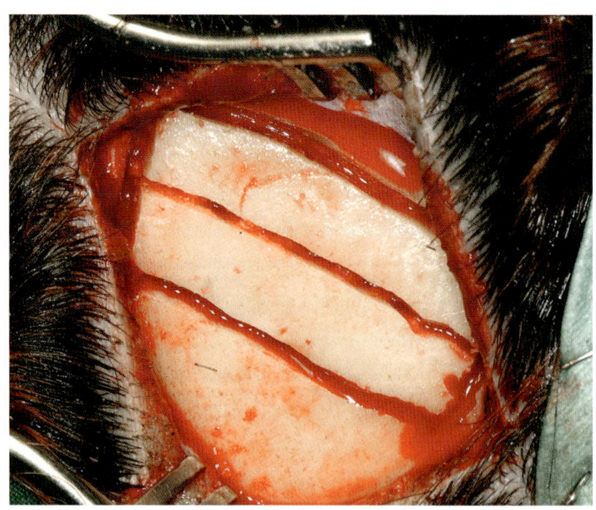

Fig 9-47 Osteotomies delimiting calvaria block grafts.

Case 5 (Figs 9-48 to 9-59)

The patient presented with Cawood and Howell's Class IV maxillary atrophy. Reconstruction was with onlay iliac crest corticocancellous bone blocks covered with collagen membranes.

Figs 9-48 to 9-59 Case 5

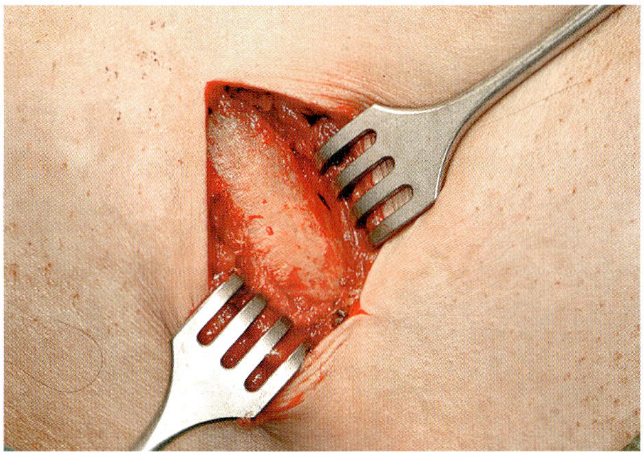

Fig 9-48 Iliac crest approach.

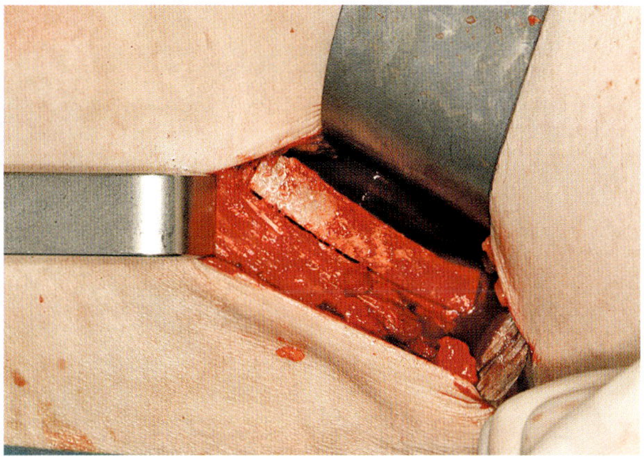

Fig 9-49 Osteotomies delimiting Iliac crest block grafts.

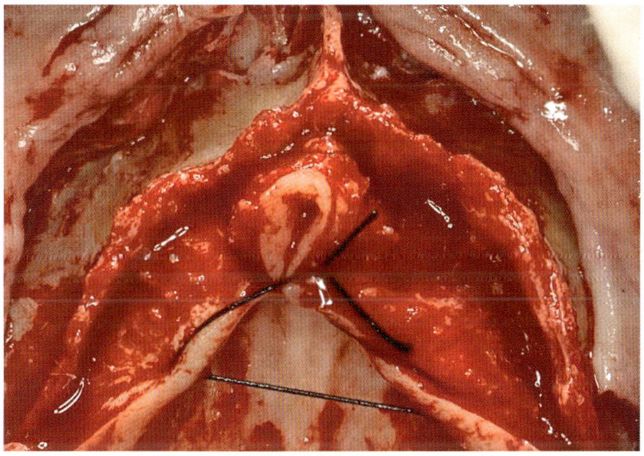

Fig 9-50 Cawood and Howell's[1] Class IV maxillary atrophy. Occlusal view.

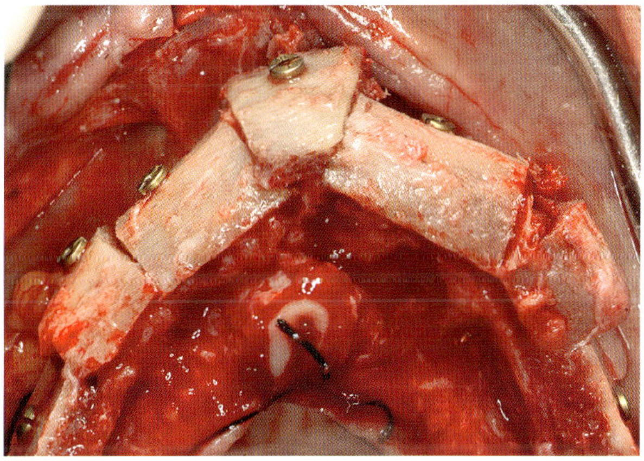

Fig 9-51 Reconstruction with onlay corticocancellous blocks covered with collagen membranes. Occlusal view.

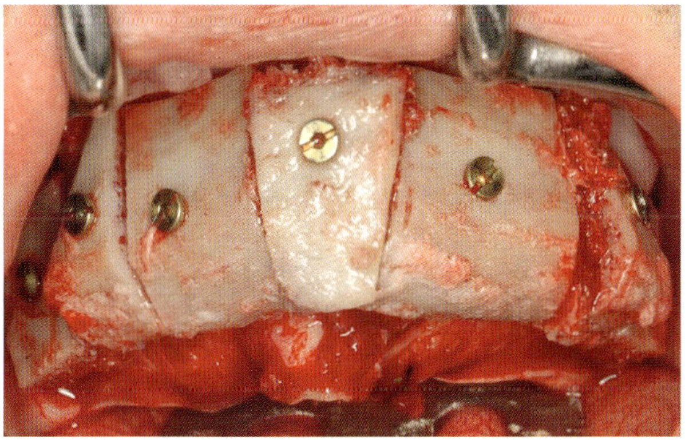

Fig 9-52 Reconstruction with onlay corticocancellous blocks covered with collagen membranes. Anterior view.

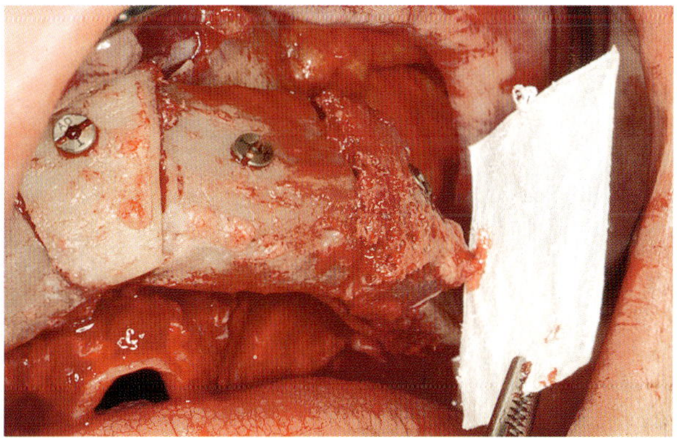

Fig 9-53 Reconstruction with onlay corticocancellous blocks covered with collagen membranes. Facing the membrane.

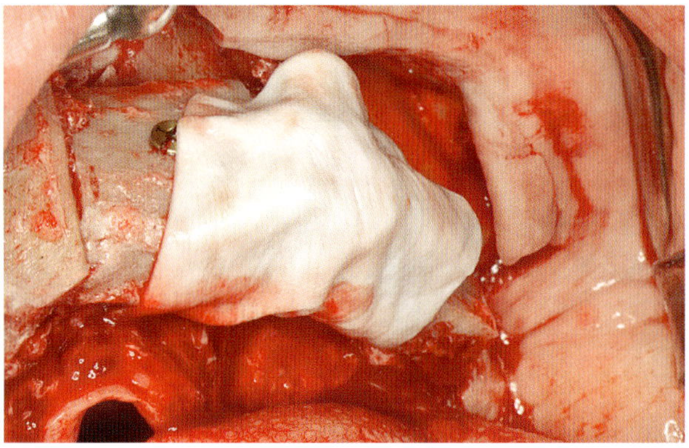

Fig 9-54 Reconstruction with onlay corticocancellous blocks covered with collagen membranes. Membrane adapted.

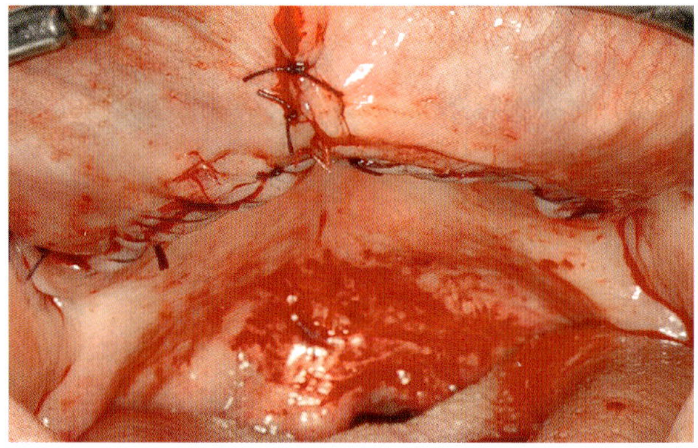

Fig 9-55 Reconstruction with onlay corticocancellous blocks covered with collagen membranes. Tension-free wound suture.

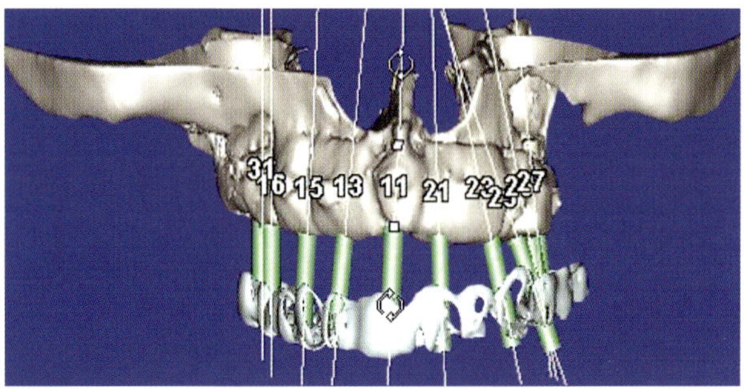

Fig 9-56 CAD/CAM (computer-aided design/computer-aided manufacturing) splint guided implant surgery at 4 months. Anterior view.

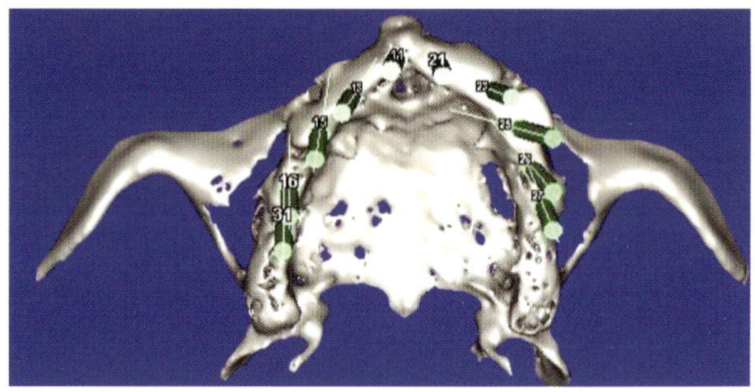

Fig 9-57 CAD/CAM (computer-aided design/computer-aided manufacturing) splint guided implant surgery at 4 months. Occlusal view.

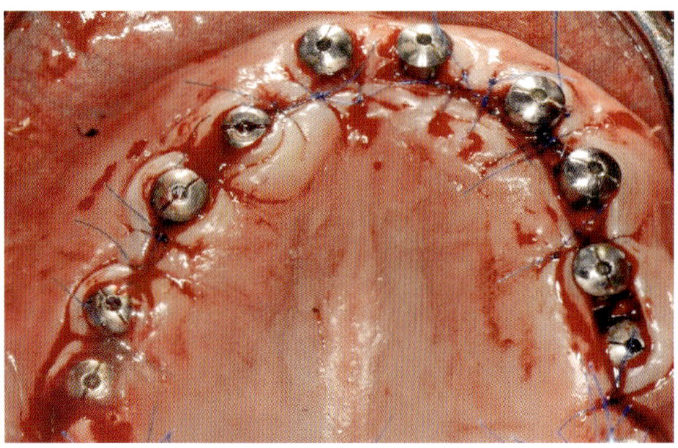

Fig 9-58 Implant placement at 4 months after integration of bone blocks.

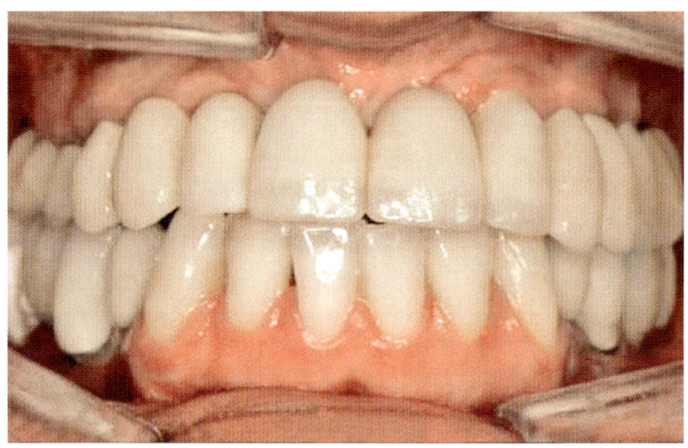

Fig 9-59 Metal-ceramic prosthetic rehabilitation.

Case 6 (Figs 9-60 to 9-75)

The patient presented with Cawood and Howell Class V maxillary atrophy. Treatment was by horizontal and vertical reconstruction of the anterior maxilla with bilateral autogenous bone block from the mandibular ramus/body, xenografts, and collagen membranes. Implant placement took place at the second stage.

Figs 9-60 to 9-75 Case 6

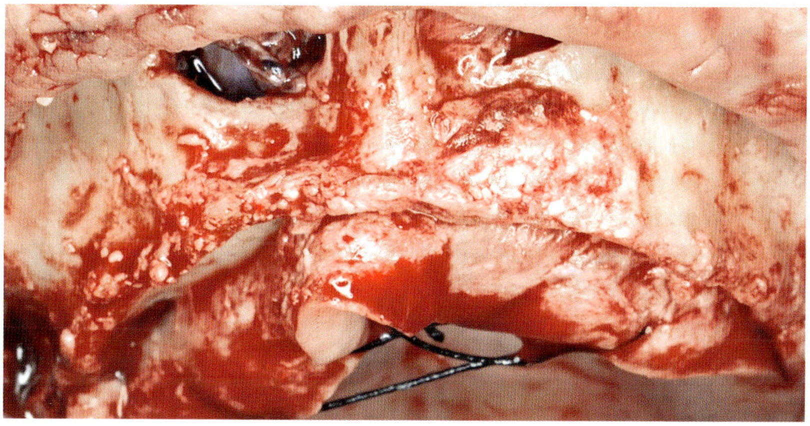

Fig 9-60 Cawood and Howell[1] class V maxillary atrophy.

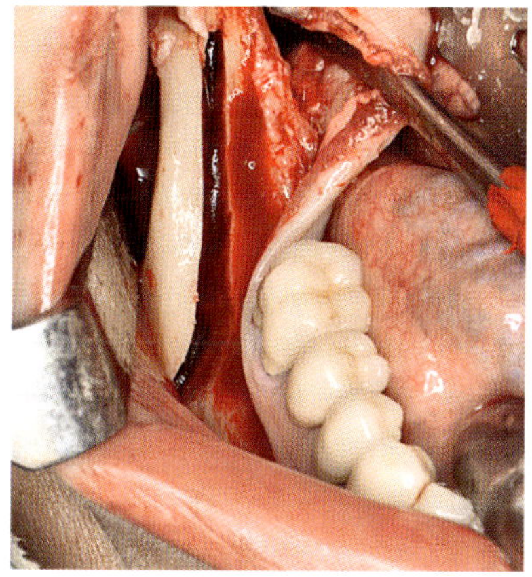

Fig 9-61 Intraoral harvesting of autogenous blocks from the right mandibular ramus/body.

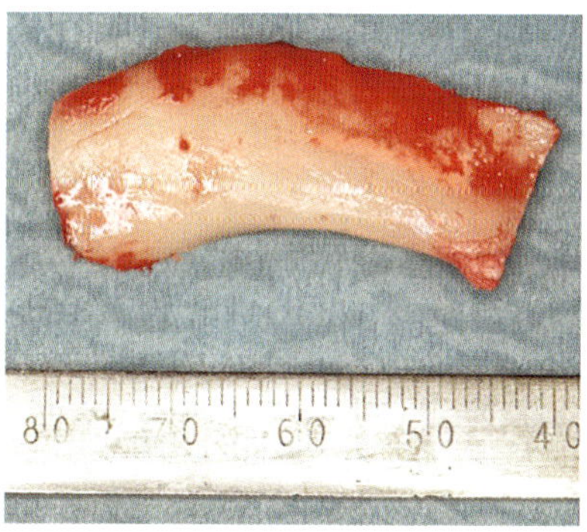

Fig 9-62 Autogenous bone block graft extracted from the mandibular ramus.

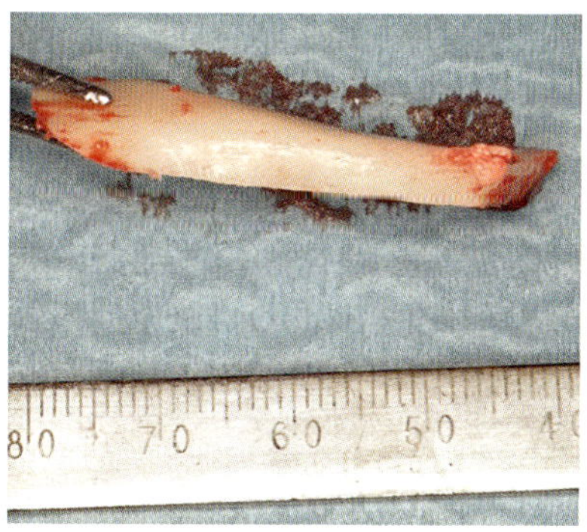

Fig 9-63 Autogenous bone block graft extracted from the mandibular ramus.

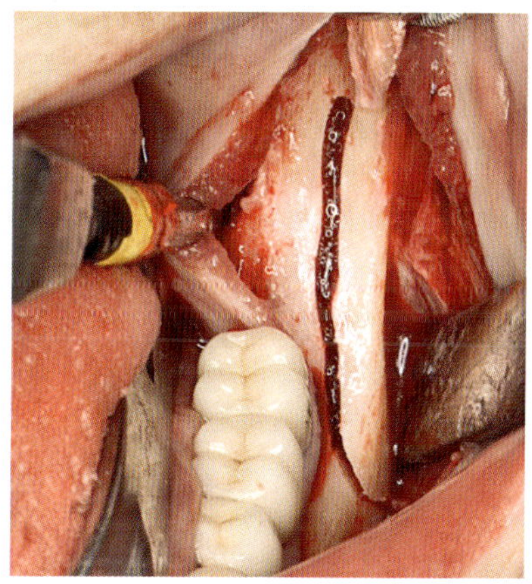

Fig 9-64 Intraoral harvesting of autogenous bone block from the left mandibular ramus.

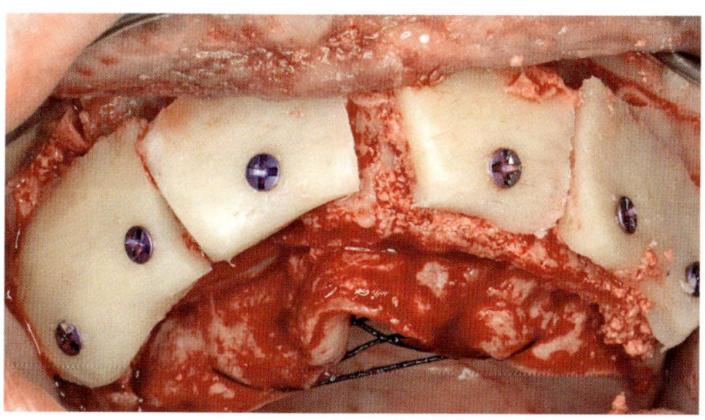

Fig 9-65 Horizontal and vertical reconstruction of the anterior maxilla with blocks, xenografts, and collagen membranes. Anterior view.

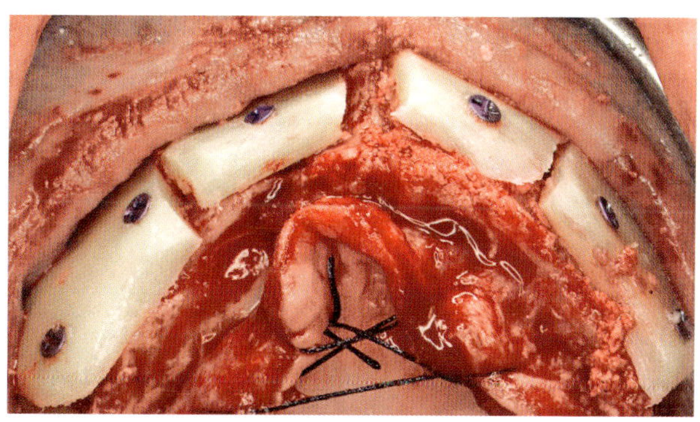

Fig 9-66 Horizontal and vertical reconstruction of the anterior maxilla with blocks, xenografts, and collagen membranes. Occlusal view.

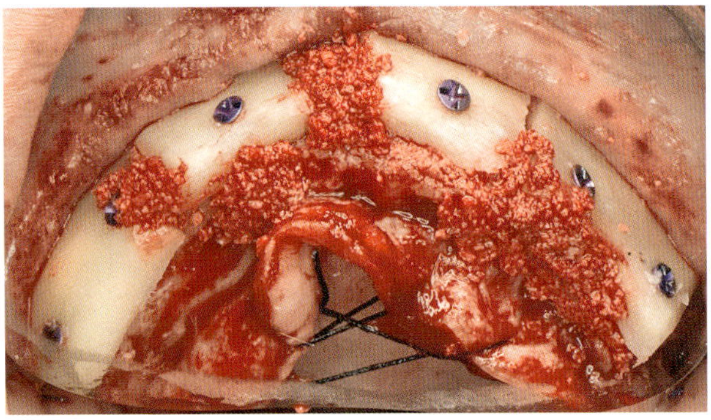

Fig 9-67 Horizontal and vertical reconstruction of the anterior maxilla with blocks, xenografts, and collagen membranes: filling of the gaps.

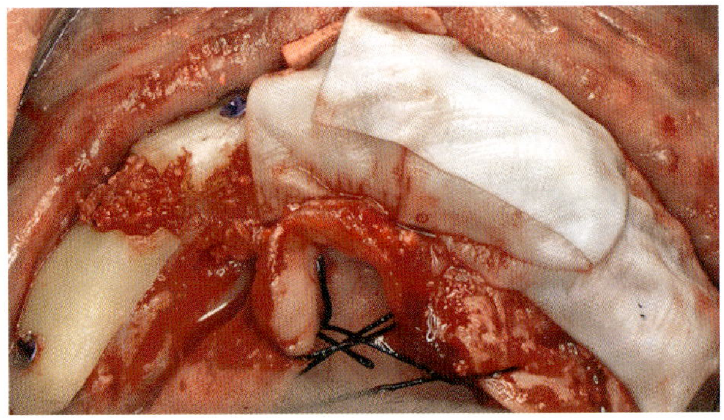

Fig 9-68 Horizontal and vertical reconstruction of the anterior maxilla with blocks, xenografts, and collagen membranes: placing the membrane.

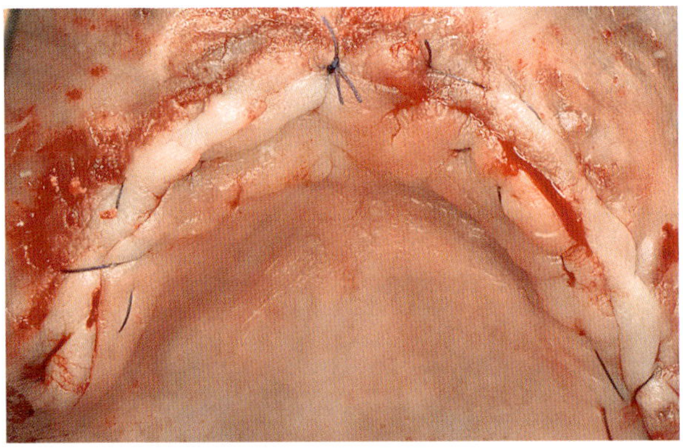

Fig 9-69 Horizontal and vertical reconstruction of the anterior maxilla with blocks, xenografts, and collagen membranes: suturing the wound.

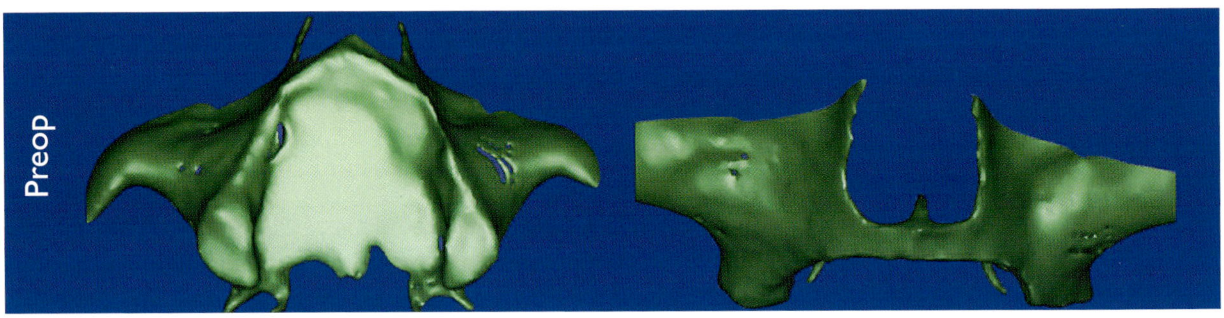

Fig 9-70 Preoperative three-dimensional reconstruction.

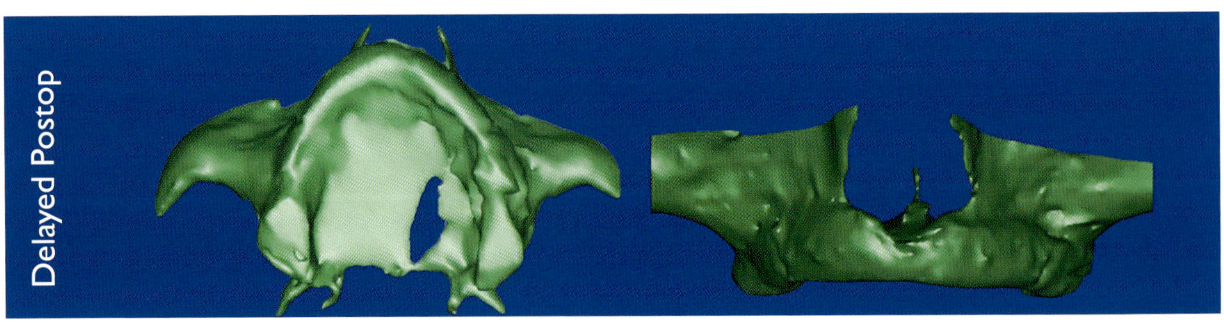

Fig 9-71 Postoperative three-dimensional reconstruction.

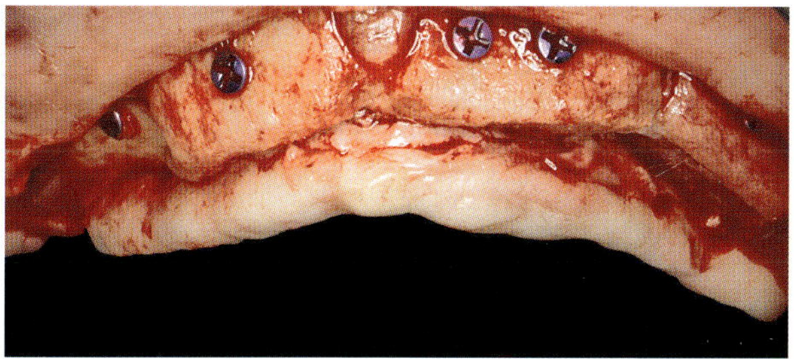

Fig 9-72 Surgical anterior view of incorporated block grafts.

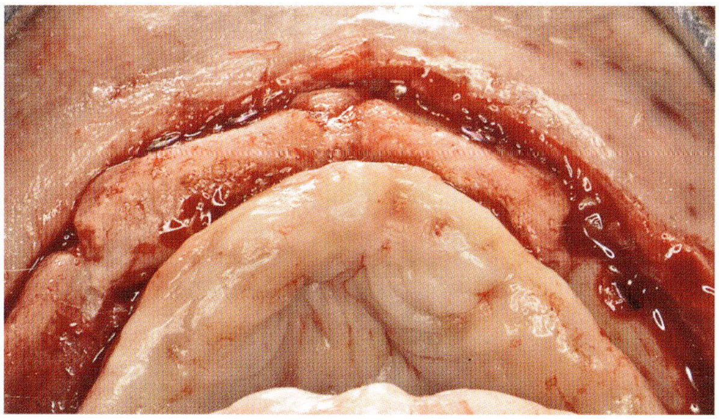

Fig 9-73 Surgical occlusal view of incorporated block grafts.

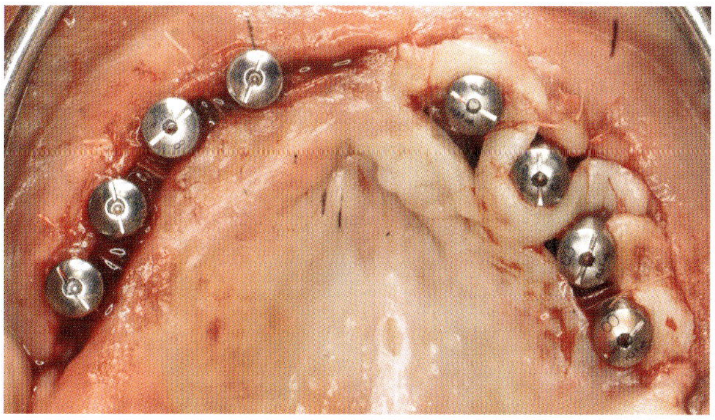

Fig 9-74 Implant placement at 4 months' osseointegration.

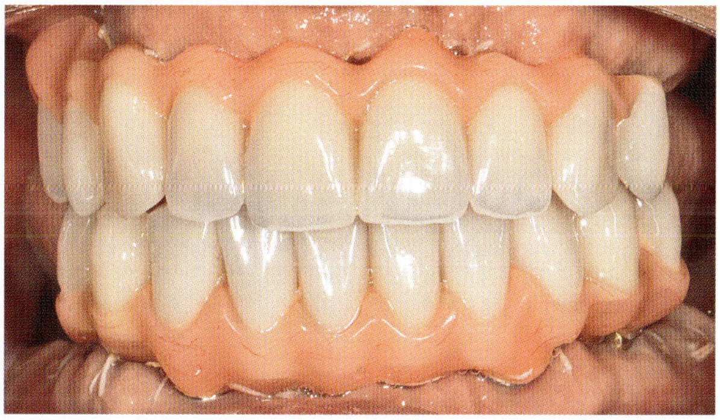

Fig 9-75 Clinical anterior view of prosthetic rehabilitation.

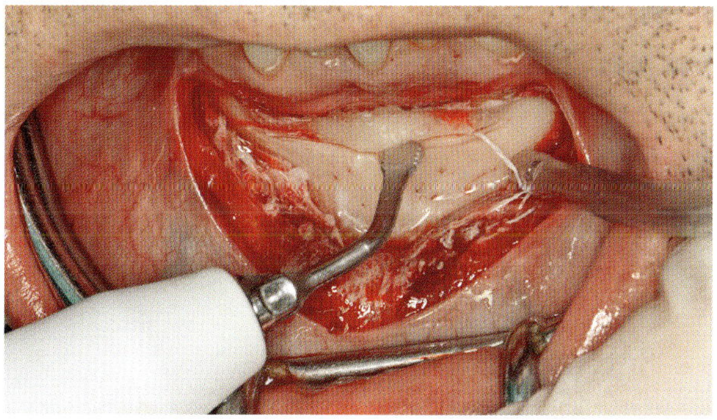

Fig 9-76 Clinical view of the mandibular symphysis as the bone grafting donor area. A piezoelectric device was used to create the osteotomies for block bone grafting.

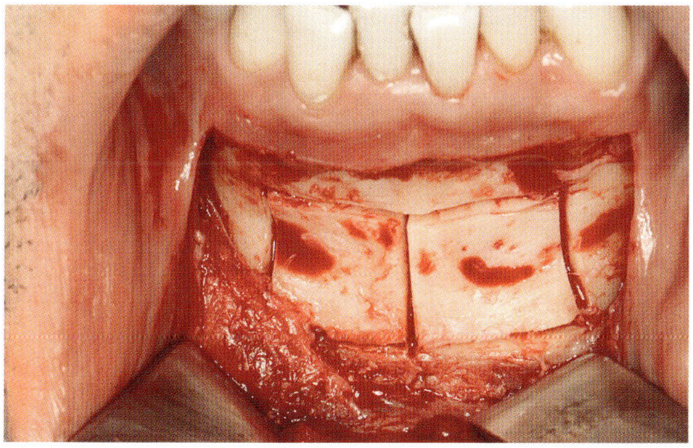

Fig 9-77 Two bone blocks from the mandibular symphysis ready to be extracted.

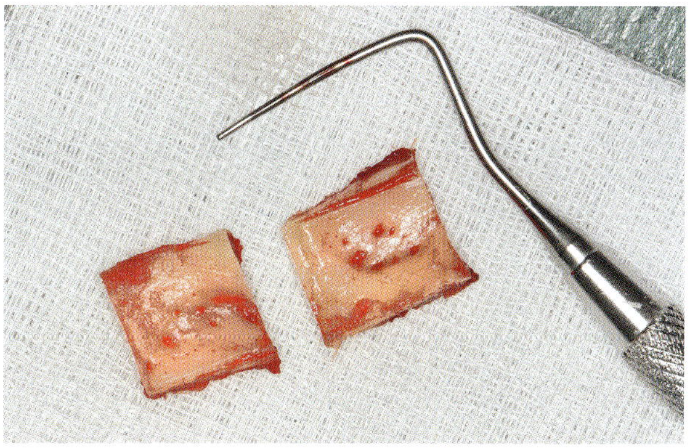

Fig 9-78 Two bone blocks from the mandibular symphysis.

References

1. Cawood JI, Howell RA. A classification of edentulous jaws. Int J Oral Maxillofac Surg 1988;17:232-236.
2. Hatano N, Shimizu Y, Ooya K. A clinical long-term radiographic evaluation of graft height changes after maxillary sinus floor augmentation with a 2:1 autogenous bone/xenograft mixture and simultaneous placement of dental implants. Clin Oral Implants Res 2004;15:339-345.
3. Tarnow DP, Wallace SS, Froum SJ, Rohrer MD, Cho SC. Histologic and clinical comparison of bilateral sinus floor elevations with and without barrier membrane placement in 12 patients: part 3 of an ongoing prospective study. Int J Periodontics Restorative Dent 2000;20:116-125.
4. Fugazzotto PA, Vlassis J. Long-term success of sinus augmentation using various surgical approaches and grafting materials. Int J Oral Maxillofac Implants 1998;13:52-58.
5. Tatum H Jr. Maxillary and sinus implant reconstruction. Dent Clin North Am 1986;30:207-229.
6. Boyne PJ, James RA. Grafting of the maxillary sinus floor with autogenous marrow and bone. J Oral Surg 1980;38:613-616.
7. Lund V. The evolution of surgery on the maxillary sinus for chronic rhinosinusitis. Laryngoscope 2002;112:415-419.
8. Underwood AS. An inquiry into the anatomy and pathology of the maxillary sinus. J Anat Physiol 1910;44:354.
9. Kim MJ, Jung UW, Kim CS, Choi SH, Kim CK, Cho KS. Maxillary sinus septa: prevalence, height, location, and morphology. A reformatted computed tromography scan analysis. J Periodontol 2006;77: 903-908.
10. Ulm CW, Solar P, Krennmair G, Matejka M, Watzek G. Incident and suggested surgical management of septa in sinus-lift procedures. Int J Oral Maxillofac Implants 1995;10:462-465.
11. Fugazzotto PA, Vlassis J. A simplified classification and repair system for sinus membrane perforations.J Periodontol 2003;74:1534-1541.
12. Hernández Alfaro F, Torradeflot MM, Marti C. Prevalence and management of Schneiderian membrane perforations during sinus-lift procedures. Clin Oral Implants Res 2008;19:91-98.
13. Tawil G, Mawla M. Sinus floor elevation using a bovine bone mineral (Bio-Oss) with or without the concomitant use of a bilayered collagen barrier (Bio-Gide): a clinical report of immediate and delayed implant placement. Int J Oral Maxillofac Implants 2001;16:713-721.
14. Peleg M, Mazor Z, Garg AK. Augmentation grafting of the maxillary sinus and simultaneous implant placement in patients with 3 to 5 mm of residual alveolar bone height. Int J Oral Maxillofac Implants 1999;14:549-556.
15. van den Bergh JP, ten Bruggenkate CM, Disch FJ, Tuinzing DB. Anatomical aspects of sinus floor elevations.Oral Implants Res 2000;11:256-265.
16. Chiapasco M, Brusati R, Ronchi P. Le Fort I osteotomy with interpositional bone grafts and delayed oral implants for the rehabilitation of extremely atrophied maxillae: a 1–9-year clinical follow-up study on humans. Clin Oral Implants Res 2007;18:74-85.
17. Stoelinga PJ, Slagter AP, Brouns JJ .Rehabilitation of patients with severe (Class VI) maxillary resorption using Le Fort I osteotomy, interposed bone grafts and endosteal implants: 1–8 years follow-up on a two-stage procedure. Int J Oral Maxillofac Surg 2000;29:188-193.
18. Malevez C, Abarca M, Durdu F, Daelemans P. Clinical outcome of 103 consecutive zygomatic implants: A 6–48 months following up study. Clin Oral Implants Res 2004;15:18-22.
19. Bedrossian E, Stumpel LJ. Immediate stabilization at stage II of zygomatic implants: Rationale and technique. J Prosthet Dent 2001;86:10-14.
20. Boyes-Varley JG, Lownie JF, Howes DG. The zygomaticus implant protocol in the treatment of severely reabsorbed maxilla. SADJ 2003;58:106-114.
21. Stella JP, Warner MR. Sinus slot technique for simplification and improved orientation of zygomaticus dental implants: A technical note. Int J Oral Maxillofac Implants 2000;15:889-893.
22. Tulasne JF. Osseointegrated fixtures in the pterygoid region. In Worthington P, Branemark PI. Advanced osseointegration surgery, applications in the maxillofacial region. Chicago: Quintessence Publishing, 1992;23:182-188.
23. Balshi S, Wolfinger GJ, Balshi TJ. Analysis of 164 titanium oxide-surface implants in completely edentulous arches for fixed prosthesis anchorage using the pterygomaxillary region. Int J Oral Maxillofac Implants 2005;20:946-952.
24. Graves SL. The pterygoid plate implant: a solution for restoring the posterior maxilla. Int J Periodontics Restorative Dent 1994;14: 513-523.
25. Antoun H, Sitbon JM, Martinez H, Missika P. A prospective randomized study comparing two techniques of bone augmentation: onlay graft alone or associated with a membrane. Clin Oral Implants Res 2001;12:632-639.
26. Chiapasco M, Abati S, Romeo E, Vogel G. Clinical outcome of autogenous bone blocks or guided bone regeneration with e-PTFE membranes for the reconstruction of narrow edentulous ridges. Clin Oral Implants Res 1999:10:278-288.
27. Misch CM. Use of the mandibular ramus as a donor site for onlay bone grafting. J Oral Implantol 2000;26:42-49.
28. Happe A. Use of a piezoelectric surgical device to harvest bone grafts from the ramus: report of 40 cases. Int J Periodontics Restorative Dent 2007;27:241-249.
29. Sohn DS, Ahn MR, Lee WH, Yeo DS, Lim SY. Piezoelectric osteotomy for intraoral harvesting of bone blocks. Int J Periodontics Restorative Dent 2007;27:127-131.
30. Capelli M. Autogenous bone graft from the mandibular ramus: a technique for bone augmentation Int J Periodontics Restorative Dent 2003;23:277-285.
31. Cranin AN, Katzap M, Demirdjan E, Ley J. Autogenous bone ridge augmentation using the mandibular symphysis as a donor. J Oral Implantol 2001;27:43-47.
32. Pommer B, Tepper G, Gahleitner A, Zechner W, Watzek G. New safety margins for chin bone harvesting based on the course of the mandibular incisive canal in CT. Clin Oral Implants Res 2008;19:1312-1316.
33. Von Arx T, Buser D. Horizontal ridge augmentation using autogenous block grafts and the guided bone regeneration technique with collagen membranes: a clinical study with 42 patients. Clin Oral Implants Res 2006;17:359-366.
34. Lindeboom JA, van den Akker HP. A prospective placebo-controlled double-blind trial of antibiotic prophylaxis in intraoral bone grafting procedures: a pilot study. Oral Surg Oral Med Oral Pathol Oral Radiol Endod 2003;96:669-672.
35. Cordaro L, Torsello F, Morcavallo S, Mirisola di Torresanto V. Effect of bovine bone and collagen membranes on healing of mandibular bone blocks: a prospective randomized controlled study. Clin Oral Implants Res 2011;22:1145-1150.

Chapter 10

Is there a way to successfully manage the posterior atrophic mandible?

Eva Salvan Garcia, Victoria Sanchez D'Onofrio, Javier Mareque Bueno, Federico Hernández Alfaro

10.1 Introduction

In the adult patient, once teeth are lost, a continuous resorptive process in the mandible takes place, accelerated by denture wear. Diminished volume and strength of residual bone, loss of facial vertical dimension, impaired masticatory function, difficulty choosing a balanced diet, speech difficulties, and facial soft tissue changes take place as a result of advanced bone resorption.[1]

Reconstruction of severely atrophic mandible to restore oral function remains a difficult surgical and prosthetic challenge because of the minimal amount of residual bony support. In addition, the presence of the dental alveolar nerve increases the challenge, reducing the available bone for implant placement.

Many surgical techniques have been described in recent decades for volume augmentation; this wide spectrum often complicates treatment election. The aim of this chapter is to provide a decision-making guide for approaching each defect type. All the mentioned techniques are thoroughly explained, complications considered, and clinical examples of treated cases presented.

Vertical, horizontal, and combined defects require different approaches. A classification system seems essential. Several classification systems of alveolar ridge deformities have been proposed.[2,3] Seibert[2] introduced his widely used classification of ridge defects in 1983. In this classification, Class I defects represent buccolingual loss of tissue and normal apico-coronal ridge dimensions, Class II defects are those with apico-coronal loss of tissue and normal buccolingual ridge dimensions, while Class III defects represent a combination of both width and height deficiencies. Treatment options and predictability of outcomes were based on the type of defect present, with width deficiencies having more predictable results, and height and combination defects being less predictable.[2] Several modifications or different classifications have been proposed since 1983. All of them are based on the same divisions: vertical, horizontal, and combined defects.

Herein, we focus on the treatment options available, and how the choice is made between them. The description of each technique is focused on its application.

Vertical defect treatment options:

- Short implants (see Chapter 2).
- Guided bone regeneration (GBR; see Chapter 7).
- Onlay and inlay block grafting.
- Distraction osteogenesis (DO).
- Dental nerve mobilization.

Horizontal defect treatment options:

- Split crest.
- Onlay block grafting.
- GBR (see Chapter 7).
- Horizontal DO.

As short implants and GBR procedures have been extensively discussed in previous chapters, we will focus our attention on the other surgical approaches:

10.2 Onlay block grafting

10.2.1 Introduction

Sykoff[4] is thought to be the first surgeon to have performed a free bone transplant. Since the 19th century this technique has been used by surgeons worldwide. Nowadays, reconstruction of vertically atrophied ridges with onlay bone grafts is well documented, but the results have not been always promising.

What types of defects are suitable to reconstruct with this technique?

To obtain favorable reconstructive results, the procedure of bone grafting needs few fundamental requisites: a suitable vascular support, a valid interface between graft and osteogenic cell lines and the mechanical stability of the graft; it also depends on revascularization from the recipient site. This revascularization is very important for the process of resorption and deposition of new bone, also called "creeping substitution."[5,6]

The advantages of using an onlay graft are the avoidance of direct damage to the inferior alveolar nerve (IAN), easy of placement of the graft, and immediate postoperative vertical augmentation (Fig 10-1).[7]

Bone grafts fall into four general categories: autografts, allografts, xenografts, and alloplasts. The use of these materials in regenerative procedures is based on the assumption that they possess osteogenic potential (contain bone-forming cells), are osteoinductive (contain bone-inducing substances), or simply are osteoconductive (serve as a scaffold for bone formation).

Does the origin of the harvested bone make any difference to the results?

Autogenous bone harvested from intraoral or extraoral sites is the most predictable osteogenic organic graft for osseous tissue regeneration. Both extraoral and intraoral donor sites have been proposed. The primary locations for harvesting intraoral block grafts include the external oblique ridge of the posterior mandible, symphysis, and ramus. Extraoral autogenous bone can be harvested from the iliac crest, cranium, or tibia.

Recent reports, however, describe the results of alveolar augmentation using autogenous bone blocks harvested from extraoral donor sites.[8-10] It must be pointed out that patients affected by partial edentulism do not accept major surgical procedures that may imply hospitalization or general anesthesia. The use of iliac or calvarial bone grafting is a cause of major patient discomfort during the immediate postoperative phase and may be considered too invasive for ridge augmentation in partially edentulous patients.[11]

Different studies have confirmed that intraorally harvested intramembranous bone grafts have less resorption, enhanced revascularization, and better incorporation at the donor site, when compared with extraorally harvested endochondral bone grafts.[9,12-14] Moreover, intraoral bone grafts offer several benefits like conventional surgical access, proximity of donor and recipient sites, lower operative and anesthesia times, no cutaneous scar, minimal discomfort, and lower morbidity compared with extraoral locations.[9,14] The better incorporation of mandibular bone in the maxillofacial region is to be attributed to a similarity in protocollagen and a higher concentration of morphogenetic proteins and growth factors.[15]

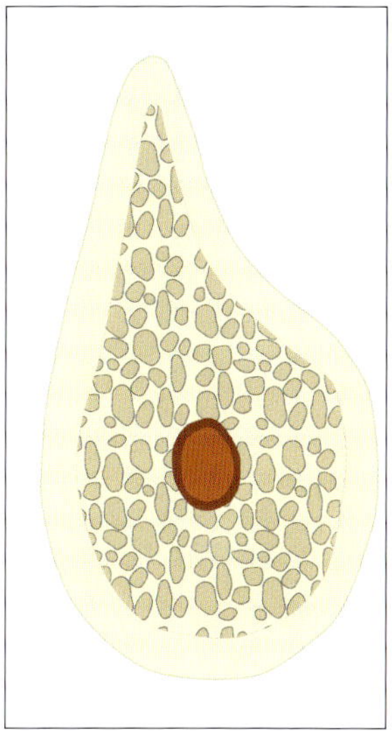

Fig 10-1a Horizontal defect.

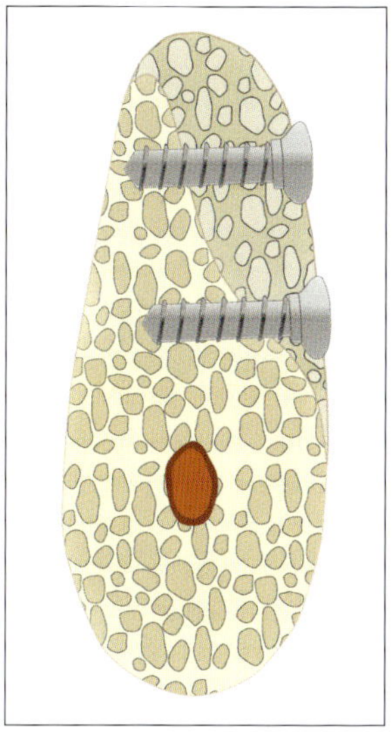

Fig 10-1b Horizontal defect corrected with an onlay graft.

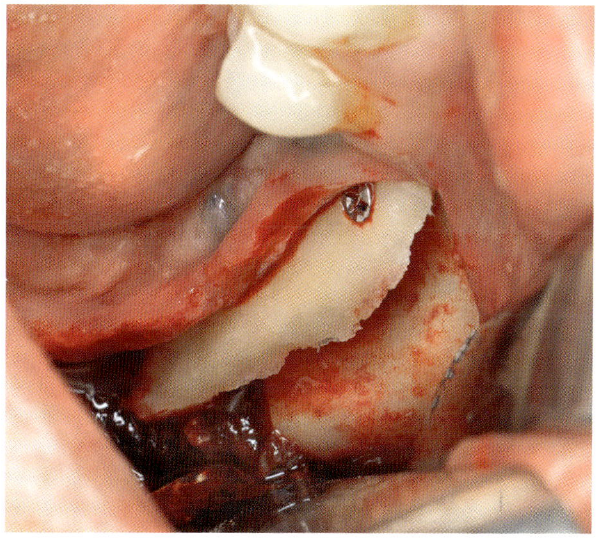

Fig 10-2 Onlay graft placed with screws.

Block grafts are harvested as corticocancellous or cortical bone autografts. The revascularization of corticocancellous block grafts takes place at a much faster rate than in cortical bone autografts and at a slower rate than particulate autografts. Revascularization of block grafts enables maintenance of their vitality, and hence reduces chances of graft infection and necrosis.

Considerations in limiting the postoperative bone resorption

The onlay technique results in higher bone resorption values before implant placement in comparison with the inlay technique. To reduce the amount of bone resorption requires a membranous bone block graft that is oversized, with respect to the desired final vertical/horizontal augmentation, and also is necessary to stabilize the graft firmly in the recipient site. The use of barrier membranes over bone grafts seems to reduce the tendency for bone graft to be reabsorbed during the healing phase.

10.2.2 Technique

How to proceed?

Onlay grafts are mostly used to correct transversal problems in the mandible. Although bone can be obtained from two different intraoral sites, we will focus our attention on ramus harvesting, as for its postsurgical behavior and amount of bone obtained it is the treatment of choice.

After infiltration a crestal incision is performed from the last remaining tooth back to the ascending ramus.

A periosteal elevator is used to mobilize the mucoperiosteal flap both vestibularly and lingually. Releasing incisions are performed at this time in order to achieve a tension-free repositioning of the flap when suturing.

The area to be grafted is measured in order to raise a correctly size graft. Then the donor site is designed with the piezoelectric device. The dimensions of the graft should be slightly bigger, because it will shrink slightly during remodeling and adaptation.

Once the osteotomies are designed the block may be raised with the help of a chisel and a hammer. Then the block is adapted to the recipient site, taking care to maximize the contact between the block and the recipient site.

Once the graft has been adapted a bur should be used to make a perforation in the block slightly larger than the diameter of the compression screw and slightly thinner in the recipient site. The graft is fixed with a screw (Fig 10-2) and the gaps may then be filled with particulate material (Fig 10-3). The reconstruction should be covered with a resorbable membrane (Fig 10-4).

Suturing with 6/0 monofilament suture is an important issue in this technique where a tension-free closure should be achieved in order to avoid wound dehiscence during the healing period.

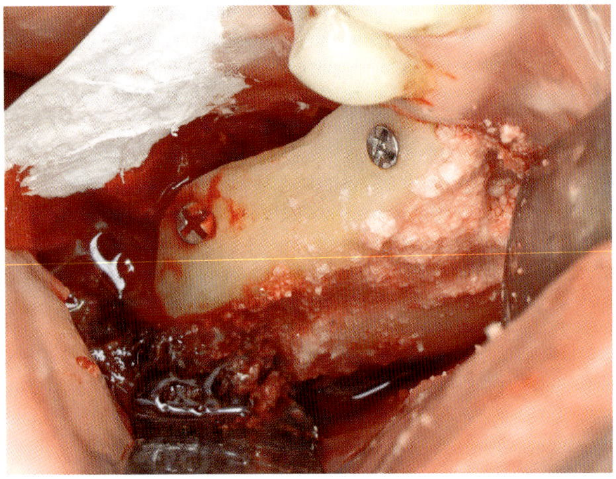

Fig 10-3 The gaps may be filled with particulate material.

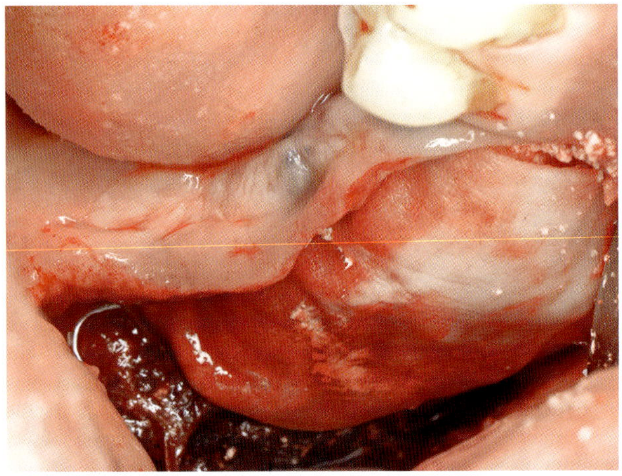

Fig 10-4 The reconstruction is covered with a resorbable membrane.

10.2.3 Complications

The most frequent complication during bone augmentation procedures with onlay grafts is wound dehiscence that leads to infection and resorption of the graft. Early exposure may result in graft necrosis, potentially because the graft has not obtained adequate vascularity to maintain its vitality. With late exposures, block autografts seemed to have adequate vascularity to maintain their vitality by the time that exposure occurred. This complication is more frequent in vertical augmentation; for transversal augmentation the incidence is much lower with correct management of the soft tissues.

Another complication may be the damage to the IAN on the donor site, in most of the cases the donor site is the ascending ramus and in this location the IAN runs close to the vestibular cortical bone. With the use of piezoelectric devices for graft raising the incidence of postoperative dysesthesia has widely decreased.

10.3 Inlay block grafting

10.3.1 Introduction

The sandwich osteotomy technique with interpositional bone grafting was first described by Schettler[16] in 1976 in the anterior totally edentulous mandible and was applied in subsequent years. Variations in the surgical technique since have been reported by Stoelinga et al.,[17] Vanassche et al.,[18] and Haers et al.,[19] who used a figure 8-shaped wire with interposed bone blocks to stabilize the cranial segment.

Interpositional graft techniques have great potential for bone graft incorporation because they ensure the blood supply, which results in low final resorption and high implant survival and success rates. However, few surveys of this procedure in this portion of the mandible have been reported.

Why is it called the "sandwich" technique?

The "sandwich" technique is a vertical bone augmentation procedure that uses vertically elevated segmented bone created from basal bone and maintains the lingual periosteum that is attached to the mobile segment. The bone graft is placed in the space between the mobile segment and the basal bone (Fig 10-5).

What are the advantages and differences compared with the onlay technique?

The alveolar basal bone sandwich osteotomy has the advantage of guaranteeing a greater vascular supply to the inlay graft than to an onlay graft. Inlay graft is less subject to resorption because the graft is surrounded by bone and periosteum on all sides, facilitating a rapid vascular connection with the surrounding tissues.

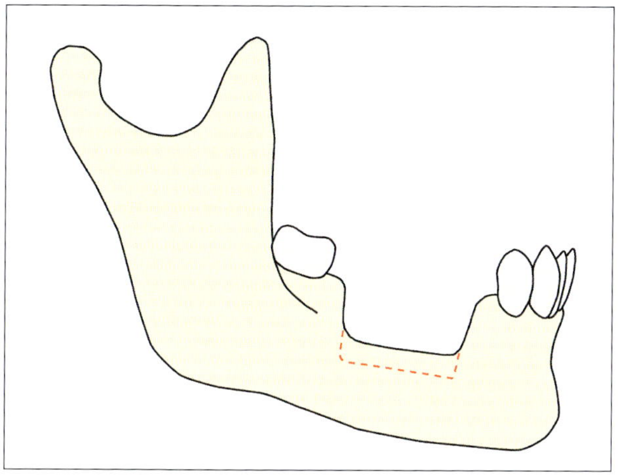

Fig 10-5a Planning of the osteotomy.

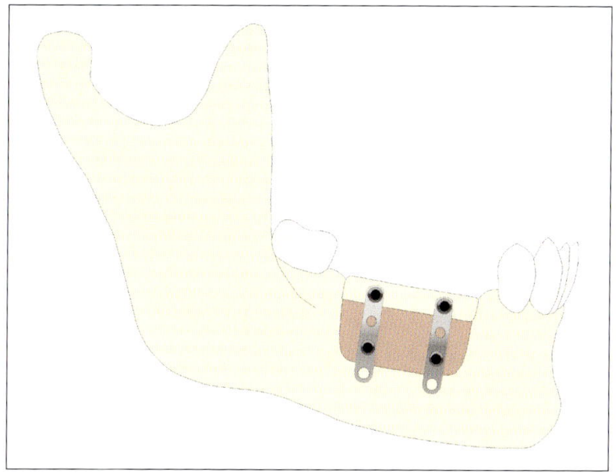

Fig 10-5b Vertical reposition of the bone and fixation with microplates.

What grafting material is appropriate?

The clinician must decide on the optimal material to graft the defect. Cancellous/particulate marrow grafts have shown more rapid vascularization and more osteogenic activity compared with autogenous block grafts. Cancellous grafts tend to repair completely with time, but cortical grafts remain as a mixture of both necrotic and viable bone.[7]

How much can be gained with this technique?

Six millimeters or more of bone gain and minimal resorption of the transpositioned bone can be achieved with this procedure.[20,21]

The rate of resorption of the grafted site decreases considerably after implant placement. Studies indicate that implant placement into a grafted area results in graft persistence and implant stability.

Are there any limitations?

There are limitations to interpositional grafting for the mandible. Interpositional grafting only corrects vertical defects, not horizontal defects. An anatomic limitation also exists to the amount of vertical gain that can be achieved with interpositional grafting. This anatomic limitation is the stretch of the soft tissue attachments to the pedicled mobilized alveolar segment of bone, which can typically only be raised 5 to 8 mm. Undue strain on the lingual soft tissue pedicle by vertically repositioning the mobilized bone can lead to a compromised blood flow, incision breakdown, graft loss, and/or accelerated graft resorption.[7]

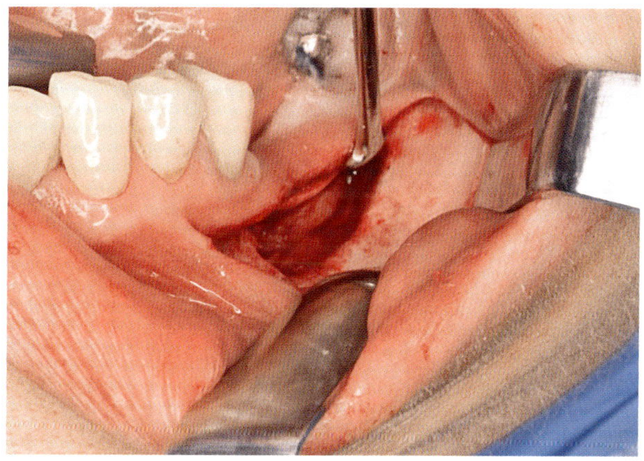

Fig 10-6 The gingiva of the bone fragment displaced must be attached to it.

The inlay technique is associated with lower bone resorption values and produces more predictable outcomes, but requires an experienced surgeon.

10.3.2 Technique

The incision should be performed vestibular to the alveolar process in the free gingiva; the incision should go deep through the periosteum.

Subperiosteal dissection is performed laterally to the alveolar process. It is important to leave the gingiva over the bone attached, because the nutrition of this bone will come through the lingual flap (Fig 10-6).

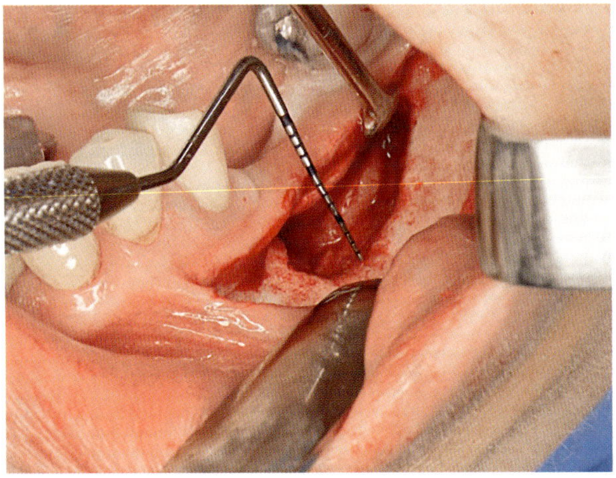

Fig 10-7 The fragment is mobilized to the planned new position, vertically and transversally.

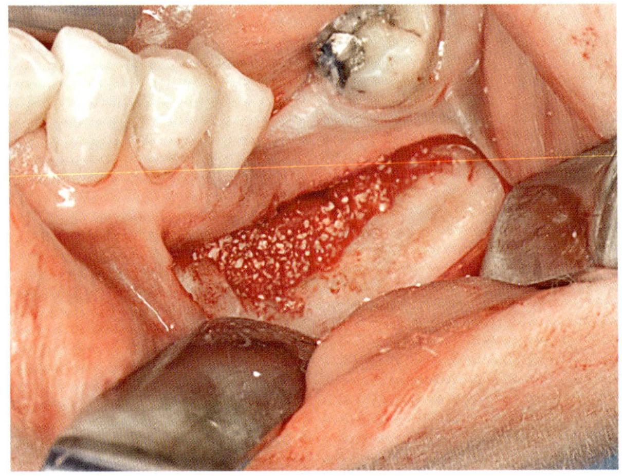

Fig 10-8 The gap is completely filled with particulate xenograft and then it is condensed.

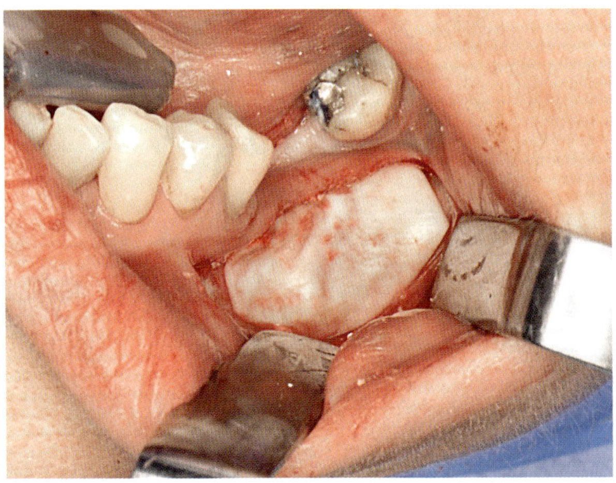

Fig 10-9 The reconstruction is covered with a resorbable membrane.

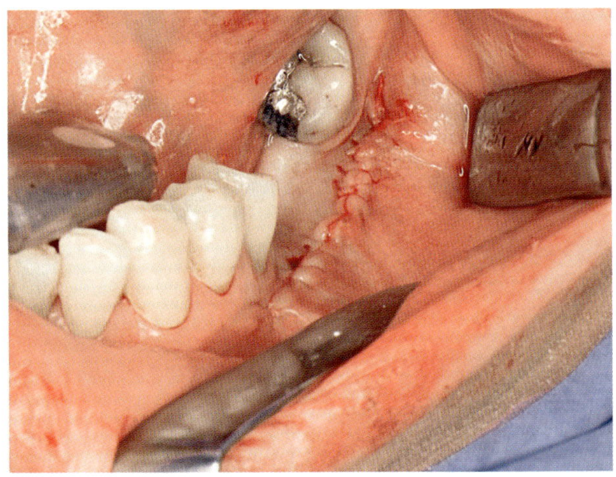

Fig 10-10 Suturing is performed with 6/0 monofilament suture.

The osteotomy is then performed on the bone over the IAN in a semilunar fashion from the last remaining tooth back to the retromolar area. The use of a piezoelectric device is recommended so that the risk of harming the nerve is reduced; the device should go deep through the vestibular cortical bone, the cancellous bone, and to the lingual cortex.

A chisel is inserted through the osteotomy and the fracture of the lingual cortex is induced in a greenstick pattern. Once the bone fragment has been released with an osteotome, the fragment should be mobilized to the planned new position, vertically and transversally (Fig 10-7). The particulate xenograft is then applied to the gap and condensed in order to completely fill the gap created (Fig 10-8). A resorvable membrane is applied laterally (Fig 10-9) and a tension-free suture is then performed with 6/0 monofilament suture (Fig 10-10).

10.3.3 Complications

Several complications may happen during the performance of inlay augmentation techniques:

- Fracture of the upper bone fragment. If the amount of bone over the IAN is small and the osteotomy is performed too high, the bone fragment over the osteotomy may have an incorrect fracture.
- Fracture of the mandible. This rare complication has been described, possibly due to incomplete osteoto-

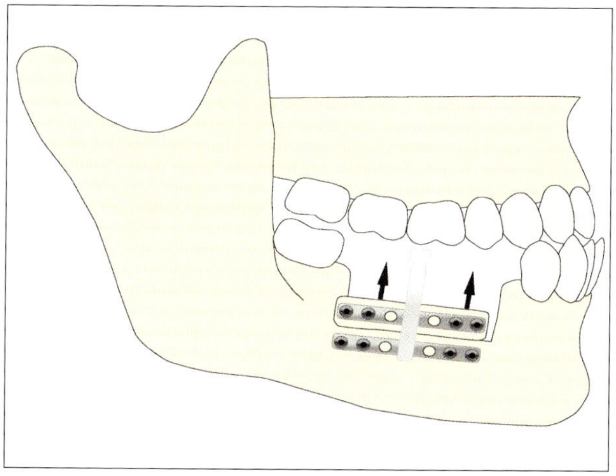

Fig 10-11a A corticotomy is used to fracture the bone into two segments, and the distraction device is placed.

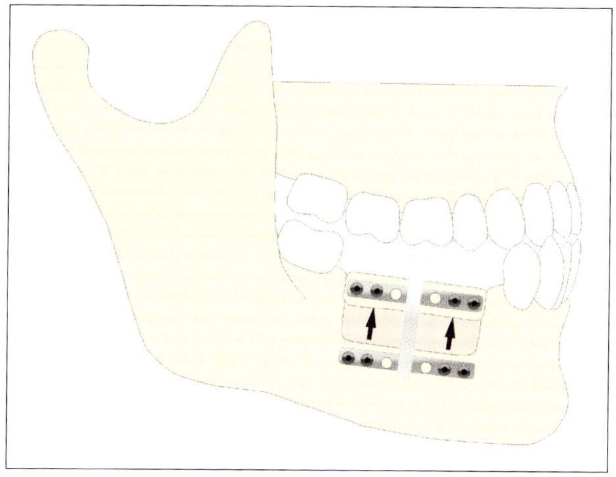

Fig 10-11b The two bone ends of the bone are gradually moved apart during the distraction phase, allowing new bone to form in the gap.

my and excessive forces when inducing the greenstick fracture.
- Another complication may be damage to the IAN. With the use of piezoelectric devices for this technique the incidence of postoperative dysesthesia has greatly decreased.

10.4 Distraction osteogenesis (DO)

10.4.1 Introduction

DO, also called callus distraction, callostasis, and osteodistraction, is a surgical process used to reconstruct skeletal deformities and lengthen the long bones of the body. A corticotomy is used to fracture the bone into two segments, and the two bone ends of the bone are gradually moved apart during the distraction phase, allowing new bone to form in the gap (Fig 10-11). When the desired or possible length is reached, a consolidation phase follows in which the bone is allowed to keep healing. DO has the benefit of simultaneously increasing bone length and the volume of surrounding soft tissues.

Since the first report of Chin and Toth[22] of alveolar DO published in 1996, numerous prospective clinical studies and case series have demonstrated the possibilities and benefits of DO for increasing height of the alveolar ridge. DO was introduced for vertical augmentation of resorbed alveolar ridges in an attempt to avoid the drawbacks and limitations of standardized treatment modalities. In recent years it has been used for the correction of horizontal defects.[23]

The technique relies on stretching the bones to achieve lengthening and new bone regeneration. Ilizarov[24] established two basic principles of DO, which are the law of tension-stress and the influence of mechanical load and vascular supply. These basic principles have three different phases: a latency phase of approximately 7 days of initial post-surgical healing, the distraction phase, consisting of the gradual incremental separation of two bone pieces at a rate of approximately 1 mm day, and the consolidation phase, when new bone is formed in the regeneration zone between the separated bone pieces.[25]

Is DO a well-documented technique with proven working protocols?

Although there are not yet established protocols for alveolar bone distraction, different authors have recommended a latency period of 5 to 7 days, a distraction rate of 0.5 to 1 mm/day, and a consolidation period of 8 to 12 weeks.[26] According to the results obtained by Robiony et al.[27] and Horiuchi et al.,[28] the optimal rate for horizontal alveolar distraction is probably about 0.5 mm/day. Meyer et al.[29] have demonstrated that the magnitude of the force applied is more important than its frequency of application. The minimum and maximum force-inducing activation and continued function of the cells contributing to osteogenesis is not accurately known.

Various distraction devices are now available for oral and maxillofacial application, including mandibular, maxillary and midfacial, cranial, and alveolar distractors. DO can be achieved by intraosseous or extraosseous devices.

Extraosseous distractors, also called juxtaosseous distractors, are placed on the buccal face of the maxillary bone. Intraosseous distractors run through the transport segment in the direction of distraction.

After all these years of extended application of alveolar DO there is still a significant divergence about various treatment parameters, such as surgical procedure, type of distractor, and minimal bone height necessary to perform the distraction. There is a lack of evidence regarding the appropriate DO protocols, maximum augmentation volume, and long-term implant success rates.[30] It remains hardly predictable to control the augmentation vector distraction in the posterior mandibular region.

10.4.2 Technique

As endosseous distractors are usually used for treatment of small defects (one absent tooth with adjacent teeth present), we will focus on the application of juxtaosseous distractors, which are more useful in the treatment of the posterior edentulous jaw.

The incision should be performed vestibular to the alveolar process in the free gingiva; the incision should go deep through the periosteum.

Subperiosteal dissection is performed laterally to the alveolar process. It is important to leave the gingiva over the bone attached, because the nutrition of this bone will come through the lingual flap.

Distractors are applied and modeled over the bone, and then the screws are placed. The device is removed and the osteotomy is performed on the bone over the IAN in an open-box shape along the area to be distracted.

The use of a piezoelectric device is advised so that the risk of harming the nerve is reduced; the device should go deep through the vestibular cortical bone, the cancellous bone, and to the lingual cortex.

A chisel is inserted through the osteotomy and the fracture of the lingual cortex is induced in a greenstick pattern. After the fracture has been finished the distraction device should be replaced and the direction of the distractor should be checked by opening the device a few millimeters to verify there was no interference during the distraction process. It is returned to the initial position and suturing is performed.

After the latency period of 5 to 7 days, the distraction process can be performed at 1 mm/day.

10.4.3 Complications

Complications that may arise during alveolar distraction have been classified by Saulic et al.[30] in three groups:

- Problems arising during surgery, generally related to osteotomy and distractor placement.
- Complications arising during distraction, including incorrect direction of distraction vector and soft-tissue complications.
- Complications arising after distraction, due to defective bone formation. Bleeding in cases of deep osteotomy, and pain and significant resorption of the distracted fragment in distractions of more than 10 mm. Gaggl et al.[26] described other complications, including dysesthesia of the mental nerve and mandibular fracture. Damage of lingual periostium and fracture of the mandible.

10.5 Dental nerve mobilization

10.5.1 Introduction

Are there treatment alternatives when those described are impossible to apply?

Sometimes severe defects are faced that are impossible to restore with short implants and where augmenting procedures would be insufficient or even impossible because of the poor bone remaining and the proximity of the IAN to the alveolar crest.

One approach to avoid nerve injury when placing implants in the severely atrophied posterior mandible is to reposition the IAN laterally and then place the implants in a medial position relative to the nerve (Fig 10-12). This technique allows placement of longer implants and better initial stabilization. In 1987, Jensen and Nock[31] presented the first documented restoration of the posterior atrophic mandible using endosseous implants in conjunction with IAN transposition; since then several modifications of the procedure have been presented.

The other method involves transpositioning the nerve by creating a window that includes the mental foramen as well as the area of implant placement, then releasing the nerve from the dental foramen and replac-

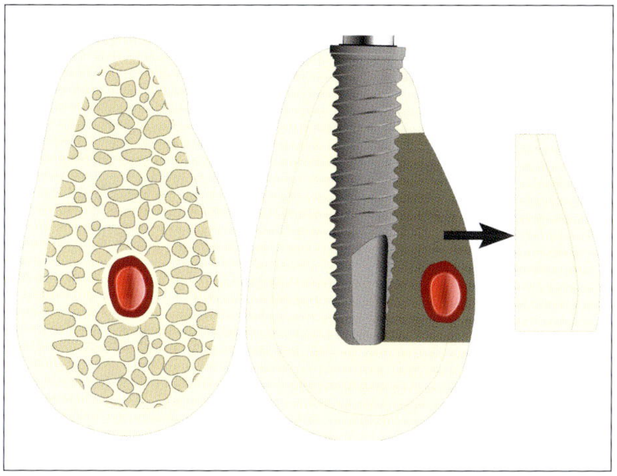

Fig 10-12 The IAN is repositioned laterally and the implants placed in a medial position relative to the nerve.

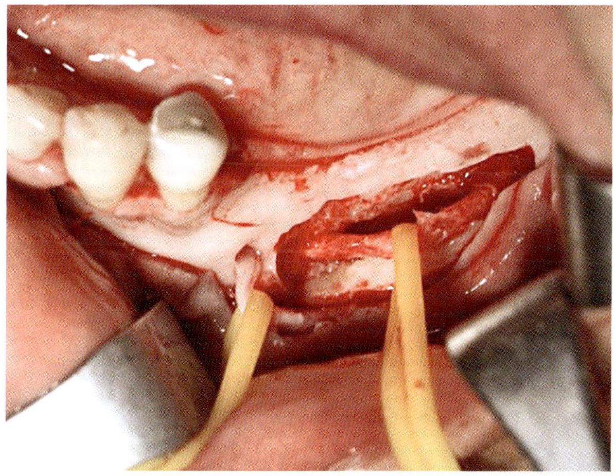

Fig 10-13 Once the nerve is widely exposed, a vessel loop is used to gently mobilize it laterally.

ing the nerve distal to its original location; the incisive nerve is severed to allow transpositioning of both the mental foramen and the IAN.[32] This technique results in the loss of sensation of its terminal incisive branch. This is of no consequence for patients who are edentulous in the anterior mandible, but it may cause some disturbance to residual dental and periodontal sensibility in any remaining anterior teeth.[33]

Is residual bone height needed?

A minimum quantity of approximately 8 mm of remaining bone above the mandibular canal is required to permit the surgical approach.[34] In situations with less bone height above the mandibular canal, autogenous bone graft before IAN transposition and implant placement must be considered. Onlay grafting or DO procedures may be considered.

10.5.2 Technique

Lateralization

After infiltration, a crestal incision is performed from the last remaining tooth back to the ascending ramus, and a releasing incision is performed mesially to the mental foramen.

A periosteal elevator is used to mobilize the mucoperiosteal flap and the mental nerve is identified.

According to the teeth to be restored, a window should be designed distally to the foramen, and the osteotomy should be performed with a piezoelectric device

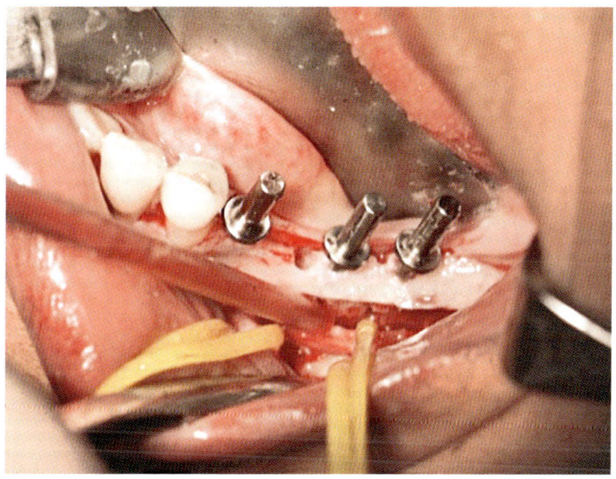

Fig 10-14 Carefully the drilling is performed and the implants are inserted.

to minimize the risk of harming the nerve. However, a round diamond bur with a straight handpiece or a reciprocating saw could be useful as well. A safe distance to the canal has to be considered, creating a window larger than needed to avoid nerve contact during the osteotomy. Once the osteotomy is complete the vestibular cortical bone is removed.

With a dissector or a scraper, the cancellous bone is carefully removed in the area where the IAN is located. Once the nerve is widely exposed, a vessel loop is used to gently mobilize it laterally (Fig 10-13).

Carefully the drilling is performed (Fig 10-14), and once the implants have been inserted a resorbable membrane should be placed before returning the nerve to its original position.

The removed cortical bone should be put back and suturing performed with 6/0 monofilament to assure good primary closure without flap tension.

Transpositioning

The procedure is exactly the same as for lateralization, except for the cortical window design.

According to the teeth to be restored the window should be designed including the foramen. Once the osteotomy is complete the vestibular cortical bone is removed. The nerve has much more mobility in this case, but in many cases the incisal branch has to be transected to achieve sufficient mobilization. When performing this technique the chances of nerve damage are higher.

10.5.3 Complications

Is this a safe procedure?

In a recent comparative study, the reported incidence of neurosensory disturbance was significantly greater for the surgical technique that released the mental nerve from the mental foramen (77.8%) than for the surgical technique that did not release the mental nerve from the mental foramen (33.3%).[35] In a study published in 2002 by Peleg et al.,[36] they proposed a variation of the osteotomies involving a technique in which two osteotomies were created (one anterior, including mental foramen, and a second more posterior). The overall incidence of transitional neurosensory disturbance was less than 8%. This is likely attributable to the fact that this technique involved first moving a large bone block. There was no movement of large bone block and mental foramen in one motion. No permanent damage was seen in this patient population.

As a negative point, this type of technique does not recover the alveolar ridge anatomy, temporarily weakens the mandible, and particularly presents the risk that eventual sensory alterations may be permanent. Inferior alveolar nerve transposition generally causes some degree of sensory alterations, like hypoesthesia (partial loss of sensitivity) and paresthesia (uncommon response to stimuli). Nerve damage occurs due to ischemia caused by distension of the nerve during the surgical procedure or by chronic nerve compression/distension after surgery.[37]

The IAN transposition method is presented as being less invasive, although it should be pointed out that this technique does not correct the increased distance between the arches, in addition to presenting high rates of permanent damage to the nerve bundle, thus being contraindicated when the ratio between the implant length and prosthetic crown is unfavorable.[38]

Nerve injury: how to proceed?

Identifying and assessing the frequency and severity of nerve damage following IAN transposition, as well as recovery potential is difficult. Clinical-neurosensory evaluations are based on the patient's own sensitivity, the stimulus-evoking technique, and the examiner's interpretation, and thus cannot yield objective results.[37]

The process of nerve regeneration after compression or less severe crush injuries usually requires several weeks to 6 months. If there is no sensory recovery during this time, permanent loss of continuity in the nerve trunk should be expected.[39] There is generally little improvement in sensation on the injured side when assessed either by objective means or subjectively by the patient 9 months after compression injury and 12 months after nerve section.

Low level laser therapy (LLLT) can be used for the treatment of nerve injuries. Because LLLT is relatively noninvasive, its ability to stimulate injured nerves without surgical intervention is desirable.[40] There have been some studies reporting the treatment of IAN paresthesia with LLLT. Clinical studies of the effects of LLLT on injured nerves have revealed an increase in nerve function and improved capacity for myelin production.[41]

Avoiding IAN damage during any surgical procedure is an important goal because of the forensic and ethical issues and the neurological sequelae, which may impair the oral function related to the nerve injury that can be expected to occur during this definitive surgical approach.

The main concern with this technique is the postoperative dysesthesia, but other complications have been described, such as mandibular fracture.

The damage to the nerve may occur while performing the osteotomy, during the release of the nerve, while mobilizing it, or during the drilling. The management of the nerve should be gentle throughout the procedure.

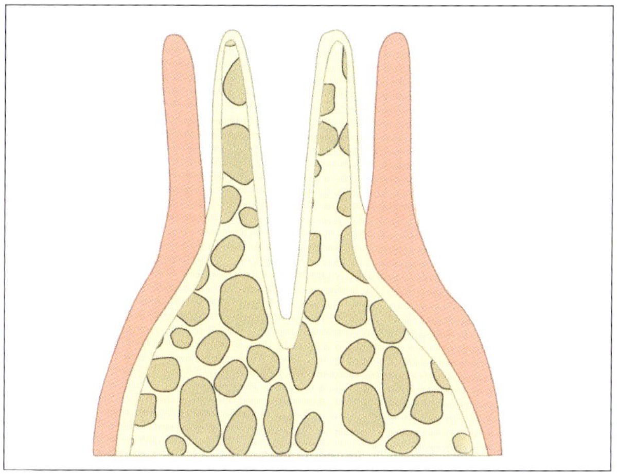

Fig 10-15a The buccal cortex is repositioned laterally by a greenstick fracture.

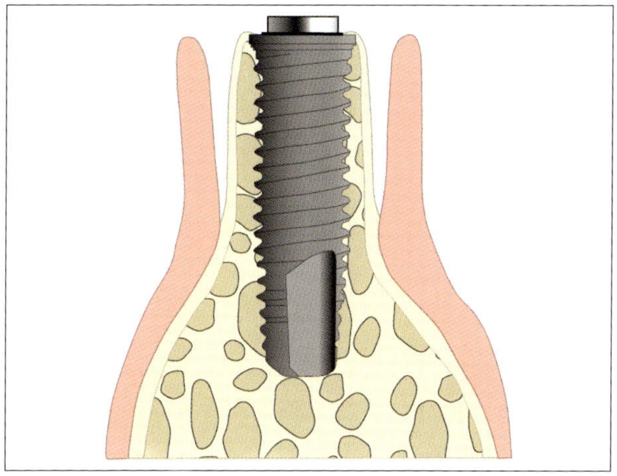

Fig 10-15b The split-crest technique creates a new implant bed by longitudinal osteotomy of the alveolar bone.

This damage can be classified as follows.

- Neurotmesis: Complete anatomic interruption of nerve, few chances for functional recovery.
- Axonotmesis: This is a nerve injury with disruption of the neuronal axon, but with maintenance of the myelin sheath. This type of nerve damage may cause paralysis of the motor, sensory, and autonomic branch. Loss in both motor and sensory spines is more complete with axonotmesis than with neurapraxia, and recovery occurs only through regeneration of the axons, a process requiring time.
- Neurapraxia: The actual structure of the nerve remains intact, but there is an interruption in conduction of the impulse down the nerve fiber. There is a temporary loss of function which is reversible within hours to months of the injury.

Before undergoing this procedure, every patient should be advised of the intervention risks and the probability of suffering posterior nerve damage and neurosensory alterations. Alternative restorative solutions should be considered.

10.6 Split crest

10.6.1 Introduction

Crestal ridge bone augmentation as ridge splitting was first introduced by Dr Hilt Tatum in the 1970s.[42] The split-crest technique is intended to create a new implant bed by longitudinal osteotomy of the alveolar bone. The buccal cortex is repositioned laterally by a greenstick fracture (Fig 10-15).

This method allows the clinician to place implants into anatomic situations involving insufficient bone thickness, moving the external cortical plate of the mandible in a labial direction to gain an increase in width so that the implants of a suitable diameter can be placed. Furthermore, bone augmentation is intended to produce an appropriate bone contour, allowing for implant placement in a proper prosthetically directed position.[43]

What are the advantages of this technique?

In comparison with onlay and inlay bone grafts, GBR, and alveolar DO, the split-crest technique does not require long periods for bone consolidation prior to implant placement and there is no morbidity of the donor site.[42] It increases precision in the positioning of dental implants and predictability in extremely thin crests that are lacking medullary.[43]

When can the technique be applied?

This ridge expansion technique is effective for the correction of moderately resorbed edentulous ridges in selected cases. In practice, this applies in situations where atrophy of the edentulous ridge has developed horizontally and cancellous bone is present between the oral and facial cortical plates, and adequate residual height exists.[44] The majority of authors consider that ridges

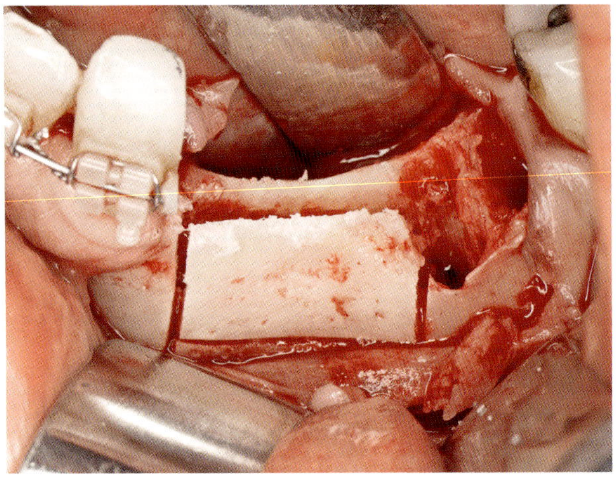

Fig 10-16 Crestal osteotomy performed with piezoelectric device.

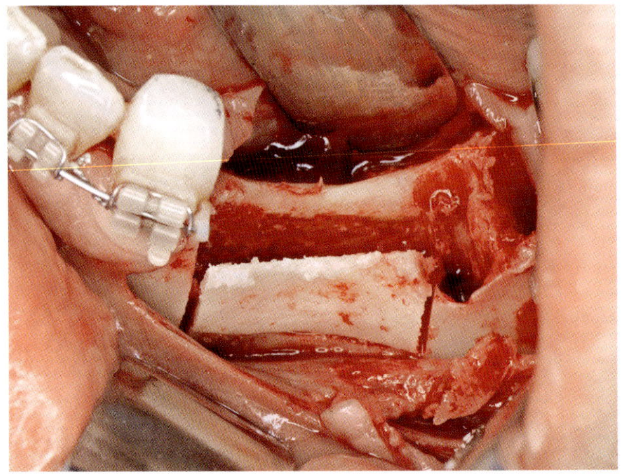

Fig 10-17 Lateral movement of the bone.

with less than 5 mm width require horizontal augmentation for placement of screw-type dental implants.[43,45,46]

The contraindications for this procedure are an excessive facial inclination of the alveolar ridge, as it may worsen the initial situation from a prosthetic point of view.

Some authors report that staged ridge splitting can be a safer technique that overcomes the complications associated with the single-stage ridge expansion without causing significant delay in treatment. In the first operation a simple corticotomy is performed at the crestal, buccal aspect but the segment is not mobilized until the second operation, when the buccal segment attached to the periosteum is lateralized and implants are placed.[44,45] This delayed lateral expansion technique is applied to ridges with a dense and thick cortex. The healing period before performing the delayed ridge expansion and implant placement is 3 to 4 weeks.[45,47]

Should the grafting material be covered?

The use of a coverage membrane in the split area is controversial. It has been suggested that fillers and membranes can only improve bone formation in the gap area. The intercortical bony gap is very similar to an extraction socket that should be left without any grafting. The use of a resorption membrane can also improve healing in soft tissue and avoids an eventual reopening of the flap.[43]

10.6.2 Technique

After infiltration, a crestal incision is performed from the last remaining tooth back to the ascending ramus.

A periosteal elevator is used to mobilize the mucoperiosteal flap gently over the crest.

The osteotomy should be performed with a piezoelectric device on the crest (Fig 10-16). Once on the cancellous bone, progressive chisel widening is continued. The lateral movement may also be performed with osteotomes (Fig 10-17).

The split length usually is grafted with autologous, allogenic, or alloplastic biomaterials depending on preference (Fig 10-18).

Also described in the literature is the approach of the membrane technique in combination with a split-crest technique for horizontal ridge augmentation associated with immediate implant placement. Carefully the drilling is performed, and once the implants have been inserted a bone graft is placed to fill the gaps and a resorbable membrane is placed to cover the implants and the reconstruction. Finally suturing is performed with 6/0 monofilament (Fig 10-19).

10.6.3 Complications

During the crestal split the main concern should be the possibility of a bad split; this happens most frequently with the vestibular bone. Should this occur, the treatment should be altered to GBR in order to completely cover the implant with bone graft.

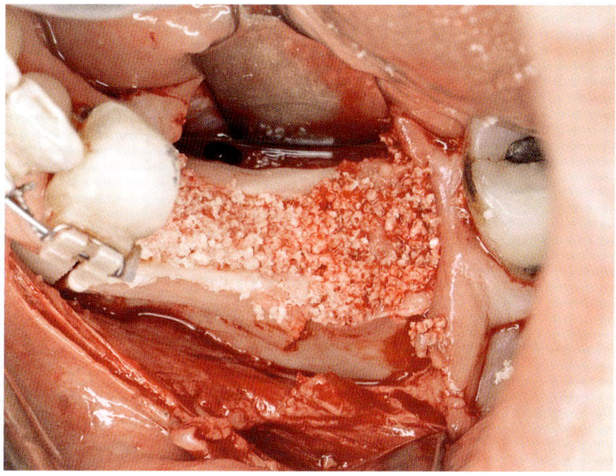

Fig 10-18 Grafting of the gap.

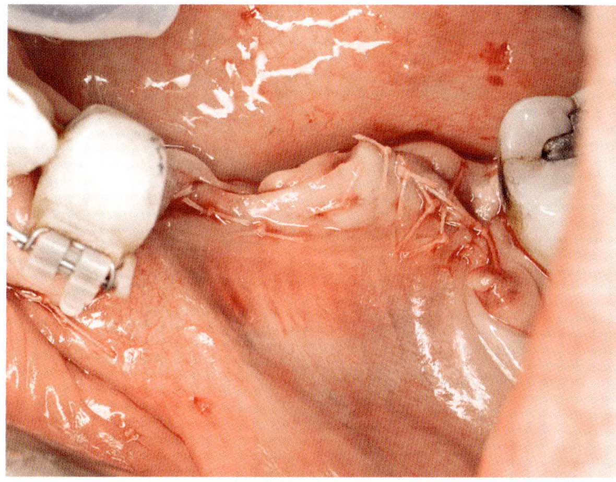

Fig 10-19 Suturing is performed with 6/0 monofilament suture.

10.7 Conclusions

Many surgical procedures have been proposed to allow dental implant placement in either a simultaneous or a staged approach. A lack of comparative studies has made it difficult to choose the most reliable and predictable augmentation technique.

10.7.1 How to make the decision?

Transposition of the mandibular nerve is technically demanding and may affect nerve bundle integrity. The placement of short implants, especially when the available bone above the inferior canal is <7 mm, is an unpredictable procedure. Furthermore, both of these techniques result in an excessive crown length with an unfavorable crown/implant ratio and poor esthetic outcomes.

The first therapeutic option to provide better functional and esthetic results is alveolar ridge augmentation by means of different grafting techniques that simultaneously provide better implant support and decreased interarch length.

10.7.2 Which is the most predictable?

The inlay technique shows great potential for bone graft incorporation, with a low resorption level and high implant survival and success rates, and recent studies into this technique have reported good outcomes. However, this technique is not simple to perform and requires at least 4 to 6 mm of residual bone above the mandibular canal.

Onlay grafting has been used successfully in the correction of vertically deficient edentulous ridges, although the reported two-stage approach results in considerable resorption of the bone graft before implant insertion.

The osteodistraction technique may not be used in all circumstances, for instance in the presence of thin ridges. It is more expensive than GBR and bone grafting, but may reduce treatment time and allow for more vertical ridge augmentation.

Although the use of iliac block graft has been advocated for augmentation of the atrophic mandible, it may be preferable to harvest block graft from an intraoral donor site to treat a limited portion of the jaws. Harvesting of iliac or calvarial bone causes major intra- and postoperative discomfort to the patient. Moreover, compared with extraoral endochondral bone grafts, intraoral membranous bone grafts undergo minimal resorption due to enhanced vascularization and better incorporation at the recipient site.

Bone substitutes, such as Bio-Oss® blocks (Geistlich, Wolhusen, Switzerland), may be a valid, cheaper alternative to autogenous bone particularly when harvested from extraoral locations, since they are associated with less postoperative morbidity.

However, the major difficulty in reconstruction of the posterior mandible is the management of soft tissues, which have a high risk of dehiscence and subsequent infection and necrosis of the graft.

Clinicians and patients should carefully evaluate the benefits and risks in relation to the desired outcome when deciding whether to use vertical ridge augmen-

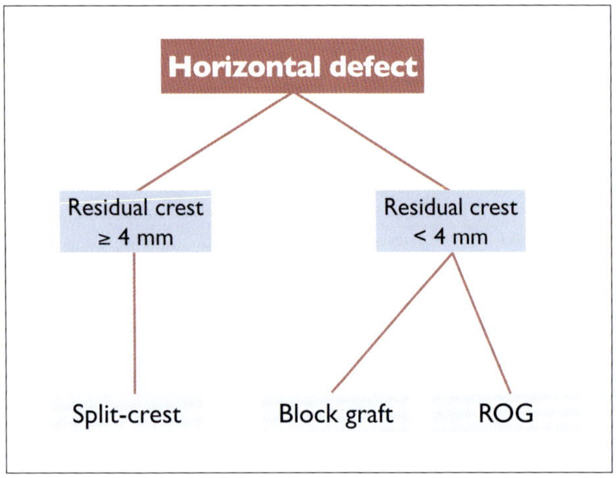

Fig 10-20 Decision-making guide for horizontal defects (see Table 10-1).

Table 10-1 Decision-making guide for horizontal defects (see Fig 10-20)

	Technical difficulty	Morbidity
Split	++	++
Block graft	++	++
GBR	+++	+

Table 10-2 Decision-making guide for vertical defects (see Fig 10-21)

	Technical difficulty	Morbidity
Short implants	+	+
Distraction	+++	++
Sandwich	+++	+
Block graft	++	++
Nerve mobilization	+++	+++
GBR	+++	+

tation techniques. In order to understand when bone augmentation procedures are needed and which are the most effective techniques, larger and well-designed trials are needed.

In order to facilitate a decision-making guide, a schematic decision process based on bone available dimensions is proposed (Fig 10-20 and Table 10-1, and Fig 10-21 and Table 10-2).

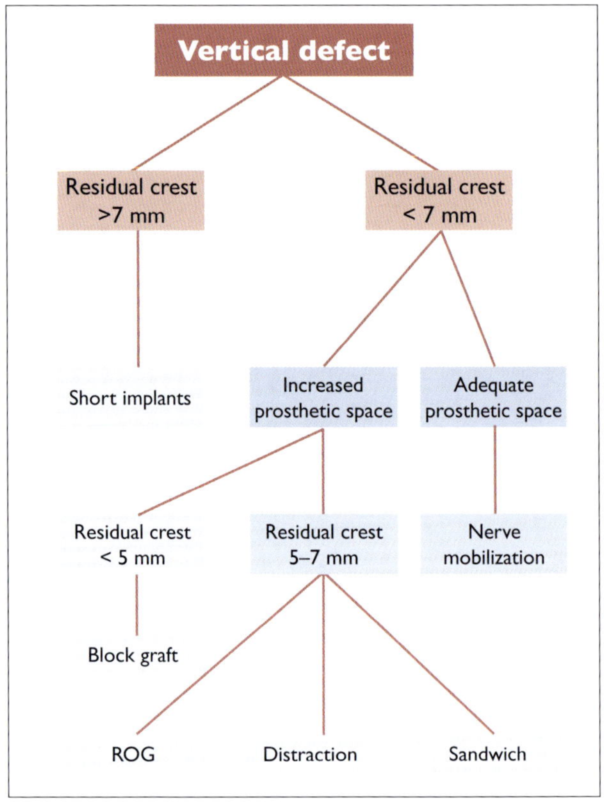

Fig 10-21 Decision-making guide for vertical defects (see Table 10-2).

References

1. Bell RB, Blakey GH, White RP, Hillebrand DG, Molina A. Stages reconstruction of the severely atrophic mandible with interpositional bloc graft and endosteal implants. J Oral Maxillofac Surg 2002;60:1135-1141.
2. Seibert JS. Reconstruction of deformed, partially edentulous ridges, using full thickness onlay grafts. Part I. Technique and wound healing. Compend Contin Educ Dent 1983;4:437-453.
3. Misch CE, Judy KW. Classification of partially edentulous arches for implant dentistry. Int J Oral Implantol 1987;4:7-13.
4. Sykoff W. Zur Frage der Knochen plastik am Unterkiefer. Zentralbl Chir 1900;35:881.
5. Tin Goh B, Lee S, Tideman H, Stoelinga P. Mandibular reconstruction in adults: a review. Int J Oral Maxillofac Surg 2008;37:597-605.
6. Polini F, Robiony M, Sembronio S, Costa F, Politi M. Bifunctional sculpturing of the bone graft for 3-dimensional augmentation of the atrophic posterior mandible. J Oral Maxillofac Surg 2009;67: 174-177.
7. Block M, Haggerty C. Interpositional osteotomy for posterior mandible ridge augmentation. J Oral Maxillofac Surg 2009;67 (Suppl 3):31-39.
8. Keller E, Van Roekel N, Desjardins R, Tolman D. Prosthetic surgical reconstruction of the severely resorbed maxilla with iliac bone grafting and tissue integrated prostheses. Int J Oral Maxillofac Implants 1987;2:155-165.
9. Raghoebar G, Batenburg R, Vissink A, Reintsema H. Augmentation of localized defects of the anterior maxillary ridge with autogenous bone before insertion of implants. J Oral Maxillofac surg 1996;54:1180-1185.

10. Lekholm U, Wannfors K, Isaksson S, Adielsson B. Oral implants in combination with bone grafts. A 3-year retrospective multicenter study using the Branemark implant system. Int J Oral Maxillofac Surg 1999;28:181-187.
11. Cordaro L, Amadè D, Cordaro M. Clinical results of alveolar ridge augmentation with mandibular block bone grafts in partially edentulous patients prior to implant placement. Clin Oral Implants Res 2002;13:101-111.
12. Proussaefs P, Lozada J, Kleinman A, Rohrer MD. The use of ramus autogenous block grafts for vertical alveolar ridge augmentation and implant placement: a pilot study. Int J Oral Maxillofac Implants 2002;17:238-248.
13. Capelli M. Autogenous bone graft from the mandibular ramus: a technique for bone augmentation. Int J Periodontics Restorative Dent 2003;23:277-285.
14. Schwartz-Arad D, Levin L. Intraoral autogenous block onlay bone grafting for extensive reconstruction of atrophic maxillary alveolar ridges. J Periodontol 2005;76:636-641.
15. Felice P, Iezzi G, Lizio G, Piattelli A, Marchetti C. Reconstruction of atrophied posterior mandible with inlay technique and mandibular ramus block graft for implant prosthetic rehabilitation. J Oral Maxillofac Surg 2009;67:372-380.
16. Schettler D. Sandwich technique with cartilage transplant for raising the alveolar process in the lower jaw. Fortschr Kiefer Gesichtschir 1976;20:61-63.
17. Stoelinga PJW, Blijdorp PA, Ross RR, de Koomen HA, Huybers AJM. Augmentation of the atrophic mandible with interposed bone graft and particulate hydroxylapatite. J Oral Maxillofac Surg 1986;44:353-360.
18. Vanassche BJE, Stoelinga PJW, de Koomen PA, Blijdorp PA, Schoenaers JHA. Reconstruction of the severely resorbed mandible with interposed bone grafts and hydroxylapatite. Int J Oral Maxillofac Surg 1988;17:157-160.
19. Haers PEJ, Van Straaten W, Stoelinga PJW, de Koomen HA, Blijdorp PA. Reconstruction of the severely resorbed mandible prior to vestibuloplasty or placement of endosseous implants. A 2- to 5-years follow-up. Int J Oral Maxillofac Surg 1991;20:149-154.
20. Marchetti C, Trasarti S, Corinaldesi G, Felice P. Interpositional bone grafts in the posterior mandibular region: a report on six patients. Int J Periodontics Restorative Dent 2007;27:547-555.
21. Sohn DS, Shin HI, Ahn MR, Lee JS. Piezoelectric vertical bone augmentation using the sandwich technique in an atrophic mandible and histomorphometric analysis of mineral allografts: a case report series. Int J Periodontics Restorative Dent 2010;30:383-391.
22. Chin M, Toth BA. Distraction osteogenesis in maxillofacial surgery using internal devices: review of five cases. J Oral Maxillofac Surg 1996;54:45-53.
23. Zvi L, Rachmiel A, Jensen O. Alveolar width distraction osteogenesis for early implant placement. J Oral Maxillofac Surg 2005;63:1724-1730.
24. Ilizarov GA. The tension-stress effect on the genesis and growth of tissues: part II. The influence of the rate and frequency of distracton. Clin Orthop Relat Res 1989;239:263-285.
25. McAllister B, Gaffaney T. Distraction osteogenesis for vertical bone augmentation prior to implant reconstruction. Periodontol 2000 2003;33:54-66.
26. Gaggl A, Schultes G, Kärcher H. Distraction implants: a new possibility for augmentative treatment of the edentulous atrophic mandible: case report. Br J Oral Maxillofac Surg 1999;37:481-485.
27. Robiony M, Polini F, Costa F, Politi M. Osteogenesis distraction and platelet rich plasma for bone restoration of the severely atrophic mandible: preliminary results. J Oral Maxillofac Surg 2002;60:630-635.
28. Horiuchi K, Uchida H, Yamamoto K, Hatano N. Anteroinferior distraction of the atrophic subtotal maxillary alveolus for implant placement: a case report. Int J Oral Maxillofac Implants 2002;17:416-423.
29. Meyer G, Fanghänel J, Proff P. Morphofunctional aspects of dental implants. Ann Anat 2012;194:190-194.
30. Saulic N, Lizuka T, Martin M, Garcia A. Alveolar distraction osteogenesis: a systematic review. Int J Oral Maxillofac Surg 2008;37:1-7.
31. Jensen O, Nock D. Inferior alveolar nerve repositioning in conjunction with placement of osseointegrated implants: a case report. Oral Surg Oral Med Oral Pathol 1987;63:263-268.
32. Ferrigno N, Laureti M, Fanali S. Inferior alveolar nerve transposition in conjunction with implant placement. Int J Oral Maxillofac Implants 2005;20:610-620.
33. Morrison A, Chiarot M, Kirby S. Mental nerve function after inferior alveolar nerve transposition for placement of dental implants. J Can Dent Assoc 2002;68:46-50.
34. Rosenquist B. Fixture placement posterior to the mental foramen with transpositioning of the inferior alveolar nerve. Int J Oral Maxillofac Implants 1992;7:45-50.
35. Kan JY, Lozada JL, Boyne PJ, Goodacre CJ, Rungcharassaeng K. Mandibular fracture after endosseous implant placement in conjunction with inferior alveolar nerve transposition: a patient treatment report. Int J Oral Maxillofac Implants 1997;12:655-659.
36. Peleg M, Mazor Z, Chaushu G, Garg A. Lateralization of inferior alveolar nerve with simultaneous implant placement: a modified technique. Int J Oral Maxillofac Implants 2002;17:101-106.
37. Ramos B, Neto A. Inferior alveolar nerve transposition. Oral Maxillofac Surg 2009;13:213-219.
38. Vasconcelos JA, Avila GB, Ribeiro JC, Dias SC, Pereira LJ. Inferior alveolar nerve transposition with involvement of the mental foramen for implant placement. Med Oral Patol Oral Cir Bucal 2008;13:722-725.
39. Tay AB, Go WS. Effect of exposed inferior alveolar neurovascular bundle during surgical removal of impacted lower third molars. J Oral Maxillofac Surg 2004;62:592-600.
40. Ozen T, Orhan K, Gorur I, Ozturk A. Efficacy of low level laser therapy on neurosensory recovery after injury to the inferior alveolar nerve. Head Face Med 2006;15:2-3.
41. Demetriades N, Park J, Laskarides C. Alternative bone expansion technique for implant placement in atrophic edentulous maxilla and mandible. J Oral Implantol 2010;37:463-471.
42. Piccinini M. Mandibular bone expansion technique in conjunction with root form implants: a case report. J Oral Maxillofac Surg 2009;67:1931-1936.
43. Chen S, Beagle J, Jensen S, Chiapasco M, Darby I. Consensus statements and recommended clinical procedures regarding surgical techniques. Int J Oral Maxillofac Implants 2009;24(Suppl):272-278.
44. Enislidis G, Wittwer G, Ewers R. Preliminary report on a staged ridge splitting technique for implant placement in the mandible: a technical note. Int J Oral Maxillofac Implants 2006;21:445-449.
45. Blus C, Szmukler-Moncler S, Vozza I, Rispoli L, Polastri C. Split-crest and immediate placement with ultrasonic bone surgery (piezosurgery): 3-year follow-up of 180 treated implant sites. Quintessence Int 2010;41:463-469.
46. Sohn D, Lee H, Heo J, Moon J, Park I, Romanos G. Immediate and delayed lateral ridge expansion technique in the atrophic posterior mandibular ridge. J Oral Maxillofac Surg 2010;68:2283-2290.
47. Simion M, Baldoni M, Zafte D. Jawbone enlargement using immediate implant placement associated with a split-crest technique and guided tissue regeneration. Int J Periodontics Restorative Dent 1992;12:463-473.

Chapter 11

Tissue engineering: how long before reality?

Punjamaporn Chatakun, Maher el Atari, Federico Hernández Alfaro

11.1 Introduction

Bone augmentation is generally carried out using autogenous bone, allograft, xenograft, or alloplastic material. The ideal bone graft incorporates three main elements: osteogenic, osteoinductive, and osteoconductive. Autogenous bone is the gold standard. The autogenous corticocancellous bone graft is a well-accepted procedure and ideal for reconstruction of alveolar bone.[1-3] The cancellous bone is rich in osteogenic cells and the cortical bone is highly osteoconductive. The advantages of autogenous bone graft are the rapid angiogenisis from the surrounding original bone,[4] and the supply of osteoblasts.[5] However, discomfort and pain at the donor site of autogenous bone grafting are unavoidable. Additionally, there is limited supply of the donor site.[6] Autogenous bone grafts contain all the essential properties, but they are not available in every situation. Alternative methods including allogeneic bone transplantation have their own limitations, such as tissue matching, the risk of disease transmission, batch variability, and an inability to survive and integrate following implantation.[7] The large variability in bone defects, the huge biological complexity of bone, the high metabolic activity of bone, and the necessary vascularization motivate the development of new treatment strategies.[8]

Alloplastic biomaterials are a commonly used option in bone reconstruction. A histological study in animal models for comparison of alloplastic material (OsteoSet®; Wright Medical Technology, Arlington, TN) and bone tissue engineering at 2 and 4 months reported that alloplastic materials have only osteoconductive properties, so healing of a grafted bone defect will take more than 4 months.[9] The bone tissue engineering (basal and complex osteogenic medium) had significantly better healing rates than the groups with alloplastic commercial biomaterial. The report emphasized the osteoconductive potential of alloplastic biomaterials and the osteogenic potential of engineered bone grafts.[9] The scaffold materials, through tissue engineering protocols, initiated angiogenesis, encouraged tissue deposition, and culminated in restoration of structure and function specific to the grafted site.[6]

Tissue engineering is another alternative method. This procedure is minimally uncomfortable and there is no donor site morbidity.[10] Tissue engineering involves regeneration of tissue and restoration of function through implantation of cells/tissue grown outside the body, or stimulating cells to grow into an implanted matrix.[11] It is an alternative to conventional methods for reconstruction.[9] The three main components of tissue engineering are growth factors, stem cells, and scaffolds (Fig 11-1).

In oral implantology, the study of tissue engineering focuses on bone regeneration. Nevertheless, soft tissue regeneration is also a subject of study. Strategies to engineer bone tissue have been developed using three components: scaffold, growth factors, and mesenchymal stem cells (MSCs). Regeneration of alveolar tissue uses several technological advances, including novel approaches that apply concepts of tissue engineering.[12]

This chapter reviews and describes how to apply tissue engineering for oral implant dentistry, by assessing the following topics:

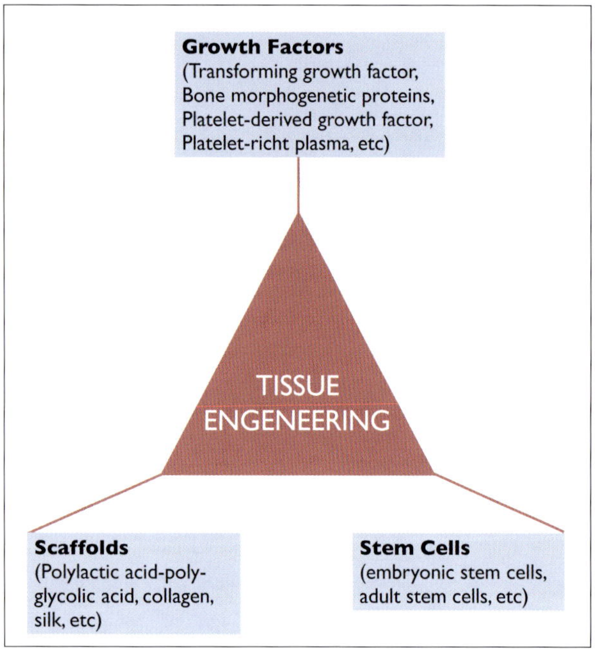

Fig 11-1 Key factors involved in tissue engineering.

- 11.2 Growth factors
  - 11.2.1 Transforming growth factor (TGF-β)
  - 11.2.2 Bone morphogenetic proteins (BMPs)
  - 11.2.3 Platelet-derived growth factor (PDGF)
  - 11.2.4 Platelet-rich plasma (PRP)
  - 11.2.5 Platelet-rich fibrin (PRF)
  - 11.2.6 Insulin-like growth factors (IGFs)
  - 11.2.7 Fibroblast growth factors (FGFs)
  - 11.2.8 Enamel matrix derivative (EMD)
- 11.3 Stem cells
  - 11.3.1 MSCs
    - Bone-marrow-derived stem cells
    - Adipose-tissue-derived stem cells (ATSCs)
  - 11.3.2 Hematopoietic stem cells (HSCs)
  - 11.3.3 Dental pulp stem cells (DPSCs)
- 11.4 Scaffold
  - 11.4.1 Synthetic polymer
    - Polylactic acid (PLA)-polyglycolic acid (PGA)
    - Polyanhydrides
    - Polycarbonates
    - Polyfumarates
  - 11.4.2 Natural polymer
    - Collagen
    - Collagen-glycosaminoglycans
    - Silk
- 11.5 Conclusions

11.2 Growth factors

Numerous growth factors have been identified that enhance various types of cell migration, adherence, and proliferation. These include TGF-β, BMPs, PDGF, PRP, PRF, IGFs, FGFs, and EMD.

11.2.1 TGF-β

TGF-βs are members of the TGF-β superfamily. So far, five subtypes have been demonstrated.[13] It exists as three different gene products: TGF-β1, TGF-β2, and TGF-β3. TGF-β1 is found in high concentrations in bone and platelets.[14] TGF-β1 is the most well-known factor involved in chondrogenic differentiation. TGF-β is produced by osteoblasts. It is stored in the bone matrix and makes bone the largest reservoir of TGF-β in the body.[15] TGF-β has a role in bone regeneration and repair. It is involved in bone and connective tissue regeneration and has chemotactic and mitogenic properties, influencing osteoblast progenitor cells and inhibiting osteoclasts and bone resorption.[16]

Mohammed et al.[17] reported the use of TGF-β1 in conjunction with guided tissue regeneration (GTR) in periodontal defects. They found that TGF-β1 encouraged bone regeneration in class II furcation defects in sheep, an effect enhanced by the presence of a barrier membrane. The combination of TGF-β1 and IGF-1 in a biodegradable poly(D,L-lactide) coating markedly increases the fixation and osseointegration of porous coated titanium implants in an unloaded 1-mm gap model.[18] Interestingly, a single application of TGF-β1 in the primate did not induce bone formation in calvarial defects, while it induced endochondral bone differentiation in heterotopic sites. *In vivo*, platelet-derived porcine TGF-β1 (pTGF-β1) induces endochondral bone in heterotopic sites of guanidinium-inactivated collagenous bone matrix as carrier-induced cartilage and bone formation.[19] Similarly, adeno-associated virus of TGF-β1 can improve cartilage repair *in vivo* of human MSCs.[20]

11.2.2 BMPs

BMPs are multifunctional proteins with a wide range of biologic activities involving a variety of cell types.[21] BMPs regulate growth, differentiation, chemotaxis, and apoptosis; and play pivotal roles in morphogenesis.[22]

Dr Marshall Urist, an orthopedic surgeon, observed and researched this protein and proposed the name "bone morphogenetic protein" in the scientific literature in the *Journal of Dental Research* in 1971.[23] In 1988, Wozney et al.[24] extracted 40 mg of inductive proteins from 40 kg of bone. Chromatography showed the extract contained several proteins, but further purification was not possible. Implantation of this protein component of bone matrix resulted in a complex series of cellular events, including mesenchymal cell infiltration, cartilage formation, vascularization, bone formation, and ultimately remodeling of the new bone tissue along with population by hematopoietic bone marrow elements.[25] There are three subclasses of BMPs followed by the derived amino acid sequences found in osteoinductive extracts of bone. The first subclass contains BMP-2 and BMP-4, highly related molecules that differ mainly in the amino terminal region. In the second subclass are BMP-5, BMP-6, and BMP-7, also known as osteogenic protein-1 (OP-1), and BMP-8 (OP-2). In the third subclass, and more distantly related to these factors, is BMP-3, also called osteogenin.[26] BMPs comprise the osteoinductive component of several tissue engineering products. They occur in late-stage development as replacements for autogenous bone graft, and for bone augmentation and repair.[26]

Many studies have shown that BMPs induce bone and cartilage formation.[27-30] BMPs have been applied in oral implant dentistry in various methods. Many studies support the use of BMP-2 and recombinant human BMP-2 (rhBMP-2).[27-29] *In vivo* osteoinductive activity of an apatite-covered titanium coated implant with BMP-2/heparin enhanced new endosteal bone formation.[30] Another study reported a positive effect of liposomal vector/BMP-2 on bone regeneration and osseointegration in peri-implant bone defect.[31] A histological, animal study on alveolar ridge augmentation using implants coated with rhBMP-2 showed strong bone formation that exceeded the implant platform. The newly formed bone joined with native bone, including cortex formation.[32] Similarly, another animal study reported that rhBMP-2-coated implants exhibited robust radiographic bone formation extending to and above the implant platform.[33] Jung et al.[34] reported no significant differences between implant placement in bone augmentation with and without rhBMP-2. Both presented excellent clinical and radiological outcomes after 3 and 5 years.[34] Lee et al.[35] showed that biodegradable membranes impregnated with BMP-2 greatly improved bone regeneration in a rabbit calvarial model, due to the osteoinductive properties of rhBMP-2 released from the membrane during healing. An rhBMP-2–collagen composite scaffold showed excellent biocompatibility and possessed bone-inducing capacity in rats within 2 weeks, and no adverse response was detected around the implanted scaffold.[36] In 2004, Warnke et al.[37] demonstrated a case of mandibular reconstruction by using a titanium mesh cage filled with bone mineral block, 7 mg of rhBMP-7 and 20 ml of the patient's bone marrow. The construction was implanted into the latissimus dorsi muscle and then was transferred to repair the mandibular defect. This technique provided a good three-dimensional (3D) outcome.[37] Regarding the safety of BMPs, there are reports of minor side effects including headaches, an increase and modification of the plasma amylase without pancreatitis, and a decrease in magnesium levels and tachycardia associated with BMPs.[38] The appearance of anti-BMP antibodies or anti-collagen antibodies has also been reported among less than 4% of the population, with no significant clinical consequences.[38]

11.2.3 PDGF

PDGF is a glycoprotein, originally identified in platelets and in serum as a mitogen for fibroblasts, smooth muscle cells, and glial cells in culture. Two PDGF polypeptides, PDGF-A and PDGF-B, were known and hence seemed to comprise the complete mammalian PDGF family.[39] PDGF is synthesized by blood platelets, monocytes, macrophages, and endothelial cells, and influences most mesodermal cells. It increases DNA synthesis, cell replication, and collagen and non-collagen protein synthesis in cultures of rat calvarial cells.[13]

PDGFs bind to and signal through two cell-surface receptor tyrosine kinases. PDGF-A only binds to PDGF-α receptor, whereas PDGF-B can bind to both α and β receptors. The PDGF molecules are bivalent, and PDGF-dependent receptor dimerization is a prerequisite for receptor autophosphorylation and subsequent signal propagation. The two receptor genes may be expressed individually or together in cells.[39] The two PDGF receptors have partially overlapping and partially distinct signaling capabilities *in vitro*.[40,41]

In 1989, Lynch et al.[42] initially reported the application of PDGF and IGF-1 for periodontal regeneration in a beagle dog. PDGF has an important role in the healing of bone and periodontium. PDGF results in intramembranous bone formation, that is, bone formation in the absence of cartilage. Purified rhPDGF-BB is a potent wound healing growth factor and stimulator of the proliferation and recruitment of both periodontal ligament and bone cells.[43] PDGF-BB is a potent mediator of tooth-supporting periodontal tissue repair and regeneration.[44] It binds to both α and β PDGF receptors, and promotes wound healing in both hard and soft tissues, such as skin and periodontium.[44] There is a report of using methylcellulose gel (4.4%) with rhPDGF-BB on rabbit calvarial bone defects; the results showed the newly formed bone had trabecular structure and an increased amount of bone marrow.[45] A study comparing bone formation around dental implants in dogs found expanded polytetrafluoroethylene (ePTFE) membranes in combination with PDGF/IGF-1 had the highest bone density compared with sites that received ePTFE membranes alone or ePTFE membranes and demineralized freeze-dried bone.[46] In a human model, the application of rhPDGF-BB incorporated in allograft improved periodontal regeneration in both class II furcations and interproximal intrabony defects.[43] PDGF-BB delivered with a chitosan/tricalcium phosphate (TCP) sponge carrier in rat calvarial defect enhanced bone regeneration by up to 4 weeks.[47]

11.2.4 PRP

PRP was first introduced to the oral surgery community by Whitman et al.[48] in their 1997 article entitled "Platelet gel: an autologous alternative to fibrin glue with applications in oral and maxillofacial surgery". PRP is an autologous source of PDGF, vascular endothelial growth factor (VEGF) and TGF-β. It is obtained by sequestering and concentrating platelets by gradient density centrifugation.[49] A natural blood clot contains 95% red blood cells, 5% platelets, less than 1% white blood cells, and numerous amounts of fibrin strands. A PRP blood clot contains 4% red blood cells, 95% platelets, and 1% white blood cells.[50] PRP plays a fundamental role in hemostasis and it is a natural source of growth factors and adhesive glycoproteins.[51,52] The use of PRP is based on the premise that the large number of platelets in PRP release significant quantities of growth factors. These growth factors promote chemotaxis of precursor cells, cell mitosis, collagen production, initiating vascular in-growth and inducing cell differentiation.[49] PRP is an easily accessible, cost-effective, and safe source of growth factors.[53] Two methods are currently available for point-of-care production of PRP: general-purpose cell separators and platelet-concentrating cell separators.[50] General-purpose cell separators require 450 ml of blood. Blood is collected into a collection bag containing citrate-phosphate-dextrose anticoagulant. It is first centrifuged at 5600 rpm to separate red blood cells from platelet-poor plasma (PPP) and PRP. It is finally centrifuged at 2400 rpm to get 30 ml of PRP.[50] Platelet-concentrating cell separators use smaller quantities of blood. Two systems are approved by the US Food and Drug Administration (FDA): Harvest SmartPRep® Platelet Concentrate System (HSPCS; Harvest Technologies, Plymouth, MA) and the 3i Platelet Concentrate Collection System (3i PCCS; 3i Implant Innovations, Palm Beach Gardens, FL).[50]

The use of PRP alone did not show benefit in rabbit cranial defects compared with other untreated defects.[54] Many studies performed addition of PRP to autogenous bone grafts or bone substitutes. Marx and colleagues demonstrated a higher maturation rate and greater radiographic bone density of 44 patients at 6 months after cancellous marrow bone grafting using platelet concentrates (PRP) as a source of autologous growth factors.[55] Another study of 6 months in an animal model compared using autologous iliac corticocancellous bone with using PRP and only autologous bone. PRP appeared to enhance early autologous graft healing. However, after 2 months this effect is no longer significant. The authors did not find a changed amount of PRP after new bone formation, and there was no increase in trabecular density.[56] Fennis et al.[57] reported that PRP enhanced healing of autologous bone grafts in a sheep mandibular continuity resection model. The benefits were especially seen at 6 and 12 weeks. Oyama et al.[53] evaluated seven alveolar cleft patients who had iliac bone grafts with PRP by using 3D computed tomography scans, and compared with controls. They concluded that the volume of regenerated bone using PRP was higher. A study to compare PRP and PRF cultured in human osteoblasts, human fibroblasts, and human osteoblast-derived osteosarcoma cells demonstrated PRP application in cell cultures leaded to higher levels of growth factors than PRF application.[58]

Tissue engineering research reports the use of autologous MSCs combined with an osteoconductive scaffold as a live bone substitute. In histomorphometric analysis,

Pieri et al.[59] investigated improving bone formation and bone-to-implant contact (BIC) in maxillary sinus grafting by comparing MSCs and PRP seeded on a fluorohydroxyapatite (FHA) scaffold and FHA alone. An animal model showed that sinus augmentation with MSCs–PRP, combined with FHA may enhance bone formation and osseointegration of dental implants compared with FHA alone.[59] However, Klongnoi et al.[60] used the same experimental design, and they concluded that the application of PRP could not reveal significant beneficial effects on the BIC, the percentage of the newly formed bone, and the remaining bone substitute. In an animal model, PRP could not promote new bone regeneration in critical size defects.[61] Bovine bone with PRP increased vertical bone augmentation *in vivo*.[62] In a recent human study of removal sites treated with PRP, it was shown to improve bone formation and the patient did not present postoperative pain, bleeding, or numbness.[63]

11.2.5 PRF

PRF is the second generation of platelet concentrate. It was first described by Choukroun et al.[50] in France. PRF consists of cytokines, glycan chains, and structural glycoproteins enmeshed within a fibrin network. These components have synergetic effects on healing processes.[64] PRF is not only a platelet concentrate but also an immune node able to stimulate defense mechanisms.[65] The preparation technique for PRF requires blood in 10 ml test tubes without an anticoagulant, immediately centrifuged at 2700 rpm for 12 min,[50] or centrifuged at 3000 rpm for 10 min.[66] A fibrin clot is then obtained in the middle of the tube, between the red corpuscles at the bottom and acellular plasma at the top.[66] The protocol is then to collect a fibrin clot charged with serum and platelet.[66] PRF can be squeezed out of the fluids for forming the membrane and can also be used in conjugation with bone grafts.[50]

From histologic evaluation, one study compared six sites of sinus lift by use of PRF mixed with freeze-dried bone allograft (FDBA) with three sites of sinus lift, and by using FDBA without PRF with three sites of sinus lift.[67] After 4 months of healing time, the group of PRF with FDBA particles showed the presence of residual bone surrounded by newly formed bone and connective tissue similar to that after 8 months of healing time of the group of FDBA without PRF.[67] However, it is necessary to perform similar large-scale studies to validate this result.[67] Another study reported implant placement using PRF as grafting material in the bone-added osteotome sinus floor augmentation. This technique presented endosinus bone gain of 3.2 mm on average. Within 2 to 3 months of healing, the implants exhibited a resistance torque of 25 Ncm, applied during abutment tightening.[68] On the other hand, scintigraphic evaluation between PRF-treated and non-PRF-treated sockets showed that PRF might not enhance bone healing in sockets 4 weeks after surgery.[69]

At present, PRF is not a popular treatment choice. Further evaluation is required to understand the benefits and to obtain predictable results.

11.2.6 IGFs

IGFs are a class of polypeptide growth factors, and are important in demineralized bone-induced heterotopic osteogenesis. IGF-1 (somatomedin-C; 7.5 kDa) and IGF-2 (skeletal growth factor; 8.7 kDa) are produced by different types of cells, including osteoblasts.[13] IGF-1 has 47% homology with insulin and it stimulates cartilage growth, bone matrix formation, and replication of pre-osteoblasts and osteoblasts.[70] Both IGF-I and -II share 62% amino acid sequence homology with proinsulin and bind to two distinct cell-surface receptors.[71,72]

Both IGF-1 and IGF-2 increase bone collagen synthesis and decrease collagen degradation in intact rat calvaria *in vitro*[73] and stimulate proliferation of osteoblasts in serum-free cultures of human bone cells.[16] An *in vivo* study of IGF-1 on bone metabolism reported IGF-1 infusion significantly increased cortical bone formation for up to 14 days, and increased by 22% trabecular bone formation; however, the infusion was for 7 days.[74] The authors concluded that IGF-1 appears to be a purely anabolic hormone for bone formation, since it significantly stimulates osteoblast proliferation and decreases the number of osteoclasts;[74] IGF-1 was also shown to be potentially useful for periodontal regeneration enhancement[75] and increased the formation of gingival attachment.[76]

Similar to other growth factors, IGF-1 combined with other growth factors may promote greater bone formation than individual factors. Cultures treated with IGF-1/TGF-β revealed synergistic increases in non-collagen protein synthesis and greater collagen content above individual factors, without significant alterations in the percentage of collagen synthesized.[77]

11.2.7 FGFs

The FGF family consists of 22 members of structurally related polypeptide growth factors.[78] Various cells synthesize FGFs, including monocytes, macrophages, osteoblasts, and chondrocytes. They affect most mesodermal and neuroectodermal cells.[13]

FGFs can enhance cell proliferation, motility, differentiation, mitogenesis, wound healing and tissue repair, and angiogenesis.[79,80] Basic fibroblast growth factor (bFGF) acts at sites of injury and stimulates similar vascular cell responses. It is released relatively slowly from the fibrin clot because of covalent binding of bFGF to fibrinogen.[81] Fibrin gel-immobilized VEGF and bFGF significantly enhanced the angiogenic response at 2 weeks, as evidenced by increased vascular density.[82] In terms of periodontal regeneration, a topical application of bFGF can enhance periodontal regeneration in inflamed class II furcation defects in non-human primates.[83] In a dog model study, a smaller dose of bFGF enhances the periodontal regeneration in class III furcation defects and leads to greater filling of these defects with both mineralized and non-mineralized tissues.[84] bFGF in combination with a biodegradable polymer coated onto titanium implants in rabbit tibiae stimulated bone formation adjacent to the surface of an implant inserted in bone after 12 weeks of healing.[85]

11.2.8 EMD

EMD is formed from amelogenins with metalloendoprotease and serine protease activity. The biologic effect of EMD is through stimulation of local growth factor secretion and cytokine expression in the treated tissues, inducing a regenerative process that mimics odontogenesis. More than 95% of EMD is amelogenins. Amelogenin structure and function has a role in biomineralization and hard tissue formation.[86]

EMD in the form of a purified acid extract of proteins from pig enamel matrix, is commercialized as Emdogain® (Straumann, Basel, Switzerland). EMD has shown positive results in stimulating periodontal regeneration,[87,88] and exhibited stimulation of angiogenesis of the periodontal wounds.[89] A recent study reported that EMD alone effectively promoted new cementum and functionally oriented connective tissue formation.[90] A human clinical trial reported that topical application of EMD onto root surface lesion can promote an increase of radiographic bone gain and clinical attachment.[91] Another study showed that the application of EMD can improve 2- and 3-wall intrabony defects.[92] The treatment of EMD combined with bovine-derived xenograft resulted in the improvement of probing pocket depth and clinical attachment level. However, there is no significant difference when comparing with sites treated only with bovine-derived xenograft.[93] One animal study reported an improvement in osseointegration of implants that were coated with EMD.[94] When EMD was applied on the trabecular bone (femurs of rats), volume was significantly greater than for implants in propylene glycol alginate (applied at 14 and 30 days post-implantation).[94] No adverse effects from application of EMD for periodontal surgery were found.[91-93] Application of EMD before tooth replantation after a dry extra-alveolar period of 60 min promotes a favorable healing of the periodontal ligament cells.[95]

11.3 Stem cells

Many tissue engineering strategies rely on rapid cell expansion while maintaining the capacity for functional differentiation. With respect to this, the cell source remains a complicating factor in the study of cell behavior in skeletal tissue engineering.[96]

Stem cells are unspecialized cells. They are classified into three categories, based on the degree of differentiation: totipotent, pluripotent, or multipotent. They are also characterized by two unique properties in one cell: their high self-renewal activity and their multilineage differentiation potential, which make them an ideal source for cellular therapy and regenerative medicine.

Stem cells can be readily isolated, expanded, and transplanted. Their application in cell-based therapies has become a major focus of research.[97,98] The pathway of stem cell differentiation is as follows:

stem cell → stem cell + progenitor cell → differentiated cell.[99]

Cells derived from different sources have been shown to fulfill those criteria, including embryonic stem cells and adult stem cells isolated from various tissues.[100] For tissue engineering applications, biomaterials often serve as scaffold for a specific cell type. Embryonic and adult stem cells are an ideal cell source for tissue engineering.

11.3.1 MSCs

MSCs are capable of differentiating into cells of mesenchymal origin (osteoblasts) and producing tissue such as bone.[9,97] They are easily isolated from bone marrow and expanded in culture through various passages while retaining their multipotent differentiation capacity.[101,102] MSCs can differentiate into several types of cells, including fibroblasts, adipocytes, osteoblasts, chondrocytes, and skeletal muscle cells.[103] As primary prospective isolation of MSCs from tissue remains difficult, clinical use of MSCs currently still depends on culture isolation followed by expansion. However, not only isolation methods, but also the culture conditions for selection and expansion of MSCs are highly variable, and the fate *in vivo* of cells following expansion is not fully studied.[100] The isolation of MSCs by density centrifugation followed by selection of the plastic adherent fraction is frequently used; the composition of expansion media differs. The type of MSC expansion media considerably influences morphology, proliferation, expansion capacity, passage number, clonogenicity, and differentiation potential.[104]

Bone substitution materials can be combined with vital cells such as MSCs to increase bone formation.[26,105-107] Under restrictive stimulation, MSCs undergo osteogenic differentiation via a well-defined pathway,[108] acquiring osteoblastic markers and secreting extracellular matrix (ECM) and calcium deposits. MSCs are low-immunogenic both *in vitro* and *in vivo*.[109,110]

Augmentation of the host cell population can be used effectively to improve the healing of bone lesions. If the soft and hard tissues of the defect site are healthy, the expansion of host cells is often successful. Four different strategies have been introduced in maxillofacial surgery:[111]

- Application of cytokines or vectors at the defect site.
- Application of mechanical loads.
- Exposure to electromagnetic fields.
- The use of separating membranes.

A main advantage of augmenting the local cell population is that the regenerate tissue can be expected to have the same biological properties as the lost tissue. The harvesting and culture technique, the implantation procedure, and immunological aspects have a major impact on the clinical outcome.

Bone marrow-derived stem cells

Friedenstein et al.[112] described the first successful isolation of bone marrow MSCs. Bone marrow stromal cells (BMSCs) are progenitors of skeletal tissue components such as bone, cartilage, the hematopoiesis-supporting stroma, and adipocytes.[113] BMSCs represent a particularly attractive osteogenic cell source due to the availability of established culture techniques to isolate and *ex vivo* expand this cell population from adult human donors.[114] In dog models, a bone defect treated with allogeneic MSCs loaded on hydroxyapatite (HA)-TCP implants had new bone formation at 16 weeks and no adverse immune response was detected without the use of immunosuppressive therapy.[115] Cultured human gingival connective tissue *in vivo* showed that it could be a reservoir of MSCs that could be used in regenerative procedures based on tissue engineering.[116]

ATSCs

ATSCs are multipotent cells and are found in mesodermally derived adipose tissue that contains a stromal population of cells.[117] ATSCs have the potential to differentiate into bone, cartilage, fat, myocardium, skin, and neuron.[118] ATSCs have a similar ability to differentiate into osteoblasts to that of BMSCs.[119] Moreover, it has been reported that only a few cells derived from ATSCs differentiate into beating cells that are thought to represent cardiomyocytes phenotypically.[120] It is easy to get a large volume of adipose tissue and a less painful procedure. A recent study of delayed implant placement in rabbit calvarium by using adipose-derived adult stem cells with anorganic bovine bone (ABB) for vertical bone regeneration, concluded that adipose-derived adult stem cells on ABB might effectively increase vertical bone regeneration and implant osseointegration, versus ABB alone.[121]

Alloderm was used as a scaffold of adult stem cells for adipose tissue engineering. The authors suggested that adipose stem cell–alloderm complexes can be used as injectable 3D soft tissue fillers.[122]

11.3.2 HSCs

HSCs can undergo self-renewing cell divisions *in vivo*, differentiate at the single cell level into all mature blood cells and functionally repopulate the hematopoietic system of a myeloablated recipient. These properties make HSCs much more valuable from a therapeutic standpoint than committed progenitors, which have limited self-renewal potential and thus cannot provide long-term reconstitution of the hematopoietic system.[123] The hematopoietic system produces many millions of cells on a daily basis, the most primitive HSC, also termed the long-term repopulating HSC (LTR-HSC) is a relatively quiescent cell during steady state hematopoiesis. The relative quiescence of HSCs protects their genomic integrity by reducing the rounds of DNA replication and thus the probability of acquiring DNA damage that might compromise multilineage differentiation potential and/or render them malignant over time.[100] HSC transplantation has long been used in the treatment of choice for various hematologic, neoplastic, and congenital disorders.[124]

11.3.3 DPSCs

DPSCs are pluripotent stem cells. They were found in the "cell rich zone" of dental pulp. Gronthos et al.[125] isolated a clonogenic and proliferated population of cells from adult human dental pulp. These dental pulp stem cells produced sporadically with densely calcified nodules, and did not form adipocytes. DPSCs also have self-renewal capability and multilineage differentiation capacity. They can form ectopic dentin and associate to pulp tissue *in vivo*. DPSCs present parameters characterizing the osteoblastic phenotype, osteoblast-like cells, alkaline phosphatase, collagen I, osteopontin and osteocalcin. Therefore, they may be a potential source of osteoblasts for bone regeneration.[126] DPSCs show good adherence and bone tissue formation on microconcavity surface textures. SBP-DPSCs are a multipotent stem cell subpopulation of DPSCs. They can differentiate into osteoblasts, synthesizing 3D woven bone tissue chips *in vitro*, and are capable of synergistic differentiation into osteoblasts and endotheliocytes.[127]

11.4 Scaffold

Biodegradable scaffolds have played an important role in tissue engineering assay over the past decade. An ideal scaffold should provide chemical stability or degradability and physical properties matching the surrounding tissue to provide cytocompatibility, support adhesion, proliferation, stability, and mechanical strength.[97] The scaffold creates a medium where the cells are able to maintain phenotype and to synthesize the necessary proteins and molecules, mandatory conditions for a scaffold as demonstrated by Lutolf and Hubbell.[128] Scaffold should be effective for transport of nutrients, oxygen, and waste.[129]

For a macroporous scaffold, the following phases can be distinguished in scaffold colonization and tissue formation:

- Attachment.
- Proliferation and migration.
- ECM production.
- Mineralization.

During this process of tissue formation, the cell shifts from essentially a 2D configuration on the scaffold surface to a 3D situation embedded in the matrix material. It is well known that there are marked differences in cell expression in 2D culture compared with the 3D situation.[96] Liu and Roy[130] demonstrated that mouse embryonic stem cells differentiated on 3D, highly porous, tantalum-based scaffolds (Cytomatrix®, Woburn, MA) have significantly higher hematopoietic differentiation efficiency than those cultured under conventional 2D tissue culture conditions. Liu and colleagues also reported that compared with 2D tissue culture plates, cells differentiated on porous, Cytomatrix® scaffolds possess significantly higher expression levels of ECM-related genes, as well as genes that regulate cell growth, proliferation, and differentiation.[131] In addition, these differences in gene expression were more pronounced in 3D dynamic culture compared with 3D static culture. 3D scaffolds provide support for cells to attach, grow, and differentiate, and define the spatial shape of the tissue engineered transplant.[97]

There are two kinds of polymer materials: synthetic polymer, and naturally derived polymers.[132] Natural polymers such as collagen and glycosaminoglycan offer good biocompatibility and bioactivity, and synthetic polymers can elaborate physicochemical features such as degradation rate, microstructure, and mechanical strength. The most commonly used synthetic materials are PLA, PGA, and their copolymers, poly(lactic-co-glycolic acid) (PLGA).[129] The main biodegradable synthetic polymers include polyesters, polyanhydrides, polyorthoesters, polycaprolactones, polycarbonates, and polyfumarates.[133,134]

Scaffolds used in oral mucosa and skin reconstruction fall into several different categories:[135]

- Naturally derived scaffolds, such as acellular dermis and amniotic membrane.
- Fibroblast-populated skin substitutes.
- Collagen-based scaffolds.
- Gelatin-based scaffolds.
- Fibrin-based materials.
- Synthetic scaffolds, such as polymers.
- Hybrid scaffolds, which are combinations of natural and synthetic matrices.

Bone tissue engineering requires porous biodegradable scaffolds combined with a non-immunogenic cell source with osteogenic potential.[136] A variety of biomaterials have been investigated for stem cells in the context of bone tissue engineering.[97] A cell-seeded scaffold is often strained *in vitro*.[137] Several methods have been developed to create porous scaffolds, including gas foaming,[138,139] fiber bonding,[140] 3D printing,[141] phase separation,[142] emulsion freeze-drying, and porogen leaching.[143] These scaffolds can be in the form of a solid foam, nanofibrous matrix, microsphere, or hydrogel.[144] The applications of synthetic and natural polymers are summarized in Table 11-1.

Table 11-1 Synthetic biodegradable polymers

Polymer	Application
Synthetic polymer	
PLA-PGA	Bone[149,150,153,156] Cartilage[153,155]
Polyanhydride	Bone[159,160]
	Drug carrier and drug delivery[157,158,161]
Polycarbonate	Bone[162]
Polyfumarate	Bone[163,165]
Natural polymer	
Collagen	Bone[170-176]
Collagen-glycosaminoglycans	Bone[181]
Silk	Bone[185]
	Soft tissue[183]

11.4.1 Synthetic polymer

PLA-PGA

PLA and PGA are aliphatic polyesters and belong to the α-hydroxy group. To synthesize high-molecular-weight PLA and PGA, ring opening polymerization of the cyclic diesters glycolide or lactide is most commonly used.[145,146] PLA undergoes hydrolytic scission to its monomeric form, lactic acid, which is eliminated from the body by the incorporation into the tricarboxylic acid cycle. The principal elimination path for lactic acid is respiration, and it is primarily excreted by lungs as CO_2.[147] Polylactides are used to make screws and plates for fracture treatment, and are safe.[148] PGA can be broken down by hydrolysis, nonspecific esterases and carboxypeptidases. The glycolic acid monomer is either excreted in the urine or enters the tricarboxylic acid cycle.[75] A rat bone cell culture model presented bone cell penetration and formation of a calcified collagenous bone-like tissue on the weave of the PGA membrane after 3 weeks in culture.[149] Similarly, histologic, biochemical, and radiographic studies of repair bone defect in white rabbit with resorbable PGA implants seeded with periosteal cells showed improved bone formation using this technique.[150]

Copolymer PLGA is a synthetic polyester with a hydrophobic and bioinert surface.[151] Fialkov et al.[152] described the development of a new method of PLGA foam processing, modifying the production of a biodegradable scaffold with similar porosity to human trabecular bone. PLA-PGA materials have been used extensively to fabricate scaffolds for engineering musculoskeletal tissue. These include scaffolds for bone, cartilage, and meniscus.[153] Thompson et al.[154] studied a 50:50 PLA/PGA under a cyclic compressive load over a 6-week period. They concluded that dynamic loading and the environment in which an implant is placed affect its biodegradation. The PLGA microspheres were compounded with the fibrin gel for enhancement of mechanical strength and stability.[151] A non-woven resorbable material consisting of PGA and poly-L-lactic acid (PLLA) in a 90:10 ratio (Ethisorb®, Ethicon, Norderstedt, Germany) is suitable for creating cartilage without risk of infection and for large defect reconstruction.[155] The biodegradable composites of ß-TCP and poly(L-lactide-*co*-glycolide-*co*-ε-caprolactone) (PLGC) is useful for guided bone regeneration and GTR membranes as well as tissue/infection barrier membranes.[156]

Polyanhydrides

Polyanhydrides inherently degrade by surface erosion without the need for the incorporation of catalysts. Furthermore, polyanhydrides have been shown to be highly sensitive to hydrolysis and degrade rapidly.[153] Polyanhydrides are a class of surface eroding biomaterials with applications in vaccine and drug delivery.[157]

They can be used as protein/drug carriers.[158] Photo-crosslinked polyanhydride networks are useful to modulate protein release and improve system properties for bone regeneration applications.[159,160] Using polyanhydride and PLA combined as carriers for antibiotics might be useful in the treatment of chronic osteomyelitis and in the prophylaxis of bone infection.[161]

Polycarbonates

Polycarbonate-based polymers are synthesized in several forms. Poly(trimethylene carbonate) is an aliphatic compound found to degrade under physiological conditions. Aliphatic polycarbonates become extremely soft in the temperature range of 40 to 60°C.[153] Nano-HA/polycarbonate composite can stimulate new bone growth in bone repair.[162]

Polyfumarates

Peter et al.[163] studied a partially saturated linear polyester based on poly(propylene fumarate) (PPF) to use in filling skeletal defects. They identified this polymer's mechanical properties as similar to those of trabecular bone. The polyfumarates showed less roughness and less porous surface than the most hydrophilic polymers.[164] A compatibilized blend of poly(ε-caprolactone) (PCL) and poly(diisopropyl fumarate) (PDIPF) found osteoblast adherence and proliferation more than on either homo-polymer, showed a greater number of cellular processes with a better organized actin cytoskeleton, and expressed more type-I collagen and mineral, both markers of osteoblast phenotype.[165]

11.4.2 Natural polymer

Collagen

Collagen is a major structural component forming the natural ECM of connective tissues and organs.[166] Type I collagen extracted from animal tissues and gelatin prepared from denaturation of collagen is capable of forming porous gel matrices, which are already commercially available as skin replacements.[167] Using *in vitro* models, Masuda first developed the technique to reconstruct the oral mucosa by seeding keratinocytes on contracted collagen gels containing fibroblasts (CCG) in a reconstruction medium at the gas–liquid interface for 10 days. The oral mucosal models were well-differentiated and histologically similar to native tissues.[168]

Animal-sourced collagens have been widely used as a biomaterial for decades in biomedical applications, such as injectable collagen formulations for soft tissue augmentation, hemostats for control of bleeding during surgery and after trauma, wound transdressings, and vascular graft coatings.[169] Recombinant collagen accumulation has been demonstrated in bioreactor-based eukaryotic production systems, mammalian cell culture, insect cell culture, yeast, and transgenic production systems.[169] Animal-derived collagen may present risk of contamination with prions and viruses and the original source material cannot be easily identified, in contrast to recombinant collagen. Additionally, animal-derived collagen is limited by intellectual property rights and customizability.[169]

In a human study, comparison between Collagraft® (Zimmer and Collagen Corporation, Warsaw, IN; consists of a mixture of porous beads composed of 60% HA and 40% TCP ceramic and fibrillar collagen) and autograft; Collagraft presented the function as well as autogenous graft when used in the treatment of acute long bone fractures at 6- and 12-month follow-up.[170] Two-stage maxillary sinus lift and implant placement in rhBMP-2/absorbable collagen sponge (ACS) had results similar to autogenous bone graft after functional loading.[171] A randomized controlled trial showed that rhBMP-2/ACS safely induced adequate bone for the placement and functional loading of endosseous dental implants in patients requiring staged maxillary sinus floor augmentation.[172] rhBMP-2/ACS can also be used for alveolar ridge preservation after tooth extraction.[173] HA and collagen composites composite have the potential of mimicking and replacing diseased skeletal bones.[174,175] The culture of osteoblast on electrospun collagen/HA nanofibers showed increasing mineralization, thus this nanofibrous scaffold may be a biomaterial suitable for bone regeneration.[175] The new bone substitute materials consisting of collagen and TCP on mandibular dog teeth defects showed good osteoconduction and biodegradable character with non-critical inflammatory symptoms.[176] Collagen (Bio-Gide®; Geistlich, Wolhusen, Switzerland) was not suitable as a matrix for organizing a 3D network of cultured cells because collagen fibers are arranged too densely to allow a homogeneous cell distribution and the establishment of a tissue-like network.[177] In another study, long bone defect in the tibial diaphysis of 16 sheep was supplied with PRP-loaded collagen scaffold and it did not increase new bone formation.[61]

Collagen-glycosaminoglycans (CG)

Glycosaminoglycans are essential components of the ECM, composed of long, non-branched polymers of repeating disaccharide units, one of which is an amino sugar.[135] Compound collagen-based matrices have been suggested to improve the function of scaffolds. The modified fabrication technique has allowed production of CG scaffolds with a more homogenous structure characterized by less variation in mean pore size throughout the scaffold (mean: 95.9 μm).[178] The fraction of viable cells attached to the CG scaffold decreased with increasing mean pore size,[179] and a mean pore size of 325 μm was deemed optimal for bone tissue engineering.[180] CG scaffolds were seeded with osteoblast and cultured. They were found to have a porosity of approximately 99%, high cell metabolic activity and cell number, and good cell infiltration over the 7 days in culture.[181]

Silk

Silk fibroin is biocompatible and provides a long-term augmentation. Moreover, its properties include good oxygen and water vapor permeability, and biodegradability.[182] It has very slow degradation with minimal negative impact on the surrounding tissues.[183] For preparing 3D porous sponges of silk, the process depends on the alteration of surface area, crystallinity, and bulk versus surface proteolytic digestion.[184] Human fibroblasts embedded in silk gel had a survival rate up to 68.4% and were able to proliferate and synthesize proteins. The soft tissue augmentation was stable at 1 month after subcutaneous implantation and a mild inflammation was found after 12 months.[183] Silk fibroin membrane has shown good biocompatibility with enhanced bone regeneration in a rabbit calvarial model, with no evidence of any inflammatory reaction.[185]

11.5 Conclusions

- Although there are numerous studies that present tissue engineering as a successful treatment, long-term results are still unclear.
- Growth factors are key components of bone regeneration.
- Healing may be improved by the administration of osteogenic agents, for example BMPs and IGFs. However, the efficacy of these agents depends on the application technique.
- Applications combining two or more growth factors may be more favorable.
- The role of stem cells and understanding of their applications are being developed for use in human oral implantology.
- Scaffold biomaterials are also being developed for supporting adhesion, growth, and differentiation of cells.
- Long-term safety of tissue engineering is still unclear.

References

1. Aghaloo TL, Moy PK. Which hard tissue augmentation techniques are the most successful in furnishing bony support for implant placement? Int J Oral Maxillofac Implants 2007;22(Suppl):49-70.
2. Del Fabbro M, Testori T, Francetti L, Weinstein R. Systematic review of survival rates for implants placed in the grafted maxillary sinus. Int J Periodontics Restorative Dent 2004;24:565-577.
3. Wallace SS, Froum SJ. Effect of maxillary sinus augmentation on the survival of endosseous dental implants. A systematic review. Ann Periodontol 2003;8:328-343.
4. Schlegel KA, Fichtner G, Schultze-Mosgau S, Wiltfang J. Histologic findings in sinus augmentation with autogenous bone chips versus a bovine bone substitute. Int J Oral Maxillofac Implants 2003;18: 53-58.
5. Yildirim M, Spiekermann H, Handt S, Edelhoff D. Maxillary sinus augmentation with the xenograft Bio-Oss and autogenous intraoral bone for qualitative improvement of the implant site: a histologic and histomorphometric clinical study in humans. Int J Oral Maxillofac Implants 2001;16:23-33.
6. Schimming R, Schmelzeisen R. Tissue-engineered bone for maxillary sinus augmentation. J Oral Maxillofac Surg 2004;62:724-729.
7. Khan SN, Cammisa FP Jr, Sandhu HS, Diwan AD, Girardi FP, Lane JM. The biology of bone grafting. J Am Acad Orthop Surg 2005;13: 77-86.
8. Frohlich M, Grayson WL, Wan LQ, Marolt D, Drobnic M, Vunjak-Novakovic G. Tissue engineered bone grafts: biological requirements, tissue culture and clinical relevance. Curr Stem Cell Res Ther 2008;3:254-264.

9. Lucaciu O, Băciuţ M, Băciuţ G, Câmpian R, Soriţău O, Bran S, et al. Tissue engineered bone versus alloplastic commercial biomaterials in craniofacial reconstruction. Rom J Morphol Embryol 2010;51:129-136.
10. Schmelzeisen R, Schimming R, Sittinger M. Making bone: implant insertion into tissue-engineered bone for maxillary sinus floor augmentation. A preliminary report. J Craniomaxillofac Surg 2003;31:34-39.
11. Vats A, Tolley NS, Polak JM, Gough JE. Scaffolds and biomaterials for tissue engineering: a review of clinical applications. Clin Otolaryngol Allied Sci 2003;28:165-172.
12. Ueda M, Tohnai I, Nakai H. Tissue engineering research in oral implant surgery. Artif Organs 2001;25:164-171.
13. Solheim E. Growth factors in bone. Int Orthop 1998;22:410-416.
14. Wirthlin MR. Growth substances: potential use in periodontics. J West Soc Periodontol Periodontal Abstr 1989;37:101-125.
15. Bonewald LF, Mundy GR. Role of transforming growth factor-beta in bone remodeling. Clin Orthop Relat Res 1990;250:261-276.
16. Mohan S, Baylink DJ. Bone growth factors. Clin Orthop Relat Res 1991;263:30-48.
17. Mohammed S, Pack AR, Kardos TB. The effect of transforming growth factor beta one (TGF-β1) on wound healing, with or without barrier membranes, in a Class II furcation defect in sheep. J Periodontal Res 1998;33:335-344.
18. Lamberg A, Schmidmaier G, Søballe K, Elmengaard B. Locally delivered TGF-β1 and IGF-1 enhance the fixation of titanium implants: a study in dogs. Acta Orthop 2006;77:799-805.
19. Duneas N, Crooks J, Ripamonti U. Transforming growth factor-β1: induction of bone morphogenetic protein genes expression during endochondral bone formation in the baboon, and synergistic interaction with osteogenic protein-1 (BMP-7). Growth Factors 1998;15:259-277.
20. Pagnotto MR, Wang Z, Karpie JC, Ferretti M, Xiao X, Chu CR. Adeno-associated viral gene transfer of transforming growth factor-β1 to human mesenchymal stem cells improves cartilage repair. Gene Ther 2007;14:804-813.
21. Ebara S, Nakayama K. Mechanism for the action of bone morphogenetic proteins and regulation of their activity. Spine (Phila Pa 1976) 2002;27(16 Suppl 1):S10-15.
22. Hogan BL. Bone morphogenetic proteins: multifunctional regulators of vertebrate development. Genes Dev 1996;10:1580-1594.
23. Urist MR, Strates BS. Bone morphogenetic protein. J Dent Res 1971;50:1392-1406.
24. Wozney JM, Rosen V, Celeste AJ, Mitsock LM, Whitters MJ, Kriz RW, et al. Novel regulators of bone formation: molecular clones and activities. Science 1988;242:1528-1534.
25. Reddi AH. Cell biology and biochemistry of endochondral bone development. Coll Relat Res 1981;1:209-226.
26. Wozney JM. Overview of bone morphogenetic proteins. Spine (Phila Pa 1976) 2002;27(16 Suppl 1):S2-8.
27. Wikesjo UM, Qahash M, Huang YH, Xiropaidis A, Polimeni G, Susin C. Bone morphogenetic proteins for periodontal and alveolar indications; biological observations - clinical implications. Orthod Craniofac Res 2009;12:263-270.
28. Herford AS, Boyne PJ. Reconstruction of mandibular continuity defects with bone morphogenetic protein-2 (rhBMP-2). J Oral Maxillofac Surg 2008;66:616-624.
29. Lan J, Wang ZF, Shi B, Xia HB, Cheng XR. The influence of recombinant human BMP-2 on bone-implant osseointegration: biomechanical testing and histomorphometric analysis. Int J Oral Maxillofac Surg 2007;36:345-349.
30. Ishibe T, Goto T, Kodama T, Miyazaki T, Kobayashi S, Takahashi T. Bone formation on apatite-coated titanium with incorporated BMP-2/heparin in vivo. Oral Surg Oral Med Oral Pathol Oral Radiol Endod 2009;108:867-875.
31. Lutz R, Park J, Felszeghy E, Wiltfang J, Nkenke E, Schlegel KA. Bone regeneration after topical BMP-2-gene delivery in circumferential peri-implant bone defects. Clin Oral Implants Res 2008;19: 590-599.
32. Wikesjo UM, Qahash M, Polimeni G, Susin C, Shanaman RH, Rohrer MD, et al. Alveolar ridge augmentation using implants coated with recombinant human bone morphogenetic protein-2: histologic observations. J Clin Periodontol 2008;35:1001-1010.
33. Leknes KN, Yang J, Qahash M, Polimeni G, Susin C, Wikesjö UM. Alveolar ridge augmentation using implants coated with recombinant human bone morphogenetic protein-2: radiographic observations. Clin Oral Implants Res 2008;19:1027-1033.
34. Jung RE, Windisch SI, Eggenschwiler AM, Thoma DS, Weber FE, Hämmerle CH. A randomized-controlled clinical trial evaluating clinical and radiological outcomes after 3 and 5 years of dental implants placed in bone regenerated by means of GBR techniques with or without the addition of BMP-2. Clin Oral Implants Res 2009;20:660-666.
35. Lee YM, Nam SH, Seol YJ, Kim TI, Lee SJ, Ku Y, et al. Enhanced bone augmentation by controlled release of recombinant human bone morphogenetic protein-2 from bioabsorbable membranes. J Periodontol 2003;74:865-872.
36. Hou LT, Liu CM, Liu BY, Chang PC, Chen MH, Ho MH, et al. Tissue engineering bone formation in novel recombinant human bone morphogenic protein 2-atelocollagen composite scaffolds. J Periodontol 2007;78:335-343.
37. Warnke PH, Springer IN, Wiltfang J, Acil Y, Eufinger H, Wehmöller M, et al. Growth and transplantation of a custom vascularised bone graft in a man. Lancet 2004;364:766-770.
38. Obert L, Deschaseaux F, Garbuio P. Critical analysis and efficacy of BMPs in long bones non-union. Injury 2005;36(Suppl 3):S38-42.
39. Betsholtz C, Karlsson L, Lindahl P. Developmental roles of platelet-derived growth factors. Bioessays 2001;23:494-507.
40. Rosenkranz S, Kazlauskas A. Evidence for distinct signaling properties and biological responses induced by the PDGF receptor alpha and beta sub-types. Growth Factors 1999;16:201-216.
41. Heldin CH, Ostman A, Ronnstrand L. Signal transduction via platelet-derived growth factor receptors. Biochim Biophys Acta 1998;1378:F79-113.
42. Lynch SE, Williams RC, Polson AM, Howell TH, Reddy MS, Zappa UE, Antoniades HN. A combination of platelet-derived and insulin-like growth factors enhances periodontal regeneration. J Clin Periodontol 1989;16:545-548.
43. Nevins M, et al. Periodontal regeneration in humans using recombinant human platelet-derived growth factor-BB (rhPDGF-BB) and allogenic bone. J Periodontol 2003;74:1282-1292.
44. Lin Z, Sugai JV, Jin Q, Chandler LA, Giannobile WV. Platelet-derived growth factor-B gene delivery sustains gingival fibroblast signal transduction. J Periodontal Res 2008;43(4):440-449.
45. Vikjaer D, Blom S, Hjørting-Hansen E, Pinholt EM. Effect of platelet-derived growth factor-BB on bone formation in calvarial defects: an experimental study in rabbits. Eur J Oral Sci 1997;105:59-66.
46. Becker W, Lynch SE, Lekholm U, Becker BE, Caffesse R, Donath K, Sanchez R. A comparison of ePTFE membranes alone or in combination with platelet-derived growth factors and insulin-like growth factor-I or demineralized freeze-dried bone in promoting bone formation around immediate extraction socket implants. J Periodontol 1992;63:929-940.
47. Lee YM, Park YJ, Lee SJ, Ku Y, Han SB, Klokkevold PR, Chung CP. The bone regenerative effect of platelet-derived growth factor-BB delivered with a chitosan/tricalcium phosphate sponge carrier. J Periodontol 2000;71:418-424.
48. Whitman DH, Berry RL, Green DM. Platelet gel: an autologous alternative to fibrin glue with applications in oral and maxillofacial surgery. J Oral Maxillofac Surg 1997;55:1294-1299.

49. Freymiller EG, Aghaloo TL. Platelet-rich plasma: ready or not? J Oral Maxillofac Surg 2004;62:484-488.
50. Sunitha Raja V, Munirathnam Naidu E. Platelet-rich fibrin: evolution of a second-generation platelet concentrate. Indian J Dent Res 2008;19:42-46.
51. Pryor ME, Polimeni G, Koo KT, Hartman MJ, Gross H, April M, et al. Analysis of rat calvaria defects implanted with a platelet-rich plasma preparation: histologic and histometric observations. J Clin Periodontol 2005;32:966-972.
52. Christgau M, Moder D, Hiller KA, Dada A, Schmitz G, Schmalz G. Growth factors and cytokines in autologous platelet concentrate and their correlation to periodontal regeneration outcomes. J Clin Periodontol 2006;33:837-845.
53. Oyama T, Nishimoto S, Tsugawa T, Shimizu F. Efficacy of platelet-rich plasma in alveolar bone grafting. J Oral Maxillofac Surg 2004;62:555-855.
54. Aghaloo TL, Moy PK, Freymiller EG. Investigation of platelet-rich plasma in rabbit cranial defects: A pilot study. J Oral Maxillofac Surg 2002;60:1176-1181.
55. Marx RE, Carlson ER, Eichstaedt RM, Schimmele SR, Strauss JE, Georgeff KR. Platelet-rich plasma: growth factor enhancement for bone grafts. Oral Surg Oral Med Oral Pathol Oral Radiol Endod 1998;85:638-646.
56. Gerard D, Carlson ER, Gotcher JE, Jacobs M. Effects of platelet-rich plasma on the healing of autologous bone grafted mandibular defects in dogs. J Oral Maxillofac Surg 2006;64:443-451.
57. Fennis JP, Stoelinga PJ, Jansen JA. Mandibular reconstruction: a histological and histomorphometric study on the use of autogenous scaffolds, particulate cortico-cancellous bone grafts and platelet rich plasma in goats. Int J Oral Maxillofac Surg 2004;33:48-55.
58. Gassling VL, Açil Y, Springer IN, Hubert N, Wiltfang J. Platelet-rich plasma and platelet-rich fibrin in human cell culture. Oral Surg Oral Med Oral Pathol Oral Radiol Endod 2009;108:48-55.
59. Pieri F, Lucarelli E, Corinaldesi G, Iezzi G, Piattelli A, Giardino R, et al. Mesenchymal stem cells and platelet-rich plasma enhance bone formation in sinus grafting: a histomorphometric study in minipigs. J Clin Periodontol 2008;35:539-546.
60. Klongnoi B, Rupprecht S, Kessler P, Zimmermann R, Thorwarth M, Pongsiri S, et al. Lack of beneficial effects of platelet-rich plasma on sinus augmentation using a fluorohydroxyapatite or autogenous bone: an explorative study. J Clin Periodontol 2006;33:500-509.
61. Sarkar MR, Augat P, Shefelbine SJ, Schorlemmer S, Huber-Lang M, Claes L, et al. Bone formation in a long bone defect model using a platelet-rich plasma-loaded collagen scaffold. Biomaterials 2006;27:1817-1823.
62. Torres J, Tamimi F, Tresguerres IF, Alkhraisat MH, Khraisat A, Blanco L, Lopez-Cabarcos E. Effect of combining platelet-rich plasma with anorganic bovine bone on vertical bone regeneration: early healing assessment in rabbit calvariae. Int J Oral Maxillofac Implants 2010;25:123-129.
63. Rutkowski JL, Johnson DA, Radio NM, Fennell JW. Platelet rich plasma to facilitate wound healing following tooth extraction. J Oral Implantol 2010;36:11-23.
64. Dohan DM, Choukroun J, Diss A, Dohan SL, Dohan AJ, Mouhyi J, Gogly B. Platelet-rich fibrin (PRF): a second-generation platelet concentrate. Part II: platelet-related biologic features. Oral Surg Oral Med Oral Pathol Oral Radiol Endod 2006;101:e45-50.
65. Dohan DM, Choukroun J, Diss A, Dohan SL, Dohan AJ, Mouhyi J, Gogly B. Platelet-rich fibrin (PRF): a second-generation platelet concentrate. Part III: leucocyte activation: a new feature for platelet concentrates? Oral Surg Oral Med Oral Pathol Oral Radiol Endod 2006;101:e51-55.
66. Dohan DM, Choukroun J, Diss A, Dohan SL, Dohan AJ, Mouhyi J, Gogly B. Platelet-rich fibrin (PRF): a second-generation platelet concentrate. Part I: technological concepts and evolution. Oral Surg Oral Med Oral Pathol Oral Radiol Endod 2006;101:e37-44.
67. Choukroun J, Diss A, Simonpieri A, Girard MO, Schoeffler C, Dohan SL, et al. Platelet-rich fibrin (PRF): a second-generation platelet concentrate. Part V: histologic evaluations of PRF effects on bone allograft maturation in sinus lift. Oral Surg Oral Med Oral Pathol Oral Radiol Endod 2006;101:299-303.
68. Diss A, Dohan DM, Mouhyi J, Mahler P. Osteotome sinus floor elevation using Choukroun's platelet-rich fibrin as grafting material: a 1-year prospective pilot study with microthreaded implants. Oral Surg Oral Med Oral Pathol Oral Radiol Endod 2008;105: 572-579.
69. Gurbuzer B, Pikdöken L, Tunali M, Urhan M, Küçükodaci Z, Ercan F. Scintigraphic evaluation of osteoblastic activity in extraction sockets treated with platelet-rich fibrin. J Oral Maxillofac Surg 2010;68:980-989.
70. Sanchez AR, Sheridan PJ, Kupp LI. Is platelet-rich plasma the perfect enhancement factor? A current review. Int J Oral Maxillofac Implants 2003;18:93-103.
71. Rinderknecht E, Humbel RE. The amino acid sequence of human insulin-like growth factor I and its structural homology with proinsulin. J Biol Chem 1978;253:2769-2776.
72. Mohan S, Jennings JC, Linkhart TA, Baylink DJ. Primary structure of human skeletal growth factor: homology with human insulin-like growth factor-II. Biochim Biophys Acta 1988;966:44-55.
73. McCarthy TL, Centrella M, Canalis E. Regulatory effects of insulin-like growth factors I and II on bone collagen synthesis in rat calvarial cultures. Endocrinology 1989;124:301-309.
74. Spencer EM, Liu CC, Si EC, Howard GA. In vivo actions of insulin-like growth factor-I (IGF-1) on bone formation and resorption in rats. Bone 1991;12:21-26.
75. Chen G, Ushida T, Tateishi T. Scaffold design for tissue engineering. Macromol Biosci 2002;2:67-77.
76. Giannobile WV, Finkelman RD, Lynch SE. Comparison of canine and non-human primate animal models for periodontal regenerative therapy: results following a single administration of PDGF/IGF- 1. J Periodontol 1994;65:1158-1168.
77. Giannobile WV, Whitson SW, Lynch SE. Non-coordinate control of bone formation displayed by growth factor combinations with IGF- 1. J Dent Res 1997;76:1569-1578.
78. Werner S, Grose R. Regulation of wound healing by growth factors and cytokines. Physiol Rev 2003;83:835-870.
79. Basilico C, Moscatelli D. The FGF family of growth factors and oncogenes. Adv Cancer Res 1992;59:115-165.
80. Boilly B, Vercoutter-Edouart AS, Hondermarck H, Nurcombe V, Le Bourhis X. FGF signals for cell proliferation and migration through different pathways. Cytokine Growth Factor Rev 2000;11: 295-302.
81. Sahni A, Odrljin T, Francis CW. Binding of basic fibroblast growth factor to fibrinogen and fibrin. J Biol Chem 1998;273:7554-7559.
82. Arkudas A, Tjiawi J, Bleiziffer O, Grabinger L, Polykandriotis E, Beier JP, et al. Fibrin gel-immobilized VEGF and bFGF efficiently stimulate angiogenesis in the AV loop model. Mol Med 2007;13: 480-487.
83. Takayama S. Murakami S, Shimabukuro Y, Kitamura M, Okada H. Periodontal regeneration by FGF-2 (bFGF) in primate models. J Dent Res 2001;80:2075-2079.
84. Rossa C Jr, Marcantonio E Jr, Cirelli JA, Marcantonio RA, Spolidorio LC, Fogo JC. Regeneration of Class III furcation defects with basic fibroblast growth factor (b-FGF) associated with GTR. A descriptive and histometric study in dogs. J Periodontol 2000;71:775-784.

85. Lee SY, Koak JY, Heo SJ, Kim SK, Lee SJ, Nam SY. Osseointegration of anodized titanium implants coated with poly(lactide-co-glycolide)/ basic fibroblast growth factor by electrospray. Int J Oral Maxillofac Implants 2010;25:315-320.
86. Lyngstadaas SP, Wohlfahrt JC, Brookes SJ, Paine ML, Snead ML, Reseland JE. Enamel matrix proteins; old molecules for new applications. Orthod Craniofac Res 2009;12:243-253.
87. Lyngstadaas SP, Lundberg E, Ekdahl H, Andersson C, Gestrelius S. Autocrine growth factors in human periodontal ligament cells cultured on enamel matrix derivative. J Clin Periodontol 2001;28: 181-188.
88. Mao JJ, Giannobile WV, Helms JA, Hollister SJ, Krebsbach PH, Longaker MT, Shi S. Craniofacial tissue engineering by stem cells. J Dent Res 2006;85:966-979.
89. Yuan K, Chen CL, Lin MT. Enamel matrix derivative exhibits angiogenic effect in vitro and in a murine model. J Clin Periodontol 2003;30:732-738.
90. Alhezaimi K, Al-Shalan T, O'Neill R, Shapurian T, Naghshbandi J, Levi P Jr, Griffin T. Connective tissue-cementum regeneration: a new histologic regeneration following the use of enamel matrix derivative in dehiscence-type defects. A dog model. Int J Periodontics Restorative Dent 2009;29:425-433.
91. Heijl L, Heden G, Svärdström G, Ostgren A. Enamel matrix derivative (EMDOGAIN) in the treatment of intrabony periodontal defects. J Clin Periodontol 1997;24:705-714.
92. Sculean A, Reich E, Chiantella GC, Brecx M. Treatment of intrabony periodontal defects with an enamel matrix protein derivative (Emdogain): a report of 32 cases. Int J Periodontics Restorative Dent 1999;19:157-163.
93. Sculean A, Barbé G, Chiantella GC, Arweiler NB, Berakdar M, Brecx M. Clinical evaluation of an enamel matrix protein derivative combined with a bioactive glass for the treatment of intrabony periodontal defects in humans. J Periodontol 2002;73:401-408.
94. Shimizu-Ishiura M, Tanaka S, Lee WS, Debari K, Sasaki T. Effects of enamel matrix derivative to titanium implantation in rat femurs. J Biomed Mater Res 2002;60:269-276.
95. Fridstrom M, Schollin J, Crossner CG. Evaluating Emdogain and healing of replanted teeth using an intra-individual experimental-control study design. Dent Traumatol 2008;24:299-304.
96.Sengers BG, Taylor M, Please CP, Oreffo RO. Computational modelling of cell spreading and tissue regeneration in porous scaffolds. Biomaterials 2007;28:1926-1940.
97. Neuss S, Apel C, Buttler P, Denecke B, Dhanasingh A, Ding X, et al. Assessment of stem cell/biomaterial combinations for stem cell-based tissue engineering. Biomaterials 2008;29:302-313.
98. Kasten P, Vogel J, Luginbühl R, Niemeyer P, Tonak M, Lorenz H, et al. Ectopic bone formation associated with mesenchymal stem cells in a resorbable calcium deficient hydroxyapatite carrier. Biomaterials 2005;26:5879-5889.
99. Nadig RR. Stem cell therapy: Hype or hope? A review. J Conserv Dent 2009;12:131-138.
100. Roobrouck VD, Ulloa-Montoya F, Verfaillie CM. Self-renewal and differentiation capacity of young and aged stem cells. Exp Cell Res 2008;314:1937-1944.
101. Neuss S, Becher E, Wöltje M, Tietze L, Jahnen-Dechent W. Functional expression of HGF and HGF receptor/c-met in adult human mesenchymal stem cells suggests a role in cell mobilization, tissue repair, and wound healing. Stem Cells 2004;22:405-414.
102. Neuss S, Stainforth R, Salber J, Schenck P, Bovi M, Knüchel R, Perez-Bouza A. Long-term survival and bipotent terminal differentiation of human mesenchymal stem cells (hMSC) in combination with a commercially available three-dimensional collagen scaffold. Cell Transplant 2008;17:977-986.
103. Prockop DJ. Marrow stromal cells as stem cells for nonhematopoietic tissues. Science 1997;276:71-74.
104. Apel A, Groth A, Schlesinger S, Bruns H, Schemmer P, Büchler MW, Herr I. Suitability of human mesenchymal stem cells for gene therapy depends on the expansion medium. Exp Cell Res 2009;315: 498-507.
105. Bruder SP, Kraus KH, Goldberg VM, Kadiyala S. The effect of implants loaded with autologous mesenchymal stem cells on the healing of canine segmental bone defects. J Bone Joint Surg Am 1998;80: 985-996.
106. Kon E, Muraglia A, Corsi A, Bianco P, Marcacci M, Martin I, Boyde A, et al. Autologous bone marrow stromal cells loaded onto porous hydroxyapatite ceramic accelerate bone repair in critical-size defects of sheep long bones. J Biomed Mater Res 2000;49:328-337.
107. Lieberman JR, Daluiski A, Einhorn TA. The role of growth factors in the repair of bone. Biology and clinical applications. J Bone Joint Surg Am 2002;84-A:1032-1044.
108. Qi H, Aguiar DJ, Williams SM, La Pean A, Pan W, Verfaillie CM. Identification of genes responsible for osteoblast differentiation from human mesodermal progenitor cells. Proc Natl Acad Sci U S A 2003;100:3305-3310.
109. Horwitz EM. Marrow mesenchymal cell transplantation for genetic disorders of bone. Cytotherapy 2001;3:399-401.
110. Newman RE, Yoo D, LeRoux MA, Danilkovitch-Miagkova A. Treatment of inflammatory diseases with mesenchymal stem cells. Inflamm Allergy Drug Targets 2009;8:110-123.
111. Meyer U, Wiesmann HP, Berr K, Kübler NR, Handschel J. Cell-based bone reconstruction therapies: principles of clinical approaches. Int J Oral Maxillofac Implants 2006;21:899-906.
112. Friedenstein AJ, Chailakhjan RK, Lalykina KS. The development of fibroblast colonies in monolayer cultures of guinea-pig bone marrow and spleen cells. Cell Tissue Kinet 1970;3:393-403.
113. Bianco P, Riminucci M, Gronthos S, Robey PG. Bone marrow stromal stem cells: nature, biology, and potential applications. Stem Cells 2001;19:180-192.
114. Bianco P, Gehron Robey P. Marrow stromal stem cells. J Clin Invest 2000;105:1663-1668.
115. Arinzeh TL, Peter SJ, Archambault MP, van den Bos C, Gordon S, Kraus K, et al. Allogeneic mesenchymal stem cells regenerate bone in a critical-sized canine segmental defect. J Bone Joint Surg Am 2003;85-A:1927-1935.
116. Mitrano TI, Grob MS, Carrión F, Nova-Lamperti E, Luz PA, Fierro FS, et al. Culture and characterization of mesenchymal stem cells from human gingival tissue. J Periodontol, 2010;81:917-925.
117. Ahn HH, Kim KS, Lee JH, Lee JY, Kim BS, Lee IW, et al. In vivo osteogenic differentiation of human adipose-derived stem cells in an injectable in situ-forming gel scaffold. Tissue Eng Part A 2009;15:1821-1832.
118. Hattori H, Masuoka K, Sato M, Ishihara M, Asazuma T, Takase B, et al. Bone formation using human adipose tissue-derived stromal cells and a biodegradable scaffold. J Biomed Mater Res B Appl Biomater 2006;76:230-239.
119. Hattori H, Sato M, Masuoka K, Ishihara M, Kikuchi T, Matsui T, et al. Osteogenic potential of human adipose tissue-derived stromal cells as an alternative stem cell source. Cells Tissues Organs 2004;178:2-12.
120. Rangappa S, Fen C, Lee EH, Bongso A, Sim EK. Transformation of adult mesenchymal stem cells isolated from the fatty tissue into cardiomyocytes. Ann Thorac Surg 2003;75:775-779.
121. Pieri F, Lucarelli E, Corinaldesi G, Aldini NN, Fini M, Parrilli A, et al. Dose-dependent effect of adipose-derived adult stem cells on vertical bone regeneration in rabbit calvarium. Biomaterials 2010;31:3527-3535.
122. Yoo G, Lim JS. Tissue engineering of injectable soft tissue filler: using adipose stem cells and micronized acellular dermal matrix. J Korean Med Sci 2009;24:104-109.

123. Bunting KD, Hawley RG. Integrative molecular and developmental biology of adult stem cells. Biol Cell 2003;95:563-578.
124. Tabbara IA, Zimmerman K, Morgan C, Nahleh Z. Allogeneic hematopoietic stem cell transplantation: complications and results. Arch Intern Med 2002;162:1558-1566.
125. Gronthos S, Mankani M, Brahim J, Robey PG, Shi S. Postnatal human dental pulp stem cells (DPSCs) in vitro and in vivo. Proc Natl Acad Sci U S A 2000;97:13625-13630.
126. Mori G, Centonze M, Brunetti G, Ballini A, Oranger A, Mori C, et al. Osteogenic properties of human dental pulp stem cells. J Biol Regul Homeost Agents 2010;24:167-175.
127. Graziano A, d'Aquino R, Laino G, Papaccio G. Dental pulp stem cells: a promising tool for bone regeneration. Stem Cell Rev 2008;4:21-26.
128. Lutolf MP, Hubbell JA. Synthetic biomaterials as instructive extracellular microenvironments for morphogenesis in tissue engineering. Nat Biotechnol 2005;23:47-55.
129. Nakashima M, Akamine A. The application of tissue engineering to regeneration of pulp and dentin in endodontics. J Endod 2005;31:711-718.
130. Liu H, Roy K. Biomimetic three-dimensional cultures significantly increase hematopoietic differentiation efficacy of embryonic stem cells. Tissue Eng 2005;11:319-330.
131. Liu H, Lin J, Roy K. Effect of 3D scaffold and dynamic culture condition on the global gene expression profile of mouse embryonic stem cells. Biomaterials 2006;27:5978-5989.
132. Kim BS, Mooney DJ. Development of biocompatible synthetic extracellular matrices for tissue engineering. Trends Biotechnol 1998;16:224-230.
133. Langer R. Biomaterials in drug delivery and tissue engineering: one laboratory's experience. Acc Chem Res 2000;33:94-101.
134. Burg KJ, Porter S, Kellam JF. Biomaterial developments for bone tissue engineering. Biomaterials 2000;21:2347-2359.
135. Moharamzadeh K, Brook IM, Van Noort R, Scutt AM, Thornhill MH. Tissue-engineered oral mucosa: a review of the scientific literature. J Dent Res 2007;86:115-124.
136. Schneider RK, Puellen A, Kramann R, Raupach K, Bornemann J, Knuechel R, et al. The osteogenic differentiation of adult bone marrow and perinatal umbilical mesenchymal stem cells and matrix remodelling in three-dimensional collagen scaffolds. Biomaterials 2010;31:467-480.
137. Ignatius A, Blessing H, Liedert A, Schmidt C, Neidlinger-Wilke C, Kaspar D, et al. Tissue engineering of bone: effects of mechanical strain on osteoblastic cells in type I collagen matrices. Biomaterials 2005;26:311-318.
138. Mooney DJ, Mazzoni CL, Breuer C, McNamara K, Hern D, Vacanti JP, Langer R. Stabilized polyglycolic acid fibre-based tubes for tissue engineering. Biomaterials 1996;17:115-124.
139. Harris LD, Kim BS, Mooney DJ. Open pore biodegradable matrices formed with gas foaming. J Biomed Mater Res 1998;42:396-402.
140. Mikos AG, Bao Y, Cima LG, Ingber DE, Vacanti JP, Langer R. Preparation of poly(glycolic acid) bonded fiber structures for cell attachment and transplantation. J Biomed Mater Res 1993;27:183-189.
141. Hutmacher DW. Scaffolds in tissue engineering bone and cartilage. Biomaterials 2000;21:2529-2543.
142. Schugens C, Maquet V, Grandfils C, Jerome R, Teyssie P. Polylactide macroporous biodegradable implants for cell transplantation. II. Preparation of polylactide foams by liquid-liquid phase separation. J Biomed Mater Res 1996;30:449-461.
143. Mikos AG, Sarakinos G, Leite SM, Vacanti JP, Langer R. Laminated three-dimensional biodegradable foams for use in tissue engineering. Biomaterials 1993;14:323-330.
144. Chung HJ, Park TG. Surface engineered and drug releasing prefabricated scaffolds for tissue engineering. Adv Drug Deliv Rev 2007;59:249-262.
145. Eling B, Gogolewski S, Pennings AJ. Biodegradable materials of poly(L-lactic acid): 1. Melt-spun and solution spun fibres. Polymer 1982;23:1587-1593.
146. Gilding DK, Reed AM. Biodegradable polymers for use in surgery. Polyglycolic/poly(lactic acid) homo- and copolymers: 1. Polymer 1979;20:1459-1464.
147. Brady JM, Cutright DE, Miller RA, Barristone GC. Resorption rate, route, route of elimination, and ultrastructure of the implant site of polylactic acid in the abdominal wall of the rat. J Biomed Mater Res 1973;7:155-166.
148. Lamberg A, Bechtold JE, Baas J, Søballe K, Elmengaard B. Effect of local TGF-β1 and IGF-1 release on implant fixation: comparison with hydroxyapatite coating: a paired study in dogs. Acta Orthop 2009;80:499-504.
149. Hatton PV, Walsh J, Brook IM. The response of cultured bone cells to resorbable polyglycolic acid and silicone membranes for use in orbital floor fracture repair. Clin Mater 1994;17:71-80.
150. Breitbart AS, Grande DA, Kessler R, Ryaby JT, Fitzsimmons RJ, Grant RT. Tissue engineered bone repair of calvarial defects using cultured periosteal cells. Plast Reconstr Surg 1998;101:567-574; discussion 575-576.
151. Zhao H, Ma L, Gao C, Shen J. A composite scaffold of PLGA microspheres/fibrin gel for cartilage tissue engineering: fabrication, physical properties, and cell responsiveness. J Biomed Mater Res B Appl Biomater 2009;88:240-249.
152. Fialkov JA, Holy CE, Shoichet MS, Davies JE. In vivo bone engineering in a rabbit femur. J Craniofac Surg 2003;14:324-332.
153. Agrawal CM, Ray RB. Biodegradable polymeric scaffolds for musculo-skeletal tissue engineering. J Biomed Mater Res 2001;55:141-150.
154. Thompson DE, Agrawal CM, Athanasiou K. The effects of dynamic compressive loading on biodegradable implants of 50-50% polylactic acid-polyglycolic acid. Tissue Eng 1996;2:61-74.
155. Rotter N, Aigner J, Naumann A, Planck H, Hammer C, Burmester G, Sittinger M. Cartilage reconstruction in head and neck surgery: comparison of resorbable polymer scaffolds for tissue engineering of human septal cartilage. J Biomed Mater Res 1998;42:347-356.
156. Kikuchi M, Koyama Y, Yamada T, Imamura Y, Okada T, Shirahama N, et al. Development of guided bone regeneration membrane composed of beta-tricalcium phosphate and poly (L-lactide-co-glycolide-co-epsilon-caprolactone) composites. Biomaterials 2004;25:5979-5986.
157. Petersen LK, Sackett CK, Narasimhan B. High-throughput analysis of protein stability in polyanhydride nanoparticles. Acta Biomater 2010;6:3873-3881.
158. Petersen LK, et al. Lipocalin-2-loaded amphiphilic polyanhydride microparticles accelerate cell migration. J Biomater Sci Polym Ed 2010;July 2. Epub ahead of print.
159. Weiner AA, Moore MC, Walker AH, Shastri VP. Modulation of protein release from photocrosslinked networks by gelatin microparticles. Int J Pharm 2008;360:107-114.
160. Weiner AA, Shuck DM, Bush JR, Prasad Shastri V. In vitro degradation characteristics of photocrosslinked anhydride systems for bone augmentation applications. Biomaterials 2007;28:5259-5270.
161. Chen L, Wang H, Wang J, Chen M, Shang L. Ofloxacin-delivery system of a polyanhydride and polylactide blend used in the treatment of bone infection. J Biomed Mater Res B Appl Biomater 2007;83:589-595.
162. Liao J, Zhang L, Zuo Y, Wang H, Li Jidong, Z-Q, Li Y. Development of nanohydroxyapatite/polycarbonate composite for bone repair. J Biomater Appl 2009;24:31-45.
163. Peter SJ, Yaszemski MJ, Suggs LJ, Payne RG, Langer R, Hayes WC, Unroe MR, et al. Characterization of partially saturated poly(propylene fumarate) for orthopaedic application. J Biomater Sci Polym Ed 1997;8:893-904.

164. Cortizo MS, Molinuevo MS, Cortizo AM. Biocompatibility and biodegradation of polyester and polyfumarate based-scaffolds for bone tissue engineering. J Tissue Eng Regen Med 2008;2:33-42.
165. Fernandez JM, Molinuevo MS, Cortizo AM, McCarthy AD, Cortizo MS. Characterization of poly(epsilon-caprolactone)/polyfumarate blends as scaffolds for bone tissue engineering. J Biomater Sci Polym Ed 2010;21:1297-1312.
166. Riesle J, Hollander AP, Langer R, Freed LE, Vunjak-Novakovic G. Collagen in tissue-engineered cartilage: types, structure, and crosslinks. J Cell Biochem 1998;71:313-327.
167. Pieper JS, Hafmans T, van Wachem PB, van Luyn MJ, Brouwer LA, Veerkamp JH, van Kuppevelt TH. Loading of collagen-heparan sulfate matrices with bFGF promotes angiogenesis and tissue generation in rats. J Biomed Mater Res 2002;62:185-194.
168. Masuda I. [An in vitro oral mucosal model reconstructed from human normal gingival cells]. Kokubyo Gakkai Zasshi 1996;63: 334-353.
169. Yang C, Hillas PJ, Báez JA, Nokelainen M, Balan J, Tang J, et al. The application of recombinant human collagen in tissue engineering. BioDrugs 2004;18:103-119.
170. Cornell CN, Lane JM, Chapman M, Merkow R, Seligson D, Henry S, et al. Multicenter trial of Collagraft as bone graft substitute. J Orthop Trauma 1991;5:1-8.
171. Triplett RG, Nevins M, Marx RE, Spagnoli DB, Oates TW, Moy PK, Boyne PJ. Pivotal, randomized, parallel evaluation of recombinant human bone morphogenetic protein-2/absorbable collagen sponge and autogenous bone graft for maxillary sinus floor augmentation. J Oral Maxillofac Surg 2009;67:1947-1960.
172. Boyne PJ, Lilly LC, Marx RE, Moy PK, Nevins M, Spagnoli DB, Triplett RG. De novo bone induction by recombinant human bone morphogenetic protein-2 (rhBMP-2) in maxillary sinus floor augmentation. J Oral Maxillofac Surg 2005;63:1693-1707.
173. Howell TH, Fiorellini J, Jones A, Alder M, Nummikoski P, Lazaro M, et al. A feasibility study evaluating rhBMP-2/absorbable collagen sponge device for local alveolar ridge preservation or augmentation. Int J Periodontics Restorative Dent 1997;17:124-139.
174. Wahl DA, Czernuszka JT. Collagen-hydroxyapatite composites for hard tissue repair. Eur Cell Mater 2006;11:43-56.
175. Venugopal J, Low S, Choon AT, Sampath Kumar TS, Ramakrishna S. Mineralization of osteoblasts with electrospun collagen/hydroxyapatite nanofibers. J Mater Sci Mater Med 2008;19: 2039-2046.
176. Takahashi K. Effect of new bone substitute materials consisting of collagen and tricalcium phosphate. Bull Tokyo Dent Coll 2009; 50:1-11.
177. Hillmann G, Steinkamp-Zucht A, Geurtsen W, Gross G, Hoffmann A. Culture of primary human gingival fibroblasts on biodegradable membranes. Biomaterials 2002;23:1461-1469.
178. O'Brien FJ, Harley BA, Yannas IV, Gibson L. Influence of freezing rate on pore structure in freeze-dried collagen-GAG scaffolds. Biomaterials 2004;25:1077-1086.
179. O'Brien FJ, Harley BA, Yannas IV, Gibson LJ. The effect of pore size on cell adhesion in collagen-GAG scaffolds. Biomaterials 2005;26:433-441.
180. Murphy CM, Haugh MG, O'Brien FJ. The effect of mean pore size on cell attachment, proliferation and migration in collagen-glycosaminoglycan scaffolds for bone tissue engineering. Biomaterials 2010;31:461-466.
181. Tierney CM, Jaasma MJ, O'Brien FJ. Osteoblast activity on collagen-GAG scaffolds is affected by collagen and GAG concentrations. J Biomed Mater Res A 2009;91:92-101.
182. Santin M, Motta A, Freddi G, Cannas M. In vitro evaluation of the inflammatory potential of the silk fibroin. J Biomed Mater Res 1999;46:382-389.
183. Etienne O, Schneider A, Kluge JA, Bellemin-Laponnaz C, Polidori C, Leisk GG, et al. Soft tissue augmentation using silk gels: an in vitro and in vivo study. J Periodontol 2009;80:1852-1858.
184. Nazarov R, Jin HJ, Kaplan DL. Porous 3-D scaffolds from regenerated silk fibroin. Biomacromolecules 2004;5:718-726.
185. Kim KH, Jeong L, Park HN, Shin SY, Park WH, Lee SC, et al. Biological efficacy of silk fibroin nanofiber membranes for guided bone regeneration. J Biotechnol 2005;120:327-339.

Index

D

E

K

L

M

N

O

P

Q

R

S

U

V

W

X

Z